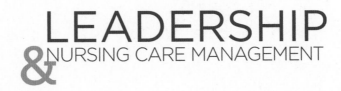

LEADERSHIP
&NURSING CARE MANAGEMENT

LEADERSHIP
& NURSING CARE MANAGEMENT

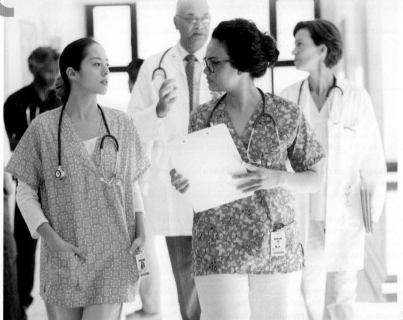

Sixth Edition

DIANE L. HUBER, PhD, RN, NEA-BC, FAAN

Professor
College of Nursing and College of Public Health
The University of Iowa
Iowa City, Iowa

ELSEVIER

ELSEVIER

3251 Riverport Lane
St. Louis, Missouri 63043

LEADERSHIP & NURSING CARE MANAGEMENT, SIXTH EDITION ISBN: 978-0-323-38966-2

Notices

Previous editions copyrighted 2014, 2010, 2006, 2000, and 1996.

International Standard Book Number: 978-0-323-38966-2

Senior Content Strategist: Yvonne Alexopoulos
Senior Content Development Manager: Laurie Gower
Associate Content Development Specialist: Laurel Shea
Publishing Services Manager: Jeff Patterson
Book Production Specialist: Bill Drone
Designer: Amy Buxton

Printed in China

Last digit is the print number: 9 8 7 6 5 4 3 2 1

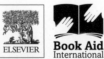

Jennifer Bellot, PhD, RN, MHSA, CNE
Associate Professor and Director, DNP Program
Jefferson College of Nursing
Thomas Jefferson University
Philadelphia, Pennsylvania

Jane M. Brokel, PhD, RN
Section Instructor, Online Nursing
Simmons College
Adjunct Faculty, College of Nursing
University of Iowa
President, NANDA International, Inc.
Registered Nurse, Parish Nursing Cluster Parishes and
    Accurate Home Care

Marie-Hélène Budworth, PhD, MS, BA
Associate Professor of Human Resource Management
Director
School of Human Resource Management
York University
Toronto, Ontario, Canada

Lynn Christensen, MSN, RN
Safety and Emergency Management Officer
Inova Loudoun Hospital
Leesburg, Virginia

Sean P. Clarke, PhD, RN, FAAN
Professor and Associate Dean
Undergraduate Program
Connell School of Nursing
Boston College
Chestnut Hill, Massachusetts

Karen S. Cox, PD, RN, FACHE, FAAN
Executive Vice President/Chief Operating Officer
V. Fred Burry, MD, and Sandra Hobart Burry Chair in
    Nursing Advocacy and Leadership
Children's Mercy Hospital
Kansas City, Missouri

Kathleen B. Cox, PhD, RN
Associate Director
School of Nursing
Radford University
Radford, Virginia

Laura Cullen, DNP, RN, FAAN
Evidence-Based Practice Scientist
Office of Nursing Research, Evidence-Based Practice
    and Quality
Department of Nursing Services and Patient Care
University of Iowa Hospitals and Clinics
Iowa City, Iowa

Cindy J. Dawson, MSN, RN, CORLN
Director
Clinical Functions Ambulatory Nursing
University of Iowa Hospitals and Clinics
Iowa City, Iowa

Elizabeth T. Dugan, PhD, RN, MBA, MSN, NEA-BC
Chief Nursing Officer
Inova Loudoun Hospital
Leesburg, Virginia

Michele Farrington, BSN, RN, CPHON
Clinical Healthcare Research Associate
Office of Nursing Research, Evidence-Based Practice
    and Quality and Ambulatory Nursing
University of Iowa Hospitals and Clinics
Iowa City, Iowa

Ellen Fink-Samnick, MSW, ACSW, LCSW, CCM, CRP
Principal
EFS Supervision Strategies, LLC
Burke, Virginia

Betsy Frank, PhD, RN, ANEF
Professor Emerita
School of Nursing
Indiana State University
Terre Haute, Indiana

Maryanne Garon, DNSc, RN
Professor and Nursing Leadership Concentration
  Coordinator
California State University, Fullerton
Fullerton, California

Gregory O. Ginn, BA, MEd, MBA, PhD
Adjunct Assistant Professor
Embry-Riddle Aeronautical University–Worldwide
Daytona Beach, Florida

Kirsten Hanrahan, DNP, ARNP
Nurse Scientist
Office of Nursing Research, Evidence-Based Practice
  and Quality
Department of Nursing and Patient Care Services
University of Iowa Hospitals and Clinics
Iowa City, Iowa

Mary G. Harper, PhD, RN-BC
Director of Nursing Professional Development
Association for Nursing Professional Development
Flagler Beach, Florida

Farinaz Havaei, PhD
PhD Candidate
School of Nursing
University of British Columbia
Vancouver, British Columbia, Canada

L. Jean Henry, PhD
Associate Professor
Public Health/Community Health Promotion
College of Education and Health Professions
University of Arkansas
Fayetteville, Arkansas

Julie A. Holt, RN, MSN, CENP
Vice President, Patient Services
Chief Nurse Executive
The Christ Hospital Health Network
Cincinnati, Ohio

Cheryl Hoying, PhD, RN, NEA-BC, FACHE, FAAN
Senior Vice President, Patient Services Division
Cincinnati Children's Hospital Medical Center
Associate Dean
College of Nursing
University of Cincinnati
Cincinnati, Ohio

Lianne Jeffs, PhD, RN, FAAN
St. Michael's Hospital Volunteer Association Chair in
  Nursing Research
Scientist, Keenan Research Centre of the Li Ka Shing
  Knowledge Institute
Associate Professor, Lawrence Bloomberg Faculty of
  Nursing and Institute of Health Policy Management
  and Evaluation
University of Toronto
Toronto, Ontario, Canada

M. Lindell Joseph, PhD, RN
Associate Clinical Professor and MSN/CNL Program
  Coordinator
College of Nursing
University of Iowa
Iowa City, Iowa

Jayne Josephsen, EdD, MS, RN, CHPN
Associate Professor
School of Nursing
Boise State University
Boise, Idaho

Susan R. Lacey, PhD, RN, FAAN
Professor
College of Nursing
Medical University of South Carolina
Charleston, South Carolina

Trudy A. Laffoon, MA, RN-BC
Nurse Manager
Pain Management and Medicine Specialty Clinics
University of Iowa Hospitals and Clinics
Iowa City, Iowa

Michael Soon Lee, DBA, MBA, BA
President
EthnoConnect®
Member
National Speakers Association
Dublin, California

Maura MacPhee, PhD, RN
Associate Professor
School of Nursing
Associate Director
Undergraduate Nursing Program
University of British Columbia
Vancouver, British Columbia, Canada

Lynn S. Muller, JD, RN, CCM, BA-HCM
Partner
Muller & Muller, Attorneys at Law
Adjunct Professor
School of Nursing
Saint Peter's University
Englewood Cliffs, New Jersey

Nathan Neis, DNP, CPNP-AC
Nurse Practitioner
PICU/CICU at Children's Hospital of Wisconsin
Milwaukee, Wisconsin

Adrienne Olney, MS
Research Associate
Children's Mercy Hospitals and Clinics
Kansas City, Missouri

Anne Gallagher Peach, RN, MSN, NEA-BC
Partner
Future Vision Group
Orlando, Florida

Luc R. Pelletier, MSN, APRN, PMHCNS-BC, FAAN, CPHQ, FNAHQ
Senior Nursing Specialist
Sharp Mesa Vista Hospital
Adjunct Professor
National University
San Diego, California

Slimen Saliba, PhD, MBA, MA, BA
Senior Vice President of Marketing
Adventist Health System–Florida Division
Orlando, Florida

Teresa Kathleen Sparks, JD, MSN, BSN, RN
Faculty
MHCA and BSN Programs
College of Health Sciences
University of Arkansas, Fort Smith
Fort Smith, Arkansas

Abdullah S. Suhemat, BScN, MSN
Lawrence S. Bloomberg Faculty of Nursing
University of Toronto
Toronto, Ontario, Canada

Linda B. Talley, MS, BSN, RN, NE-BC
Vice President and Chief Nursing Officer
Children's National Health System
Washington, DC

Diane H. Thorgrimson, MHSA, BS
Executive Director
Workforce Planning, Special Projects, and Productivity
  for Patient Services
Children's National Health System
Washington, DC

Teresa M. Treiger, RN-BC, MA, CHCQM-CM/TOC, CCM
Principal and Case Manager
Ascent Care Management, LLC
Quincy, Massachusetts

Kathleen A. Vertino, DNP, PMHNP-BC, CARN-AP
Board-Certified Nurse Practitioner
Psychiatry
Buffalo, New York

Carol A. Wong, PhD, RN
Associate Professor
Arthur Labatt Family School of Nursing, Faculty of
  Health Sciences
Western University
London, Ontario, Canada

REVIEWERS

Karen E. Alexander, PhD, RN, CNOR
Director, RN-BSN, and Assistant Professor
Department of Clinical Health and
    Applied Sciences—Nursing
University of Houston Clear Lake
Houston, Texas

Barbara B. Blozen, EdD, MA, RN, BC, CNL
Associate Professor
Department of Nursing
New Jersey City University
Jersey City, New Jersey

Lori Jo Bork, PhD, RN, MS, BSN, CCRN
Professor of Nursing
Department of Nursing
Dakota Wesleyan University
Mitchell, South Dakota

Karen Brown-Fackler, RN, EdD, NEA-BC, CNL, CNE
Associate Professor of Nursing
Department of Nursing
Saginaw Valley State University
University Center, Michigan

Beverly Waller Dabney, PhD, RN, CCM
Associate Professor of Nursing
Department of Nursing
Southwestern Adventist University
Keene, Texas

Rebecca M. Davidson, PhD, MSN, RN
Instructor of Nursing
Caylor School of Nursing
Lincoln Memorial University
Knoxville, Tennessee

Richard C. Meeks, DNP, RN, COI
Assistant Professor
School of Nursing
Middle Tennessee State University
Murfreesboro, Tennessee

Barbara J. Pinekenstein, DNP, RN-BC, CPHIMS
Clinical Professor
Richard E. Sinaiko Professor in Health Care Leadership
University of Wisconsin, Madison
Madison, Wisconsin

Darlene M. Rogers, MSN, BS, RN-BC
Clinical Instructor
Georgia Baptist College of Nursing
Mercer University
Atlanta, Georgia

Strong leadership and care management are imperatives for nursing. Highlighted by a series of reports from the prestigious Institute of Medicine (IOM; now called the National Academies of Sciences, Engineering, and Medicine, Health and Medicine Division)—most recently *The Future of Nursing: Leading Change, Advancing Health*—it is clear that nurses matter to health care delivery systems. Yet the United States is in the midst of a continuing and projected nurse shortage. Strong nurse leaders and managers are important for clients (and their safety), delivery systems (and their viability), and payers (and their solvency). Pressures remain to balance cost and quality considerations in a complex, chaotic, and turbulent health care environment.

Although society's need for excellent nursing care remains the nurse's constant underlying reason for existence, nursing is in reality much more than that. Because nurses offer cost-effective expertise in solving problems related to the coordination and delivery of health care to individuals and populations in society, they have become a crucial linchpin in health care delivery and are highly valued. Nurses are well prepared to lead clinical change strategies and effectively manage the coordination and integration of interdisciplinary teams, population needs, and systems of care across the continuum. This has been especially important following implementation of the 2010 Patient Protection and Affordable Care Act (ACA), and nurses are needed to address care coordination and integration across the health care delivery system.

It can be argued that nursing is a unique profession in which the primary focus is caring—giving and managing the care that clients need. Thus nurses are both health care providers and health care coordinators; that is, they have both clinical and managerial role components. Beginning with the first edition of *Leadership & Nursing Care Management*, it has been this text's philosophy that these two components can be discussed separately but in fact overlap. Because all nurses are involved in coordinating client care, leadership and management principles are a part of the core competencies they need to function in a complex health care environment.

The turbulent swirl of change in this country's health care industry has become a paradigm shift that has provided both challenges and opportunities for nursing. Nurses need a stronger background in nursing leadership and care management to be prepared for contemporary and future nursing practice. As nurses mature in advanced practice roles and as the health care delivery system restructures, nurses will become increasingly pivotal to cost-effective health care delivery. Research is bearing this out. Leadership and management are crucial skills and abilities for complex and integrated community and regional networks that employ and deploy nurses to provide health care services to clients and communities.

Today's nurses are expected to be able to lead and manage care across the health care continuum—a radically different approach to nursing from what has been the norm for hospital staff nursing practice. In all settings, including both nurse-run and interdisciplinary clinics, nursing leadership and management are complementary skills that add value to solid clinical care and patient- and client-oriented practice. Thus there is an urgent need to advance nurses' knowledge and skills in leadership and management. In addition, nurses who are expected to make and implement day-to-day management decisions need to know how these precepts can be practically applied to the organization and delivery of nursing care in a way that conserves scarce resources, reduces costs, and maintains or improves quality of care. This is the emphasis on adding value, innovation, and prevention interventions.

The primary modality for health care in the United States has moved away from acute care hospitalization. As prevention, wellness, and alternative sites for care delivery become more important, nursing's already rich experiential tradition of practice in these settings is emerging. This text reflects this contemporary trend by blending the hospital and nonhospital perspectives with an eye toward systems leadership and management.

PURPOSE AND AUDIENCE

The intent of this text is to provide both a broad introduction to the field and a synthesis of the knowledge base and skills related to both nursing leadership and nursing care management. It is an evidence-based blend of practice and theory that breaks new ground by explaining the intersection of nursing care with leading people and managing organizations and systems. It highlights the evidence base for care management. It combines traditional management perspectives and theory with contemporary health care trends and issues and consistently integrates leadership and management concepts. These concepts are illustrated and made relevant by practice-based examples.

The impetus for writing this text comes from teaching both undergraduate and graduate students in nursing leadership and management and from perceiving the need for a comprehensive, practice-based textbook that blends and integrates leadership and management into an understandable and applicable whole.

Therefore the main goal of *Leadership & Nursing Care Management* is twofold: (1) to clearly differentiate traditional leadership and management perspectives and (2) to relate them in an integrated way with contemporary nursing trends and practice applications. This textbook is designed to serve the needs of nurses and nursing students who seek a foundation in the principles of leading and coordinating nursing services in relation to client care, peers, superiors, and subordinates.

ORGANIZATION AND COVERAGE

This sixth edition continues the format first used with the third edition. The first two editions were Dr. Huber's single-authored texts. The edited book approach draws together the best thinking of experts in the field—both nurses and non-nurses—to enrich and deepen the presentation of core essential knowledge and skills. Beginning with the first edition, a hallmark of *Leadership & Nursing Care Management* has been its depth of coverage, its comprehensiveness, and its strong evidence-based foundation. This sixth edition continues the emphasis on explaining theory in an easily understandable way to enhance comprehension.

The content of this sixth edition has been reorganized and refreshed to integrate leadership and care management topics with the nurse executive leadership competencies of the 2015 American Organization of Nurse Executives (AONE) while revamping, refocusing, and synthesizing the content. AONE has identified the evidence-based core competencies in the field, and

the content of this book has been aligned accordingly to reflect the knowledge underlying quality management of nursing services. This will help the reader develop the crucial skills and knowledge needed for core competencies.

The organizational framework of this book groups the 27 chapters into the following five parts:

Part I: Leadership aligns with the AONE competency category of the same name and provides an orientation to the basic principles of both leadership and management. Part I contains chapters on Leadership and Management Principles, Change and Innovation, and Organizational Climate and Culture.

Part II: Professionalism aligns with the AONE competency category of the same name and addresses the nurse's role and career development. The reader is prompted to examine the role of the nurse leader and manager. Part II discusses the content areas of Managerial Decision Making, Managing Time and Stress, and Legal and Ethical Issues.

Part III: Communication and Relationship Building aligns with the AONE competency category of the same name. Part III focuses on Communication Leadership, Team Building and Working With Effective Groups, Delegation in Nursing, Power and Conflict, and Workplace Diversity. These are essential knowledge and skill areas for nurse leaders and managers as they work with and through others in care delivery.

Part IV: Knowledge of the Health Care Environment covers the AONE competency category of the same name and features a broad array of chapters. Part IV encompasses Organizational Structure, Decentralization and Shared Governance, Strategic Management, Professional Practice Models, Case and Population Health Management, Evidence-Based Practice: Strategies for Nursing Leaders, Quality and Safety, and Measuring and Managing Outcomes. This discussion highlights the importance of understanding the health care organizational structures within which nursing care delivery must operate. This section includes information on traditional organizational theory, professional practice models, and the dynamics of decentralized and shared governance.

Part V: Business Skills aligns with the AONE competency category on business skills and principles and contains an extensive grouping of chapters related to Prevention of Workplace Violence; Confronting the Nursing Shortage;

Staffing and Scheduling; Budgeting, Productivity, and Costing Out Nursing; Performance Appraisal; Emergency Management and Preparedness; Data Management and Clinical Informatics; and Marketing. These chapters discuss the opportunities and challenges for the nurse leader-manager when dealing with the health care workforce. The wide range of human resource responsibilities of nurse managers is reviewed, and resources for further study are provided. The significant share of scarce organization budgets consumed by the human resources of an institution makes this area of management a key challenge that requires intricate skills in leadership and management. This section examines some of the important factors that nurse leader-managers must consider in the nursing and health care environment. Also in this section are chapters that build on organizational theory and demonstrate the importance of integrating organizations and systems with the current technology and theory applications, including data management and informatics, strategic management, and marketing.

The 27 chapters in this text are organized in a consistent format that highlights the following features:
- Concept definitions
- Theoretical and research background
- Leadership and management implications
- Current issues and trends
- Case Studies and Critical Thinking Exercises
- Research Notes

This format is designed to bridge the gap between theory and practice and to increase the relevance of nursing leadership and management by demonstrating the way in which theory translates into behaviors appropriate to contemporary leadership and nursing care management.

TEXT FEATURES

This book contains several interesting and effective aids to readers' comprehension, critical thinking, and application.

Critical Thinking Exercises

Found at the end of each chapter, this feature challenges readers to inquire and reflect, analyze critically the knowledge presented, and apply it to the situation.

Research Notes

These summaries of current research studies are highlighted in every chapter and introduce the reader to the liveliness and applicability of the available literature in nursing leadership and management.

Case Studies

Found at the end of each chapter, these vignettes introduce the reader to the "real world" of nursing leadership and management and demonstrate the ways in which the chapter concepts operate in specific situations. These vignettes show the creativity and energy that characterize expert nurse administrators as they tackle issues in practice.

LEARNING AND TEACHING AIDS

For Students

The Evolve Student Resources for this book include the following:
- *NCLEX Review Questions*, including rationales and page references

For Instructors

The Evolve Instructor Resources for this book include the following:
- *TEACH for Nurses* lesson plans, based on textbook chapter Learning Objectives, serve as ready-made, modifiable lesson plans and a complete roadmap to link all parts of the educational package. These concise and straightforward lesson plans can be modified or combined to meet your particular scheduling and teaching needs.
- *Test Bank* in ExamView format, featuring over 650 test items, complete with correct answer, rationale, cognitive level, nursing process step, appropriate NCLEX label, and corresponding textbook page references. The ExamView program allows instructors to create new tests; edit, add, and delete test questions; sort questions by NCLEX category, cognitive level, and nursing process step; and administer and grade tests online.
- *PowerPoint Presentations* with more than 650 customizable lecture slides.
- *Audience Response Questions* for i-clicker and other systems with two to three multiple-answer questions per chapter to stimulate class discussion and assess student understanding of key concepts.

ACKNOWLEDGMENTS

This book is dedicated to my husband, Bob Huber. He made this book a reality and was the text and graphics support behind it through the fifth edition. For his love, caring, and support I am eternally grateful. To my children, Brad Gardner and Lisa Witte, and their spouses, Nonalee Gardner and John Witte, for their enthusiasm and love. I am forever privileged that they are in my life. I thank them for the gifts of Kathryn Anne Gardner (the Princess), Anthony James Gardner (A.J.), Logan Thomas Witte, and Olivia Morgan Witte. I love being Grandma to these wonderful people. Also special are Chris Huber; Beth Nau and grandchildren Brandon, Danielle, Creighton, Chloe, and the late Cameron Nau; and Von and Kirk Danielson and Kory, Ryan, and Sean Danielson.

To my professional colleagues who inspired me and served as examples of excellence in nursing, I am grateful that you are in my life. To my nursing students, past and future, my thanks for being a source of continual intellectual stimulation and challenge. To all of you who have read and used this book, thank you. It is so very humbling and heartwarming when you mention this to me as we intersect on professional pathways. I am glad it is of use to you.

This book's first two editions evolved under the tender care of Thomas Eoyang, former editorial manager at W.B. Saunders Company, whose guidance, support, and caring were invaluable. To the editors in the Elsevier Nursing Division who worked so hard to facilitate everything related to the sixth edition, and to the excellent staff at Elsevier, a sincere thank you.

Diane L. Huber

PART I Leadership

1 Leadership and Management Principles, 1
Diane L. Huber
  Definitions, 2
  Leadership and Care Management
    Differentiated, 2
  Leadership Overview, 3
  Background Related to Leadership, 6
  Leadership: Five Interwoven Aspects, 6
  Leadership Theories, 8
  Contemporary Leadership: Interactional and
    Relationship-Based, 14
  Effective Leadership, 17
  Followership, 17
  Leadership and Management Roles, 18
  MANAGEMENT OVERVIEW, 18
  Definitions, 18
  Background: The Management Process, 19
  Management in Organizations, 22
  Leadership and Management Implications, 28
  Current Issues and Trends, 28

2 Change and Innovation, 32
Maryanne Garon
  Definitions, 33
  Background, 33
  Change Theories/Models, 34
  The Process of Change, 36
  Leadership and Change, 40
  Power and Politics, 40
  Innovation Theory, 41
  Leadership and Management Implications, 44
  Current Issues and Trends, 45
  Best Practice Suggestions for Nurse
    Leaders, 46

3 Organizational Climate and Culture, 49
Jennifer Bellot
  Definitions, 49
  Background, 51
  Research, 51
  Leadership and Management Implications, 54
  Current Issues and Trends, 55

PART II Professionalism

4 Managerial Decision Making, 60
Betsy Frank
  Definitions, 60
  Background, 61
  Decision-Making Process, 64
  Clinical Decision Making, 64
  Managerial and Organizational Decision
    Making, 65
  Decision-Making Tools, 67
  Leadership and Management Implications, 69
  Current Issues and Trends, 70

5 Managing Time and Stress, 74
Susan R. Lacey, Karen S. Cox, Adrienne Olney
  Definitions, 75
  The Relationship Between Time and Stress, 75
  Moral Distress, 76
  Resilience, 77
  Leadership and Management Implications, 77
  Current Issues and Trends, 81

6 Legal and Ethical Issues, 85
Lynn S. Muller
  Definitions, 86
  Background, 87
  The Legal System and Sources of Law, 87
  Licensure, Multi-State, and Distance
    Practice, 92
  Legal Documents and the Nurse, 93
  Ethical Components, 95
  Leadership and Management Implications, 96
  Current Issues and Trends, 99

PART III Communication and Relationship Building

7 Communication Leadership, 102
Kathleen A. Vertino
  Definitions, 102
  Background, 102
  Communication Theories and Models, 103
  Organizational Culture and Climate, 108

Holistic and Spiritual Health Care, 109
Leadership and Management
   Implications, 110
Communication to Facilitate Change:
   Kotter, 113
Current Issues and Trends, 114
Communication Issues, 114

8   Team Building and Working With Effective
    Groups, 118
    Anne Gallagher Peach
    Definitions, 119
    Background, 120
    Why Groups Are Formed, 121
    Advantages of Groups, 122
    Disadvantages of Groups, 123
    Group Decision Making, 124
    Working With Teams, 125
    Committees, 128
    Effective Meetings, 129
    Constructive Group Roles and Behaviors, 132
    Disruptive Roles and Behaviors, 133
    Managing Disruptive Behavior in Groups, 134
    Leadership and Management
       Implications, 134
    Current Issues and Trends, 135

9   Delegation in Nursing, 140
    Jayne Josephsen
    Definitions, 141
    The Process of Delegation, 142
    Prioritization, 144
    Barriers to Delegation, 145
    Ethical and Legal Issues Concerning
       Delegation, 147
    Leadership and Management
       Implications, 149
    Current Issues and Trends, 149

10 Power and Conflict, 153
    Kathleen B. Cox
    POWER, 153
    Definitions, 153
    Authority and Influence, 155
    Sources of Power, 156
    The Power of the Subunit, 158
    Power Theories, 159
    Leadership and Management
       Implications, 160

CONFLICT, 161
    Definitions, 162
    Views of Conflict, 162
    Types of Conflict, 163
    Models of Conflict, 164
    Bullying and Disruptive Behavior, 166
    Conflict Scales, 167
    Conflict Management and Alternative Dispute
       Resolution, 167
    Conflict Resolution, 169
    Leadership and Management
       Implications, 171
    Current Issues and Trends, 172

11 Workplace Diversity, 175
    Michael Soon Lee
    Definitions, 175
    Background, 176
    The Impact of Culture, 176
    The National CLAS Standards, 178
    Gaining a Competitive Edge in the
       Marketplace, 180
    Decreasing the Risk of Liability, 180
    Communication, 181
    Generational Diversity, 181
    Leadership and Management
       Implications, 182
    Current Issues and Trends, 184

PART IV   Knowledge of the Health Care Environment

12 Organizational Structure, 187
    Carol A. Wong
    Definitions, 187
    Organization Theory, 187
    Key Theories of Organizations as Social
       Systems, 189
    Key Organizational Design Concepts, 191
    Organizational Charts, 198
    Organizational Shapes, 198
    Structural Power, 201
    Leadership and Management Implications, 201
    Current Issues and Trends, 203

13 Decentralization and Shared Governance, 206
    Cheryl Hoying
    Definitions, 206
    Background, 206

Shared Governance, 208
Leadership and Management
    Implications, 209
Current Issues and Trends, 212

14 **Strategic Management, 216**
    Mary G. Harper
    Definitions, 217
    Strategic Planning Process, 217
    Elements of a Strategic Plan, 221
    Implementation of the Strategic Plan, 222
    Leadership and Management
        Implications, 222
    Current Issues and Trends, 222
    Conclusion, 223

15 **Professional Practice Models, 225**
    Maura MacPhee, Farinaz Havaei
    Definitions, 226
    Background, 226
    Types of Care Delivery Models, 230
    Evolving Models, 234
    Innovative and Future Models, 234
    Leadership and Management
        Implications, 236
    Current Issues and Trends, 236

16 **Case and Population Health Management, 240**
    Ellen Fink-Samnick, Teresa M. Treiger
    Definitions, 240
    Background, 241
    Case Management, 242
    Disease Management, 254
    Leadership and Management
        Implications, 262
    Current Issues and Trends, 263

17 **Evidence-Based Practice: Strategies for Nursing
    Leaders, 268**
    *Laura Cullen, Kirsten Hanrahan, Nathan Neis,
    Michele Farrington, Trudy A. Laffoon, Cindy J. Dawson*
    Definitions, 268
    Models, 270
    Steps for Performing Evidence-Based
        Practice, 270
    Implementing and Sustaining Evidence-Based
        Practice Changes, 271
    An Evidence-Based Practice Exemplar, 274

Organizational Infrastructure and Context, 276
Leadership Roles in Promoting
    Evidence-Based Practice, 279
Leadership and Management
    Implications, 280
Current Issues and Trends, 280
Conclusion, 282

18 **Quality and Safety, 286**
    Luc R. Pelletier
    Definitions, 286
    Health Care Quality in the Twenty-First
        Century, 288
    Collaboration and Health Care Quality as
        Professional Nursing Imperatives, 290
    Industrial Models of Quality, 290
    Standards of Quality, 291
    Emerging Models of Health Care Performance
        and Quality Management, 293
    Costs Associated With Poor Health Care
        Quality, 296
    Leadership and Management
        Implications, 297
    Current Issues and Trends, 303

19 **Measuring and Managing Outcomes, 317**
    Sean P. Clarke, Lianne Jeffs, Abdullah S. Suhemat
    Definitions, 317
    Influences on Outcomes, 320
    Measurement of Outcomes, 320
    Elements of Outcomes Research, 320
    Leadership and Management
        Implications, 321
    Current Issues and Trends, 322

PART V   Business Skills

20 **Prevention of Workplace Violence, 328**
    Gregory O. Ginn, L. Jean Henry, Teresa Kathleen Sparks
    Definitions, 328
    Background, 329
    Parameters of Violence, 330
    Regulatory Background, 330
    Leadership and Management
        Implications, 334
    Current Issues and Trends, 335
    Conclusion, 337

21 Confronting the Nursing Shortage, 340
Julie A. Holt
  Definitions, 340
  Background, 341
  Factors Contributing to the Nursing
    Shortage, 344
  American Nurses Association's Call to
    Action, 354
  The Future of Nursing: Leading Change,
    Advancing Health, 355
  Recruitment, 356
  Retention: New Graduates and Experienced
    Registered Nurses, 361
  Leadership and Management
    Implications, 364

22 Staffing and Scheduling, 369
M. Lindell Joseph
  Definitions, 370
  Framework for Staffing Management, 371
  Strategies Influencing Staffing
    Management, 371
  Leadership and Management
    Implications, 376
  The Staffing Management Plan, 377
  Organizational Outcomes, 383
  Current Issues and Trends, 384

**23 Budgeting, Productivity, and Costing Out
Nursing, 388**
Linda B. Talley, Diane H. Thorgrimson
  Background, 388
  Definitions, 389
  The Budget Process, 389
  Tracking and Monitoring of Budgets, 393
  Leadership and Management
    Implications, 394
  Productivity, 397
  Current Issues and Trends, 398

24 Performance Appraisal, 401
Marie-Hélène Budworth
  Definitions, 401
  Purposes of Performance Appraisal, 401
  Issues in Performance Appraisal, 402
  Leadership and Management
    Implications, 407
  Current Issues and Trends, 407

25 Emergency Management and Preparedness, 410
Elizabeth T. Dugan, Lynn Christensen
  Transitioning Theory Into Practice for
    All-Hazards Preparedness, 410
  Definitions, 411
  Getting Started: First Steps, 411
  Crisis Standards of Care, 421
  Leadership and Management
    Implications, 421
  Current Issues and Trends, 422

26 Data Management and Clinical Informatics, 428
Jane M. Brokel
  Definitions, 429
  Nursing's Data Needs, 431
  Nursing Informatics, 433
  Electronic Health Records, 436
  Health Information Exchanges, 438
  Effectiveness, 439
  Standardized Clinical Terminology, 439
  Nursing Management Minimum Data Set, 440
  Leadership and Management
    Implications, 442
  Current Issues and Trends, 443

27 Marketing, 447
Slimen Saliba
  Definitions and Core Concepts, 448
  Background, 450
  Marketing Strategy, 450
  The Marketing Process: Focus on Marketing
    Mix, 451
  Leadership and Management
    Implications, 453
  Current Issues and Trends, 455
  Summary, 456

References, 460
Index, 501

Leadership and Management Principles

Diane L. Huber

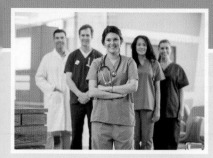

http://evolve.elsevier.com/Huber/leadership

Health care is predicted to be in for a "bumpy ride" in the near future (Curtin, 2016). Both the practice of health care professionals and the effectiveness of organizations are affected by change, complexity, and environmental turbulence. The twin skills of leadership and management are crucial to nurses' effectiveness and organizational survival. There is an evidence base of knowledge about leadership and management, and both can be learned.

Issues of cost, access, methods and structures of care delivery, and quality form the broader context of health care. The effect on nursing is an urgent need for leadership and management at all levels and places where nurses work. With 2.9 million licensed registered nurses (RNs) in the United States (Bureau of Health Professions [BHPr], 2014), RNs are the largest segment of the health care workforce. Strong and prepared leaders are needed to guide their practice. Leading and managing are essential skills, made more acutely urgent given health care system characteristics of rapid change, complexity, and chaos.

The BHPr (2014) noted that the rapidly changing health care delivery system is redefining both how care is delivered and the role of the nursing workforce. Emerging care delivery models, with a focus on managing health status and preventing acute health issues, will likely contribute to new growth in demand for nurses as they assume new and/or expanded roles in preventive care and care coordination. Supply and demand for nurses will continue to be affected by

Photo used with permission from FatCamera/Getty Images.

numerous factors, including population growth and the aging of the nation's population, overall economic conditions, aging of the nursing workforce, and changes in health care reimbursement.

Leaders guide and motivate nurses to achieve their care provision goals as they practice nursing. Managers organize and guide nurses' work in organizations where they practice. Together the result is structures and processes that deliver desired outcomes. For the health care system, there are two predominant sets of desired outcomes. The first is the six aims for improvement of the Institute of Medicine (IOM, called the National Academies of Sciences, Engineering, and Medicine, Health and Medicine Division, since 2016) (IOM, 2001): Health care needs to be safe, effective, patient centered, timely, efficient, and equitable. The second is the Institute for Healthcare Improvement's (IHI, 2016) Triple Aim: Health care needs to simultaneously improve the health of the population, enhance the experience and the outcomes of the patient, and reduce per capita cost of care to benefit communities. The major national leadership initiatives in nursing are the IOM's (2011) report *The Future of Nursing: Leading Change, Advancing Health* and the Magnet Recognition Program® (American Nurses Credentialing Center [ANCC], 2016a). As nurses seek to embed themselves and grow in jobs and careers within health care services, leadership and management knowledge, skills, and abilities are important to overall effectiveness.

In nursing, leadership is studied as a way to increase the knowledge, skills, and abilities that nurses need to facilitate clinical and administrative outcomes while working with people across a variety of situations, settings, and sites. Effective leadership can also increase understanding and control of nurses' professional work settings. There is a long history, rich literature, and evidence base regarding leadership theories, much of it from outside of nursing. Nursing has drawn from both classic and contemporary thinkers.

For example, Bennis (1994) made a strong argument for leadership, stating that quality of life depends on the quality of leaders. He noted three reasons why leaders are important: the character of change in society, the de-emphasis on integrity in institutions, and the responsibility for the effectiveness of organizations. Fiedler and Garcia (1987) argued that leadership is one of the most important factors determining the survival and success of groups and organizations. *Effective* leadership is also important in nursing, specifically because of its impact on the quality of nurses' work lives, because it functions as a stabilizing influence during constant change, and because it underpins nurses' productivity and quality of care delivery.

Nurse leaders and managers are responsible for designing, developing, implementing, and sustaining the organizational infrastructure and environment that enable both large- and small-scale interventions for quality and safety. Research has shown that there are organizational and cultural factors that mediate hospital or system-wide interventions. These include the prevailing culture, such as being patient centered and having available effort and resources; human relationships, including leadership styles and teamwork; and an approach used for routine monitoring of systems and services (Clay-Williams et al., 2014; Stetler et al., 2014).

This chapter presents definitions and a detailed overview of both leadership and management. Theories are reviewed and important elements are discussed. Leadership and management implications and issues for nurses are presented, and practical examples are used to explain the content.

DEFINITIONS

There are a variety of definitions of **leadership,** one of which is the process of influencing people to accomplish goals. Key concepts related to leadership are influence, vision, communication, group process, goal attainment, and motivation. Hersey and colleagues (2013) defined

leadership as a process of influencing the behavior of either an individual or a group, regardless of the reason, in an effort to achieve goals in a given situation. Burns (1978) noted that leadership occurs when human beings with motives and purposes mobilize in competition or conflict with others to arouse, engage, and satisfy motives. Leaders "mobilize others to want to make extraordinary things happen in organizations" (Kouzes & Posner, 2012, p. 2).

Most leadership definitions incorporate the two components of an interaction among people and the process of influencing. Thus leadership is a social exchange phenomenon. At its core, leadership is about influencing people. In contrast, management involves influencing employees to meet an organization's goals and is focused primarily on organizational goals and objectives. Bennis (1994) listed a number of distinctions between leadership and management. He noted that the leader focuses on people, whereas the manager focuses on systems and structures. The leader innovates and conquers the context or situation. Another distinction is that a leader innovates, whereas a manager administers. Kotter (2001) noted that managers cope with complexity, whereas leaders cope with change.

Management is defined as the coordination and integration of resources through planning, organizing, coordinating, directing, and controlling to accomplish specific institutional goals and objectives. Hersey and colleagues (2013, p. 3) defined management as the "process of working with and through individuals and groups and other resources (such as equipment, capital, and technology) to accomplish organizational goals." They identified management as a special kind of leadership that concentrates on the achievement of organizational goals.

LEADERSHIP AND CARE MANAGEMENT DIFFERENTIATED

Leadership theory is often discussed separately from management theory. Some say leadership and management are two very different things. Yet clearly there is overlap in that an individual can be *both* leading and managing in some cases. The area of overlap may not be clear or explained. The premise of this book is that leadership and management are not identical ideas. This can be seen in their distinct definitions, yet sometimes they occur together or via multitasking.

If the delivery of nursing services involves the organization and coordination of complex activities in the human services realm, then both leadership and management are important elements. The leader's focus is on people; the manager focuses on systems and structure (Bennis, 1994). Thus, although both are used to accomplish goals, each has a different focus. Management is focused on task accomplishment, and leadership is focused on human relationship aspects. They may be sequential, and they are interrelated. Clearly, a balance of the two is necessary. Leadership and management have some shared characteristics. There is a "gray area" in which the focus of their outcomes overlap. In this area of overlap, the processes and strategies look similar and may be employed for a similar outcome or blended together to accomplish goals. This overlap occurs where the two processes are integrated or synthesized to accomplish goals and where the same strategies are employed even though the goals may differ. For example, a nurse may use leadership strategies or management strategies to motivate others, but the desired outcome of the motivation is likely to be different. For example, leadership may be used to empower nurses and management to reduce costs.

Leadership and management are equally important processes. Because they each have a different focus, their importance varies according to what is needed in a specific situation. Hersey and colleagues (2013) thought that leadership was a broader concept than management. They described management as a special kind of leadership. This view would position management as a part of leadership, not as a distinct concept. However, according to the definitions, characteristics, and processes, the concepts of leadership and management are different; but at the area of overlap they look similar. For example, directing occurs in both leadership and management activities (the area of overlap), whereas inspiring a vision is clearly a leadership function. Both leadership and management are necessary. Mintzberg's (1994) idea was that nursing management occurred in an interactive model rather than through a stepwise linear process. The interactive nature of both leadership and management make relationships and relationship building fundamental elements. "Transformational change happens one relationship at a time" (Koloroutis, 2004).

Jennings and colleagues (2007) took an evidence-based approach to differentiating nursing leadership from management to identify discrete competencies through an integrative content analysis of the literature base. In 140 articles reviewed, they found 894 competencies, of which 862 (96%) were common to both leadership and management. Thus the overlap area appeared to be larger than previously thought. However, leadership and management do serve distinct purposes. Perhaps it is time to apply leadership and management concepts and competencies by setting, level of role responsibility, career stage, and social context to more fully apply the evidence base to practice. For example, the American Organization of Nurse Executives (AONE) (2015) has begun this work by promulgating two levels of administrative competencies: nurse manager and nurse executive.

LEADERSHIP OVERVIEW

Leadership is an activity of human engagement and a relationship experience founded in trust, communication, inspiration, action, and "servanthood." The leadership role is so important because it embodies commitment and forward-reaching action. Arising from a drive to make things better, leaders use their power to bring teams together, spark innovation, create positive communication, and drive forward toward group goals.

Leadership is important to study, learn, and practice in today's complex, rapidly changing, turbulent, and chaotic health care work environment. Such an environment generates challenges to the nurse's identity, coping skills, and ability to work with others in harmony. It also presents the opportunity to lead, challenge assumptions, consolidate a purpose, and move a vision forward. Leadership is important for nurses because they need to possess knowledge and skills in the art and science of solving problems in work groups, systems of care, and the environment of care delivery. The effectiveness of an individual nurse depends partly on that individual's competence and partly on the creation of a facilitating environment that contains sufficient resources to accomplish goals. This is an underappreciated reality when it is assumed that results occur from only individual competence and effort. However, health care delivery is a team effort.

The nurse leader combines clinical, administrative, financial, and operational skills to solve problems in the care environment so that nurses can provide cost-effective care in a way that is satisfying and health promoting for patients and clients. Such an environment does not simply happen; it requires special skills and the courage and motivation to move a vision into action. For example, it may be easier to continue on the way things have always been done, but this strategy would not capture the advantages of new innovations. Thus the study of nursing leadership and care management directs critical thinking toward what it takes to be a nursing "environment architect," transition leader, and manager of care delivery services.

Strong evidence for the nurse leader's critical role both in the business of a health care organization and in the quality and safety of service delivery has been laid out by the IOM (2004), the ANCC's Magnet Recognition Program® (ANCC, 2016a), and the AONE (2015). The IOM focuses on the following five areas of management practice:

- Implementing evidence-based management
- Balancing tensions between efficiency and reliability
- Creating and sustaining trust
- Actively managing the change process through communication, feedback, training, sustained effort and attention, and worker involvement
- Creating a learning environment

The ANCC's Magnet program acknowledges excellence in nursing services and leadership based on five components: transformational leadership, structural empowerment, new knowledge, exemplary professional practice, and empirical outcomes (ANCC, 2016b). The Magnet Recognition Program® focuses specifically on nursing, is considered the "gold standard" in nursing, and is addressed in several chapters in this book because of its centrality to the evidence-based management practice called for by the IOM (2004). AONE's 2015

nurse executive competencies are described as falling within the following five domains of skill: communication and relationship management, leadership, business skills and principles, knowledge of the health care environment, and professionalism. Taken together, these source documents overlap and converge on the primary attributes, knowledge domains, abilities, and skills that nurse leaders need to lead people and manage organizations in health care.

The Two Roles of a Nurse

Nursing is a service profession, the core mission of which is the care, restoration of health, and nurturing of human beings in their experiences of health and illness. Nurses have two basic roles (McClure, 1991): care providers and care coordinators/integrators. The first role is the one that is recognized more often. The acute care medical model in hospitals over time came to be the primary focus of attention and jobs for nurses. In this illness-focused model, the nurse's care provider or "doing" role was the most important and valued aspect of nursing. Little reward came from the "thinking" and integrating skills nurses were capable of. The second role, the coordinator/integrator role, is a complementary function that arises from nursing's central positioning in the day-to-day coordination of service delivery and central location at the hub of information flow regarding care and service delivery. This linkage relationship is shown visually in Fig. 1.1.

With the shift to primary care and care coordination, the nurse's care management role has become more prominent, needed, and valued. The delivery of nursing services involves the organization and coordination of complex activities. Nurses use managerial and leadership skills to facilitate delivery of quality nursing care. A current example is the shift to population health

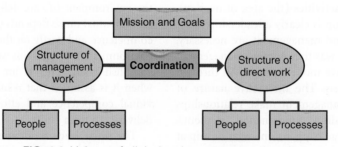

FIG. 1.1 Linkage of clinical and management domains.

management (PHM), which is responsive to the IHI's Triple Aim. Nurses have emerged as well-prepared practitioners, especially at the clinical nurse leader (CNL) and nurse practitioner levels of preparation (Joseph & Huber, 2015).

The Leadership Role

Leadership is a unique role and function. It can be part of a formal organizational managerial position, or it can arise spontaneously in any group. Certain characteristics, such as being motivated by challenge, commitment, and autonomy, are thought to be associated with leadership. Effectiveness is a key outcome of leadership efforts in health care. It has been suggested that there is a scarcity of leaders and a crisis in leadership in nursing. In times of chaos, complexity, and change, leadership is essential to provide the guidance, direction, and sense of stability needed to ensure followers' effectiveness and satisfaction. Nurses are challenged to respond with leadership and can best respond by demonstrating vision, using innovativeness (Joseph, 2015; Joseph et al., 2016), adapting to changes, seeking new tools for dealing with the new health care environment, and leading the way with client-centered strategies. Effective leaders are change agents and promote innovation. Innovation is seen as a viable mechanism to address care delivery complexity and is further discussed in Chapter 2.

Leadership Skills

Leadership is a natural element of nursing practice because the majority of nurses practice in work groups or units. Possessing the license of an RN implies certain leadership skills and requires the ability to delegate and supervise the work of others. Leadership can be understood as the ability to inspire confidence and support among followers, especially in organizations in which competence and commitment produce performance.

Leadership is an important issue related to how nurses integrate the various elements of nursing practice to ensure the highest quality of care for clients. Every nurse needs two critical skills to enhance professional practice. One is a skill with interpersonal relationships. This is fundamental to leadership and the work of nursing. The second is skill in applying the problem-solving process. This involves the ability to think critically, identify problems, and develop objectivity and a degree of maturity or judgment. Leadership skills build on professional and clinical skills. Hersey

and colleagues (2013) identified the following three skills needed for leading or influencing:

1. *Diagnosing:* Diagnosing involves being able to understand the situation and the problem to be solved or resolved. This is a cognitive competency.
2. *Adapting:* Adapting involves being able to adapt behaviors and other resources to match the situation. This is a behavioral competency.
3. *Communicating:* Communicating is used to advance the process in a way that individuals can understand and accept. This is a process competency.

Emotional Intelligence

Among the important personal leadership skills for nurses is emotional intelligence (EI). Based on the work of Goleman (2007), relational and emotional integrity are hallmarks of good leaders. EI traits are emotional factors consisting of five defining attributes: self-awareness, self-regulation or discipline, motivation, social awareness, and relationship management. EI can be understood as a constellation of self-perceptions of the person's empathy, impulsivity, and assertiveness, also including elements of social and personal intelligence. EI has been studied in nursing and shown to be related to transformational leadership (Spano-Szekely et al., 2016), nursing team performance and cohesiveness (Quoidbach & Hansenne, 2009), quality of care (Adams & Iseler, 2014), and as a moderator of stress-burnout (Görgens-Ekermans & Brand, 2010). Spano-Szekely and colleagues recommended that EI characteristics be considered during the hiring of nurse managers.

Adaptive thinking abilities are needed for leadership in the complex, volatile, and unpredictable environment of health care (Spano-Szekely et al., 2016). This is because the leader operates in a crucial cultural and contextual influencing mode within the organizational environment. The leader's behavior, patterns of actions, attitude, and performance have a special impact on the team's attitude and behaviors and on the context and character of work life. Followers observe and respond to all aspects of what leaders say and do (or do not do). Followers need to be able to depend on role consistency, balance, and behavioral integrity from the leader. The four EI skill sets needed by good leaders are as follows:

1. *Self-awareness:* Ability to read one's own emotional state and be aware of one's own mood and how this affects staff relationships

2. *Self-management:* Ability to take corrective action so as not to transfer negative affect to staff relationships
3. *Social awareness:* An intuitive skill of empathy and expressiveness in being sensitive and aware of the emotions and moods of others
4. *Relationship management:* Use of effective communication with others to disarm conflict and the ability to develop the emotional maturity of team members

Relationship Management and Relational Coordination

High performance, organizational health, and effectiveness are organizational goals. Relationship-based care has been proposed as a model for nursing care that promotes organizational health, thus resulting in positive outcomes (Koloroutis, 2004). Relationship-based care focuses on the care provider's three crucial relationships: relationship with patients and families, with self (nurtured by self-knowing and self-care), and with colleagues (commitment to healthy interpersonal relationships).

Gittell (2009) emphasized the centrality of relationship management because patient care is a coordination challenge. She noted that relational coordination drives quality and efficiency outcomes and health care performance. Relational coordination is defined as "coordinating work through relationships of shared goals, shared knowledge, and mutual respect" (p. xiii). Relational coordination focuses on *relationships among roles* rather than between individuals.

These interpersonal relationship skills are crucial to the work of leadership. The chaos and complexity of the seismic shifts in health care structure, delivery, form, technology, and knowledge have made visible the urgent need for leaders to emerge, mobilize, and encourage followers. Leaders are pivotal for connecting the efforts of followers to organizational goals in order to produce outcomes. However, good leaders are anchors to the vision and the larger mission, guides to coping and being productive, and champions of energy and enthusiasm for the work.

BACKGROUND RELATED TO LEADERSHIP

Terms related to leadership are *leadership styles, followership,* and *empowerment.* **Leadership styles** are defined as different combinations of task and relationship behaviors used to influence others to accomplish goals. **Followership** is defined as an interpersonal process of

participation. **Empowerment** means giving people the authority, responsibility, and freedom to act on their expert knowledge and skills.

Leadership can be best understood as a process. Much attention has been focused on leadership as a group and organizational process because organizational change is heavily influenced by the context or environment. Nurses need to have a solid foundation of knowledge in leadership and care management at all levels, although the depth and focus of care management roles and skills may vary by level. For example, the clinical nurse care provider or direct care ("bedside") nurse concentrates on the coordination of nursing care to individuals or groups and is a leader and manager within his/her scope of practice. This may include such activities as arranging access to services, providing direct care, doing referrals, and supporting a patient's family.

Nurses without formal positional authority are **informal leaders**. They influence peers and administrators and function in an influence sphere within interdisciplinary teams. Downey and colleagues (2011) described informal leaders as the hidden treasure of nursing leadership. They have varying forms of power, but they are a part of the shadow organization that operates behind the scenes of the formal chain of command in informal networks of people. They serve as advocates for the work being done and heighten the contributions of themselves and others through influence, relationship building, knowledge, and expertise. These nurses can be developed and empowered to affect unit performance and culture.

At the next level, the nurse manager concentrates on the day-to-day administration and coordination of services provided by a group of nurses. The nurse executive's role and functions concentrate on long-term administration of an institution or program that delivers nursing services, focusing on integrating the system and building a culture (Mintzberg, 1998). CNLs and advanced practice registered nurses (APRNs) provide leadership in the care and care transitions of individuals and populations while providing expertise to the organization in specialty areas.

LEADERSHIP: FIVE INTERWOVEN ASPECTS

Hersey and colleagues (2013) noted that the leadership process is a function of the leader, the followers, and

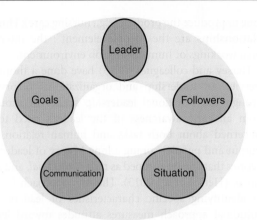

FIG. 1.2 Components of a leadership moment.

other situational variables. The leadership process includes five interwoven, connected but distinct, aspects: (1) the leader, (2) the follower, (3) the situation, (4) the communication process, and (5) the goals. Fig. 1.2 shows how these components relate to one another. All five elements interact within any given leadership circumstance.

Process Part 1: The Leader

The values, skills, and style of the leader are important. His or her internalized pattern of basic behaviors influences actions and the ability to lead. Leaders' perceptions of themselves, their roles, and their expectations also have an impact on their followers. Self-awareness is crucial to leadership effectiveness. Among the internal forces in leaders that impinge on leadership style are values, energy level, confidence in employees, leadership inclinations, motivation for leadership, and sense of security in uncertainty. Interpersonal, emotional, and social intelligence skills also contribute to the effective leadership of knowledge workers (Goleman, 2007).

Process Part 2: The Follower

Followership is the flip side of leadership. It is likely that without followers there is no leadership. Followers are vital because they accept or reject the leader and determine the leader's personal power (Hersey et al., 2013). Followership is underappreciated. "Leaders can be leaders only if they have followers" (Grossman & Valiga, 2013, p. 43). Followership can be learned and consciously developed. There are types of followers, ranging from being vital to the success of the group to being passive and unthinking. Using the variables of performance initiative (high to low) and relationship initiative (high to low), Grossman and Valiga (2013) developed a grid of four followership styles: subordinate, contributor, partner, and politician. Effective followers show characteristics of assertiveness, determination, willingness to challenge ideas, an ability to act, and openness to new ideas. Followers also need self-awareness to know themselves and their expectations. Situations in which members of a group are not accustomed to working together or do not hold shared expectations frequently lead to conflict. Followership is based on trust. Groups have personalities that include a discernible level of trust. The wise leader assesses the trust and readiness to change levels of the group. Followership is not as simple as it seems.

Process Part 3: The Situation

The specific circumstances surrounding any given leadership situation will vary. Elements such as work demands, control systems, amount of task structure, degree of interaction, amount of time available for decision making, and external environment shape the differences among situations (Hersey et al., 2013). For example, in acute care hospitals, staffing levels and policies strongly influence many aspects of a nurse's work life. Organizational culture and ethos are also important factors in the situation. For example, in one setting the culture may resemble one big happy family, with an emphasis on teamwork and morale boosting. The cultural aspects of that leadership situation are different from those of an organization where there is a fast-paced tempo and people seem too busy. Environmental or cultural differences also cause the leadership situation to vary. The leadership situation in a group that is knowledgeable and experienced in solving problems is very different from the leadership situation in a group that is not experienced at the task or at working together. The personality styles of both superiors and subordinates have an influence on the situation, the work demands, and the amount of time and resources available.

Process Part 4: Communication

Communication processes vary among groups regarding the patterns and channels used and the degree to which the communication flow is open or closed. Communicating is basic to the process of influencing and thus to leadership. Almost every issue or problem contains a communication aspect. Through communication, the leader's vision and message are received by the followers. After choosing a channel, the sender transmits a message, but the message is filtered through the receiver's perception. Communication is transmitted through both verbal and nonverbal modes. Organizations include a variety of communication structures and flows. These may be downward, upward, horizontal, grapevines, or networks. Communication may be formal or informal (Hersey et al., 2013). Certain acts performed by leaders have positive effects and make people feel more respected; listening and informal chatting are prime examples because they foster interpersonal and relational trust and social cohesion.

Process Part 5: Goals

Organizations have goals, and individuals working in organizations also have goals. These goals may or may not be congruent. For example, the goal of the organization may be to decrease costs or increase revenue. In contrast, the goal of the individual nurse may be to spend time counseling and teaching clients because that is what is seen by the nurse as the most important activity. Goals may thus be in conflict, in which case there is tension and a need for leadership.

Clearly, leadership is a complex and multidimensional process. Nurses need to be aware of the interacting elements in any leadership situation. Critical thinking can be applied to diagnosing and analyzing the five elements, adapting to the situation, and communicating for effectiveness. For example, if a nurse works in a situation in which there is a high level of frustration, it may be time to step back and analyze the basic five elements. Doing so sets the stage for better decision making about change strategies and strategic management.

LEADERSHIP THEORIES

Leadership is so critical that it has been studied for a very long time, especially in the business literature. Leadership theories are presented here because the review of the development of thought about what leadership is helps the nurse to critically analyze perspectives and alternative approaches to skills and choices about one's own leadership style in any given situation. Leadership in fundamentally about the two basic elements of tasks and relationships. **Tasks** are the job aspects that must be done to produce the product (e.g., nursing care). Human **relationships** are the "people element": the interpersonal workings of humans in a job environment.

Hersey and colleagues (2013) have done a thorough overview of leadership and organizational theory up through the situational leadership school of thought. From an early awareness of the leader's need to be concerned about both tasks and human relationships (output and people) sprang a long history of leadership theories that can be grouped as *trait, attitudinal,* and *situational* (Hersey et al., 2013). The trait approach focuses on identifying specific characteristics of leaders. The attitudinal approach measures attitudes toward leader behavior. The situational approach focuses on observed behaviors of leaders and how leadership styles can be matched to situations. Leadership theories have evolved away from an early focus on the traits or characteristics of the leader as a person because it was found that it is not possible to predict leadership from clusters of traits, yet interest remains in the characteristics to look for in good leaders. Major theories will be discussed.

Trait Theories: Characteristics of Leadership

In the trait approach, theorists have sought to understand leadership by examining the characteristics of leaders. Presumably, leaders could be differentiated from nonleaders. The trait approach has generated multiple lists of traits proposed to be essential to leadership. Bennis (1994) identified a recipe for leadership that contained six ingredients: a guiding vision, passion, integrity (including self-knowledge, candor, and maturity), trust, curiosity, and daring. Leaders arise in a context, and they are said to be made, not born. They appear to learn leadership skills in stages (Bennis, 2004). Thus leadership skills can be both taught and learned. It is important for nurses to recognize that they can learn, practice, and improve their personal leadership competencies.

Leaders need to ask the right questions, such as these: What needs to be done? What can I do to make a difference? What are the goals? What constitutes performance and results? Leaders are active, not passive. Leaders engage their environment with behaviors of doing, influencing, and moving. These are action terms that need to be melded with expertise and empathy. Leaders are those who talk about adventures into new territory and take the risks inherent in innovation (Kouzes & Posner, 2012). Leadership means giving guidance and using a focused vision.

Research by Bennis and Thomas (2002) indicated that extraordinary leaders possess skills required to overcome adversity and emerge stronger and more committed. Great leaders possess the following four essential skills: the ability to engage others in shared meaning, a distinctive and compelling vocal tone, a sense of integrity, and a combination of hardiness and ability to grasp context, called "adaptive capacity."

Characteristics such as knowledge, motivating people to work harder, trust, communication, enthusiasm, vision, courage, ability to see the big picture, and ability to take risks are associated with important leadership qualities in research findings. Kouzes and Posner (2012) found that for people to be willing followers, the leader needs to be honest, forward-looking, competent, and inspiring. They identified the Five Practices of Exemplary Leadership that correlate with leadership excellence:

1. *Model the way:* Leaders set an example and structure events so that incremental progress is celebrated as small wins.
2. *Inspire a shared vision:* Leaders envision the future and enlist others in sharing the dream.
3. *Challenge the process:* Leaders go beyond the status quo to search for opportunities, experiment, and take risks to achieve lofty goals.
4. *Enable others to act:* Leaders foster collaboration and develop and strengthen others so that the whole team performs well.
5. *Encourage the heart:* Leaders appreciate and recognize individual contributions and formally celebrate accomplishments.

This model of leadership has been used in nursing research looking at staff nurse clinical leadership (Patrick et al., 2011).

Vision and Trust

Although the lists of leadership characteristics and competencies vary somewhat, the functions of visioning, setting the direction, inspiration, motivation, and enabling systems and followers are at the core of leadership activity. Bennis (1994) discussed what has come to be called "the vision thing." The one specific defining quality of leaders is vision: the ability to create a vision and put it into operation.

Leadership is founded on trust: "Trust is the emotional glue that binds leaders and employees together and is a measure of the legitimacy of leadership" (Malloch, 2002, p. 14). Organizations that focus on sustaining a healing culture rebuild organizational trust by focusing on trust in relationships with employees. Behaviors that build trust include sharing relevant information, reducing controls, and meeting expectations. Trust-destroying behaviors include being insensitive to beliefs and values, avoiding discussion of sensitive issues, and encouraging competition via winners and losers. Trust goes both ways and needs to be nurtured. Nurses can start by examining their own behaviors and then taking deliberative actions to strengthen trust in the environment.

Leadership Styles Theories

As leadership theories evolved, leadership came to be viewed as a dynamic process and an interaction among the leader, the followers, and the situation. Leadership theory began to move beyond a focus on traits to explore the concept of leadership styles. Styles of leadership range from authoritarian to permissive to democratic and from transactional to transformational. The individual nurse's task is to determine in which environments he or she functions best and is most comfortable or where he or she most likely will succeed. This facilitates placement for success and a better match between leader and follower.

Leadership styles are defined as different combinations of task and relationship behaviors used to influence others to accomplish goals. They are sets or clusters of behaviors used in the process of effecting leadership. Hersey and colleagues (2013) defined these terms as follows:

- *Task behavior:* The extent to which leaders organize and define roles; explain activities; determine when, where, and how tasks are to be accomplished; and endeavor to get work accomplished
- *Relationship behavior:* The extent to which leaders maintain personal relationships by opening communication and providing psycho-emotional support and facilitating behaviors

Hersey and colleagues (2013) said that leadership styles are the consistent behavior patterns exhibited in influencing the activities of others by working with and through them, as perceived by those others. Different styles evoke variable responses in different situations. A leader's leadership style is some combination of task and relationship behavior.

Tannenbaum and Schmidt (1973) suggested that a leader might select one of many behavior styles arrayed

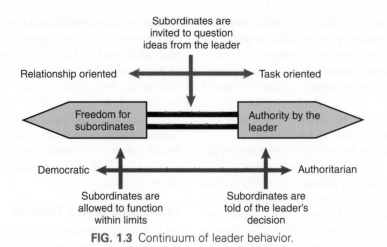

FIG. 1.3 Continuum of leader behavior.

along a continuum. The continuum ranges from democratic to authoritarian (or subordinate centered to leader centered). Their work suggested that there are a variety of leadership styles (Fig. 1.3) or points along the continuum. They discussed three distinct styles: authoritarian, democratic, and laissez-faire. Some individuals are able to integrate styles and flexibly match to the situation at hand, but this is rare.

Authoritarian

The authoritarian leadership style primarily uses directive behaviors. Decisions of policy are made solely by the leader, who tends to dictate tasks and techniques to followers. Leaders tell the followers what to do and how to do it. This style emphasizes a high concern for task. Authoritarian leaders are characterized by giving orders. Their style can create hostility and dependency among followers; it may also stifle creativity and innovation. On the other hand, this style can be very efficient, especially in a crisis or during a code situation.

Democratic

This approach implies a relationship and person orientation. Policies are a matter of group discussion and decision. The leader encourages and assists discussion and group decision making. Human relations and teamwork are the focus. The leader shares responsibility with the followers by involving them in decision making. In nursing, interdisciplinary teamwork is a major element in effectiveness. The democratic style may appear to move more slowly and is thought to

take longer than using an authoritarian style. This is because group consensus needs time and facilitation to be fostered. Furthermore, the needs of disenfranchised minority groups must be balanced. Intergroup cohesion is a focus with this style. The challenge of the democratic style is to get people with different professional backgrounds, personal biases, and psychological needs together to focus on the problem and next action steps. Motivating participation is a constant challenge.

Laissez-Faire

This style promotes complete freedom for group or individual decisions. There is a minimum of leader participation. A leader using this style may seem to be apathetic. Because the style is based on noninterference, a clear decision may never be formulated. The laissez-faire style results in a decision, conscious or otherwise, to avoid interference and let events take their own course. The leader is either permissive and fosters freedom or is inept at guiding a group. Followers may need greater structure than the leader gives them. Despite its potential drawbacks, this style has advantages when used with some circumstances involving groups of fully independent care providers or professionals working together.

Overall, one style is not necessarily better than another. Each has advantages and disadvantages. There are situational and contextual factors to consider when choosing a style. Styles should vary according to the appropriateness of the situation with reference to an evaluation of effectiveness. Flexibility is important. For example, if a nurse prefers to operate in a democratic style yet suddenly a code situation occurs, then the nurse must rapidly switch from a democratic to an authoritarian style. Some democratic leaders cannot vary their style sufficiently to handle crises. On the other hand, in a staff meeting, an authoritarian leader may be ineffective with a group of professionals and would need to be flexible enough to switch to a democratic or laissez-faire style, depending on the circumstances. The basic needs are for leader self-awareness and knowledge of the group's ability and willingness levels before examining the situational elements and choosing a leadership style. Self-awareness is key to strategically using leadership styles.

Feminist Leadership Perspective

Leadership styles appear to have a gender component. The feminist perspective on leadership was presented by Helgeson (1995a, b). She identified female leadership as a web-like structure that is dynamic and continuously expanding and contracting. It is characterized by a concern for family, community, and culture. The inclination is for a democratic power style, and the emphasis is on the importance of establishing relationships, maintaining connections with others, and deriving strength from empowering others. By contrast, leadership approaches described by men, as a generalization, tend to be influenced by the military and participating in team sports. Men tend to spend their time on meetings and tasks requiring immediate attention, focusing on completion of tasks and achievement of goals. Women tend to focus on process; men tend to focus on achievement and closure. Women tend to be more flexible and value cooperation, connectedness, and relationships. Exploring the feminist perspective on leadership is valuable in that it provides food for thought as health care organizations and the nurses working in them struggle with not wanting to let go of the familiar hierarchical management style yet need to reconfigure to the circular or web structure to be effective. It is not known whether gender differences are permanent characteristics or are culturally mediated artifacts that blur with time.

Reynolds (2011) explored the thesis that servant leadership is a gender-integrative, partnership-oriented approach to leadership, using the feminist ethic of care. Leadership is a system for organizing activity, and gender is a system for organizing meaning. Yet mainstream leadership theory has ignored gender-related aspects of power. Scholars of communication and leadership have identified the management of meaning as one of the significant acts of leadership. Barker and Young (1994) saw transformational leadership as providing a favorable environment and a feminist connection for nurse leaders.

Situational Leadership Theories

A third phase of leadership theories grew out of a group of contingency theories whose central idea was that organizational behavior is contingent on the situation or environment. This means that which theory or style is the best all depends on the situation at hand. What is needed by the leader is diagnostic ability. The leader observes and analyzes which abilities and motives are present in the followers. With sensitivity, cues in the environment can be identified and used to make choices regarding leadership style. One choice a leader has is to alter his or her own behavior and the leadership style used. Personal flexibility and leadership skills are needed to vary one's style when the followers' needs and motives change or vary. The ability to diagnose, choose, and alter behavior to implement a leadership style best matched to the situation is a critical skill needed for effective leadership. Thus no one leadership style is optimal in all situations. The nature of the situation needs to be considered. Styles can be chosen to match the situation (Hersey et al., 2013).

In situational leadership theories, leadership in groups is never a static circumstance. The situation is dynamic and subject to change. In a very difficult situation, relationships may be the leader's preferred emphasis. However, if interpersonal relationships are not an immediate problem or if the group is on the verge of collapse, then strong authoritative direction is needed to get the group moving and accomplishing. For this situation, the task-oriented leader is a more effective match between leader and job. However, groups do not remain static; they move back and forth through stages. When the problem is no longer just the need to get the group moving but also includes solving numerous interpersonal conflicts, a relationship-oriented leader is better matched to the situation. Eventually, as the situation progresses, a relationship-oriented leader can become less effective. This occurs because once the group has less conflict, individuals may begin to coast along, and positive motivation may be lost as individuals become apathetic. Once again, a task-oriented style is called for to challenge individuals by using the motivation they need to continue to produce. Because of the factor of constant change, maintaining good leadership is complicated for any group.

The Situational Leadership® Model

The Situational Leadership® Model of Hersey and colleagues (2013) focuses on the interplay among three elements: the amount of guidance and direction (task behavior) a leader gives; the amount of socioemotional support (relationship behavior) a leader provides; and the Performance Readiness® Level that individuals or teams (followers) exhibit in performing specific activity, task, or job. Using a grid that results from task and relationship axes ranging from high to low, task behavior is plotted on the horizontal axis, and relationship behavior is plotted on the vertical axis (See the grid on The Center for Leadership Studies website: *https://situational.com/situational-leadership/about-situational-leadership/*). This makes it possible to describe leader behavior in four quadrants: (1) high task, low relationship (S1, telling); (2) high task, high relationship (S2, selling); (3) high relationship, low task (S3, participating); and (4) low task, low relationship (S4, delegating) (Hersey, 2009). As applied to the continuum of authoritarian versus democratic styles, telling would be authoritarian and participating would be democratic.

To choose an appropriate style, the leader needs to be knowledgeable about the Performance Readiness® level of the followers. This leads to the third dimension of effectiveness: the situation, which determines the effectiveness of a leader's behavior style. "In reality the third dimension is the environment" (Hersey et al., 2013). Thus the difference between effective and ineffective styles often will not be the actual behavior of the leader but rather the appropriateness of the leader's behavior as matched to the environment in which it is used.

Found below the basic grid is a continuum of Performance Readiness® ranging from low to high. The Performance Readiness® level of an individual or group is determined by both ability and willingness. The first consideration regarding readiness is the followers' ability. *Ability* is the demonstrated knowledge, experience, and skill that a follower brings to a task or activity. *Knowledge* is demonstrated understanding of the task. *Skill* is the demonstrated proficiency in the task. *Experience* is the demonstrated ability gained from performing a task (Hersey et al., 2013).

The other part of readiness is *willingness*. Willingness is the extent to which a follower has demonstrated confidence, commitment, and motivation to accomplish a specific task. *Confidence* is demonstrated self-assurance in the ability to perform a task. *Commitment* is demonstrated dedication to perform a task. *Motivation* is demonstrated desire to perform a task (Hersey et al., 2013). Both ability and willingness need to be assessed; then they can be plotted on the grid to determine readiness.

Hersey and colleagues (2013) combined the aspects of ability and willingness and showed them displayed on the grid in four levels of readiness: (1) R1: both unable and unwilling or insecure; (2) R2: unable but willing or confident; (3) R3: able but unwilling or insecure; and (4) R4: both able and willing or confident. The Situational Leadership® Model correlates the four different levels of Performance Readiness® to the four basic leadership styles. The result is a visual display and model that provides the opportunity for the leader to assess a follower's behavior and identifies a way to understand and select the leadership style that has the highest probability of effectively influencing a specific person for a specific task (Hersey, 2009).

Thus at the Situational Leadership® Model's core, Hersey and colleagues (2013) emphasized the importance of the readiness of followers. Any leader behavior is predicted to be more or less effective depending on the Performance Readiness® of the followers that the leader is attempting to influence. The leader's chosen leadership style would have to take into account where the followers are in terms of their Performance Readiness® level. The principles of the Situational Leadership® Model can be applied to a work group. The leader begins with assessment and analysis. Have the members worked together for a long time in the job, or are they new employees? The culture is more solidified in a work group that has worked together for many years on a unit. Using the Situational Leadership® Model, leaders (1) identify the specific job, task or activity, (2) assess current Performance Readiness®, and (3) match and communicate by selecting and exhibiting the appropriate leadership style: S1, S2, S3, or S4 (Hersey et al., 2013). For example, telling is an appropriate leadership style to use with followers who are at the novice level and with followers who are unable, unwilling, or insecure. An example is when a nurse is appointed as chair of a committee. The nurse needs to assess and then adapt his or her leadership style to match the Performance Readiness® level of the followers in order to be most effective.

Thus in this view of leadership, it is situational or contingent and concerned with what produces effectiveness. Hersey and colleagues (2013) noted that the common themes include the following: the leader needs to be flexible in behavior, able to diagnose the leadership style appropriate to the situation, and able to apply the appropriate style given the Performance Readiness® of followers.

Transactional and Transformational Leadership

After the eras of trait, attitudinal, and Situational Leadership® theories, an interest arose in how leaders produced quantum results. Burns (1978) and Dunham and Klafehn (1990) broadened the concept of leadership styles to include two types of leaders: the transactional leader and the transformational leader.

A *transactional leader* is defined as a leader or manager who functions in a caregiver role and is focused on day-to-day operations. Such leaders survey their followers' needs and set goals for them based on what can be expected from the followers. A transactional leader is focused on the maintenance and management of ongoing and routine work. Transactional leadership is a social exchange: One thing is exchanged for another, generally to accomplish daily work (Bass & Riggio, 2006; Steaban, 2016).

A *transformational leader* is defined as a leader who motivates followers to perform to their full potential over time by influencing a change in perceptions and by providing a sense of direction. Transformational leaders use charisma, individualized consideration, and intellectual stimulation to produce greater effort, effectiveness, and satisfaction in followers. Transformational leaders grow and develop others by empowering them (Bass & Riggio, 2006; Steaban, 2016). Fig. 1.4 distinguishes between transactional and transformational leadership.

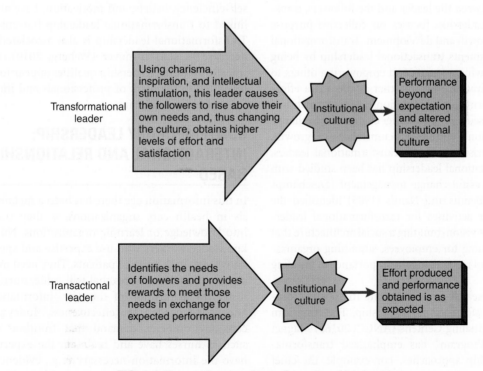

FIG. 1.4 Transactional and transformational leadership.

The transactional leader is more common. This type of leader approaches followers in an exchange posture, with the purpose of exchanging one thing for another, such as a politician who promises jobs for votes. Burns (1978) said that transactional leadership occurs when the leader takes the initiative in contacting others for the exchange of valued things. Therefore transactional leadership is comparable to a bargain or contract for mutual benefits that aids the individual differences of both the leader and the follower. The transactional leader works within the existing organizational culture and is an essential component of effective leadership at the level of task accomplishment. Examples would be the exchange of a salary for the services of a nurse to provide care or when a leader offers release time or paid time to entice staff members to do project or committee work. Continuous or incremental change, the first order of change, can be handled well at the transactional level.

Transformational leadership occurs when persons engage with others so that leaders and followers raise each other to higher levels of motivation and ethical decision making (Burns, 1978). Instead of emphasizing differences between the leader and the followers, transformational leadership focuses on collective purpose and mutual growth and development. Transformational leadership augments transactional leadership by being committed, having a vision, and empowering others to heighten motivation in a way that attains extra effort beyond performance expectations. Transformational leadership is used for higher-order change and to change the organization's culture. Circumstances of growth, change, and crisis call forth transformational leaders, and transformational leadership has been studied with regard to successful change management (Deschamps et al., 2016). Bennis and Nanus (1985) identified the following four activities for transformational leadership: creating a vision, building a social architecture that provides meaning for employees, sustaining organizational trust, and recognizing the importance of building self-esteem.

There is research to demonstrate the positive outcomes of transformational leadership. The American Nurses Credentialing Center's (ANCC, 2016a) Magnet Recognition Program® has emphasized transformational leadership approaches. For example, the chief nursing officer of Magnet-designated organizations'

transformational leadership style has been shown to have a positive impact on the work environment (Buck & Doucette, 2015). Transformational leadership was the type of leadership most often reported in Magnet research studies (Upenieks, 2003a, b). A transformational leadership style has been shown to generate greater follower commitment, follower satisfaction, and overall effectiveness (Kleinman, 2004). In nursing homes, the most transformative style of top managers (consensus managers) was found to be associated with better quality outcomes (Castle & Decker, 2011). Deschamps and colleagues (2016) found that leadership is an important factor in implementing changes, but justice is also a crucial factor. The positive impact of transformational leadership is mediated by organizational justice.

Transformational leaders have been shown to have an impact on both organizations and individuals. Organizational impacts include increased organizational citizenship, stronger organizational culture, and clearer organizational vision (Thomson et al., 2016). Improvements in outcomes for individuals, including empowerment, job satisfaction, commitment, trust, self-efficiency, beliefs, and motivation, have also been linked to transformational leadership (Givens, 2008). Transformational leadership is also associated with a decrease in staff turnover (Weberg, 2010). Overall, transformational leadership qualities appear to be better suited to the work of professionals and important for leadership in nursing.

CONTEMPORARY LEADERSHIP: INTERACTIONAL AND RELATIONSHIP-BASED

In this information age there has been a metamorphosis in health care organizations as they transform into knowledge or learning organizations. Nurses are knowledge workers who use expertise and specialized knowledge in the care of patients. They need matching organizational structures that will value, nurture, and foster the acquisition of the data, information, and knowledge needed for effectiveness. Today's health care environments demand that frontline workers such as nurses have and maintain the expertise and have the information necessary (e.g., evidence-based practice) to take action to solve problems. They need leadership that is interactional, relational, and transformational at all levels.

Arising in conjunction with the application of complexity theory and chaos theory (as discussed under Management in Organizations), leadership was described by Wheatley (2006) as being simpler, less stressful, and more appropriate to complex organizations in the midst of chaos. Her view of leadership emphasized the importance of connectedness and relationships within self-organizing systems. Nursing has a natural niche within interactional and relationship leadership theories. Optimal health care delivery is truly interdisciplinary, holistic, and highly team based. When connections and relationships are strong, patients benefit. Contemporary definitions of leadership describe leadership as being the result of a relationship between leaders and followers where a distinct set of competencies is used to allow the relationship to achieve shared goals. This is complex and requires nurses to be creative and flexible. Old ways of leading and managing are insufficient to present circumstances. Thus it is proposed that "quantum" leadership is needed to produce results in today's health care environment. Quantum leadership is about discovering. It is an ongoing process of exploration, curiosity, and asking questions (McCauley, 2005). Driven by organizational stress and the feeling that something more and different in work life is needed, quantum leadership is one type of leadership strategy that helps nurses focus on the future, stretch and break boundaries, and encourage breakthrough thinking to solve problems in a complex and fluid care environment. Quantum approaches build on feminist and transformational leadership perspectives and dive more deeply into the behavioral, relational, and interactional elements that form the activities and functions of a leader.

Complexity Leadership

Traditional leadership theories were developed during the industrial era and describe traits, situations, and a role with power concentrated in a position in the organization. The focus is on maximizing production and reducing variance. Linear models assume input will yield a proportional output (linear processes). Weberg (2012) argues that a focus on linear systems requires management, not leadership, because it removes the capacity for the system to change and innovate. Using complexity science principles and systems thinking,

Weberg advocated for complexity leadership because it gives a context for organizational operations whereby the behaviors of leadership foster interaction, increase network strength, and generate stability in order to create the energy for constant change, growth, and adaptation. Interconnectedness and change become normal operating conditions. Complexity leadership is a new type of leadership "based on adaptive capacity, understanding the external environment and connecting with the internal organizational culture and thriving in situations where groups need to learn their way out of unpredictable problems" (Weberg, 2012, p. 271). In health care, this will require a shift toward complexity behaviors that embrace complex systems and continually search for value-added innovations. Leaders need to develop innovation competence.

Servant Leadership

Another popular contemporary leadership concept is called *servant leadership.* Greenleaf (2002) used the term to describe leaders who choose first to serve others and then to be a leader, as opposed to those who are leaders first (often because of a power drive or need to acquire material possessions) and later choose to serve. Servant leaders put others first. They choose to make sure that other people's highest-priority needs are being served in a way that promotes personal growth and helps others become freer and more autonomous. When applied to health care, servant leadership is an attractive alternative to the traditional bureaucratic environment experienced by nurses. The servant leadership model draws attention to the necessity for leaders to be attentive to the needs of others and is a model that enhances the personal growth of nurses, improves the quality of care, values teamwork, and promotes personal involvement and caring behavior. Reynolds (2011) melded the feminist and servant leadership perspectives, calling servant leadership gender-integrative leadership that values equally the masculine and feminine dualities, qualities, activities, and behaviors. Hanse and colleagues (2016) studied the impact of servant leadership dimensions on leader–member exchange among health care professionals and found that servant leadership dimensions are likely to help develop stronger exchange relationships between nurse managers and individual subordinates. A servant leader culture involves interpersonal interaction and promotes strong relationships and trust between leaders and followers.

Authentic Leadership

Following from the IHI's Triple Aim, focus has now turned to the importance of employees thriving in organizations for organizational performance. Thriving at work—defined as a state where individuals at work experience both a sense of vitality and a sense of learning (Mortier et al., 2016)—is an understudied yet important aspect of work life and nurse vitality. Mortier and colleagues found that nurse managers' authentic leadership enhances nurse thriving.

Authentic leadership was described by Avolio and Gardner (2005) as a leadership style rooted in the concept of authenticity ("to thine own self be true"), where the leader is a fully functioning person in tune with themselves and their basic nature, self-actualizing, and having strong ethical convictions. Authentic leaders are "those who are deeply aware of how they think and behave and are perceived by others as being aware of their own and others' values/moral perspectives, knowledge, and strengths; aware of the context in which they operate; and who are confident, hopeful, optimistic, resilient, and of high moral character" (Avolio & Gardner, 2005, p. 321).

There are four aspects of authentic leadership:

- Self-awareness: how the leaders perceive themselves in comparison with the world and with their understanding of their own strengths and weaknesses
- An internal moral perspective: leaders align their beliefs with their actions and are not often persuaded by external pressures
- Balanced processing: their decision making is based on analyses of all relevant data, being positive or confirming information or negative clues
- Relational transparency: how openly the leader presents him- or herself to others

The authentic leadership style is seen as fair and supportive and one that provides a healthier and more ethical work environment (Avolio & Gardner 2005; Mortier et al., 2016). This style has been studied in nursing and shown to have a positive effect on nurse job satisfaction and performance (Wong & Laschinger, 2013).

Clinical Leadership

All nurses in all positions exhibit leadership. For example, the "bedside" nurse uses informal leadership to influence high quality care delivery. Mannix and colleagues (2013) used an integrative review of literature on clinical leadership to elicit defining attributes of contemporary clinical leadership in nursing. The technical and practical skills necessary for competent clinical practice and leading a team emerged. The data were grouped into three categories of clinical leadership with either a clinical, follower/team, or personal qualities focus. "Clinical leaders who demonstrate clinical competence, possess effective communication and are supportive of colleagues have been linked to building healthy workplaces" (Mannix et al., 2013, p. 19). For example, one staff nurse who worked on a surgical and neuroscience intensive care unit recognized that there was incomplete and incorrect spinal cord injury/surgical patient assessment and documentation, which is critical when a patient's condition declines so that the degree of change is known. She took the initiative and contacted the nurse manager, invited other staff nurses to join her, set up a small committee, updated and simplified the assessment tool, and led the education of the staff on the revised tool with positive outcomes. This is clinical leadership.

There is a renewed focus on clinical leadership models at the point of care. Typically aimed at a hospital unit where care is delivered, the crucial role played by nurses in quality, safety, care coordination, and related aims of the IOM and IHI are the centerpiece. Stimulated by the Affordable Care Act, nursing roles of care coordinator, CNL, and APRN have emerged and show continued growth. Joseph and Huber (2015, p. 56) defined clinical leadership as "the process of influencing point-of-care innovation and improvement in both organizational processes and individual care practices to achieve quality and safety of care outcomes." Previous definitions focused on hospital-based staff nurses, where clinical leadership was defined as "staff nurse behaviors that provide direction and support to clients and the health care team in the delivery of patient care" (Patrick et al., 2011, p. 450). Patrick and colleagues (2011) viewed every registered staff nurse as a clinical leader and used Kouzes and Posner's (1995) model of transformational leadership as a framework to describe and measure clinical leadership practices. Their review of literature identified five key aspects of clinical leadership: clinical expertise, effective communication, collaboration, coordination, and interpersonal understanding. Empowering work environments create a supportive structure for staff nurses as clinical leaders to achieve the best outcomes of care. "Clinical leadership uses the skills of the RN and adds components of general leadership skills, skills in management of care delivery at the point of care, and focused skills in using evidence-based practice for problem solving and outcomes management. There is clearly a need for clinical leadership in nursing because of the many and varied point-of-care implementation problems that arise" (Joseph & Huber, 2015, p. 56).

EFFECTIVE LEADERSHIP

Effective leadership is an integrated blend of leadership principles and characteristics with management principles and techniques. Nurses can grow such skills by knowledge and awareness (e.g., through assessment tools) and then may put knowledge and skills to work through guided exercises and mentored experiences. This is especially true for succession planning and the development of nurse managers (Mackoff et al., 2013).

Leadership effectiveness is based on the ability to adapt in a complex and chaotic environment. Adaptive problems arise from change and chaos and are often systems problems that affect people, planning, institutional operations, or work processes. Effective leaders first have strong self-awareness of their leadership strengths and weaknesses as well as preferred or most comfortable leadership styles and flexibility. Then they expand this to a grasp of themselves, their team, their goals, nursing and health care, and important evaluative data for "dashboards." They use their personal style, vision, and energy to focus on goal attainment and group satisfaction. Starting with whatever natural talent a nurse possesses, essential leadership skills can be practiced over time for greater effectiveness. Effective leadership uses empowerment. For nurses, empowering means that the power over clinical practice decisions is invested in staff nurses, enabling them to do what they do best. This process is similar to nurses empowering clients. Leadership involves elements of vigor and vision and can be understood as a dynamic combination of competence, willingness to take responsibility, and strength of character to do what is right because it is the right thing to do. See Chapter 10 for further discussion of sources of power.

FOLLOWERSHIP

Leaders do not operate in isolation. Instead, leadership involves cooperation and collaboration. The basic nature of leadership is interactive; it revolves around the interpersonal relationships among leaders and followers. Therefore cooperation and collaboration between the leader and followers enhance the group's effectiveness. Although it may seem obvious, followership quality is important. There is a dynamic relationship between leaders and followers, and both are important.

Followership is an interpersonal process of participation. It implies an engagement of the follower with the leader, and possibly a group, by which the follower takes guidance and direction from the leader to accomplish group goals. The importance of followership is emphasized because leadership requires the presence of followers. The relationship between the leader and the followers defines leadership. The corollary to leadership is followership, or helping to get the job done. A good leader clearly needs good followers. Bennis (1994) noted that followers need three things from leaders: direction, trust, and hope. Kouzes and Posner (2012) noted that for people to follow willingly, they need to believe the leader is honest, forward looking, competent, and inspiring. With these three elements in place, followers are empowered in their participation efforts. Any situation can be analyzed to determine whether the desired leader attributes are present and to what extent.

Types of Followers

There are several typologies that distinguish types of followers. Kelley (1992) explored followership style and plotted styles along the two axes of passive to active and dependent to independent. The five styles of followership are alienated, exemplary, conformist, passive, and pragmatist. Chaleff's (2003) grid used axes of low to high challenge and low to high support, resulting in four quadrants: implementer, partner, individualist, and resource. Kellerman (2008) aligned followers on the single dimension of engagement and divided them into five types: isolate, bystander, participant, activist, and diehard. Isolates are completely detached/not engaged. Bystanders, participants, activists, and diehards are engaged to some degree with leaders, other followers, the group, or the organization. Bystanders observe, participants engage, activists feel strongly and act, and diehards are prepared to die for the cause. Grossman and

Valiga (2013) similarly discussed types of followers and identified them on dimensions of activity and independence: effective or exemplary, alienated, yes people, and sheep.

Understanding types of followers is as important as understanding types of leaders: It creates the ability to match leadership style to effectiveness in care delivery. Effective followers are an asset to be nurtured, developed, and valued. Effective followers contribute to success in organizations. Nurses can and should examine their own behavior and ask themselves the question, "In this situation, what kind of follower am I?"

Self-awareness is an important aspect of both leadership and followership. This means that nurses can assess themselves to better understand their own style and leadership characteristics. Self-assessment tools are available to assist nurses in awareness of both leadership and followership behaviors. Examples are the LEAD instruments developed by Hersey and colleagues (2013), the Multifactor Leadership Questionnaire (MLQ) (Bass & Avolio, 1990), and multiple training instruments. Leadership-related research instruments were identified, compared, and evaluated by Huber and colleagues (2000). Some instruments are useful for research and others for leadership training or self-diagnosis. A wide variety of tools are available to help individuals increase their effectiveness through greater awareness and subsequent honing of both their leadership and followership skills.

LEADERSHIP AND MANAGEMENT ROLES

A distinction can be made between leadership and management roles, yet leaders and managers find that their activities often overlap. Leadership is concerned with influencing individuals and groups and activities of change management and human resources management. Management activities are concerned with managing the resources and the operations of an organization. This may translate into a focus on tasks and processes. In an environment that is constantly changing, the ability to shift back and forth among roles, sometimes by multitasking or integrating efforts toward goal achievement, is a valuable skill.

Certain pressures influence the role of the manager and demand new skill sets to facilitate clinical work. Examples include when technology changes more quickly than clinicians are able to learn and adapt to it, when management duties extend to include temporary workers employed by others (e.g., outsourced functions and agency nurses), and when a radical organizational shift, such as to an accountable care organization (ACO), is necessary. The demands of management work are increasing in amount, scope, complexity, and intensity, especially under conditions of constrained resources. This may increase role stress and leave less time to plan. Thus nurses are challenged to acquire knowledge, skills, and abilities that help them manage effectively under pressure.

MANAGEMENT OVERVIEW

Along with an array of opportunities such as instantaneous communication across vast distances, health care organizations and the people in them struggle with an ever-accelerating rate of change, knowledge explosion, and information flow. The recruitment, development, deployment, motivation, and leveraging of human capital (nurses) as scarce resources and prime assets are critical management issues for service industries in general and specifically for nursing and health care. At the core, managers manage people and organizations. People's time and effort—as well as organizations' money, facilities, and supplies—need to be directed in a coordinated effort to achieve best results and meet objectives. If leaders inspire and motivate, then managers focus on getting the work done.

Because nurses are the central hub of care delivery and information flows, it is helpful to think of the work of nurses as having both care delivery and care coordination aspects. Although the coordination of care has always been a key nursing function, it is becoming more visible and valued in health care and as nurses assume care coordination roles that focus on integrating clinical care. However, the relative proportion of the nurse's role that is devoted to management and coordination functions varies within nursing according to the job category. Nurse managers balance two competing needs: the needs of the staff related to growth, efficiency, motivation, morale, and accomplishment with the outcome of staff satisfaction and the needs of the employer for productivity, quality, and cost effectiveness with the outcome of productivity.

DEFINITIONS

Management is defined as the process of coordination and integration of resources through activities of planning, organizing, coordinating, directing, and controlling to accomplish specific institutional goals and objectives. Management has been viewed as an art and a science related to planning and directing both human effort and scarce resources to attain established objectives. Another definition of management is a process by which organizational goals are met through the application of skills and the use of resources.

Management, then, applies to organizations. The definition of leadership emphasizes actions that influence toward group goals; the definition of management focuses on organizational goals. The achievement of organizational goals through leadership and manipulation of the environment is management. In a systems approach to management, the inputs would be represented by human resources and physical and technical resources. The outputs would be the realization of goals through task accomplishment, culture development, removal of barriers, and efficiency optimization.

Thus management is a separate function with a specific purpose and related roles but one that is focused on organizations and operations. It is associated with important day-to-day functions geared toward maintenance and stability and associated with transactional leadership or "doing things right" via task accomplishment. To achieve organizational goals, managers are involved in activities such as analyzing issues, establishing goals and objectives, mapping out work plans, organizing assets and supplies, developing and motivating people, communicating, managing technology, handling change and conflict, measurement, analysis, and evaluation. Without talent and attention to these functions, effectiveness and morale drop. Effective managers are thought to be those who can weave strategy, execution, discipline, inspiration, and leadership together as they unite an organization toward achieving its goals.

BACKGROUND: THE MANAGEMENT PROCESS

Drucker (2004) suggested that effective executives do not need to be leaders. "Great managers may be charismatic or dull, generous or tightfisted, visionary or numbers oriented. But every effective executive follows eight simple practices" (Drucker, 2004, p. 59). These eight practices are divided into the following three categories:
A. Practices That Give Executives the Knowledge They Need
   1. They asked: "What needs to be done?"
   2. They asked: "What is right for the enterprise?"

B. Practices That Help Executives Convert Knowledge to Action
   3. They developed action plans.
   4. They took responsibility for decisions.
   5. They took responsibility for communicating.
   6. They were focused on opportunities, not problems.
C. Practices That Ensure That the Whole Organization Feels Responsible and Accountable
   7. They ran productive meetings.
   8. They thought and said "we," not "I."

Effective management also appears to be a result of artful balancing, because managers need to function at the point at which reflective thinking combines with practical doing. This is described as managerial mind-sets within the bounds of management practice. Managers interpret and deal with their world from the following five perspectives (Gosling & Mintzberg, 2003):
1. *Reflective mind-set:* Managing self
2. *Analytic mind-set:* Managing organizations
3. *Worldly mind-set:* Managing context
4. *Collaborative mind-set:* Managing relationships
5. *Action mind-set:* Managing change

These five mind-sets were described as being like threads for the manager to weave. The process is as follows: analyze, act, reflect, act, collaborate, reanalyze, articulate new insights, and act again.

Management is central to the work of nursing. **Nursing management** is defined as the coordination and integration of nursing resources by applying the management process to accomplish nursing care and service goals and objectives.

An organization can be any institution, agency, or facility. Working to achieve an organization's goals involves the process of management. The principles that guide the process of management were formulated by Fayol a very long time ago (1949). He said that managers perform unique and discrete functions: They plan, organize, coordinate, and control. Thus management was seen as a unique and separate activity from the work of producing a product. Workers labor to produce the product; managers manage organizations toward goal achievement. Someone needs to monitor financial indicators; hire, train, and evaluate personnel; improve quality; coordinate work and effort; fix systems problems; and ensure that goals are met. In nursing, this means that nurses do the work of providing nursing care while nurse managers coordinate and integrate the work of individual nurses with the larger system. These are distinctly different activities.

The four steps of the management process are planning, organizing, directing, and controlling (Fayol, 1949). These functions make up the scope of a manager's major effort. Planning involves determining the long-term and short-term objectives and the corresponding actions that must be taken. Organizing means mobilizing human and material resources to accomplish what is needed. Directing relates to methods of motivating, guiding, and leading people through work processes. Controlling has a specific meaning closer to the monitoring and evaluating actions that are familiar to nurses. The management process can be compared with an orchestra performing a concert or a team playing a football game. There is a plan and an organized group of players. A director manages the performance and controls the outcome by making corrections and adjustments along the way but does not play an instrument or a position. Management is discrete and separate work. The management process is a rational, logical process based on problem-solving principles.

Planning

Planning is the managerial function of selecting priorities, results, and methods to achieve results; setting the direction for a system; and then guiding the system. **Planning** is defined as "A basic management function involving formulation of one or more detailed plans to achieve optimum balance of needs or demands with the available resources. The planning process (1) identifies the goals or objectives to be achieved, (2) formulates strategies to achieve them, (3) arranges or creates the means required, and (4) implements, directs, and monitors all steps in their proper sequence" (BusinessDictionary.com, 2016a). Planning can be detailed, specific, and rigid, or it can be broad, general, and flexible. Planning is deciding in advance what is to be done and when, by whom, and how it is to be done. It is traditionally thought of as a linear process. Hersey and colleagues (2013) described planning as involving the setting of goals and objectives and developing "work maps" to show how they are to be accomplished. Planning activities include identifying goals, objectives, methods, resources, responsible parties, and due dates. There are two types of planning: strategic and tactical.

Strategic planning: More broad ranged, this approach means determining the overall purposes and directions of the organization. This is often focused on mission, vision, and major goal identification (see Chapter 14).

Tactical planning: More short ranged, this type means determining the specific details of implementing broader goals. Examples are project planning, staffing planning, and marketing plans.

Planning heavily depends on the decision-making process. Part of planning is choosing among a number of alternatives. Thus in nursing, the manager often must balance the needs of patients, staff, administrators, and physicians under conditions of limited resources.

Planning involves considering systems inputs, processes, outputs, and outcomes. The process of planning in its larger context means that planners work backward through the system. Starting with the results, outcomes, or outputs desired, they then identify the processes needed to produce the results and the inputs or resources needed to carry out the processes. Typical planning phases include the following:

- Identify the mission.
- Conduct an environmental scan.
- Analyze the situation (e.g., SWOT analysis of strengths, weaknesses, opportunities, and threats).
- Establish goals.
- Identify strategies to reach goals.
- Set objectives to achieve goals.
- Assign responsibilities and timelines.
- Write a planning document.
- Celebrate success and completion.

The nurse is engaged in a constant mental planning operation when deciding what specific things are to be accomplished for the patient. The same is true for the nurse manager who is deciding how to devise, implement, and maintain a positive and productive work environment for nurses.

Planning is a function that assumes stability and the ability to predict and project into the future. Yet the current environment is turbulent, making planning difficult. Learning and adapting are important abilities in a changeable environment. Interactive planning has been suggested as an approach to planning in complex situations and changing environments (Foust, 1994). Interactive planning takes a developmental approach. Problems are viewed as interrelated. Interactive planning principles emphasize the importance of participation among participants, a nonlinear view of relationships called *systems thinking,* and a focus on creating a desired future outcome. Interactive planning can contribute to effective care planning and to effective care management by nurses (Foust, 1994). This may be due in part to the phenomenon of an environment of chaos and complexity.

Organizing

Organizing is a management function related to allocating and configuring resources to accomplish preferred goals and objectives. It is the activities done to collect and configure resources to implement plans effectively and efficiently. **Organizing** can be defined as "assembling required resources to attain organizational objectives" (BusinessDictionary.com, 2016b), thus it is the mobilizing of the human and material resources of the institution to achieve organizational objectives. Fayol (1949) noted that the organizing function was concerned with building up the material and human structures into a working infrastructure. Authority, power, and structure are used for influence. The goal is to get the human, equipment, and material resources mobilized, organized, and working. Organizing so that the goals and objectives can be accomplished includes forging and strengthening relationships between workers and the environment. The first step is to organize the work, then the people are organized, and finally the environment is organized.

Organizing closely follows the planning process. In fact, these terms are often referred to together: *planning* and *organizing.* Organizing encompasses activities designed to bring together an array of various resources including personnel, money, and equipment in a manner that is the most effective for accomplishing organizational goals. There are a number of ways to do this, but the essence of organizing is the integration and coordination of resources (Hersey et al., 2013).

There are a wide variety of topics related to organizing, which is considered to be one of the major functions of management. For example, organizing can be thought of as a process of identifying roles in relationship to one another. Thus organizing involves activities related to establishing a structure and hierarchy of jobs and positions within a unit or department. Responsibilities are assigned to each job. The complexity of this aspect of organizing is related to the size of the organization and the number of employees and jobs. Organizing in nursing also relates to the activities of budget management,

staffing, and scheduling and to other human resources and personnel functions such as developing committees and bylaws, orientation, and staff in-service. Institutions organize by establishing a structure, such as a hierarchy with divisions or departments, and by developing some method for division of labor and subsequent coordination among subunits.

Directing

Directing is the managerial function of establishing direction and then influencing people to follow that direction. Directing is defined as "a basic management function that includes building an effective work climate and creating opportunity for motivation, supervising, scheduling, and disciplining" (BusinessDictionary.com, 2016c). Directing can also be called *leading* or *coordinating.* **Coordinating** is defined as motivating and leading personnel to carry out the desired actions.

Along with communicating and leading, motivation is often included with the description of the activities of directing others. Motivating is a major strategy related to determining the followers' level of performance and thereby to influencing how effectively the goals of the organization will be met. The amount of employee effort that can be influenced by motivation is thought to be from 20% to 30% at the low end and as high as 80% to 90% for highly motivated people (Hersey et al., 2013). A wide range of effort can be affected through motivation.

On a day-to-day basis, coaching is used as a technique to direct and motivate followers. The manager delegates activities and responsibilities when making assignments. The function of directing involves actions of supervising and guiding others within their assigned duties. The use of interpersonal skills is required to delicately balance the need to direct and supervise for task accomplishment with the need to create and maintain a motivational climate with high participation and positive outcomes.

Within nursing there is a legal aspect to the managerial directing function. Under some state licensing laws, supervision is a defined and regulated legal element of nursing practice. Because delegation and supervision are viewed legally as a part of the practice of nursing, nurses have a specific need to know and understand this area of nursing responsibility within their scope of practice. Nurses carry responsibility and accountability for the quality and quantity of their supervision, as well as for the quality and quantity of their own actions in regard to care provision. Nurse managers carry the added responsibility and accountability for the coordination of groups of nurse providers and assistive or ancillary personnel, sometimes across settings and sites of care. Nurse managers also have an overall responsibility to monitor and provide surveillance or vigilance regarding situations that can lead to failure to rescue, patient safety errors, or negligence. Too many hours worked, nurse fatigue from stress, too heavy a patient workload, and other systems problems are situations to monitor with regard to legal accountability (see Chapter 6).

Controlling

Controlling is the management function of monitoring and adjusting the plan, processes, and resources to effectively and efficiently achieve goals. It is a way of coordinating activities within organizations by systematically figuring out whether what is occurring is what is wanted. The controlling aspect of the managerial process may seem at first to carry a negative connotation. However, when used in reference to management, the word *control* does not mean being negatively manipulative or punitive toward others. Managerial controlling means ensuring that the proper processes are followed. In nursing, the term *evaluation* is used to refer to similar actions and activities. Control or evaluation means ensuring that the flow and processes of work, as well as goal accomplishment, proceed as planned. **Controlling** is defined as "the basic management function of (1) establishing benchmarks or standards, (2) comparing actual performance against them, and (3) taking corrective action, if required" (BusinessDictionary.com, 2016d). Thus it is concerned with comparing the results of work with predetermined standards of performance and taking corrective action when needed. This means ensuring that the results are as desired and, if they are not up to standards, taking some action to modify, remediate, or reverse variances.

The coordination of activities of a system is one aspect of managerial control, along with financial management, compliance, quality and risk management, feedback mechanisms, performance management, policies and procedures, and research and trend analysis. These control activities are used by managers to communicate to reach a goal, track activities toward the goal, guide behaviors, coordinate efforts, and decide what to do. They are important to the success of

any organization. Ongoing, careful review using standardized documents, informatics systems, and standardized measures prevents drift and the waste of time and resources that occur when direction is vague. Well-exercised, managerial control is flexible enough to allow innovation yet present enough to effectively structure groups and organizations toward goal attainment. This is an artful balance.

The management function of controlling involves feeding back information about the results and outcomes of work activities, combined with activities to follow up and compare outcomes with plans. Appropriate adjustments need to be made wherever outcomes vary or deviate from expectations (Hersey et al., 2013). For example, when a standardized clinical practice protocol is used in nursing to track client care, the variances are analyzed and corrected as a function of managerial control. The controlling function of management is a constant process of internal reevaluation.

MANAGEMENT IN ORGANIZATIONS
The Nature of Managerial Work

Managers manage people and the environment. One view of management suggests that the manager's behavior, the role, and the situation created for people to work in actually trigger or cause followers' behavior. Thus the manager's role is distinct and important for individual and organizational outcomes because of its direct impact on how and what gets done.

Mintzberg (1975) described the manager's job in terms of 10 roles or sets of behaviors. Derived from the formal authority and status of the position are three interpersonal roles: figurehead, leader, and liaison. As the nerve center of the organizational unit, information processing is a key part of the role. Informational roles are monitor, disseminator, and spokesperson. Information is the basic input to decision making. The decisional roles are entrepreneur, disturbance handler, resource allocator, and negotiator (Fig. 1.5). Mintzberg suggested a number of important managerial skills as follows:
- Developing peer relationships
- Carrying out negotiations
- Motivating subordinates
- Resolving conflicts
- Establishing information networks and disseminating information

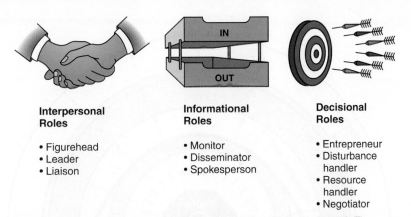

Interpersonal Roles

- Figurehead
- Leader
- Liaison

Informational Roles

- Monitor
- Disseminator
- Spokesperson

Decisional Roles

- Entrepreneur
- Disturbance handler
- Resource handler
- Negotiator

FIG. 1.5 Mintzberg's 10 managerial roles. (Data from Mintzberg, H. [1975]. The manager's job: Folklore and fact. In M. Matteson, & J. Ivancevich [Eds.], *Management classics* [3rd ed., pp. 63–85]. Plano, TX: Business Publications.)

- Making decisions in conditions of extreme ambiguity
- Allocating resources

If management is important to achieving organizational goals, then the skills, abilities, functions, actions, and strategies used by managers to manage are important to know and understand. Mintzberg (1994) elaborated his earlier work on the nature of managerial work by expanding it to an interactive model (Fig. 1.6). The model uses concentric circles. At the core is a person who is in a job. The person has some unique set of values, experiences, knowledge, and competencies. The combination of the person and the job creates a frame composed of the job's purpose, the person's perspective about what needs to be done, and selected strategies for doing the job. The frame can range across two continua: from vague to very specific and from person-selected to externally imposed. The frame results in an agenda of work issues and time scheduling. Placed at the center of the figure, these elements form the core of the job of a manager. Managerial roles and behaviors at this level include conceiving the frame and scheduling the agenda.

Growing out of the core are three concentric circles—from abstract to concrete. These are called the *information, people,* and *action levels* of managerial work. At the most abstract level, the manager processes information and uses it to drive the action. At the next level, the manager works with people to encourage work activities. At the most concrete level, the manager manages the action.

At the information level, the associated managerial roles are communicating information and controlling by using information to control the work of others. At the people level, the managerial roles are leading and linking. Leading involves encouraging and enabling individuals (by mentoring and rewarding), groups (by team building and conflict resolution), and the whole organization (by building a culture). The linking roles have the manager relating to the external environment by building networks of contacts and acquiring information from the environment to transmit back to the unit. At the action level, the associated managerial role is called *doing* or *supervising*. Behaviors include doing, handling disturbances, and negotiating (Mintzberg, 1994). This model could be used as a basis for self-assessment and can be applied to specific managerial jobs. Nurses who strive to apply the concepts to their managerial work could use the model to examine and analyze managerial styles, behaviors, and roles.

Contemporary Management Theories

Human organizations are complex in nature. It is tricky to provide overall direction for an organization in times of rapid environmental change. The recent focus of leadership theory has been on interactional, relational, and transformational leadership to guide organizations through successful change and chaos. However, less attention has been focused on how to advise managers who are working toward the organization's goals and trying to use resources effectively and efficiently under conditions of change, scarcity, and complexity. Forces such as technology, the Internet, social media, increasing diversity, and a global marketplace create pressure to be more sensitive, flexible, and adaptable to stakeholders' expectations and demands.

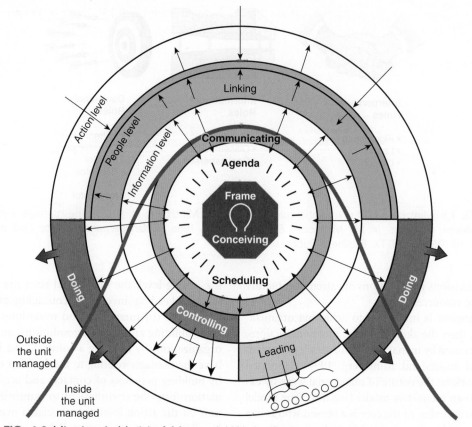

FIG. 1.6 Mintzberg's Model of Managerial Work. (Redrawn from Mintzberg, H. [1994]. Managing as blended care. *Journal of Nursing Administration, 24*[9], 30.)

The result has been a reconfiguration or restructuring of many organizations from the classic hierarchical, top-down, rigid form to a more fluid, organic, team-based, collaborative structure. This has had an impact on how managers manage. Managers cannot control continued rapid change. Old familiar plans and behaviors no longer provide clear direction for the future. Managers now need to focus on two major aspects of management: managing change through constant assessment, guidance, and adaptation and managing employees through worker-centered teams and other self-organizing and self-designing group structures. Bureaucratic management is out; organic and virtual management is in.

A variety of contemporary theories of management have arisen to help organize management thought. Four major management theories now predominate: contingency theory, systems theory, complexity theory, and chaos theory. Each one contributes principles useful for nursing management and administration and for nurse managers working to coordinate and integrate health care delivery.

Contingency Theory

Contingency theory is considered a leadership theory, but it also applies to management. The basic principle is that managers need to consider the situation and all its elements when making a decision. Managers need to act on the key situational aspects with which they are confronted. Sometimes described as "it all depends" decision making, contingency theory is most often used for choosing a leadership or management style. The "best" style depends on the situation. This relates to concepts of situational leadership theory.

Systems Theory

Systems theory has helped managers to recognize their work as being embedded within a system and better understand what a system is. Managers have learned that changing one part of a system inevitably affects the whole system. General systems theory is a way of thinking about studying organizational wholes. A system is a set of interrelated and interdependent parts that are designed to achieve common goals. Systems contain a collection of elements that interact with each other in some environment. The elements of an open system and related examples in health care are shown in Table 1.1.

A key principle of systems theory is that changes in one part of the system affect other parts, creating a ripple effect within the whole. Using systems theory implies a rational approach to common goals, a global view of the whole, and an emphasis on order rather than chaos. The input–throughput–output model exemplifies this linear thinking aspect of general systems theory.

Systems theory is easy to understand but difficult to apply in bureaucratic systems or organizations with strong departmental "silos." This is because coordinators and integrators with sufficient organizational power to cross the system are needed but often not deployed. Without integrators, systems parts tend to make changes without consideration of the whole system. Shifting to systems theory thinking helps managers view, analyze, and interpret patterns and events through the lens of interrelationships of the parts and coordination of the whole.

One application of systems theory to theories of quality management is found in the work of W. Edwards Deming's System of Profound Knowledge with its four parts: appreciation for a system, knowledge of variation, theory of knowledge, and psychology of change (W. Edwards

Deming Institute, 2016). Deming "defined a system as a network of interdependent components that work together to try to accomplish the aim of the system. The aim for any system should be that everybody gains, not one part of the system at the expense of any other" (W. Edwards Deming Institute, 2016). This is a management framework grounded in systems theory. "It is based on the principle that each organization is composed of a system of interrelated processes and people which make up system's components. The success of all workers within the system is dependent on management's capability to orchestrate the delicate balance of each component for optimization of the entire system" (Berry, n.d., p. 1).

In health care, concepts such as interrelatedness and interdependence fit well with multidisciplinary teamwork and shared governance professional models. However, concepts of attaining a steady state and equilibrium are difficult to reconcile with the reality of uncertainty, risk, change, and ambiguity that characterize the turbulence of the change occurring in the health care delivery environment. An example of the use of systems theory is basing an analysis of a planned change, such as implementing a new program, on systems concepts by identifying inputs, throughputs, outputs, and feedback loops to more effectively plan how the new program fits into the existing system. Sometimes this process is used for short time frame or rapid response team projects.

Complexity Theory

Complexity theory is a more general umbrella theory that encompasses chaos theory. Arising in scientific fields such as astronomy, chemistry, biology, geology, and meteorology and involving disciplines such as engineering, mathematics, physics, psychology, and economics, the body of literature on the behavior of complex adaptive systems has been growing since the late 1980s. Complexity theory explains the behavior of the whole system. Complex systems are networks of people exchanging information and are self-organizing. Complexity theory core concepts are self-organization, interaction, emergence, system history, and temporality (Chandler et al., 2015). The focus of complexity theory is the behavior over time of certain complex and dynamically changing systems. The concern is about the predictability of the behavior of systems that perform in regular and predictable ways under certain conditions but in other conditions change in irregular and unpredictable ways, are

TABLE 1.1 Open System Elements and Health Care Examples

Open System Elements	Health Care Examples
Inputs to the system (resources)	Money, people, technology
Transforming processes and interactions (throughputs)	Nursing services, management
Outputs of the system	Clinical outcomes, better quality of life
Feedback	Customer and nurse satisfaction, government regulation, accreditation, lawsuits

unstable, and move further away from starting conditions unless stopped by an overriding constraint. What is most intriguing is that almost undetectable differences in initial conditions will lead to diverging reactions in these systems until the evolution of their behavior is highly dissimilar. Thus stable and unstable behavior is the focus of interest (Rosenhead, 1998).

Stable and unstable behavior can be thought of as two zones. In the stable zone, a disturbed system returns to its initial state. In the unstable zone, any small disturbance leads to movement away from the starting point and further divergence. Which subsequent type of behavior will occur depends on environmental conditions. The area between starting and divergence is called *chaotic behavior*. This refers to systems that have behavior with certain regularity yet defy prediction based on that regularity. The classic example of this is weather prediction before sophisticated computer modeling programs (Rosenhead, 1998).

Before the formulation of complexity theory, the unpredictability of systems was attributed to randomness that was measured by statistical probability. It is now understood that a small difference in starting conditions can result in apparently random, quite different trajectories that are highly irregular but not without some form. Plotted over time, the apparently random meanderings of these systems can show a pattern to the movements, but the variation stays within a pattern that repeats itself (Rosenhead, 1998).

Complexity theory has informed classical management theories. Previous management theories heavily emphasized rationality, predictability, stability, setting a mission, determining strategy, and eliminating deviation. Discoveries from complexity and chaos theories include the fact that the natural world does not operate like clockwork machinery.

Managers need to alter their reflexive behaviors, put an emphasis on "double-loop learning" that also examines the appropriateness of operating assumptions, foster diversity, be open to strategy based on serendipity, welcome disorder as a partner, use instability positively, provoke a controlled ferment of ideas, release creativity, and seek the edge of chaos in the complex interactions that occur among people. Change management takes on a noticeably different form when complexity theory is used. Complexity theory is being used in health care to explain the complexity of the social context in order to better explain the organization of health care and

patterns of professional behavior (Chandler et al., 2015). "A new style of leadership is required in complex adapting organizations. This style is one in which the leader serves their people with vision and guidance to see the interconnectedness of the whole system. The leaders must first gain and communicate a shared identity and then be able to allow the organization ownership of that identity" (Berry, n.d., p. 2).

Chaos Theory

Most would agree that one characteristic of nursing is its unpredictability, its chaos and complexity. To use a theory about chaos and complexity is intuitively attractive. Sometimes no matter how hard nursing leaders try to maintain consistency and control, things do become chaotic. Projects seem to take off on their own and defy direction. Chaos is commonly known as disorganization and disorderliness, but the meaning for this concept in chaos theory is quite different. It refers to behavior that is unpredictable in spite of certain regularities. As described by Lorenz (1993), the chaos phenomenon differs from the predictable swinging of a pendulum of a clock. Instead, it is more like the unpredictable random patterns of weather. A meteorologist, Lorenz was preparing for presenting the weather report when he decided to run the numbers through the computer once more to update the information. He initiated the program a short time later than his original run, and the outcome was quite different. This illustrates a fundamental observation of chaos theory: Changing the starting point of a computer analysis of the weather can result in a change in the outcome. Lorenz (1993) presented a paper titled "Does the Flap of a Butterfly's Wing in Brazil Set Off a Tornado in Texas?" describing this phenomenon of chaos. This "butterfly effect" label is often referred to in the literature when discussing chaos theory.

Chaos has become one concept of complexity theory. Over the past three or four decades, complexity theory has been the focus of scientific disciplines such as astronomy, chemistry, physics, evolutionary biology, geology, and meteorology. Systems studied in these disciplines have phenomena in common, which seem to pass from an organized state through a chaotic phase and then emerge or evolve into a higher level of organization. Examples of this emergence are not unlike Darwin's evolutionary theory of natural selection. Pediani (1996) pointed to examples from the sciences, such as pharmacology, in which chaos theory and complexity theory seem relevant to some patients' responses to drugs. Thus chaos theory may have broad application in relation to clinical practice.

In management, the traditional focus for leaders is to identify organizational goals and to make decisions facilitating goal achievement. Control is central to logical management processes, but in complexity theory, the idea of control is considered a delusion because uncertainty and deviations would be denied and disregarded. The natural world, according to this theory, does not operate this way and is continually evolving to a higher level of complexity. In complexity theory, the future is so unpredictable that long-term planning is not helpful. Rather, it is suggested that managers need to look for instability and complex interactions among people so that learning occurs and the best result "emerges." The idea of the interconnectedness of the parts (people) of the whole suggests that communication among the parts (people) is a key feature of complexity theory.

Chaos is seen as a particular mode of behavior within the more general field of complexity theory (Rosenhead, 1998). Sometimes the two are used together: chaos and complexity. Chaos, as used in complexity theory, is not utter confusion and disorder but rather a system that defies prediction despite certain regularities. Chaos is the boundary zone between stability and instability, and systems in chaos exhibit bounded instability and unpredictability of specific behavior within a predictable general structure of behavior. They may pass through randomness to evolve to a higher order of self-organized complex adaptive structures (Rosenhead, 1998). At first, this seems to make no sense. However, chaos theory principles can be applied in health care. For example, managerial planning for an evidence-based practice change such as bedside reporting can produce chaos and unpredictable results.

As many health care organizations move away from bureaucratic models and recognize organizations as whole systems, more organic and fluid structures are replacing the older ones. Sometimes referred to as "learning organizations," these structures are tapping into the inherent capacity for individuals to exhibit self-organization. In the transition, experiences of change, information overload, entrenched behaviors, and chaos reflect human reactions to organizations as living systems that are adapting and growing (Wheatley, 2006). Complexity and a sense of things being beyond one's control create a search for a simpler way of understanding and leading organizations.

Randomness and complexity are two principal characteristics of chaos. There is a paradox in the fact that even in the simplest of systems, it is extraordinarily difficult to accurately predict the course of events, yet some order arises spontaneously even in these simple systems. Patterns form in nature. Some are orderly, and some are not. Concepts of nonlinearity and feedback help explain situations of complexity without randomness (with order). Chaos theory suggests that simple systems may give rise to complex behavior, and complex systems may exhibit simple behavior. At the essence of chaos is a fine balance between forces of stability and those of instability. Two examples are snowflake formation and the behavior of the weather.

It is difficult for minds trained in linear thinking to grasp chaos theory. In the past, the effects of nonlinearity were discounted. Much of scientific thought was based on assumptions of linearity and beliefs that small differences averaged out, slight variances converged toward a point, and approximations could give a relatively accurate picture of what could happen. It was assumed that predictability would come from learning how to account for all variables and a greater level of detail. However, the wholeness of systems resists being studied in parts. Both chaos and order are important elements in the powerful and unpredictable effects created by iteration in nonlinear systems (Wheatley, 2006). An example of chaos theory in action is when a seemingly small change, such as using assistive personnel instead of professionals, in effect creates ripples and larger impacts on the system than preplanning would seem to indicate. This is why organizations use small tests of change.

The manager's job is to reveal and handle the mostly hidden dynamics of the system and forge a direction for the organization as a complex adaptive system. The goal is for a self-managed system with people capable of engaging in cooperative behavior, using feedback to learn and adapt, self-organizing, and operating with flexibility.

Chaos theory can be used in nursing for research, health care strategy, or statistical modeling (Haigh, 2008) and can be applied to management in health care organizations. For example, chaos was used to model nursing service outcomes by applying a simple population growth equation to an acute pain service (Haigh, 2008). Forward planning for service development was possible by tracking and manipulating the trajectory of the service. Peake and McDowall (2012) investigated midcareer transitions in nursing and found midcareer success outcomes were shaped by chance, unplanned events, and nonlinearity of outcomes.

LEADERSHIP AND MANAGEMENT IMPLICATIONS

It can be argued that all nurses are managers. Staff nurses are the employees at the most critical point in fulfilling the purpose of health care organizations: They are in close and frequent contact with the patient at the point of care, and they coordinate the delivery of health care services.

As nurses work in a rapidly changing practice environment, leadership is important because it affects the climate and work environment of the organization. It affects how nurses feel about themselves at work and about their jobs. By extension, leadership affects organizational and individual productivity. For example, if nurses feel goal-directed and think that their contributions are important, they are more motivated to do the work. Important for the professional practice of nurses is how they feel about themselves and how satisfied they are with their jobs. Both aspects have implications for how well nurses are retained and recruited. Leadership cannot be overlooked because leaders function as problem finders and problem solvers. They are people who help everyone else overcome obstacles. The leadership role is one of bridging, integrating, motivating, and creating organizational "glue."

Leadership in nursing is crucial. *First,* it is important to nurses because of the size of the profession. Nurses make up the largest single health care occupation and one that is experiencing critical shortages. Pressures in the health care environment, including costs, are rapidly thrusting nurses into leadership roles in highly complex and stressful work situations.

Given the challenges of cost containment, an aging population needing more health care services, and issues of access and quality of care, nurse leaders are experiencing greater pressure to perform and produce more effective alignment of key processes, functions, and resources. Organizations have underinvested in nursing leadership skill development, leaving them at risk of underperforming, especially in the three strategic challenges of finance, workforce, and patient safety (O'Neil et al., 2008). Thus there is a call for structured transition management and leadership development programs for nurses assuming leadership and management responsibilities in organizations (Campbell, 2016).

Research has brought to light the gaps, barriers, and needs related to developing nursing leaders as a human capital asset. The top five competencies identified by nurse leaders were: building effective teams, translating vision into strategy, communicating vision and strategy internally, managing conflict, and managing focus on the patient and customer (O'Neil et al., 2008).

Second, nursing's work is complex, often conducted in complex and chaotic settings. Tremendous changes in nursing have occurred in the past 25 years. Leadership is needed to guide and motivate nurses and health care delivery systems toward positive achievements for better patient care. Leadership in nursing is needed to influence the organizational context of care for greater effectiveness and productivity because leaders establish norms and values, define expectations, reward behaviors, and reinforce culture. Authenticity and caring are valued in nurse leaders and are exhibited by people who are genuine, trustworthy, reliable, and believable and who create a positive environment (Pipe, 2008; Shirey, 2006).

Third, nurses are knowledge workers in an information age. Knowledge workers respond to inspiration, not supervision. Although professionals require little direction and supervision, what they do need is protection and support (Mintzberg, 1998). This is best manifested in the covert leadership of the unobtrusive actions that permeate all the things the leader does. Inspiration can also come from a focus on results. Leaders need to model what they want. The good news is that leadership can be taught and learned. Nurses can read, learn, and practice effective leadership and followership.

CURRENT ISSUES AND TRENDS

Current issues and trends that have significance for leadership in nursing include the dramatic US demographic data related to both the aging of the baby boom generation and the demographic profile of nursing in the United States. A major societal and public policy issue related to the aging of a large demographic bulge of baby boomers is beginning to reach a critical point. Called the "2030 problem" (Bahrampour, 2013; Knickman & Snell, 2002), this socioeconomic and demographic phenomenon is real, looming, urgent, and fraught with health care challenges. Statistics show that there are approximately 40.3 million Americans ages 65 years and older, representing 13% of the population, or 1 in 8 Americans (US Census Bureau, 2014). The percentage of Americans 65 years of age and older has tripled since 1900. Issues related to health burdens and chronic illness are characteristic of older adults. In fact, persons 85 years of age and older may spend up to half of their remaining lives inactive or dependent.

US population and health trends are assessed and monitored by governmental agencies such as the US Census Bureau, Centers for Disease Control and Prevention, Bureau of Labor Statistics, and Health Resources and Services Administration. The statistics related to the baby boom generation are impressive. Born between 1946 and 1964, baby boomers in 2030 will be between the ages of 66 and 84 years, are projected to number 60 million people, and one in five (20%) Americans will be 65 or older. In addition to baby boomers, the US population in 2030 is projected to also include 9 million people born before 1946. The projected population of people 65 years and older in 2050 is 88.5 million (US Census Bureau, 2014). This predictable tidal wave will make chronic illness and long-term care a huge economic burden. Knickman and Snell (2002) suggested that there are four key "aging shocks": (1) noncovered costs of prescription medications, (2) noncovered medical care costs, (3) private insurance costs for Medigap, and (4) costs of long-term care. They projected that there will be an overwhelming economic burden if tax rates need to be raised dramatically, economic growth is retarded because of high service costs, or future generations of workers have worse general well-being because of service costs or income transfers. Nurses and the health care system will be challenged to find evidence-based care delivery and service systems models and strategies that address the projected growth industry in chronic illness. One response has been the emphasis on prevention and wellness, targeting behavior change upstream from the development of chronic illness.

Examining the demographic profile of nursing in the United States offers a clue about nursing followership. There are 2.9 million RNs in the United States, making up the single largest health profession. Distribution patterns show that shortages exist and may persist or worsen in a number of states (BHPr, 2014). The average age of an RN in the United States was 50 years in 2014; 9% are male; 55% hold a bachelor's or higher degree (American Nurses Association, 2014). There has been a slowdown in the aging trend in nursing due to an increase in 2008 in the number of employed RNs who are less than 30 years of age.

Leadership is considered key to the success of health care organizations. Nurses are pressed to demonstrate the outcomes of their care and provide evidence of the effectiveness of their service delivery. The link between leadership style and staff satisfaction highlights the importance of leadership in times of chaos. A nurse leader needs to be dynamic, show interpersonal skills, and be a visionary for the organization and the profession. The ability to inspire and motivate followers to carry out the vision is crucial. Effective leadership has a profound impact on nurse recruitment and retention.

The classic notions of management and managerial work were developed in a sociopolitical era of industrialization and bureaucratization. Competitive pressures and economic forces now are compelling organizations to adopt new flexible strategies and structures. Organizations are being urged to become leaner, more entrepreneurial, and less bureaucratic. This trend has created levels of complexity and interdependency that challenge nurse leaders and managers.

Traditional sources of power are eroding, and some motivational tools are less effective than they used to be. The erosion of power from hierarchical positions is perceived as a loss of authority and may create confusion about how to mobilize and motivate staff (Kanter, 1989). Kanter noted that in a leaner and flatter corporation there are many more channels for action, and managers need to work synergistically with other departments. Managers' strategic and collaborative roles become more important as they serve as integrators and facilitators, not as watchdogs and interventionists.

Current and emerging issues in health care are complex and ethically challenging for managers. The "big three" issues of access, cost, and quality continue to be persistent themes that affect any organization's internal operations. Insurance coverage is an issue of access, as is the geographical location of facilities, providers, and services. Increased complexity and technology prompt provider specialization and affect cost. Consumer preferences and increased health care awareness affect both cost and quality. Critical medical errors and patient safety issues create pressure related to the need for quality. Complexity, randomness, and chaos created by change call for new management and leadership strategies.

As health care reconfigures, health care delivery settings will likely be knowledge-based organizations composed primarily of specialists whose performance is directed by organized feedback from colleagues, patients, and data analytics. Nurses are positioned at the care coordination intersection and have needed skills for facilitating flow and integrating care delivery. Nurses' roles may change, but their need for leadership inspiration and managerial competence will remain. Nurses are well prepared to serve as leaders, care providers, integrators, and facilitators of patient care. This is the age of the nurse as leader and manager.

RESEARCH NOTE

Source
Read, E.A., & Laschinger, H.K.S. (2015). The influence of authentic leadership and empowerment on nurses' relational social capital, mental health and job satisfaction over the first year of practice. *Journal of Advanced Nursing, 71*(7), 1611–1623.

Purpose
The combination of authentic leadership and structural empowerment has been shown to be associated with higher job satisfaction among new graduate nurses, but the added value of positive interpersonal relationships at work (relational social capital) is unknown. The purpose of this study was to test a model of the effects of authentic leadership, structural empowerment, and relational social capital on new graduate nurses' mental health and job satisfaction over their first year of practice.

Discussion
The mediating role of relational social capital was examined and tested. A longitudinal survey design was used with 191 new graduate nurses in Canada. A theoretical model was developed, and path analysis using structural equation modeling was used to test the model. Nurse manager authentic leadership behavior has a positive influence on new graduate nurses' perceptions of structural empowerment, which then has a positive influence on relational social capital. These positive work environment conditions enhance job satisfaction and reduce mental health symptoms. This is important because new nurses have been shown to place importance on feeling that they belong and experiencing a strong sense of community. Study participants were mostly female and worked full time in medicine/surgery or critical care. Path analysis supported the model; structural empowerment mediated the relationship between authentic leadership and relational social capital. This then had a positive effect on job satisfaction and a negative effect on mental health symptoms.

Application to Practice
Leaders can have a positive impact on new graduate nurses' retention and mental health by using authentic leadership and empowerment strategies. Creating empowering workplaces and enhancing new graduates' relational social capital through quality of relationships and a strong sense of community may be especially important. Leadership training for nurse managers is a recommended strategy to help support new graduate nurses and affect positive retention and health outcomes.

CASE STUDY

Nurse Maria Rodriguez just graduated with her baccalaureate degree and landed her ideal job as a new staff nurse on the neuroscience unit of the flagship hospital of the We Care Health System. The system has a nurse residency program to support new nurses in their first year of work, and Maria is in this program, but within 3 months she realizes that her unit work environment is chaotic and divisive. Job satisfaction among the staff nurses is low, and turnover is high. This creates constant churn, a high proportion of staff on orientation, and nurses assuming charge and leadership roles with barely a year's experience. Now the nurse manager has resigned. Maria is asked to be on the search committee for the nurse manager replacement. Maria reviews the literature for best practices and the evidence base on nurse manager effectiveness. She reads that nurses leave managers, not organizations, and that emotional intelligence, authentic leadership, relationships with support, and structural empowerment characteristics are important for nurse satisfaction. Clearly, there are identifiable leadership styles and behaviors of nurse managers that promote satisfaction and retention of nurses. Maria composes questions to be used for the nurse manager interview process that will help identify candidates with the strongest potential for positive leadership qualities.

■ CRITICAL THINKING EXERCISE

It was the end of another long, hectic, and frustrating day in Ambulatory Clinic A for Nurse John Folkrod. There were daily issues with sluggish patient flow and long wait times for patients in the waiting room. John's usual reaction was to bottle up the frustration, causing personal health issues, or to vent it by complaining to colleagues. Neither method influenced a positive change in the situation. Fortunately, the nurse manager is a visionary, authentic leader. However, John has not approached her, assuming that the situation was obvious to the manager and not desiring to "make waves" or be seen as a troublemaker.

1. What is the problem?
2. Whose problem is it?
3. What are John's followership role and options for followership strategies to resolve the situation?
4. What leadership behaviors and styles might be effective?
5. How might the situation be analyzed using relationship-based care principles?

2

Change and Innovation

Maryanne Garon

http://evolve.elsevier.com/Huber/leadership

Change is a pervasive element of society, of today's health care environment, and of life. The prevalence of change is especially evident in 21st-century health care. Wheatley's (2007, p. 84) quote could describe the changes in health care in the last decade:

> We participate in a world where change is all there is. We sit in the midst of continuous creation, in a universe whose creativity and adaptability are beyond comprehension. Nothing is ever the same twice, really.

Nurses today are accustomed to change in their environments. Many have seen changes in the acuity of patients, changes in practice models and skill mixes, a change to evidence-based practice, changes in educational requirements, and changes within their own roles. Some nurses report that changes in practice are so frequent that they are taken for granted (Copnell & Bruni, 2006). Yet the nursing profession struggles to maintain its emphasis on humanism and healing in the face of some of the mandated changes (Clarke, 2013). Nurses want to ensure that the very basis of nursing, providing care and support for patients, does not change (Copnell & Bruni, 2006).

The changes in 21st-century health care have been described as "revolutionary" (Longenecker & Longenecker, 2014). From new laws and regulations from the Affordable Care Act, increased focus on both cost cutting and indicators of quality, and staffing challenges, leaders are under constant pressure to change in order to meet goals and improve outcomes. Other changes, including increased numbers of aging baby boomers, strain on emergency

services, "never events," accountable care organizations, pay for performance, the Human Genome Project, and nurse shortages followed by a flood of new nurses have all affected and led to changes in the health care system over the last decade.

The pace of change is only accelerating, and continuous change is becoming the new normal. All these changes demand the time and attention of nurses, who can choose to resist and ignore or who can decide to participate actively in the change process. Those who must implement these changes are most likely to be at the point of care: the staff nurses. Ongoing and perpetual change can be very stressful for the staff nurse and lead to change fatigue (Vestal, 2013).

Change is seldom easy. It can be complex and irrational. Even when it is the individual's own decision to make a change, it can be difficult. When someone makes a change, such as deciding to stop smoking, to lose weight, or to go back to school, then the initiating, following through, and sustaining of that change is challenging. Initiating and sustaining organizational change adds unique challenges. When change is seen as unnecessary, imposed from above, or threatening workers' sense of security, the process is even more difficult. To guide the change process, nurse managers and leaders need a thorough understanding of change grounded in theory, applicable research, and reports of successful change processes.

Although there are multiple approaches or models of change in the literature, most fall into the realm of either planned change theories or models and emergent models (Shanley, 2007). Critiques of the planned approach highlight the prominence of its top-down approach and overemphasis on the role of managers in the

Photo used with permission from Portra/Getty Images.

process. In addition, the emphasis on cookbook-like approaches portrays change itself as linear rather than complex and multidimensional.

In emergent approaches, the complex and multidimensional view of change is central. The emphasis is on principles or processes of change because there has been little support for one particular strategy or number of steps being more effective than another (Longenecker & Longenecker, 2014; Shanley, 2007). Emerging views of change also emphasize the importance of the participatory process in change. Therefore, in this model it is essential for nurse leaders to understand the role of recipients in creating and sustaining change. Viewing change and resistance as two opposing forces can result in *stereotyping* one group as irrational resisters rather than as partners in and co-creators of change.

DEFINITIONS

Concepts related to change and innovation include change, planned change, innovation, transformation, resistance, and change agent.

Change is an alteration to make something different, a complex process that occurs over time and is influenced by any number of unpredictable variables. **Planned change** is a decision to make a deliberate effort to improve the system. **Innovation** is the use of a new idea or method. **Transformation** means the use of new ideas, innovations, and creativity to change fundamental properties or the state of a system. **Resistance** means to refuse to accept or be changed by something, a force that acts to stop the progress of something or make it slower. **Change agent** is a person or thing that encourages people to change their behavior or

opinions. The term has come to be used for a person who functions as a change facilitator (Cambridge Dictionary, 2016).

BACKGROUND

Change has long been a topic of interest to individuals and organizations. Yet few have questioned either the success of change efforts or why they have so often failed. Implementing change is a complex problem that is often unsuccessful. Studies suggest that 70% of organizational change initiatives do not succeed (Axelrod et al., 2006). Too often organizational change efforts have emphasized a top-down planned change strategy. In most of these cases, the focus was on the role of administrators and top managers in the change process. Change was seen as initiated by administrators who formulate a plan for the change and communicate it to middle managers and others. Strategies for disseminating the change, informing staff, and dealing with resisters (often viewed as stubborn and irrational) are developed and implemented (Table 2.1 displays contrasting views of change).

Alternative views have emerged that promoted the idea that top-down change is not just undesirable; it does not work (Balogun, 2006; Longenecker & Longenecker, 2014). Porter-O'Grady and Malloch (2015, p. 79) conceptualize this as "moving from the center [the point of service] outward." Staff and other "recipients" of change at the point of service must be viewed as integral to the process rather than as potential obstructions to be influenced and acted upon. All levels and parts of the system need to be involved in planning for and sustaining change, and ideas for change can come from all

TABLE 2.1   Contrasting Views of Change

	Planned Change (Traditional View)	Emergent View
Direction	Top-down, linear	Multidirectional, multidimensional
Initiator	Leader initiated	Diffuse
Process	Planned, step-by-step process	Principles to guide process
Organizational culture	May be considered	Essential to consider
Power issues	Not considered or not spoken	Essential to consider
Role of staff/recipients of change	Resisters	Participants in change process
View of the change recipients	May be assessed so they can be changed or manipulated	Essential to process

levels. In addition, when considering the processes of change, issues of power and how individuals make sense of the change are essential.

Evidence supports this emergent view of change (Shanley, 2007). Although there is little evidence in the literature showing whether any of the specific approaches to planned change actually work (Hallencreutz & Turner, 2011), there is some evidence about what *does* work (Balogun, 2006; Packard & Shih, 2014). The literature points to the decreased importance of executives and increased importance of those affected by any change. The planned approach is too simplistic, takes too much for granted, and does not allow for the analysis of the complex aspects of change over time. Because organizations and the change process are so complex, change efforts must be localized and incorporate a variety of approaches (Hallencreutz & Turner; 2011).

Theories of change that focus on the human side of change are important to consider. The leader-collaborator relationship needs to be central to the process. In addition, leaders must assess and understand the participants' responses to change, political and power issues that affect initiation of change, and how to develop organizational or unit cultures that facilitate and sustain change (Longenecker & Longenecker, 2014).

Along with communication, change management is a critical leadership competency for nurses. The American Organization of Nurse Executives' (AONE) Nurse Executive Competencies (2015) emphasize the need for change management knowledge, skills, and abilities. In addition, in its 2011 report, *The Future of Nursing: Leading Change, Advancing Health,* the Institute of Medicine (IOM) (now called the National Academies of Sciences, Engineering, and Medicine, Health and Medicine Division) has called upon nurses to use their numbers and adaptive capacity to take leading roles in health care change.

Organizational Change

Organizational change has been defined as "an alteration of a core aspect of an organization's operation" (Mills et al., 2009, p. 4). Most often it refers to management efforts to move an organization from a current state to "some desired future state to increase organizational functioning" (Weimer et al., 2008, p. 381). These efforts are often described as planned change and involve top-down conception, communication, and implementation. However, organizational change is a complex process that is not necessarily linear (Jansson,

2013). In addition, newer approaches to organizational change that are consistent with the emergent views can be found in the literature.

Leaders are called upon to focus on the importance of human relationships in the change process. The traditional hierarchical mind-set of relying on power and control and top-down, manager-driven approaches has not been successful (Anderson & Anderson, 2009). Instead, leaders learned that they had to focus more on the process of change and human relationship aspects. Anderson and Anderson (2009) called the old way of viewing change as the industrial mind-set and note that organizational leaders need to move toward an emerging mind-set. The industrial mind-set is a mechanistic worldview, relying on power and control, certainty, and predictability. Anderson and Anderson (2009) identified the emerging mind-set, like other complexity views, as one grounded in wholeness and relationship, embracing co-creation and participation. A component of this emerging mind-set is that leaders need to move to what they call *conscious change* leadership. Conscious change leaders are aware of the dynamics of change and learn to lead from the principles of the emerging mind-set. Conscious change leaders must be willing to look internally to transform their own mind-set, expand their thinking about process, and evolve their own leadership style.

Systems theory, complexity theory, and chaos theory are all models or worldviews that influence organizational change and that are more consistent with the foundations of the emerging mind-set (see Chapter 1). These are not prescriptive models; instead the focus is on interrelationships, processes, and systemic behavior. These models suggest that the behaviors of complex systems are nonlinear, spontaneous, and self-organizing. Small changes can often produce larger dynamic (and sometimes unintended) effects. These models help us promote a different understanding of changes in complex systems and how systems adapt to change (Porter-O'Grady & Malloch, 2015).

CHANGE THEORIES/MODELS

Nurse leaders, from the bedside to the executive suite, need to understand and be able to apply a variety of change theories, individualizing them to their organization and situation. The majority of change theories originate from the work of Kurt Lewin. Most nurses

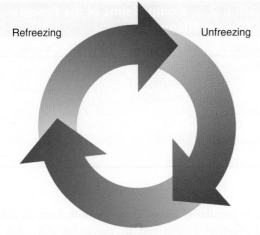

FIG. 2.1 Elements of a successful change. (Data from Lewin, K. [1947]. Frontiers in group dynamics: Concept, method, and reality in social science; social equilibrium and social change. *Human Relations, 1*[1], 5–41; Lewin, K. [1951]. *Field theory in social science: Selected theoretical papers.* New York, NY: Harper & Row.)

have heard of Lewin and his three elements for a successful change: (1) unfreezing, (2) moving, and (3) refreezing (Fig. 2.1). It might be tempting to consider his ideas more consistent with the older, more traditional views of planned change (Burnes, 2004)), but his model is also meant to help increase understanding about how groups and organizations change, and not as a rigid strategy to impose change. Lewin's basic change process is still useful and applicable today and is the basis for many newer theories.

Lewin's Change Process

Lewin coined the term *planned change* to distinguish the process from accidental or imposed change (Burnes, 2004). Lewin's (1947, 1951) theory of change used ideas of equilibrium within systems. *Unfreezing*, the first stage of change, can be characterized as a process of "thawing out" the system and creating the motivation or readiness for change. An awareness of the need for change occurs. This first stage is cognitive exposure to the change idea, diagnosis of the problem, and work to generate alternative solutions. The unfreezing stage is considered to be finalized when those involved in the change process understand and generally accept the necessity of change.

The second change stage is *moving*. This means proceeding to a new level of behavior, which implies that the actual visible change occurs in this stage. When the individuals involved collect enough information to clarify and identify the problem, the change itself can be planned and initiated. Lewin (1951) observed that a process of "cognitive redefinition"—or looking at the problem from a new perspective—happens. As a first step to launch a change, a pilot test may be done so that the change can be pretested and a transition period launched.

The final change stage is *refreezing*. In this stage, new changes are integrated and stabilized. Reinforcement of behavior is crucial as individuals integrate the change into their own value systems. It is important to reward change behavior. Leadership strategies of *positive feedback*, *encouragement*, and *constructive criticism* reinforce new behavior. Leaders point the way throughout the process of change.

Lewin's (1947, 1951) planned change process stages can be compared with the nursing process and the generic problem-solving process (Table 2.2). Unfreezing is like assessing in the nursing process and like problem identification and definition in the problem-solving process. Moving is similar to planning and implementing in the nursing process and similar to problem analysis and seeking alternative solutions in the problem-solving process. Refreezing is like evaluation in the nursing process and like implementation and evaluation in the problem-solving process.

Individuals and systems naturally strive for equilibrium. Lewin (1951) saw this as a balance between driving forces that promote change and restraining

TABLE 2.2 Similarities of Change, Nursing Process, and Problem Solving

Change	Nursing Process	Problem Solving
Unfreezing	Assessing	Problem identification and definition
Moving	Planning and implementing	Problem analysis and seeking alternatives
Refreezing	Evaluation	Implementation and evaluation

Data from Workman, R., & Kenney, M. (1988). The change experience. In S. Pinkerton, & P. Schroeder (Eds.), *Commitment to excellence: Developing a professional nursing staff* (pp. 17–25). Rockville, MD: Aspen.

forces that inhibit change. Both driving and restraining forces impinge on any situation. The relative strengths of these forces can be analyzed. To create change, the equilibrium is broken by altering the relative strengths of driving and restraining forces. A force field analysis facilitates the identification and analysis of driving and restraining forces in any situation. Unfreezing occurs when disequilibrium is introduced into the system to disrupt the status quo. Moving is the change to a new status quo. Refreezing occurs when the change becomes the new status quo and new behaviors are frozen.

The process of change may flow back and forth among stages. It is not a simple linear process in which one step follows the preceding one. The process may move rapidly, or it may stall in any one phase. The goal of planned change is to plan, control, and evaluate the change.

Lewin's (1947, 1951) work forms the classic foundation for change theory. Other change theorists have elaborated further understanding and application of change theory. Bennis and colleagues (1961) assembled a book of readings on planned change that emphasized planner–adopter cooperation and high levels of adopter participation. Because actually implementing planned change is more dynamic and complex than Lewin's model, Lippitt (1973) refined and expanded Lewin's (1947, 1951) work on unfreezing, moving, and refreezing to identify the seven phases of the change process that more fully describe planned change:

1. Diagnosis of the problem
2. Assessment of motivation and capacity to change
3. Assessment of the change agent's motivation and resources
4. Selecting progressive change objectives
5. Choosing an appropriate role for the change agent
6. Maintaining the change once it is started
7. Termination of the helping relationship with the change agent

The first three steps can be compared with Lewin's unfreezing (1947, 1951). Steps 4 and 5 match moving, and steps 6 and 7 are comparable to refreezing.

Kotter's Model of Change

Kotter introduced his change management model in 1996. It was based on his experiences as a consultant with businesses undergoing change. Similar to other change models, Kotter's has not been empirically tested,

TABLE 2.3 Comparisons of the Process of Change Theories

Lewin	Rogers	Lippitt	Kotter
Unfreezing	Awareness, interest, evaluation	Steps 1, 2, 3	Stages 1–6
Moving	Trial	Steps 4, 5	Stage 9
Refreezing	Adoption	Steps 6, 7	Stage 10

but its popularity seems to derive both from its direct and practical format and its successful utilization in multiple settings (Appelbaum et al., 2012). His model consists of these eight steps:

1. Establish a sense of urgency.
2. Create a guiding coalition.
3. Develop a vision and strategy.
4. Communicate the change vision.
5. Empower employees for broad-based action.
6. Generate short-term wins.
7. Consolidate gains and produce more change.
8. Anchor new approaches in the culture.

Kotter's model is inclusive of employees and focuses on both engaging them in the change process and empowering them to be involved. Its emphasis is on helping others to see the need for the change and to embrace it. One potential shortcoming is that Kotter (2012) insisted that the eight steps be implemented in order, without substantial overlap. Because studies have suggested that organizations prefer to use change strategies that best fit their culture, such strict adherence to the plan may be harder to adapt. After reviewing the work of Lewin, Lippitt, and Kotter, it is evident that the various conceptualizations of the stages of the process of change bear similarity to one another but vary in emphasis (Table 2.3).

THE PROCESS OF CHANGE

Change in health care has been shown to be continuous and rapid. It may appear to be like a continuum from haphazard drift at one end to a structured, planned change at the other. Van Woerkum and colleagues (2011, p. 148) acknowledged that "change happens" and that there are three ways it happens: by the emergence of events—essentially change by chance; by the use of language—how we arrive at new interpretations and ideas, by talking with one another about them; and by the development of practices—the result of a chain of activities, purposeful and planned.

Within nursing and health care, change is sometimes forced on us by events, whether it be changing disaster policies because of lessons learned from a fire, flood, tornado, or hurricane or changing the way patient records are handled after the Health Insurance Portability and Accountability Act of 1996 (HIPAA) was passed. Through language, which may include meetings, journal stories, and interpretations of reports, nurses make conscious efforts to change to meet the latest accreditation requirements or safety standards. The development of new practices in response to new evidence or best practices occurs regularly and falls under planned change. One example is the broad adoption of evidence-based protocols and practices as a way of making sure that desirable outcomes are achieved.

Change Management

To ensure that the process of change is effective, it is important to understand how unintended consequences can result from top-down planning or ineffective communication. Based on her extensive research on organizational change, Balogun (2006) noted the following implications for leaders managing the process of change:

- Executives and administrators do not direct change, but they do initiate and influence the direction of change.
- The recipients of change (middle managers and staff) translate and edit plans for change.
- The main method by which recipients interpret what the change is all about is through informal communication with peers (not top-down or official information channels).
- Senior managers need to monitor these communications and learn to engage in lateral, informal communications. Some of this can be accomplished using "management by walking about."
- More explicit attention must be given to open discussions and storytelling in communication about change.
- The recipients of change will mediate the outcomes, so senior managers need to acknowledge this and actively engage with them.

- In large organizations, using change ambassadors to help with the engagement/discussion process may be helpful.
- Finally, senior managers need to "live the changes" they want others to adopt. The recipients of change are quick to notice inconsistencies among the actions, words, and deeds of the leaders.

Balogun (2006) asserted that the meaning of "managing" change needs to be reconsidered. The focus needs to change from one of top-down control to one of participation and communication.

Assessing readiness for change could be helpful when preplanning the management of change. A number of tools exist that purport to do this. However, like so many other areas of the study of organizational change, there is limited evidence of reliability and validity of most of the published tools for assessing readiness for change (Weimer et al., 2008). Therefore the change agent/leader needs to proceed with caution in selecting and using a tool, seeking one that is consistent with organizational culture and using judgment in the application of the findings. Open communication within the change process, early involvement of staff, listening to their input and concerns, and engaging them in the change may be the most effective means to assess readiness for change.

Change Management: Small Scale

In today's health care environment, with the emphasis on patient safety and quality goals, there is a need to make small rapid changes to improve care. Two related models can be used to make these small rapid changes. They are rapid cycle change and Transforming Care at the Bedside (TCAB) (Robert Wood Johnson Foundation [RWJF], 2015). Both use the plan-do-study-act (PDSA) model as a basis. Rapid cycle change is based on the idea that changes should first be tried on a small scale to see how they work. TCAB was a program created by RWJF that ran from 2003 through 2008. Its goal was to improve quality and safety on medical–surgical acute care units by engaging in changes to improve practice. The idea was to create a small test, evolve the idea, get feedback, and proceed. RWJF has a downloadable toolkit on its website to help organizations use the process. Numerous projects were implemented and carried out between 2003 and 2008. They included the creation of rapid response teams, the initiation of multidisciplinary rounds at the bedside, and planned interventions to decrease patient falls. One of the key features of TCAB is that it was not a top-down approach but engaged clinicians at the bedside in the design and implementation of new work practices and systems (RWJF, 2015). TCAB also emphasized that the improvement process was continuous, not a one-time occurrence.

Rapid cycle change, a methodology adapted from Toyota Production System principles, uses a small, focused, rapid process to make process improvements (Agency for Healthcare Research and Quality, 2012). Rather than initiating long research studies, in rapid cycle change staff are encouraged to brainstorm new ideas, try a potential change, and test its effectiveness. This can be done with one nurse, one shift, and one patient. Demonstrating the effectiveness of small change encourages nurses to try others. Rapid cycle change is often discussed and used in conjunction with TCAB (Valente, 2011).

The Human Factor: Resistance

Resistance to change has attracted considerable attention in the management literature (Thomas & Hardy, 2011). Resistance is of concern because it is seen to interfere with the change process, but resistance should be expected as integral to the whole process of change. Although the old ways may need to be changed, the natural fear of what will replace them may cause people to cling to the old. People may fear being disorganized or having their routines interrupted. Some may have a vested interest in the status quo. Others may believe that a change may diminish their own status or disrupt their network of interpersonal relationships.

Almost all changes encounter some resistance as a natural phenomenon. Resistance may be rooted in anxiety or fear. For example, some individuals fear expenditure of the energy needed to cope with change. Some fear a loss of status, power, control, money, or employment. Misconceptions and inaccurate information about what the change might mean and individuals' emotional reactions create resistance to change. Although resistance is characterized as a challenge, a negative behavior, or something to be overcome, not all resistance is bad. It may be a warning to the change agent to reevaluate the change, clarify the purpose, or increase communication. The leader or change agent may need to re-conceptualize his or her approach to the change, anticipate resistance,

determine why it is occurring, and better understand the perspective of the resisters.

Leaders also need to understand that resistance is an adaptive response to power (Thomas & Hardy, 2011). When those affected by change have played a part in negotiating the process of change, there is more likelihood they will buy into the change. In addition, when it is understood that power and resistance act together, the focus can change. It shifts the question to: "how do relations of power and resistance operate together in producing change?" (Thomas & Hardy, 2011, p. 326). Leaders who understand the power-resistance relationship will be better able to guide change in their settings. Another way to understand the concept of resistance is to re-conceptualize staff nurses as the solution in initiating change rather than as the problem. Too often nurses have been characterized as the targets of change, irrational resisters, and problems to overcome rather than as co-creators of change. Nurses are central to change within health care. They are the largest group of health care providers. They play a key role in the initiation, planning, and sustenance of change (Leeman et al., 2007). In fact, because of their numbers and their key role in the process, nurses were found to be the only viable agents of sustaining change (Balfour & Clarke, 2001).

Resistance Reframed

One way to reframe perceptions of resistance is to consider the positive effect that resisters and resistance have played in history and in the development of the United States. From the actions of the rebels in the Boston Tea Party to the antislavery abolitionists in the 19th century to the civil rights activists of the 1960s, resistance has shaped our history. Furthermore, some individuals have contributed to our views on resistance. They include Thoreau, who in 1849 wrote his classic essay *Civil Disobedience* and contributed the underlying idea that acting from principle, on the belief of what is right, is above the law. John Woolman, a Quaker, spent his life convincing other Quakers to give up slavery by personally visiting them one by one and discussing their views of morality. Sojourner Truth, an African-American woman born as a slave, worked tirelessly for the rights of African Americans. Martin Luther King, Jr. led the Civil Rights Movement in the 1960s and inspired with his words on passive resistance. All of these resisters were leaders who inspired others to work for change. So, as leaders, how do we inspire others to work for change rather than impose organizational change from above? This is the challenge.

Re-conceptualizing staff and others as the co-creators of change instead of resisters not only provides an alternative view of change and resistance but also can point to new strategies for moving organizations toward change. In viewing resistance from the emergent view, it is important not to dichotomize initiators and recipients of change. Involving everyone is essential to the change process. The success and sustainability of the change depends on the commitment to the change by those at the level of the change.

Nurses live with change daily. The common belief that nurses resist change is just not accurate. Instead, nurses have reported that changes occur so frequently that they could not remember all of them (Copnell & Bruni, 2006). Falk-Rafael (2000) found that the nurses in her qualitative study had six different orientations to change. Three of these were ways they ended up accepting change: critical approval, insidious assimilation, and wounded acquiescence. She found that nurses used judicious circumvention and constructive opposition when they believed that changes could jeopardize their clients' health (Falk-Rafael, 2000). The final orientation was nurses initiating change themselves through what she labeled "visionary transformation" (Falk-Rafael, 2000, p. 336). Her findings countered some commonly held beliefs about nurses' resistance to change and highlighted positive effects.

Emotional Responses to Change

Dealing with change evokes emotional responses for all involved. Although individuals must devote personal resources and energy to accomplish change, organizations tend to overlook the human emotions associated with an organizational change. Change is more successful as the intellectual and emotional issues involved in change phases are recognized and addressed.

Managers often find it difficult to manage change and experience a host of negative emotions themselves (Shanley, 2007). Employees also exhibit emotional responses to change, ranging from fear, sadness, outrage, stress, and disorientation to eroded loyalty, lack of commitment, and low risk taking (Shanley, 2007). Organizational leaders need to be aware of the potential fallout from these emotional responses when undertaking change.

Managers can provide emotional support to staff in periods of stress and change. Some of the effective strategies are: active listening, promoting action steps and solutions, keeping staff informed of decisions, soliciting input and encouraging participation, and reframing difficult messages.

The meaning that a change has for the individual is important and influences how they view that change. The meaning that the initiator of change intends is not always what the recipient of change perceives. For example, Bartunek and colleagues (2006) studied those on the receiving end of change in a hospital implementing shared governance. Although the change agents saw shared governance as an opportunity for increased empowerment for the staff, many of those on the receiving end saw it as an increase in workload. Any perceived positive gain was negated by the personal feelings of added work. Additional factors influencing this implementation were the role of emotional contagion and "inadequate, infrequent and poorly timed education about it" (Bartunek et al., 2006, p. 203). These researchers noted that emotion did play a strong role in this change effort, and the associated emotions differed between units. Emotional contagion was due to the staff influencing one another.

Although most people inherently distrust change, change can be viewed either positively or negatively. To facilitate the change process, leaders or change agents need to actively involve the recipients of change, work to understand their view, and plan adequate, timely education on the change. An additional intervention might be to monitor unit-level reactions and understanding, because it appears that individuals who understand the change better view it more positively.

Like so much in leadership, learning to lead and manage change must be a mutual process between leaders and followers. Leaders need to listen, understand, validate feelings, instruct, and encourage—and then go back and do it again. Followers need to engage with the change in good faith, allowing for a reasonable chance for success.

Transtheoretical Stages of Change Model (TTM)

Starting in 1983, Prochaska and DiClemente presented a model of the stages and processes of self-change for persons attempting smoking cessation. This model took an integrative biopsychosocial view of how to approach the process of intentional behavior change and how people move toward deciding and changing behavior in everyday life. Called the Transtheoretical Stages of Change Model (TTM), it used research that shows that people move through a series of stages when modifying their behavior. Readiness to change is a key aspect. The time an individual spends in each stage is variable; the tasks in each stage are not. The five stages are precontemplation, contemplation, preparation, action, and maintenance. The stage a patient is in has been correlated to specific health care provider actions (stage-matched interventions) to facilitate desired behavior change. Since the original work in smoking cessation, there has been widespread application of this model in a wide variety of health care, behavioral health, and rehabilitation areas, such as weight loss and alcoholism. Although TTM is more relevant to health promotion changes, it provides an interesting juxtaposition to organizational change theories.

LEADERSHIP AND CHANGE

> Never doubt that a small group of thoughtful, committed citizens can change the world. Indeed, it is the only thing that ever has.
>
> *-Margaret Mead*

Leaders are an essential part of the change process. The approach, skills, and values that individual leaders bring to change efforts are integral to its success. Some authors have even used change as part of the definition for leadership. Burns (1978), credited with introducing the idea of transformational leadership, emphasized that leadership is about transformation, and transformational leadership is a model of leadership that embodies change. Rost (1994) conceived leadership not as positional but as a process that moves people to work together to make real change in their lives or in organizations. The value of Rost's definition is that leaders do not depend on an organizational position, and the leader role may rotate depending on the change desired and the approach taken. Despite their earlier formulation, these views of leadership are more consistent with the emergent view of change.

Despite the fact that change is ever present and necessary, leaders/managers still find it one of the most difficult aspects of their role. In fact, managers often report that their reactions to change and the need to

initiate change are emotions similar to and as strong as those associated with disasters, catastrophes, and even abuse (Shanley, 2007). Change can be positive but also have multiple negative outcomes, including low morale, stress, and low self-esteem. The key lies in the management of change and human reactions through the process.

Leadership Roles in Change

Nurse leaders may take a number of roles in the process of change. Nurse executives and administrators are essential for providing the vision of a preferred future, initiating change, and helping guide the direction of change. Middle-level and first-level managers and staff, as the recipients of change, may also take roles in initiating and sustaining change. In addition, nurses in a variety of roles, from educators to clinical specialists to staff nurses, may take on roles of change agents, opinion leaders, and early adopters of innovations. This often resembles a brokering or buffering role.

Change agents can follow a number of steps in the process of change, as follows:

- Articulate a clear need for the change.
- Have the group participate by leaving details to those who have to implement the change.
- Provide reliable information and details to those who are to implement the change.
- Motivate through rewards and benefits to help the change along.
- Do not promise anything that cannot be delivered.

For example, when implementing a planned change to a new care delivery system, the change agent would need to be clear about the need for and the benefits of the change. This might include greater autonomy for nurses, greater safety and quality, or improved effectiveness. The details of implementation should be left to the group, but only after reliable and detailed information is communicated to them. Rewards and benefits—not threats about performance scrutiny—should be the basis of the motivation to change. Participation itself may be motivating. Promised benefits from the change should be limited to what the change agent can reasonably deliver.

POWER AND POLITICS

Power issues and politics are central in considering change and too often have been overlooked. Leaders need to consider power issues when planning for change.

Shanley (2007) suggested that change initiators ask, "Whose needs are being met by the change, and whose interests are being served by the change?" In addition, many of the usual approaches to planned change reinforce hierarchical managerial practices and top-down control, thus making change more difficult to implement. Understanding power can also help leaders to reframe their views of resistors and engage them as co-creators of change. Powerful change can occur through shared governance mechanisms that enhance empowerment and sustainability.

Some past changes in health care, such as the restructuring efforts of the 1990s, created change that was negative for nurses and, eventually, organizations and patients. These changes were externally imposed, reportedly for cost containment because of reimbursement changes. The top-down destructive influences of those changes were demoralizing to nurses and had long-term, unintended consequences, including changed staffing ratios, increased usage of unlicensed personnel, and possibly even contributed to the nursing shortage of the early 2000s.

In implementing change, considerations of power may be one of the most difficult areas for nurse leaders. Powerful economic or political interests may pressure nurse leaders to make organizational changes or enact restructuring to alleviate immediate problems. Unfortunately, the long-term effects of these changes may be difficult to foresee or to quantify. Nurses at all levels must learn to speak up, articulate, and support the value of their role and evaluate change for the long term. As nurses become more involved in leadership roles in the health care system, as suggested in the IOM report *The Future of Nursing* (2011), they can use their own positional influence to chart nursing's own destiny and, hopefully, prevent destructive practices like those that emerged in the 1990s.

INNOVATION THEORY

Change and *innovation* are companion terms, but many authors have differentiated innovation from change. An **innovation** is defined as something new, the introduction of a new process or new way of doing something. Innovation implies creativity and doing things differently, but it also has been described as a process with steps that can be utilized (Hernandez et al., 2013).

Innovation is a complex phenomenon. It is of interest in many fields from business to science; and, of course, in health care. Innovation is "a process involving several steps from the creation of a novel idea to its adoption, implementation and spread (diffusion) within or across organizations" (Hernandez et al., 2013, p. 167). To some, innovation is systematic, takes hard work, and has little to do with genius and inspiration (Drucker, 1992). In nursing, leaders need to promote innovation in order to address the issues and pressures for change. Leaders need to consider both how to encourage cultures of innovation and what processes are needed to implement successful cultures for innovation in health care. Organizations may innovate to incorporate the most effective evidence-based practice to meet needs of providers and patients and to gain or maintain a competitive advantage (Hernandez et. al., 2013). It is therefore important for leaders to understand and encourage innovation in their settings.

Research on innovation in nursing is beginning to emerge (Joseph, 2015). To solve complex problems in care delivery such as quality and safety, nurses need to adopt behaviors of innovativeness and be rewarded for innovative solutions. For example, Tonges and colleagues (2015) used the Kaiser Permanente Innovation Model of improve, transform, and spread as a framework for developing an Innovations Unit on an inpatient nursing unit where operational and process innovations were trialed.

Rogers' Innovation Theory

The late Everett M. Rogers is considered the "inventor" of the best-known theory on innovation (Kapoor et al., 2014). He first published his theory in 1962 and produced four editions of his book, the last in 2003. Rogers (2003) described a cognitive innovation-decision process through which individuals and groups pass.

The five stages of the innovation-decision process (Rogers, 2003) are (1) first knowledge of an innovation's existence and functions, (2) persuasion to form an attitude toward the innovation, (3) decision to adopt or reject, (4) implementation of the new idea, and (5) confirmation to reinforce or reverse the innovation decision.

The innovation-decision process is a series of actions, behaviors, and choices over time as a new idea is evaluated and a decision is made whether to incorporate this into practice. The perceived newness and associated uncertainty are distinctive aspects of the innovation.

According to Rogers (2003), most change agents concentrate on creating awareness-knowledge. However, a more important role could be played by concentrating on how-to knowledge, which adopters need to test out an innovation. Using Hersey and colleagues' (2013) four levels of change concept, the change agent would first work on awareness-knowledge, then address attitudes and emotions, and then work on how-to skills to create a change in individual behavior.

Individual members of a group or social system will adopt an innovation at different rates. This time element of the adoption of an innovation usually follows a normal, bell-shaped curve when plotted over time on a frequency basis. However, if the cumulative number of adopters is plotted, an S-shaped curve appears (Rogers, 2003). The normal adopter frequency distribution was segmented into the following five categories of innovators, early adopters, early majority, late majority, and laggards (Rogers, 2003).

Change agents can anticipate these five categories as an expected phenomenon, identify followers as to likely adopter category, and target interventions accordingly. This means that for effective change, nurse leaders can recognize that there will be individual variance in "warming up" to an innovation, plan for this with targeted strategies to decrease resistance, and capitalize on the power of innovations and early adopters.

Individuals need to be interested in the innovation and committed to making change occur. The outcomes of change are either that the change is accepted or adopted or that the change is rejected. If the change is accepted, it can be either continued or eventually dropped. If the change is rejected, it can remain rejected or be adopted later in some other form. Rogers' theory (2003) described change as more complex than Lewin's (1947, 1951) three stages. Rogers (2003) identified the following five factors as determinants of successful planned change:

1. *Relative advantage:* The degree to which the change is thought to be better than the status quo.
2. *Compatibility:* The degree to which the change is compatible with existing values of the individuals or group.
3. *Complexity:* The degree to which a change is perceived as difficult to use and understand.
4. *"Trialability":* The degree to which a change can be tested out on a limited basis.
5. *"Observability":* The degree to which the results of a change are visible to others.

Kapoor and colleagues (2014) conducted an extensive meta-analysis of research on innovation. They found that of the five factors that Rogers (2003) identified, only *relativity* and *compatibility* could be positively correlated with successful change and that complexity was *negatively* correlated. None of the other factors were found significant in those studies. Simply stated, if members of an organization perceive a change to be better than the status quo, consistent with their values and relatively easy to understand, there will be a much better chance of adoption.

Rogers (2003) was also interested in how acceptance of a new idea spread. He used the term *diffusion of innovations* to describe the adoption of a new idea or process. Innovations create consequences. To move a new idea to the level of dissemination and adoption requires information, enthusiasm, and authority (Romano, 1990). Four elements to consider in innovation diffusion are the innovation itself, communication channels, time, and the members of the social system (Romano, 1990).

Innovation in Health Care

The problems and issues facing nurses in practice are complex and multidimensional, requiring the participation of nurses in being a part of solutions. With constrained resources, this means using the evidence base and finding new methods or techniques to try out via innovation. Innovation in health care requires creativity and ownership of practice solutions. Two government agencies, the Centers for Medicare & Medicaid Services (CMS) and the Agency for Healthcare Research and Quality (AHRQ), and private organizations such as the Center for Creative Leadership (CCL, 2014) have developed resources useful to nurses and health care providers wishing to innovate.

CMS (n.d.) has created the CMS Innovation Center (*https://innovation.cms.gov/*), which supports the development and testing of innovative health care payment and service delivery models. They have webinars and forums and offer reports and datasets to the community of health care innovators, data researchers, and policy analysts. AHRQ has the AHRQ Health Care Innovations Exchange (*https://innovations.ahrq.gov/*) that offers Innovation Profiles and quality tools, articles and collections, and sponsored learning communities on high-priority topic areas such as Advancing the Practice of Patient- and

Family-Centered Care in Hospitals, Reducing Non-Urgent Emergency Services, and Promoting Medication Therapy Management for At-Risk Populations. The CCL (2014) offers a white paper, *Innovation Leadership: How to Use Innovation to Lead Effectively, Work Collaboratively, and Drive Results.* They noted that underlying the pressure on individuals and organizations to adapt is the need to innovate. Their six innovative thinking skills are paying attention, personalizing, imaging, serious play, collaborative inquiry, and crafting. To begin experimenting with innovation they recommend reframing the challenge, focusing on the customer experience, and rapid prototyping. Nurses can use these resources to apply innovative thinking to the solution of problems.

Hughes (2006) presented a review of innovations developed by nurses worldwide. She believed that reporting the number of innovations created by nurses will help promote a better understanding of the role that nurses take in innovation. The examples given were grouped in categories of historical examples, research, clinical practice, business, education, technology, public health, and policy. The following are some examples:

- Development of hospital-based coaches, MSN-prepared nurses, to assist nurses in developing process-improvement projects to enhance geriatric care (Agency for Healthcare Research and Quality [AHRQ], n.d.). Adapting an evidence-based "bundle," reducing ventilator-acquired pneumonia and lowering costs (AHRQ).
- Multidisciplinary team–generated interventions to improve medication reconciliation and patient safety (AHRQ).
- An Interdisciplinary Neighborhood Team project, which developed teams of public health nurses and community outreach workers to mobilize community-driven, population-based projects (Hughes, 2006).

How might leaders best identify, support and promote innovators? First, they need to seek out people who are not afraid to take risks (Cullen, 2015). According to Cullen, "innovators tend to be:

- frequently questioning common beliefs and practices,
- comfortable with uncertainty,
- knowledgeable experts,
- comfortable with occasional failures,
- able to identify and screen innovations for application in their organization, and

- connected with other innovators through their professional network" (p. 430).

Leaders therefore must be prepared to create environments that support innovation. They might provide opportunities for staff to brainstorm and help to prioritize ideas for implementation. Space and resources also help support innovators, as is seen in the Innovations Unit (Tonges et al., 2015). Staff nurses can help promote innovation by sharing ideas with colleagues both within and outside of health care, observing the clinical area for problems needing solutions and embracing ambiguity and opportunities (Cullen, 2015). All of these innovation-promoting behaviors may seem outside the realm of usual expectations of nurses, but the value to the organization of having direct caregivers contribute to meaningful innovation is immeasurable.

Disruptive Innovation

In contrast to system-related views of innovation, Professor Clayton M. Christensen of the Harvard Business School described "disruptive innovation." Disruptive innovation is a process wherein a simplifying technology takes root and displaces more established technologies or business practices that are slower to change, rooted in tradition, or constrained by regulation and the status quo (Christensen et al., 2000). As an example, he described a portable low intensity x-ray machine that can be used in clinics, doctors' offices, and in the field. This new technology was said to cost 10% of traditional x-rays, but it never gained acceptance or a market. In the view of Christenson and colleagues, this is because it threatened current business models. Regulators would hold on approval of the technology; insurance companies might not pay for these x-rays; and hospitals, already invested in more expensive equipment, would also join in resisting this innovation. Christensen and colleagues (2000) also identified other disruptive innovations that could positively improve health care in the United States, including increasing the use of nurse practitioners for primary care and moving more care from acute care hospitals to clinics and homes (already occurring). An example of a disruptive innovation is shown in Box 2.1. In his opinion, health care needs creative leaders and flexible organizations to incorporate new ideas and innovations and to move forward.

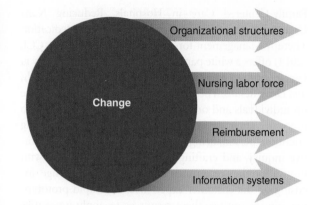
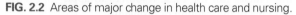

FIG. 2.2 Areas of major change in health care and nursing.

LEADERSHIP AND MANAGEMENT IMPLICATIONS

Change is implied in the definition of leadership. If leadership is defined as influencing others, then the activity of influencing is directed toward some change. The ability to envision and communicate a changed future is part of the definition of leadership. Numerous authors have noted that change is an inevitable fact of life, but leaders and managers can cope by developing processes that allow them to initiate and influence change. The essentials of leadership that are needed are an ability to envision the change needed, reflection on the issues inherent in the change, positive communication skills, an ability to promote cultures that encourage creativity and change, and showing that they actually "walk the talk."

Transformational change is a part of organizational transformation. To produce strategic change, transformational leaders work with others to ignite a vision, change structure and culture, change mind-sets and power structures, and empower others (Robbins & Davidhizar, 2007). Both leaders and managers can be effective in initiating and influencing organizational change. Anyone in the organization can be the focal point for making appropriate and effective change, but the employees in staff positions need to enlist the cooperation and support of the administrative hierarchy.

Because of constant change, nurses and health care systems have had to learn and adapt. To view the scope of change surrounding nursing in perspective, four areas of major change can be identified: organizational structures, nursing labor force, reimbursement, and information systems (Fig. 2.2). First, organizational structures have been changing and reconfiguring in response to the environment and financial pressures. For example, population-based care, case management, patient- and family-centered care, and patient safety initiatives are elements reflecting change in regard to the redesign of patient care systems.

In health care, bureaucratic systems endured for a long time but were not well suited to the work of professionals. The change to structures that empower staff was driven by the goal of improving quality outcomes. Clearly, the Affordable Care Act (ACA) of 2010 created uncertainty and change throughout the health care delivery system and its organizations because it triggered a change process that is ongoing and possibly transformative. Changes are also occurring in health care as integrated networks form and care increasingly is moved into community settings. Changing organizational structures are occurring in the midst of a nurse shortage. The complexion of the nurse workforce is changing; and recruitment and retention, education, and staff deployment alternatives are being explored. Thus nurse leaders and managers are needed who have the knowledge, skills, and abilities to effectively spark and manage change and innovation.

Learning Organizations

Because of the complexity and extent of change, knowledge and skill in applying systems principles are needed by nurses who are leading and managing change. An organization that is committed to changing itself needs continuous learning and adaptation as a systems value. Porter-O'Grady and Malloch (2015) moved away from discussion of structural components of change and emphasized the following four practices for current workplaces that foster learning organizations: empowerment, shared decision making, self-direction, and shared governance.

The concept of the learning organization was popularized by Senge, who said "Every organization is a product of how its members think and interact" (Senge et al., 1994, p. 48). A learning organization uses systems thinking, mental models, personal mastery, team learning, and shared vision when intending to change the behavior of the organization using the ability to learn. The focus is to embed a culture with the ability to continuously adapt and learn. Learning is infused through all levels. Essentially the creation, acquisition, and transference of knowledge is used to adapt behavior to reflect new evidence, new knowledge, and new insights. The learning organization is seen as key to facilitating change by using an infrastructure that supports ongoing learning and knowledge acquisition (Estrada, 2009).

CURRENT ISSUES AND TRENDS

At the end of the last century, multiple authors identified future trends in health care. They predicted that these amounted to major paradigm shifts. In 1996 Issel and Anderson identified the following six interconnected transformations that are major areas of change still influencing health care today:

1. From person-as-customer to the population-as-customer
2. From illness care to wellness care and prevention
3. From revenue management to cost management
4. From autonomy of professionals to their interdependence
5. From client as nonconsumer to consumer of cost and quality information
6. From continuity of provider to continuity of information

There have been continual shifts toward those changes. For example, the ACA (2010) is not just a payment or insurance program; its aims are to guide the United States to shift health care priorities to wellness and prevention.

Another area of important change in health care is reimbursement. For example, reimbursement (payment) for physicians has been changing, driven previously by the federal government's relative value units determinations, pay for performance, pay based on outcomes, and now value-based purchasing and population health management. Reimbursement for nurse practitioners currently is allowed under Medicare/Medicaid. Payment reforms are likely to continue and change. The cost areas include physician payment, already being ratcheted down; pharmaceutical costs; and equipment and technology costs. The government will continue to review and explore the amount of dollars spent and the way those dollars are spent in an effort to reduce a huge national budget deficit fueled partly by health care costs.

Present and future changes will bring an increasing use of computerized information systems. A massive increase in computerization is underway with the electronic health record (EHR) and meaningful use initiatives. Powerful computers and sophisticated software programs have a pattern of undergoing updates and generational changes frequently, which creates challenges of compatibility, archival retrieval, maintaining currency, and staff training. Compatibility among systems, such as relational databases, remains challenging.

These changes have and will continue to alter the health care delivery system. They present both opportunities and challenges, and nurses need to be able to anticipate and monitor trends for their immediate and long-term effects on practice. Nurses can participate in and even lead some of these trends, as they create new environments or establish new organizational forms to shape the direction of health care. It is a question of which courses of action are the best and what is the best way to direct the transformations.

The health care environment has been described as turbulent because of the rapid rate of change and the perceived constancy of change. However, change can be growth producing, renewing, and invigorating for individuals and organizations. This occurs as individuals and organizations enlist creativity to derive an innovation that improves the environment or client care delivery. "Leadership *is* the leading of creativity which leads to creative change" (Kerfoot, 1998, p. 99).

BEST PRACTICE SUGGESTIONS FOR NURSE LEADERS

There are multiple models and approaches to change, but little evidence on what works or what will work for a particular setting. This is understandable, as organizational change is decidedly difficult to research. There are multiple confounding variables and differences in settings (from systems to specific units to individual nurses). The literature on change condensed here shows that change does not happen easily, that there are multiple approaches/models of change, and that there are few studies that validate the "best way" to proceed in implementing a change.

Here are a few "take-aways" for best practice in considering the information presented in this chapter:

- Assess your particular setting and the type of change proposed.
- There is no ONE best model/theory to follow: Find a model or process (or combination of several) suited to your specific setting.
- Communicate the vision for the change.
- Avoid top-down implementation (evidence has shown that it does not work).
- Involve those at the point of care (of the change).
- Engage the "early adopters"; have them help you to influence others.
- Remember that power and resistance go hand-in-hand and that it is important to include and give voice to those affected by the change.
- Reassess and reevaluate frequently, and change the strategy if needed.
- Maintain the change by making it part of the new culture.
- Communicate, communicate, communicate.
- Listen, listen, listen.

RESEARCH NOTE

Source
Joseph, M.L. (2015). Organizational culture and climate for promoting innovativeness. *Journal of Nursing Administration*, 45, 172–178. doi:10.1097/NNA.0000000000000178

In her introduction, Joseph (2015) quoted from the International Council of Nurses (ICN) that "nursing innovation is a fundamental source of progress for healthcare systems around the world" (p. 172). Because nurses are so important in developing innovations that affect patient care, it is important to understand how they can best be supported to innovate.

Purpose
There were two purposes to this qualitative study. First, the author wanted to find out more about the experiences of nurses and nurse leaders in a hospital with a mission to support innovation. Additionally, the author had a goal to generate a thematic map of the experience.

Discussion
The study consisted of two phases: the first phase was semistructured interviews of six staff nurses and six nurse leaders, and the second phase involved interviews of focus groups to validate the model that was developed. The qualitative data were analyzed using content analysis methods, which entail reading and rereading the data, immersion in the data to gain sense of the whole, identifying commonalities that led to codes and labels, and sorting into categories. A model demonstrating innovativeness in nursing was developed from the analysis (see Fig. 2.3).

Results
Joseph identified five concepts as preconditions for innovativeness: organizational values, workplace relationships, organizational identification, organizational support, and relational leadership. Six additional concepts emerged that revealed a social process for innovativeness: trust, inquiry, idea generation, support, trialing, and learning. Joseph found that three key concepts related to innovativeness in nursing emerged from this study: relationships, leadership style, and context.

Application to Practice
Joseph's study further supports the need for supportive organizational culture and the importance of the leader and his/her relationship with staff in creating climates for innovation.

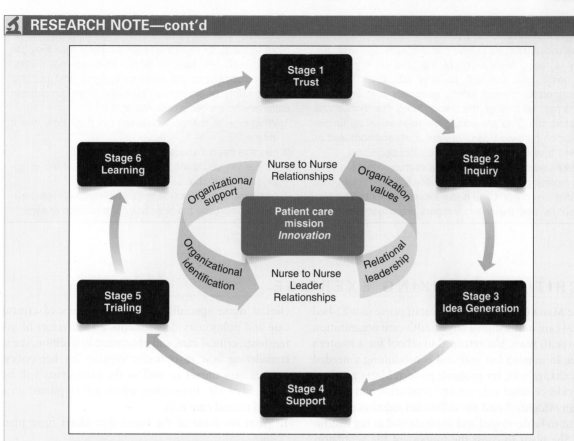

FIG. 2.3 Innovativeness in nursing. (Reprinted with permission from M. Lindell Joseph.)

Nurse leaders need to recognize the importance of their role in creating the culture for innovativeness. For nurses to be innovative, they need to have support, positive relationships with their leaders and one another, and congruence with the organizational values. Leadership style is also important in sustaining the culture for innovativeness. Joseph noted that leaders have an impact on innovativeness at all levels and can provide the culture to foster innovativeness.

CASE STUDY

Nurses Maria Robles and Adolfo Valencia work as diabetic case managers (DM) attached to family practice and internal medicine departments in a large community health care system. The department is undergoing several process changes. In an effort to improve efficiency and comply with the National Committee for Quality Assurance, the diabetes case management and education department is restructuring some of the departmental processes.

In the midst of these changes, researchers from the local university approached the department administrators to seek assistance in recruiting qualified patients for a

blood pressure research study they are conducting. The administrators decided that the DMs should be the ones to take on the recruitment responsibilities, but Maria and Adolfo were not consulted about the change, nor was their workload discussed.

This responsibility to recruit participants for a research study was presented to the nurse case managers as an addition to their current responsibilities, which include contacting patients postdischarge, monitoring the patients in their case load, educating diabetic patients, checking their blood sugars, and monitoring their medications,

Continued

CASE STUDY—cont'd

The case managers believe that this additional responsibility is taking away some of the time currently spent on their current role with patients' education. They are concerned for patient safety, especially that some patients may fall through the cracks. Since this change was initiated, the DMs are finding themselves falling further behind on their workload. They are upset and confused as to why they were not consulted on this decision.

There was no discussion or collaboration within the work unit regarding this new responsibility and who might best be able to monitor it and discuss it with patients. The consensus is that the case managers are already receiving more requests for recruitment for the study than they can keep up with. The result so far has been unhappy nurses, slow recruitment to the research protocol, and possible patient safety or satisfaction concerns (from the diabetic patients who are being case managed).

1. What type of change would you call this? How was it initiated?
2. Has this been a successful change so far?
3. Where do you think the leaders went wrong in approaching this change?
4. List three strategies that the administrators might have used to increase the possibility of a positive change.

▐ CRITICAL THINKING EXERCISE

Nurse Maria Costales has been a staff nurse in a 22-bed critical care unit within a large health care organization for over 10 years. She returned to school for a master's degree in nursing last year and is combining a needed work change with her graduate project. Maria gathered the evidence about sedation and intubation and decided that an evidence-based nurse-directed sedation protocol needed to be developed and implemented at her institution. She plans to enlist the support of the ventilator-associated pneumonia (VAP) committee, which includes members of the interdisciplinary team and frontline health care workers.

Maria wants to initiate policies and procedures, including order sets based on clinical guidelines and existing sedation protocol used by other hospitals for benchmarking. She also anticipates that there are a variety of stakeholders who need to be involved, including intensivists, clinical nurse specialists (CNS), managers of critical care and pulmonary departments, and directors of intensivists, critical care, and pharmacy. In addition, she is considering how to optimize support for her policy. Critical care nurses as well as the intensivists will be educated on this innovation, which will be piloted on a 22-bed critical care unit.

1. What are some of the issues that Maria must plan for?
2. What theory or model might be useful?
3. Who should be involved in the committee to plan this change?
4. What might Maria's first step be in planning for this innovation?
5. How might she or the committee prevent or decrease resistance of other staff—nurses, doctors, and other health care professionals involved?

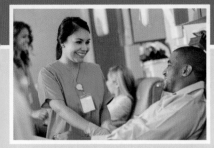

Organizational Climate and Culture

Jennifer Bellot

http://evolve.elsevier.com/Huber/leadership

Since the 1960s, health care organizations have systematically responded to economic, social, and financial challenges that have ultimately caused a transformation in health care delivery. Health care organizations now compete in a marketplace based on their ability to demonstrate lean performance, increased efficiency, and quality health outcomes. Particularly since the implementation of the Affordable Care Act (ACA) in the United States, the payment structure for health care has largely shifted from fee-for-service to prospective payment to pay-for-performance and outcomes.

Crossing the Quality Chasm (IOM, 2001), a landmark report of the Institute of Medicine (IOM, now called the National Academies of Sciences, Engineering, and Medicine, Health and Medicine Division), described the challenge of care provision in the 21st century and was one of the first publications to detail the shift from provider-centered care to patient-centered care. Inclusion of patient and family values, norms, customs, and family/caregiver participation are now dominant factors in treatment decisions. Furthermore, recent inquiry regarding patient safety has emphasized patient outcomes as well as the processes and behaviors that lead to safe care. An explosion in information technology capacity is altering the speed and transparency of communication and information delivery. Interprofessional care is gaining prominence, showing mixed to positive evidence that teamwork leads to better patient outcomes (Reeves et al., 2013). The impact of a nurse shortage, the increasing demand

for nursing care, and the drive to incorporate evidence-based practice are changing the face of nursing care. Taken together, these issues have transformed health care structures and delivery, creating a fast-paced and ever-changing practice environment for nurses to negotiate. There is an inevitable impact on organizational climate and culture.

An appreciation for workplace culture is critical for today's nurse leader. In the perfect storm, nurses may wonder how the issues detailed here link with organizational culture, the professional role of the nurse, and nurse leaders. Nurses' insight into organizational culture enables them to understand staff behaviors and relationships, norms, change processes, expectations, and communications. This holds true for all levels of nurses—from novice to expert practitioner and from direct care provider to administrator. This chapter provides an overview of culture, focusing on the factors that affect the culture within an organization. This chapter also discusses organizational culture and climate and their relationship to the nursing work environment, workforce, and practice.

DEFINITIONS

Culture

Organizational culture is rooted in anthropology, psychology, sociology, and management theory. It first appeared in the academic literature in 1952. **Culture** is the set of values, beliefs, and assumptions that are shared by members of an organization. An organization's culture provides a common belief system among its members. Culture provides a common bond so that members

Photo used with permission from asiseeit/Getty Images.

know how to relate to one another and how to show others who are outside of the organization what is valued. For example, organizational culture can encompass things like the mission statement, policies, procedures, organizational positions, the way people dress, and the language they use. Additionally, culture encompasses what is implicit in the organization, such as the unwritten rules and customs that pervade the work environment. Collectively, these variables define the character and norms of the organization.

Culture is represented in several ways. One example is the care delivery model that guides nursing practice helps interpret the culture. For instance, when a relationship-based nursing care model is used, it represents an underlying belief in patient-centered care. Open visiting hours in the intensive care unit convey the importance of family as partners in care delivery. How new nurses are oriented expresses values about the socialization of new nurses. Many visible aspects of culture reflect the underlying values of the organization.

Culture is a multifaceted phenomenon, difficult to comprehend and unravel. The health care system is incredibly complex. High-quality health care delivery is dependent on good communication and collaboration between providers, patients, and their families. One way to better understand such relationships is to appreciate how the hospital culture affects nursing units, nursing practice, and patient outcomes. For a nurse to function effectively in an organization, a solid grasp of organizational culture, characteristics, and operations is essential.

Culture has been measured both quantitatively and qualitatively. Initially it was thought that something as diffuse and intangible as culture could only be measured using qualitative techniques. Bellot (2011, p. 33) stated that "early culture researchers believed that standardized, quantitative instruments were inappropriate for cultural assessment because they would be unable to capture the subjective and unique aspects of each culture." A strictly qualitative approach to cultural assessment can be time consuming, expensive, less generalizable, and difficult to interpret. Thus various quantitative tools have been developed to more quickly assess culture and allow for comparison across different work environments. In reality, it is likely that a combination of qualitative and quantitative measures are best for capturing organizational culture (Bellot, 2011). As with any selection of a measurement tool, the choice of a measurement instrument

should be directed by definition, purpose, and context for cultural assessment.

Because of the confusion around the tendency to use organizational culture and climate interchangeably and definitional confusion, measuring these two can be difficult. Gershon and colleagues (2004) searched the literature and identified and described 12 organizational climate and culture instruments. They described the dimensions and subconstructs of each instrument and then displayed five major dimensions of leadership, group behaviors and relationships, communications, quality of work life, and health care worker outcomes by instrument. Recommendations for use were presented. A rigorous assessment of the organizational culture and climate sets the stage for planned change. Choosing the right instrument is important.

Climate

Organizational climate is a concept that is closely linked to the organization's culture and is often confused with it. Although many people use *culture* and *climate* interchangeably, the terms are not the same. **Climate** is an *individual* perception of what it feels like to work in an environment (Snow, 2002). It is how nurses perceive and feel about practices, procedures, and rewards (Sleutel, 2000). People form perceptions of the work environment because they focus on what is individually important and meaningful to them. This explains why some aspects of culture may be interpreted differently. A key feature of culture is its *group* orientation.

Climate can be easier to identify than culture. Researchers who study climate describe various components of the work environment that influence behaviors (Sleutel, 2000). Some characteristics that are used to study climate are decision making, leadership, supervisor support, peer cohesion, autonomy, conflict, work pressure, rewards, feeling of warmth, and risk (Litwin & Stringer, 1968; Stone et al., 2005). Within organizations, it is common to identify subclimates that focus on very specific aspects of the organizations (e.g., climates related to patient safety, ethics, and learning). For example, some organizations have adopted principles of a learning organization to establish an organizational culture change using knowledge and learning (see Chapter 2).

Culture–Climate Link

Climate research has formed the basis for the definition and research surrounding organizational culture, and the two are closely linked (Bellot, 2011). Regardless of the practice setting, a link exists between culture and climate. That link is what is important to understanding attitudes, motivations, and behavior among nurses (Stone et al., 2005). The common links between culture and climate can be described as the interaction of shared values about what things are important, beliefs about how things work, and behaviors about how things get done (Uttal, 1983).

Nurse Practice Environment

Although organizations usually have a single, overarching culture, many climates can exist within that culture—from unit to unit, for instance. Groups and organizations exist within society and develop a culture that has a significant effect on how members think, feel, and act. Culture becomes a learned product of the group experience. In general, nurses work together in a group such as on a nursing unit, in home care, in long-term care, or in communities. The nursing unit is a small geographical area within the larger organization where nurses work interdependently to care for patients. Nursing work groups naturally spend time together and set up their own norms, values, and ways to communicate with each other. These factors contribute to that work group having its own climate, or perception of what it feels like to work within a geographical area, contributing to the **nurse practice environment.**

Climate is evident in staff perceptions of policies, practices, and goal achievement. Some authors have described this as an organizational subculture (Hatch & Cunliffe, 2013). Understanding organizational culture from the perspective of individual nurse practice environments can offer an unprecedented view of nurses' work. Creating an environment with a culture and climate that empowers nurses to practice in ways that support a positive professional practice environment can maximize both nurse and patient outcomes.

Using the strict social science definitions, the predominance of nursing organizational research focuses on *organizational culture*—or employs the more general term *work environment*—rather than climate. For the purposes of the everyday nurse leader, the terms are interchangeable, although "organizational culture" or "work environment" are typically distinguished more precisely in the research literature.

BACKGROUND

Organizational culture has been studied as both something an organization *has* and something an organization *is* (Mark, 1996). Peters and Waterman's (1982) *In Search of Excellence* fueled a renewed business focus on culture as the means to achieve organizational success and competitive advantage. Industry leaders in the corporate world quickly realized that the philosophy and values of an organization could determine success and secure market advantage (Wooten & Crane, 2003). The health care industry has been slower than the corporate world to embrace culture as a means to optimize organizational performance.

In what may be the most widely cited definition, Schein defined **organizational culture** as "a shared value system, developed over time, that guides members on how to problem solve, adapt to the external environment, and manage relationships." (1996, p. 229). The mission statement for an organization offers a snapshot of strategic priorities and is an important way to get a sense of organizational values. Schein suggested that a deeper understanding of cultural issues in organizations is necessary to understand what goes on and, more importantly, to affect outcomes. This is particularly important in the area of health care, given the recent shift to payment based on patient outcomes.

Organizational culture affects the quality of nursing care and patient outcomes. Shared meanings—the taken-for-granted practice and assumptions of a work group—can exert a significant effect on performance and outcomes. Basic underlying assumptions are those that are never questioned and make up an integral part of the fabric of an organization that extends to the unit work level, such as a commitment to excellence and to the surrounding community. Each organizational unit and work group has cultural norms and values that blend the social realities and features that shape interactions among staff, patients, and families. The manner in which the staff perceives organizational culture, manages boundaries, and translates implied values to the unit level has a direct effect on patient care (Carthon et al., 2015).

RESEARCH

Since the mid-1990s, a growing body of research has confirmed that the relationship between nurse staffing and patient outcomes is influenced by culture or climate and the organizational characteristics of the structure in which nurses practice. More recently, studying the impact of culture has shifted from the organizational level to the unit level, where caregiver relationships, communication, and autonomy intersect to inform care decisions that affect individual outcomes. To understand how the culture of the organization and climate of a unit are related to professional practice, five contemporary trends in achieving a culture/climate of quality are discussed here: the Magnet Recognition Program®, the professional practice environment, patient safety culture, healthy work environments, and just culture.

Magnet Recognition Program®

In 1983, the American Academy of Nursing's Task Force on Nursing Practice in Hospitals studied nursing service best practices by surveying 163 hospitals. The goal was to identify and describe those factors that, when present, created an environment that attracted and retained qualified RNs who delivered quality care. The 41 best hospitals were called "Magnet hospitals" because of their clear ability to attract professional nurses. The 14 original characteristics they displayed were identified and called "Forces of Magnetism." Now administered by the American Nurses Credentialing Center (ANCC, 2016), the Magnet Recognition Program® has become the gold standard for excellence in nursing.

Magnet hospitals are an example of a positive culture that affects nurse and patient outcomes. Today, hospitals and long-term care facilities wanting to achieve Magnet Recognition Program® status must meet five key components identified by the ANCC (2016): transformational leadership; structural empowerment; exemplary professional practice; new knowledge, innovations, and improvements; and empirical outcomes. In 1998 the Magnet recognition was expanded to include long-term care facilities, although Magnet designation still largely applies to the acute care, hospital environment.

In Magnet-designated organizations, a strong visionary nurse leader nurtures a professional nursing environment and advocates for, and is supportive of, excellence in nursing practice. Magnet-designated hospitals have been recognized over the years for excellence in patient care, strong nursing practice environments, and the ability to attract and retain nurses. The advancement of professionalism, autonomy, and nursing's knowledge base are hallmarks. Periodically, the ANCC queries Magnet-designated facilities to establish an official national research agenda that is current and germane to ongoing professional development.

Aiken and colleagues have transformed the initial Magnet hospital work into a program of research congruent with quality of care and organizational effectiveness through study of the links between hospital organizational culture and care outcomes. Magnet hospitals were conceptualized as those institutions that have a specific organizational culture with characteristics of autonomy, practice control, and collaboration. In a seminal work, Aiken and colleagues (1994) examined mortality rates in 39 Magnet hospitals and 195 control hospitals using multivariate matched control sampling. Magnet hospitals had a significantly lower mortality rate (4.6% lower) for Medicare patients than did control hospitals. The Magnet-designated hospitals' cultures provided higher levels of autonomy and control of practice for nurses and fostered stronger professional relationships among nurses and physicians than did non–Magnet-designated hospitals.

Magnet research and an organizational framework developed by Aiken and colleagues (1997) provide the means to better understand the link between unit culture characteristics and adverse events. A nursing unit culture that supports and values nurse autonomy and the provision of adequate resources and effective communication among providers most likely constitutes an environment where practice excellence is the norm. Examples of recent research regarding Magnet-designated hospitals show associations with lower central-line-associated bloodstream infections (Barnes et al., 2016), lower selected-cause readmissions (McHugh & Ma, 2013), lower rates of hospital-acquired pressure ulcers (Ma & Park, 2015), and multiple other nurse and patient outcomes (Kutney-Lee et al., 2015). A repository of research references on Magnet research can be found at *http://www.nursecredentialing. org/Magnet/ResourceCenters/MagnetResearch/Magnet References.htm.*

Professional Practice Environment

In the journey toward Magnet designation, research and evidence-based practice become important in meeting the core criteria and representing a culture and climate of learning that is supportive of a professional practice environment that involves continuous learning and professional nursing development. A **professional practice environment** is characterized by a shared and positive perception of the value of learning to enhance practice, quality, and outcomes. This may be reflected in principles of a learning organization (see Chapter 2).

Cultures in which continuous learning is valued are less likely to become outdated and stale. In the past, it was not unusual to hear nurses say in relation to their practice, "We have always done it this way." Today, a professional practice environment encourages nurses to propose new ideas and adopt and implement evidence-based practices to promote clinical excellence. Moving new research findings into practice has historically taken many years. In a culture that supports professional practice, nurses are challenged to ask, "How can this be done better?" Nurses interact with many patients on a daily basis. Patients are experts about themselves, and nurses are experts about nursing practice. Blending these areas of expertise puts nurses in the best position to ask the question, "How can practice and the environment in which practice occurs be improved?" Nursing practice then becomes a vehicle for generating questions that are important to practice. This idea, along with creating a culture of lifelong learning, is one cornerstone of the IOM report *The Future of Nursing: Leading Change, Advancing Health* (IOM, 2011).

The formation of the team at the unit level holds a collective vision for continuous learning and professional practice. In turn, the norm for learning intersects with the desire for good practice and forms a cohesive unit that shares a value for learning that generates excitement for moving beyond traditional practice. Cultures in which knowledge is freely shared can have a groundswell effect. Examples of outward and visible signs that support nurses' shared values for professional practice include activities such as journal clubs, unit presentations, poster displays, and participation in evidence-based practice teams.

Patient Safety Culture and Climate

An emphasis on an organization's patient safety culture and climate has driven an avalanche of research and change in hospital practices since the publication of the IOM's (2000) report *To Err Is Human: Building a Safer Health System,* which suggested that 98,000 persons die annually in hospitals because of errors. A safety culture is an outgrowth of the larger organizational culture and emphasizes the deeper assumptions and values of the organization toward safety, whereas the safety climate is the shared perception of employees about the importance of safety within the organization (DeJoy et al., 2004). Like organizational climate, the safety climate has a number of different components, including leadership, involvement, blameless culture, communication, teamwork, commitment to safety, beliefs about errors and their cause, and others (Blegen et al., 2005).

Safety climate refers to keeping both patients and nurses safe. Strong surveillance skills regarding patients are at the heart of safety. Because they are on the front line of patient care, nurses are in an optimal position to monitor patients to prevent adverse events or near misses of adverse events. The ability of nurses to understand a patient's baseline status and recognize early, critical warning signs or changes in health status is a skill derived from having a strong nursing knowledge base. It is not simply task application. Astute recognition of deviations from normal and timely intervention signify that nurses understand the patient's baseline status and are capable of intervening to prevent or remediate an adverse event. Knowledge of the patient and the patient's baseline status is derived through subjective, objective, and intuitive observations that are honed as nurses develop a level of expertise in working with specific patient populations. Factors that influence a nurse's ability to watch over patients to avoid errors and adverse events include managerial leadership, communication style and clarity, staffing levels, excess fatigue, and lack of education and experience (Higgins, 2015; McHugh et al., 2016; Van Bogaert et al., 2014). Other aspects of a safety climate and culture, such as Six Sigma and lean health care organizations, are techniques related to creating quality and are discussed in Chapter 18.

Healthy Work Environments

Included in the concept of a safety culture/climate is a focus on nurses' health and safety. Nurses working in hospitals have one of the highest rates of work-related injuries, including back injury, needlesticks, and chemical exposures (Stokowski, 2014). When fewer nurses are working, less help is available to provide care to patients. This results in more work needing to be done in a shorter time and can lead to taking shortcuts, also known as workarounds, which can result in injury to the nurse and/or poor patient outcomes. To address these issues, the American Nurses Association (2016) has created a variety of resources, position papers, and compiled research on a healthy work environment (HWE) (*http://nursingworld.org/MainMenuCategories/WorkplaceSafety/Healthy-Work-Environment*). They defined a HWE as one that is safe, empowering, and satisfying. Paramount is a culture of safety for both patients and health care workers. General workplace improvements such as in decision making, communication, and collaboration, along with provision of authentic leadership and meaningful recognition are needed. In addition, an HWE would have programs in place to address specific workplace issues such as fatigue management, safe handling of patients, bullying and violence, infection control and prevention, sharps injury, environmental health, and disaster preparedness to demonstrate the organization's commitment to partnership with nurses.

Regardless of whether the focus of safety is on the patient or the nurse, the likelihood of injury can be lessened where there is a cohesive team. When there is a shared perception among a group of care providers about the value and importance of safety, they are more likely to work together effectively toward common goals. Espousing the values of a safety climate and endeavoring to prevent, detect, and mitigate the effect of errors and injuries increases the likelihood of improved outcomes. As nurses work together as a team, they share information, can anticipate events, and are more likely to respond appropriately to unanticipated events.

Just Culture

One major shift in an organization's safety culture/climate is the move from a punitive and reactive culture to a fair and just culture. The concept of a **just culture** was first developed by John Reason in 1997. A just culture represents the middle ground between patient safety and a culture that supports error reduction (Reason, 1997). In a fair and just culture, expectations for system and individual learning and accountability are transparent. Underlying these beliefs, the overall organizational strategy must effectively implement a fair and just culture. When an organization can freely discuss mistakes with the intention of learning from them, and when it takes the time and resources needed to understand the mistakes using root cause analysis, the organizational culture changes from punitive to respectful and open to learning. For example, within a systems-oriented approach, learning from adverse events can encourage error reporting, rather than concealment, and lead to new wisdom and improved ways of doing things. This is called a just culture. In 2010 the American Nurses Association published a position statement, formally endorsing the creation of a just culture for nurses across the health care work environment (American Nurses Association, 2010).

LEADERSHIP AND MANAGEMENT IMPLICATIONS

Nurses work in a wide variety of health care organizations, such as clinics, educational organizations, health insurance organizations, health care associations, home health care, hospitals, long-term care facilities, physician practices, mental health organizations, public health departments, rehabilitation centers, and research institutions. These organizations vary as to their business configuration, ownership, and mission, such as for-profit, not-for-profit, or governmental. The type of organization in which the nurse works has an impact on the differences seen in organizational culture and climate.

Culture is characterized by complexity and is relatively enduring, making it hard to change. Climate, on the other hand, can be easier to change. Regardless, the basic elements that constitute culture and climate must be understood before any change. Change that begins at the unit level may be most influenced by nursing leadership. Nurses have the ability to create or change a work culture, climate, or environment to accomplish a change that may affect productivity and satisfaction and promote safe, high-quality, patient-centered care. For example, units experiencing high turnover can make strategic and evidence-based decisions about processes and relationships in order to convert to a more satisfying work environment that attracts and retains nurses.

A key role of a nursing leader is to influence the culture and the climate. A primary task of the leader is to create a convincing vision that inspires and engages the entire team to move it forward. Values drive behaviors. The leader communicates this vision by influencing norms and values and creating a shared perception through role modeling and ensuring role clarity, accountability, and a nurse practice environment that promotes safe patient- and family-centered care.

Unit-based nurse managers serve as bridges between the senior nursing leadership and direct care nursing staff. Nurse managers are instrumental in shaping and managing the core values of their staff. There are a multitude of tools available to document the relationship between nursing management behavior and registered nurse job satisfaction (Feather et al., 2015). Professional organizations such as the American Organization of Nurse Executives and the American Nurses Association have long campaigned for healthy work environments that reflect positive nurse management. Increasingly, studies are showing that the nurse manager is important in retention (Al Hamdan et al., 2015), stress management (Parry et al., 2014), and work environments (D'ambra & Andrews, 2014).

Key areas within the leader's scope of control are recruiting and retaining staff, welcoming new staff, providing orientation, celebrating and recognizing staff accomplishments, facilitating change, and promoting a just culture and professional practice environment. Climate is evident in how policies are enacted, unit norms, dress code and appearance, environment, communication, and teamwork. The nurse manager can articulate the vision, mission, and goals of the organization and work with staff to translate them into unit-level values for performance, thus linking the context of the organization to clinical practice.

Values drive the way resources are distributed. They contribute to a general attitude and sense about the quality of work life and reflect the organization's core goals. Clues can be gleaned from organizational documents such as philosophy statements and meeting minutes. Caring values of the organization are reflected in the way the organization treats its staff. Organizational values may not mirror professional values. The leader's role is to bridge such values with the values of individual team members to shape the individual unit climate. Values support the mission and the related vision, which, in turn, support strategies and action plans. The key platform is shared values. Given the complexity and diversity of the nursing workforce, developing and sustaining a set of shared values is no easy task and requires leadership skill.

Leaders are expected to chart a clear course for change and mobilize staff to accomplish organizational goals. This means implementing change effectively. Effective cultural change requires communication, passion, and clear understanding of the existing culture. The nurse manager can create such opportunities by using focus groups, holding team meetings, coaching and mentoring, posting minutes from staff meetings, using clear and directive communication, and empowering staff by soliciting their input. The value of communication cannot be overstated.

In their landmark organizational behavior research, Peters and Waterman (1982) stressed that the greatest professional need people have is to find meaning in their work life. The job of managers is to help create meaning through the use of stories, slogans, symbols, rituals, legends, and myths that convey the values, beliefs, and meanings shared among the staff. Managers should function as passionate leaders to motivate staff.

The challenges of leadership belong to every nurse, not just those in formal administrative or management roles. Leadership at the staff level may be informal and simply take a different form. For example, a staff nurse adapting to a challenging patient assignment, taking initiative to change practice through performance improvement, or challenging the status quo is participating in unit culture construction. Informal clinical leadership is manifested among peers, for example, when a staff nurse sees an area for improvement and mobilizes peers or the unit-based council to pursue a solution. This can create a positive unit climate with a "can do" attitude. Further, staff nurses are critical to founding and maintaining a Magnet-designated organization.

Nurse leaders with an accurate and comprehensive assessment of culture and climate can identify strategic areas for change. A thorough understanding of organizational culture and climate is a powerful diagnostic tool that may be used to identify both troubled and high-performance areas. An effective organizational culture empowers nurses to practice to the full extent of their education and training (IOM, 2011). The culture of a nursing unit practice environment may exert a significant and independent effect beyond that of staffing and skill mix by enhancing or impeding interventions once problems are detected. Nurses serve as the surveillance system for early detection of adverse events.

CURRENT ISSUES AND TRENDS

At the beginning of the chapter, a number of forces were identified that have had significant influence in changing the culture of health care delivery. Several of these forces have particular impact on nursing care, and a brief discussion of patient- and family-centered care, generational diversity, and the Quality and Safety Education for Nurses (QSEN, 2014) initiative follows to exemplify current issues and trends related to organizational climate and culture.

Patient-Centered Care and the Patient-Centered Medical Home

Beginning in 2001 with the IOM's landmark report *Crossing the Quality Chasm*, it has been widely promulgated that the culture of patient care must transition from care that is driven by providers to care that is patient centered and family centered, in which patient and family norms, values, and preferences are respected. Shortly thereafter, the Agency for Healthcare Research and Quality (AHRQ) agreed with these recommendations and discussed four other features of optimal primary care (comprehensive care, coordinated care, accessible services, and quality and safety) to create national recognition for the patient-centered medical home (PCMH) model of primary care delivery. In this model, nurses work as part of an interprofessional team to deliver care that helps to improve patient outcomes, the patient experience, and value. Beginning research on the PCMH model shows small to moderate effects on nurse outcomes and experiences (Jackson et al., 2013).

Culture Change in Long-Term Care

After the passage of the Nursing Home Reform Act legislation (OBRA 1987) a series of quality improvement programs were implemented in nursing homes. By the mid-1990s, the culture change movement had begun to gain popularity and continues to spread today. Culture change is distinguished from typical quality improvement activities in its attempt to simultaneously alter multiple aspects of care and caregiving in the nursing home. Culture change is so named because of its aim to adopt an entirely new philosophy in long-term elder care. There is no universal operational definition of what specific elements constitute culture change programming. Instead, culture change refers to the movement to reorganize nursing home care completely. Included under this umbrella are several different initiatives that address staff, resident, environmental, or behavioral outcomes or some combination of these factors. Most culture change initiatives are focused upon resident-directed (patient-centered) care, providing services that are directed by the strengths and preferences of the individual resident and/or family.

Research has been done to evaluate various culture change initiatives, but some models have been promulgated and replicated more than others. Early culture change initiatives, although generally dedicated to the same principles of resident-directed care and homelike social structures, were unique from organization to organization. Despite the wide range of programming, research has found that nursing homes that have engaged in culture change activities report declines in avoidable hospitalizations and 30-day hospital readmissions (Zimmerman et al., 2016), declines in bedfast residents (Afendulis et al., 2016), and decreased Medicare spending (Grabowski, et al., 2016).

In 1995, at a meeting of the National Citizens' Coalition for Nursing Home Reform (NCCNHR), a panel of administrators whose nursing homes were engaged in culture change initiatives was convened. This group grew in size and strength and became known as the Pioneer Network. Today, the Pioneer Network is an organization of facilities engaged in many diverse culture change initiatives dedicated to a common set of values. These values include returning the locus of control to residents, enhancing the capacity of frontline staff to be responsive, and establishing a homelike environment that values choice, dignity, respect, self-determination, and purposeful living (http://www.pioneernetwork.net). Some of the most prominent culture change models include the Eden Alternative, the Green House Project, and the Wellspring Program.

Development of a new model or culture change must be preceded by comprehensive assessment of the organization culture, an understanding of the patient population, what members of the staff need to care for them, and what roles are required to form the change team. There is no one right model, nor does one size fit all settings. The work entails a deliberative process to facilitate change that will improve outcomes. Culture development must be an essential component of any new culture change. Transparency and frequency of clear communication is critical for cultural transformation and buy-in from all staff (Bellot, 2012).

Generational Diversity and the Nursing Shortage

The importance of a positive work climate on organizational, patient, and nurse outcomes is firmly established and evidence-based. However, creating a work environment for nurses that meets their personal and professional values can be a challenge. In 2008 for the first time since the inaugural National Sample Survey of Registered Nurses, the numbers of nurses working who were under age 30 years and over age 60 years were almost equal (US Department of Health and Human Services, 2010). Because nurses from each of these generations were raised with a different set of priorities and values, a work environment supportive to each generation is an important retention strategy. For example, baby boomer nurses value rewards. Recognition and pay may be motivators for them. In contrast, Generation X nurses are concerned with a better balance of work and life. Further, Generation Y (sometimes called Millennials), the newest generation to enter the nursing workforce, has shown indications of increased mobility and higher willingness to move to another job when dissatisfied with the work environment and culture (Tourangeau et al., 2013). Tailoring the work environment to meet generational and life-stage needs is a recurrent theme in being able to address successfully the impending nursing shortage.

Quality and Safety Education for Nurses

In 2005, Quality and Safety Education for Nurses (QSEN, 2014), a joint project of the Robert Wood Johnson

Foundation and the National League for Nursing, was announced. The purpose of QSEN is "to address the challenge of preparing future nurses with the knowledge, skills and attitudes necessary to continuously improve the quality and safety of the health care systems in which they work" (QSEN, 2014, p. 1). Widespread rollout of the QSEN program has resulted in extensive nursing faculty education that is designed to create nursing curriculum that emphasizes organizational culture attributes such as the implementation of patient-centered care, emphasis on teamwork and collaboration, integration of evidence-based practice, and creation of a culture that supports quality improvement, safety, and

informatics. To this end, QSEN's key tenets are geared toward teaching nursing students the competencies they will need to affect organizational culture and create an environment that maximizes patient safety and health outcomes.

By incorporating these elements into nursing education, it is believed that nurses will enter the workforce with the tools necessary to help create an organizational culture that fosters high-quality nursing care. QSEN has now expanded to target nurses both prelicensure and at the advanced practice level and is permeating into practice at the direct care level. This initiative is an example of how to make large-scale cultural change in nursing.

RESEARCH NOTE

Source
Carthon, J.M.B., Lasater, K.B., Sloane, D.M., & Kutney-Lee, A. (2015). The quality of hospital work environments and missed nursing care is linked to heart failure readmissions: A cross-sectional study of US hospitals. *BMJ Quality & Safety, 24*(4), 255–263.

Background
It stands to reason that when patients do not receive necessary care, they are likely to experience worse health outcomes. There has been little research, however, to provide an empiric foundation for this supposition.

Purpose
The purpose of the study was to examine the relationship between missed nursing care and hospital readmissions.

Discussion
Design: This study linked results from three surveys using data from 2005 to 2006, the University of Pennsylvania Multi-State Nursing Care and Patient Safety Survey of registered nurses (RNs), administrative patient discharge records, and the American Hospital Association's (AHA) Annual Survey. Part of the University of Pennsylvania Multi-State Nursing Care and Patient Safety Survey included the Practice Environment Scale of the Nursing Work Index (PES-NWI) to measure characteristics of the work environment.

Sample: The sample consisted of large random samples of nurses (n = 20,605) from Pennsylvania, New Jersey, and California. Hospital data were composed of 419 adult, nonfederal, acute care hospitals in the same states. The study also included patients ages 65 to 90 who had a primary diagnosis of heart failure and who were seen at the participant hospitals (n = 160,930).

Results
Using cross-sectional analysis, it was determined that 23.9% of patients were readmitted within 30 days of discharge. Over one third of the hospitals in the sample (39.1%) were characterized by good work environments, whereas 37.7% of hospitals had poor work environments. The remaining 23.3% of work environments were of mixed quality. The distribution of patients across work environment types revealed a similar pattern of poor (39%) and good environments (8.3%). The average number of nurse-reported items of care missed during a shift was 1.92 out of 10. In poor—compared with good—working environments, a greater percentage of nurses reported being unable to talk to their patients, complete care plans for their patients, or teach. Nurses were less apt to report missing medical treatments or pain management in good (as opposed to poor) environments.

Results revealed an association between missed nursing care and heart failure readmissions. This relationship was largely contingent, however, on the quality of the nurse work environment such that nurses working in favorable conditions were less apt to report missing care. Improvements in nurses' working conditions may be one strategy to reduce care omissions and improve patient outcomes.

Application to Practice
Chronically ill patients, including those with heart failure, require comprehensive care management that must begin during a hospitalization. However, increasing demands on staff nurses, paired with increasing patient acuity and complexity, may result in patient clinical needs outpacing nurses' ability to meet them. The finding that nurses are less apt to miss care in hospitals with more supportive environments suggests that affording nurses the time and resources to attend to these various needs may prove beneficial in reducing readmissions.

CASE STUDY

The Caring for You Health Care System made a strategic decision to transform a 12-bed rehabilitation unit into a new unit that could meet emergency geriatric medical patients' care needs. The unit had operated for 30 years and was a recognized leader in excellent multidisciplinary care for rehabilitation patients and families. It had experienced nursing staff, low turnover, and enjoyed strong partnerships with physicians, social workers, physical therapists, and occupational therapists. However, the financials just did not work.

The new unit was designed to meet the acute care needs of older patients with medical diagnoses. The change introduced an entirely new patient population and called for development of a new model of care for acutely ill older patients who would experience a significantly shorter length of stay than would a rehabilitation patient population. A new team of caregivers had to be identified and new processes of care had to be designed and implemented to ensure effective outcomes. The system's chief nursing officer had concerns about the effect of this change-over on nursing staff and interdisciplinary teamwork and interactions. The chief nursing officer pondered the effect of climate and culture disruption.

1. What is the problem?
2. Identify challenges faced by the chief nursing officer and staff.
3. What steps would you take to define the new model of care?
4. How will the culture of this unit change?
5. What can the staff do?

CRITICAL THINKING EXERCISE

The Magnet Recognition Program's® website offers case studies about Magnet designation that showcase culture change. One example of multiple Magnet designations is the Carle Foundation Hospital/Carle Physician Group of Urbana, Illinois (retrieved from *http://www.nursecredentialing.org/Magnet/Resources/MagnetFreeResources/Case-Studies/CarleFoundation.pdf*).

In presenting their case study, the Carle Foundation Hospital noted that it launched its first Magnet® journey as a strategy to improve nurse recruitment and retention. The process involved nursing leaders reviewing the Magnet standards. They realized that Magnet is focused on doing the right thing, including for nurses, the organization, and patients. They achieved their initial designation with great pride of accomplishment in 2009.

This pride drove their re-designation journey 4 years later. Because Magnet status put the hospital among the nation's elite, everyone was determined to maintain Magnet designation at the time of re-designation. However, there was a new environmental and cultural change to account for: the recent integration with Carle Physician Group. The integration of a hospital with a physician group posed some challenges. The climate and culture of the physician's group clinic differed from the hospital. For example, certification rates in the ambulatory clinic were low, and nurses showed little enthusiasm to pursue specialty credentials. To address this situation, nursing leaders developed and implemented a policy of paying the certification fee in advance for registered nurses. Rates for certification skyrocketed from 14% to 36% in just 8 weeks.

Other benefits to Carle from Magnet designation include a bolster to its mission to provide high-quality, world-class health care that garners national recognition. It is an important recruitment and retention tool. Physicians and nurses cite the hospital's Magnet status when choosing to work for Carle. Employees are proud to say they work for a Magnet organization.

Magnet appraisers named their New Nurse Residency Program an exemplar during their most recent site visit because the program boasted a 96% retention rate its first year.

Pursuit of Magnet standards improved outcomes. For example, implementation of CHG (basinless) bathing in the cardiovascular intensive care unit significantly reduced surgical site infection rates, with no deep/organ space infections for more than a year. This successful program has been expanded to other surgical areas.

Evidence of a culture of Magnet, with resources and programs to support nurses in enhanced competence, is seen in providing tuition assistance (rather than reimbursement) to nurses to pursue educational goals. This initiative produced a steady increase in Bachelor of Science in nursing (BSN) rates since the hospital's first designation in 2009. Now 46% of nurses have BSNs, and there is a clear plan to get to 80% by 2020 as recommended by the IOM (2011).

Carle's nursing leaders call Magnet an "indispensable roadmap" for success because it directs the organization to where they need to focus and pinpoints what they need to do to achieve desired outcomes. The Magnet journey is seen as a continuous, evolving process. Clearly, their pursuit of excellence is not a once-every-4-year goal, but rather it is an integral part of the organization's daily work.

1. What are three examples of a professional practice environment for nurses at Carle Foundation Hospital/Medical Group?

2. Based on the information provided in the case study, what are likely some prominent features of Carle's culture? Climate?

3. Based on the information provided in the case study, how might Carle continue to capitalize on their successes innovatively?

4. What steps would you take to implement one of Carle's programs in your own work environment?

5. What are some barriers you might anticipate to culture change in your work environment?

6. How might you think about planning proactively to address barriers to culture change in your work environment?

Managerial Decision Making

Betsy Frank

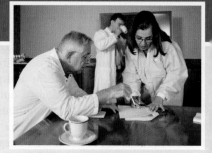

(e) http://evolve.elsevier.com/Huber/leadership

All nurses make decisions. Decisions can be categorized as clinical, involving direct care, or managerial, and they range from managing groups of patients at the unit level to the organization or community or health care delivery system levels (see Fig. 4.1). In order for nurses to make effective decisions, they need the analytical skills that take into account individual staff and patient care needs and an understanding of ethical frameworks and human resource and financial considerations. Whether at the point-of-care, unit, or organizational level, all decisions affect the level of quality and safe care that is delivered and the climate of the work environment in which nurses and other health professionals work.

In an era of changing reimbursements, value-based purchasing, and expanded roles for nursing in the health care delivery system, decision making is an important skill for nurses caring for patients and for nurse leaders and managers. Both the American Nurses Association's (2016) and the American Organization of Nurse Executives' (2015) standards for practice and competencies for nurse administrators and executives support the fact that in a fast-paced health care delivery environment, staff nurses, leaders, and managers all must be able to analyze and synthesize a large array of information, make decisions to deliver effective day-to-day patient care, and solve multifaceted problems that occur in complex health care delivery systems. Furthermore, the Magnet Recognition Program® and the *Future of Nursing* report (2011) of the Institute of Medicine (IOM, now called the National Academies of Sciences, Engineering, and

Medicine, Health and Medicine Division) highlight the need for nurses to be able to be fully involved and even take the lead in decision making from the unit level to the larger health care delivery system, including on health care institution governing boards (Altman et al., 2015).

DEFINITIONS

Decision making is the process of making choices from several courses of action in order to solve problems (Lankarani et al., 2015). For example, if a nurse calls in sick, staff coverage decisions have to be made immediately. However, if a unit is chronically short staffed, a decision will have to be made regarding long-term solutions. Decisions about staffing assignments greatly affect nurses' work life. These include skill mix, patient-to-nurse ratios, and specific patient assignments.

The process of selecting one course of action from alternatives forms the basic core of the definition of decision making. Braaten (2015) has noted that all decisions are bounded by constraints within the environment, such as the complexity of clinical cues. In a chaotic health care delivery environment, where regulations and standards of care are always changing, any decision may cause an unanticipated future problem. For example, a decision may be made to implement bedside report as an evidence-based practice. However, if this is a new technique, the implementation details—such as privacy concerns in rooms with two beds or when the patient has not been told the diagnosis—create unanticipated problems.

Decision-making environment is the context in which decisions are made. The complexity of patient care needs, staffing expertise, budget allotted to care for patients,

Photo used with permission from TerryJ/Getty Images.

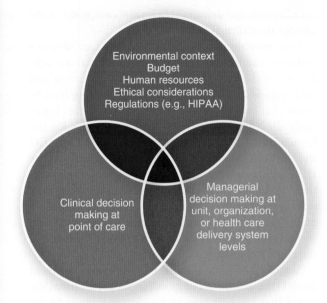

FIG. 4.1 The relationship between clinical and managerial decision making.

reimbursement regulations, and leadership styles all affect the decisions that are made. Ultimately all these factors affect the quality of the patient care that is delivered.

Clinical judgment is the interpretation of the information of patient problems and needs (Tanner, 2006),

Clinical reasoning is the process of analyzing and synthesizing both objective and subjective cues about patients (Johansen & O'Brien, 2015). The nurse's level of analysis is influenced by experience and education (Johansen & O'Brien, 2015; Tanner, 2006).

Clinical decision making involves decisions made at the point of care. The decisions are a result of clinical reasoning and clinical judgments (Cappelletti et al., 2014; Sedgwick et al., 2014).

Managerial and organizational decision making involves decisions for groups of patients at the unit, organizational, or health system levels.

BACKGROUND

Decision-Making Models

All nurses, whether managers or not, use models to help them make decisions. Many of the models include step-by-step frameworks that can guide decision making. In reality, however, decision making is an iterative process that may include an intuitive component (Benner, 1984; Tanner, 2006). Yet models can help the staff nurse and manager make some sense of the complex environment in which all decisions are made.

Such models are more than just for immediate problem solving. Decision making may also be the result of opportunities, challenges, or more long-term leadership initiatives as opposed to being triggered by an immediate problem. In any case, the processes are virtually the same, but their purposes may be slightly different. Nurse managers use decision making in managing resources and the environment of care delivery. All decision making involves an evaluation of the effectiveness of the outcomes that result from the decision-making process itself.

The nursing process is an example of one well-known model for clinical decision making. However, the nursing process does not truly capture the important component of how the staff nurse or nurse manager makes the choice between competing alternatives for action. Other models may be more appropriate.

Moving beyond the nursing process, Tanner's (2006) model has formed the basis for understanding how clinical decisions are made. Her clinical judgment model involves noticing patient cues, interpreting those cues and responding to (acting on) them, and finally reflecting on the course of action chosen so that clinical learning occurs. Goudreau and colleagues (2015) also stated that reflection was key to refining one's clinical judgment capabilities. Furthermore, Tanner (2006) and Stec (2016) have stated that clinical experience helps one to refine clinical judgments. As a nurse gets more experience, the intuitive component of judgment allows the nurse to grasp the cues more quickly (Sadler-Smith & Burke-Smally, 2015). Clinical reasoning expertise is a continuing endeavor that combines analysis and reflection (Koharchik et al., 2015). In fact, Lasater and colleagues (2015) assessed the clinical competencies of all newly hired nurses, no matter their years of experience. Using a case-study approach they found that nurses with less than 3 years of experience were the least developed in their clinical judgment.

Levett-Jones and colleagues (2010) defined five steps for clinical reasoning. They stated that clinical reasoning involved five rights: the right cues or clinical data, the right patient or setting priorities, the right time or capability of identifying high risk patients, the right action or clinical decision that results from the clinical reasoning process, and the right reason. The right reason incorporates legal and ethical considerations. For example the clinical process may lead a nurse to recommend that a patient needs respiratory support in the form of a ventilator. However, the patient may have an advance directive that would cause the clinician to make a different decision. A nurse manager might need to cut his or her staffing budget, but patient census and acuity might cause the nurse manager not to cut the budget because doing so would compromise patient quality and safety (see Chapter 6).

The DECIDE Model is a model that is useful for managerial as well as clinical situations (Guo, 2008; Stiegler & Ruskin, 2012). Using this model can help prevent cognitive errors in high-stress environments because it can help prevent missing cues and thus choosing the wrong course of action. The model outlined here is a combination of Guo's (2008) and Stiegler and Ruskin's (2012) application of the model:

- **D**efine the problem, determine why anything should be done about it, and explore what could be happening. Critical to this step is detecting that the situation has changed (Stiegler & Ruskin, 2012).
- **E**stablish desirable criteria for what you want to accomplish. What should stay the same and what can be done to avoid future problems? Predict how long it will take to respond to the changing environment.
- **C**onsider all possible alternative choices that will accomplish the desired goal or criteria for problem solution. In other words, what is a desirable outcome?
- **I**dentify the best choice or alternative based on experience, intuition, experimentation.
- **D**evelop and implement an action plan for problem solution.
- **E**valuate decision through monitoring, troubleshooting, and feedback. This step involves the reflective process emphasized by Tanner (2006).

Notice how these steps are somewhat similar to the nursing process well known by nurses and nurse managers. Thus decision making is used to solve problems. Table 4.1 displays the use of the DECIDE model to analyze whether to form an accountable care organization (ACO). According to the Centers for Medicare and Medicaid Services (CMS, 2015), an ACO is formed by a group of hospitals, health care providers, and other organizations in order to provide high-quality, coordinated care to a group of patients, most notably the chronically ill. If the ACO saves money through the

coordination and delivers high quality care, some of the savings are returned to the ACO.

One notable fact of the US health care delivery system is the lack of available services for those who live in rural areas. ACOs formed between urban and rural providers achieve the goal of delivering quality, lower-cost care to those in rural areas who are chronically ill. Nurses are critical in the planning for the formation of ACOs. The initial formation of an ACO should have nursing input from the beginning. The DECIDE model depicted in Table 4.1 shows information to consider in making a decision regarding whether a rural health clinic that is 100 miles from a major hospital and regular access to specialty care should seek to join an ACO with providers outside of the clinic's county.

Vestal (2015) has outlined a somewhat different model that is a bit more global in its perspective. She stated that the first step in decision making is to ask how one can make a situation better—or what the problem is—and who can assist in the decision-making process. The manager and clinician rarely act alone. So next desired outcomes are defined with the help of a team. Brainstorming occurs to come up with potential solutions. Once potential solutions are identified, the implications and consequences of the course of action must be analyzed. Once the implications and consequences have been analyzed, the best solution is chosen. An implementation plan is outlined, and outcome criteria are identified. Many decisions in organizations must be approved by someone else. Thus the final step in Vestal's model (2015) is to present the solution in a concise manner to the next level in the organization.

The person at the next level may look at the chosen alternative in a different context. For example, the chief executive officer may frame issues as a competitive struggle not unlike a sports event. The marketing staff may interpret problems as military battles that need to be won. Nurse executives may view concerns from a care or family frame that emphasizes collaboration and working together. Learning and understanding which analogies and perspectives offer the best view of a problem or issue are vital to effective decision making. It may be necessary for nurse managers to expand their frame of reference and be willing to consider even the most outlandish ideas. Effectiveness is

TABLE 4.1	Possible Formation of an Accountable Care Organization Using the DECIDE Model				
D—Define the Problem	**E—Establish the Criteria**	**C—Consider All the Alternatives and Steps to Be Taken**	**I—Identify the Best Alternatives**	**D—Develop and Implement the Action**	**E—Evaluate and Monitor the Solution**
Lack of access to high-quality complex care in rural areas Chronic illness in rural populations	The ACO must be consistent with health care clinic's mission, vision, and culture The clinic must be willing to be accountable for CMS for costs and quality and provide required reporting data The clinic providers must be willing to use evidence-based practice when setting standards for care	Discussions should be patient and family centered and emphasize benefits Discussions should engage physicians, other care providers, and leaders across all organizations in the possible ACO Is the ACO in line with the organizations' strategic plan an in line with all regulatory requirements?	TCPI—this alternative provides assistance in transforming practices in line with value-based purchasing	Determine patients to be served and define service area. Plan sessions with key stakeholders such as patients, providers, and other health care organizations that could be a part of the ACO Improve organizational processes using the plan-do-study-act model Develop methods to assess quality metrics and create integrated network to coordinate care between primary care provider and specialists.	Use data analysis techniques Use best practice research and stakeholder assessment Conduct a pilot project to evaluate the effectiveness and efficiency of potential ACO

ACO, Accountable care organization; *CMS,* Centers for Medicare and Medicaid Services; *TCPI,* Transforming Clinical Practice Initiative.

Acknowledgements: Amanda Fruggerio, RN, RN-BSN student; Sarah Glasscock, RN, BS; Stephanie Laws, RN, MS; and Paula Price, RN-MSN student, who assisted in developing the case study and scenarios.

tied to mirroring and messaging language that fosters shared understanding.

Baghbanian and colleagues (2012) have developed a similar model, but their model has incorporated the complexity of the environment in which decisions take place. They added ethical criteria, economic criteria, clinical criteria (quality and safety), and institutional criteria to the outcome criteria, thus the broader systems perspective is incorporated.

One note of caution is that no matter the model used or the organizational level where the decision is made, cognitive errors can occur. According to Stiegler and Ruskin (2012), decision makers may fixate on some aspect of the process, ignore important cues, bias the process, and allow emotions to get in the way of looking at the data—and thus make a decision too quickly, communicate to others selected data that they want to emphasize, judge the outcome on incomplete data, and hamper full and complete evaluation. Fig. 4.2 is an illustration of what can happen in a faulty decision process when data are ignored or biases are present in the process.

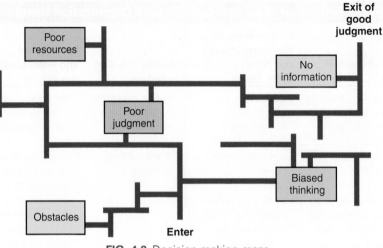

FIG. 4.2 Decision-making maze.

DECISION-MAKING PROCESS

Decisions are the visible outcomes of the leadership and management process. Decision making is essentially the process of selecting one course of action from alternatives. Decisions are made at all levels, but it is important to know who the decision maker is and what the process and timeline of decision making is. Nurses' control over decision making may vary as to amount of control and where in the process they can influence decisions. The basic elements of decision making are identifying the goal for decision making and making the decision.

The process follows the basic problem-solving process but also involves an evaluation of the effectiveness of the outcomes that result from the decision-making process itself. The seven steps of the problem solving process are (1) define the problem, (2) gather information, (3) determine the overall goal or desired outcome, (4) develop solutions, (5) consider the consequences, (6) make a decision, and (7) implement and evaluate the solution. The decision-making process adds a final step of testing or assessing the solution and the decision-making process itself. Nurses may be sole decision makers or may facilitate group decision making. Decisions are often made within the structure of shared governance or by using interprofessional teams for problem solving and decision making.

CLINICAL DECISION MAKING

Clinical decision making is the heart of nursing practice. Point-of-care decisions ultimately have an impact on the total organization's performance and, consequently, its financial viability. Delivering quality and safe patient care is a goal for all health care organizations. Thus effective clinical decisions must be made.

Clinical reasoning is a career-long development process. This process must carry over from skills learned during a nurse's education to the workplace. Nurse residency programs are one way to help newly licensed nurses develop their clinical decision making abilities. Kramer and colleagues (2012) found that newly licensed nurses identified that autonomous decision making and prioritization were challenging for them. New graduates often felt that they needed to verify their decisions with others more competent than themselves. The graduates noted they could identify what care needed to be implemented but needed support to develop confidence in making the right decisions regarding care. The use of preceptors and/or coaches and didactic presentations in the residency program helped the new graduates develop their confidence to make autonomous decisions. Staff nurses must continually make autonomous decisions regarding patient care delivery. Therefore nurse residency programs could promote the new graduate's ability to make the necessary decisions when delivering nursing care autonomously. Some examples of decisions nurses make involve such day-to-day activities as documentation, medication administration, intravenous drug therapy, and prioritization for what care is delivered to a group of patients such as by triage.

Documentation is critical for safe patient care. If the patient's medical record contains errors, then incorrect therapies could result. Since the advent of computerized documentation of care, charting by exception has become the norm (Kerr, 2013). Therefore nurses must decide what exceptions must be noted in the chart—in other words, what about the patient's status is so important that the nurse must make sure that others are aware. For example, has a patient's level of consciousness changed slowly over the past 12 hours? It might not be enough just to note the level of consciousness, but exactly how the level of consciousness has changed needs to be fully described.

When making decisions nurses know that they are responsible for accurate documentation and that they must protect the patient from adverse events; however, they must also protect themselves by showing fully what actions they took in response to a change in the patient's status (Kerr, 2013). The types of documentation are also influenced by whether a patient is newly admitted to the hospital, stable, or ready for discharge (Tower et al., 2012). Patients in each of these three phases of care have different needs, therefore nurses need to learn to pay attention to different cues and circumstances surrounding the patient's care. For example, Tower and colleagues' study showed that a more thorough documentation of the patient's ability to perform activities of daily living would be noted upon admission, but not necessarily on a day-to-day basis if the patient's condition was stable.

Medication administration involves many decisions. In order to protect the patient, the nurse must deliver medications safely while managing the environment in order to preserve safe medication administration (Dickson & Flynn, 2012). According to Dickson and Flynn's study, medication administration involves decisions regarding managing distractions, interpreting orders, and documenting errors and near misses. In addition, Sitterding and colleagues (2012) found that workflow interruptions can interrupt the cognitive processes necessary for decision making. Nurses must also educate patients, coordinate care with the prescriber, advocate for the patient to ensure pharmacy delivers medications promptly, and verify doses with colleagues (Dickson & Flynn, 2012). It is no wonder medication administration involves many more decisions than just the five "rights."

Intravenous medication delivery carries with it more risk than the usual oral medication administration because the medication is delivered directly to the bloodstream. Although nurses know the five rights of medication administration, nurses sometimes make the decision not to check the patient's identity. In their study, Dougherty and colleagues (2012) found that nurses knew they should check the identity but at the same time believed that they knew the patient. Part of their decision making was predicated on the fact that patients do not always want to keep saying their name. Such a decision by nurses is perhaps understandable, but it does carry risk. Therefore nurses must make a conscious effort to make decisions in the best interest of patient safety and not short-cut safe practices even when expert pattern recognition might be a factor in their decision.

Triage decisions occur in a very complex environment. Triage decisions are often made according to protocols (Ek & Svedlund, 2015). Not only are protocols used, but so is the nurse's knowledge and expert intuition. Nurses, however, often fear they have made wrong decisions if those decisions result in conflict with colleagues. According to Ek and Svedlund's study of Swedish nurses in an emergency dispatch center, nurses also feared wrong decisions could have an adverse impact on the patient.

Prioritization occurs not only in triage situations but also across the care spectrum. Thus decisions have to be made regarding what care has to be delivered and when the care is to be delivered. For example, nurses implicitly make decisions to ration care when time and staffing are short (Jones, 2015). On a day-to-day basis, nurses must decide if such things as routine hygiene activities are omitted in favor of administering critical treatments, including medications (Jones, 2015). Ethical frameworks may be unconsciously used when making decisions (see Chapter 6). Some patient care activities can be delegated (see Chapter 9), but on a busy day even thinking about delegation can be challenging.

Clinical decision making is complex and step-by-step processes are helpful, but not all situations lend themselves to such processes. A more holistic approach is often needed as priorities can rapidly change (Benner et al., 2010). Therefore leaders and managers at all levels of an organization must foster a culture where effective clinical decision making can occur.

MANAGERIAL AND ORGANIZATIONAL DECISION MAKING

All nurse managers and leaders need to consider the implications of their decisions. Each decision made involves financial, ethical, and human resources. Furthermore, reimbursement and other regulations must be taken into account. Nurse managers, for example, make staffing decisions and thus commit financial resources for the purpose of delivering patient care. Hospital administrators may decide to add additional services to keep up with external forces. These decisions subsequently have financial implications related to reimbursement, staffing, and personnel deployment.

Nurse managers work in a complex environment that causes stress that may ultimately hamper their cognitive decision-making abilities (Shirey et al., 2013). In any situation, a nurse manager's experience, level of work complexity, and situation factors such as uncertainty and role overload influence how he or she recognizes environmental patterns and cues and the subsequent questions asked. The decisions that result have wide impact on the organization. If a manager is stressed, important factors in the cognitive decision-making process may be missed and organizational outcomes adversely affected.

Ethical decision making is inherent in the role of the nurse manager. When decisions involve an ethical dilemma, nurse managers may experience stress (Ganz et al., 2015). Some ethical dilemmas often encountered include lack of resources and incivility in the work environment, both of which can affect the quality of the care delivered. How the nurse manager deals with these dilemmas has an effect on the quality of the work environment.

One way to deal with ethical dilemmas is through moral case discussions between staff and managers (Weidema et al., 2015). In an open and safe environment, a case study is presented for full debate, analysis, and sharing of possible action steps for resolution. However, using this participatory management technique is hard to incorporate in the workflow when there is a heavy day-to-day workload. Furthermore, conducting case discussions between staff and managers could inhibit free discussion between the two groups just because of the presence of hierarchal relationships (Weidema et al., 2015). Weidema and colleagues suggest that if staff nurses feel empowered to make autonomous decisions, communication in the case discussions could actually occur without the presence of the manager.

A nurse manager's leadership style may affect how decisions are made throughout the organization. Decisions about the safety culture are a part of a nurse manager's role. Merrill (2015) found that a transformational leadership style (see Chapter 1) contributed to a positive safety culture. Praising employees affects a nurse's job satisfaction (Sveinsdóttir et al., 2016). This in turn contributes to a healthy work environment wherein nurses are free to make autonomous decisions that contribute to positive patient outcomes. Earlier research by Van Bogaert and colleagues (2013) showed that unit-level managers had a direct impact on the level of autonomous decision making by the staff and, in turn, the quality of care delivered.

Leadership style also influences ethical decision making. Zydziunaite and colleagues (2013) found that the more experience a nurse manager had the more transformation leadership styles were used in making ethical decisions. One interesting finding was the more frequent the ethical decisions made, the more autocratic the decision-making style was. One should note, however, that Zydziunaite and colleagues conducted their study in Lithuania, which has a recent history of little decision-making autonomy because of the political system under the former Soviet Union.

Patient Acuity and Staffing: An Example of Decision Making

An example of decision making in nursing practice is staffing and assignment decisions. Patients need nursing care. Needs for care are not uniform. The need severity (physical and psychological) is called *patient acuity,* which is a rating of the complexity of the patient's condition. The degree of work needed for any patient is called *nursing intensity* and is a combination of the severity of illness, the patient's dependency, the complexity of care, and the amount of time needed. The organization staffs a set number of nurses and assistants to deliver care to patients. Both patients' needs for nursing care and the amount of nurse time that is required to meet patients' needs for care must be matched up and caregivers deployed, sometimes 24/7.

Nurses are responsible for the decision making about patient acuity and nursing intensity. Managers are responsible for the decision making about staffing and scheduling (see Chapter 22). The individual nurse experiences this decision making as workload (nursing work activities), nurse-to-patient ratios, and patient assignments. In theory, the nursing interventions required to support the patients' needs should be in proportion to the levels of severity and degrees of intensity (Craig, 2010). However, for a variety of reasons, decision making around staffing, scheduling, and patient assignments is imprecise and creates tension and stress for both nurses and managers. With decisions that may have unanticipated consequences, such as if staffing is reduced, what adverse events might occur?

DECISION-MAKING TOOLS

Both nurses at the point of care and nurse managers need a variety of tools to facilitate effective decision making. For example, there are a variety of clinical decision-making tools such as algorithms, policies, procedures, clinical protocols, standard order sets, and smart alerts.

Although trial and error or a shoot-from-the-hip approach can work, direct patient care nurses and managers have a variety of other approaches that can be used to make decisions that promote quality and safe care. For example, by analyzing the data in Table 4.2, the nurse can help decide if a computerized physician-order entry system and electronic health record should be implemented in a small clinic. Or, on the other hand, should the clinic forgo the cost and pay any penalties to the federal government for not computerizing records (CMS, 2016)?

Shared Governance

Another decision-making approach is shared governance. Although this topic will be discussed more fully in Chapter 13, a brief discussion is warranted here. Shared governance is an organizational structure that promotes empowerment and autonomous decision making at the point of care, accountability that is shared among all parties in a decision, and organizational processes that promote an egalitarian environment in decision-making processes. Structural relationships between the decision-making committees and the entire organization are well defined (Dunham-Taylor & Pinczuk, 2015). For example, a committee within a shared governance organization could develop and test a new fall-prevention protocol, exhibiting nursing practice empowerment. Having staff nurses participate in decision making is not truly shared governance if administration views the staff participation as merely seeking input rather than active engagement in solving problems in the practice of nursing (Graham-Dickerson et al., 2013).

Evidence-Informed Decision Making

All nurses are familiar with evidence-based practice for clinical standards of practice. In the management realm, using evidence to make decisions is as important as is using evidence for clinical decisions. One example is the evidence-based protocol that is widely used by staff nurses to prevent catheter acquired urinary infections (American Nurses Association, n.d.). But what about managers? Jansson and Forsberg's study (2016) revealed that nurse managers have a critical role in facilitating use of evidence at the point of care. If managers provided staff nurses with evidence-based facilitators and scientific evidence, rather than using local knowledge, patients were more involved in the decision making.

Specific interventions at the organizational level can promote evidence-informed decision making (Gifford et al., 2014). Following a 20-week intervention that included a workshop, support from evidence facilitators, and access to library resources, the majority of the staff nurses and managers were able to search for and use evidence for decision making. However, barriers did exist for using the evidence in clinical and managerial decision making, including lack of time to search for and appraise evidence and competing organizational priorities that stretched the participants thin. Gifford and colleagues (2014) suggested that the use of advanced practice nurses could facilitate evidence-informed decision making.

Pilot Projects

Pilot projects are critical for implementation for evidence-informed decision making. Pilot projects or carefully

---

TABLE 4.2 Desired Objectives Analysis

Objective	Alternative A	Alternative B	Alternative C	Alternative D
Reduces the number of medication transactions	5	4	2	3
Enables medication administration through automation	5	4	2	2
Meets or exceeds net present value target	3	2	5	3
Meets regulatory standards	3	3	3	3
Improves accuracy	4	4	5	4
Total Score	20	17	17	15

1, Does not meet objective; *2,* meets some aspects of objective; *3,* meets objective; *4,* exceeds objective; *5,* significantly exceeds objective.

defined trials are used to experiment by trying out a solution alternative on a small or restricted basis to reduce risk and to see whether major problems will occur. Pilot project strategies may resemble research projects, and these projects may also be linked to quality improvement initiatives.

SBAR

SBAR is a communication technique that helps members of the health team communicate effectively so that appropriate decisions can be made. Because hands-off communication is so crucial to decision making about patient care, SBAR is used to clarify and organize essential but complex patient care information (see Chapter 7). The acronym stands for **S**ituation, **B**ackground, **A**ssessment, **R**ecommendation (Lancaster et al., 2015). Teaching SBAR to students helps them to develop their clinical judgment skills and can also be used to help new nurses further develop their autonomous decision making. SBAR has been demonstrated to be particularly useful in long-term care settings (Renz et al., 2013). Patients in this setting can have subtle changes that can predict a worsening condition. Therefore all providers need a way to communicate in order to guide effective clinical decision making. Nurses using a tool designed by Renz and colleagues (2013), found it helpful in organizing information to be communicated. Most physicians expressed satisfaction with the way the nurses communicated information to them.

Simulation

Simulation is a well-known technique for developing and maintaining clinical decision making. It is used to teach skills and verify competencies. Simulation could also be used to improve management decision making. Endacott and colleagues (2012) used simulation to assess rural hospital nurses' clinical decision-making skills. The investigators found that nurses made decisions in four ways. They conducted a complete assessment and took proper actions, conducted a complete assessment but decisions resulted in incorrect actions, conducted an incomplete assessment but nevertheless took proper actions, or conducted an incomplete assessment and made incorrect clinical decisions. The investigators noted that nurses recognized the need for continuing education with simulation, especially with feedback so they could learn from their mistakes (Endacott et al., 2012.

Sedgwick and colleagues (2014) also used simulation to study clinical decision making in nurses who worked in rural settings. The results of their study showed that, like Endacott and colleagues (2012), nurses need to reflect on their actions if clinical reasoning skills are to develop. One interesting finding was that nurses did not exhibit the use of hospital policies and/or decision algorithms in their decision-making process. Continued use of simulation at periodic intervals could help individual nurses and teams further develop their decision-making abilities, including incorporating policies and other forms of evidence in their decisions.

Data Analytics and Decision Support Systems

Decisions need to be data driven. Nurses and nurse managers have a wide array of data—including electronic health records, human resource data, and financial data—available to them for use in making decisions (Murphy et al., 2013). Making sense of that data is necessary but often a challenge. Managers in particular can use the data to develop a balanced scorecard that assesses financial, quality, and other operational performance measures. This scorecard should be available to all staff so that organizational performance can improve (Dunham-Taylor & Pincznk, 2015).

Data analytics can be used to develop decision support systems (Nickitas & Mensik, 2015). Decision support systems use critical data to help nurse managers make decisions that affect the short-term and long-term effectiveness of the care-delivery system.

Decision support systems can allow nurse managers to use current data to conduct simulations where staffing, patient acuity, and environmental variables are manipulated in order to detect pitfalls of actions before the action is taken (Frith & Anderson, 2012). It is critical that disparate data sources be integrated if data are to be used effectively through decision support systems (Kontio et al., 2013).

Specific examples of using decision support systems include using data analytics in order to build staffing models that incorporate the full array of contextual variables, including the environment of care, patient and provider variables, and desired quality and safety outcomes (Nickitas & Mensik, 2015). Making shift-by-shift patient assignments for the nursing care team is often a time-intensive activity for the shift charge nurse. However, a data-driven decision support system can be built to lessen the time required to make patient assignments (Van Oostveen et al., 2014).

Six Sigma is a quality and decision support technique that uses data to build process-improvement models. The goal is to eliminate defects in safety and quality in health care delivery (American Society for Quality Improvement, n.d.). Essentially Six Sigma is a variant of the plan-do-study-act (PDSA) cycle promoted by the Institute for Healthcare Improvement (Satyadi, 2013). For example, data may be used to identify strengths and limitations in a patient flow process. In addition to quality and safety data, an interprofessional team may visually depict a patient care delivery process, such as postanesthesia care (Haenke & Stichler, 2015) and emergency room wait times (Molpus, 2013) in order to identify bottlenecks in the processes of patient flow. Thus Six Sigma and lean quality improvement techniques are used for clinical and managerial decision making as well (see Chapter 18).

Data analytics are most useful in assisting in decision-making, and an expanded discussion of the use of data analytics is found in Chapter 26. However, use of data to make decisions can have unintended consequences. Rambur and colleagues (2013) reported on a case study where a patient had an advance directive, but that directive was not honored because the performance measure—30-day mortality rate——would have been negatively affected. As Rambur and colleagues noted, all data must be used for the patient's benefit and not for the sake of the data itself.

LEADERSHIP AND MANAGEMENT IMPLICATIONS

All health care is delivered in complex and sometimes chaotic organizations. Decisions made using a variety of tools and strategies can lead to safer care-delivery environments. However, the rapid pace of decision making may hamper the use of available evidence to assist in that decision making. Furthermore, the time for reflection about clinicians' and managers' actions may hamper development of clinical judgment and managerial decision-making abilities.

Strategies for Decision Making

The focus of leadership and management decision making is more closely related to the nurse's role as care coordinator and systems problem solver. Some decisions, such as those requiring disciplinary action, do require the manager's *direct intervention*. In conflicts between staff members or between family and staff members, the manager might use negotiation and other forms of conflict management that could be viewed as *indirect intervention* because the manager does not

actually decide what should be done to deal with an issue but rather persuades others to solve the problem themselves. The nurse manager might *delegate* the decision making to others. For example, a unit manager might ask a team of staff nurses and the unit secretary to figure out when the best time is to order supplies for the unit.

Sometimes the nurse manager might choose *watchful waiting*. A particular staff member might be causing some interpersonal difficulties. If the staff member has submitted his or her resignation, dealing with the behavior might not be worth the energy.

Most decision making should take place within the confines of *collaboration and consultation*. That collaboration often takes place within an interprofessional context. Patient care requires a team approach between nursing, medicine, and other disciplines such as physical therapy. Working in an interprofessional context is an essential skill for both clinicians and managers (Interprofessional Education Collaborative, 2011).

Shared governance initiatives have shown that collaboration and consultation result in high-quality patient care delivery systems. Therefore a critical role for nurse managers and leaders is *facilitation* by fostering a climate that encourages creativity and interdependence.

Modeling desired decision-making behaviors is also important. For example, in hospitals, nurse leaders and managers can use change-of-shift reports to promote deep clinical reasoning using the Socratic method and asking who, what, when, and where questions such as "What nursing interventions have been effective?" or "What will happen if this course of action is chosen?" Another strategy for promoting clinical reasoning is to create a climate where mistakes can be made and then analyzed without fear of punishment (Kagan & Barnoy, 2013). Fig. 4.3 summarizes global strategies used for decision making that contribute to quality and safe patient care.

Clearly all nurses are on information overload. Ways to capture the available data and use it for effective problem solving and decision making are critical. The use of computerized informatics applications to aid decision making is on the rise. For example, hospital information systems can be used to capture data such as length of stay, skill mix, case mix, patient and employee job satisfaction, and other variables that can be important when decisions need to be made (Westra et al., 2015). Refinements such as smart alerts show promise to ease the complexity and information overload of care delivery and thus reduce errors.

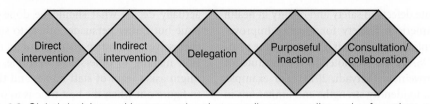

FIG. 4.3 Global decision-making strategies that contribute to quality and safe patient care.

Nurse managers and leaders solve problems in complex systems where all decisions carry some amount of risk (Shirey et al., 2013). Understanding a manager's cognitive workflow has the potential for use in decision support tools (Effken et al., 2011). Cognitive workflow analysis includes work domain, decision-making procedures, personnel skill level, and social organization and collaboration patterns. The complexity of the workflow makes it difficult to operationalize computerized decision support tools that take into account all these factors, however (J. Effken, personal communication, April 14, 2016).

The "good old days," when life was more predictable, less chaotic, and patients routinely stayed 3 to 5 days as inpatients, have disappeared. Coordination of care must begin at the first patient encounter into a system for care. For example, discharge teaching must now begin *before* admission, not after the patient is admitted for surgery. Patients may be at the hospital or surgery center for only 1 to 2 hours after the surgery has ended, thus they are still under the influence of anesthetics or analgesics and cannot comprehend or remember the instructions that were given. Because change is occurring so rapidly, past practices that exhibit any sense of permanence may provide managers with a feeling of security.

Just like complex patient-care scenarios, complex social organizations such as hospitals produce patterns that can be difficult to recognize (Wheatley, 1999) unless one is an expert at decision making. Expert nurse leaders can quickly and intuitively grasp organizational patterns without going through a step-by-step analysis of a situation, yet this skill may take time and experience to develop (Linderman et al., 2015; Shirey et al., 2013).

Inevitably some mistakes will be made, but nurse managers and leaders who view mistakes as learning opportunities help promote effective organizations. Such an attitude fosters the concept of a learning organization (see Chapter 2) where organizations stay vital by learning and growing. Leaders can foster a climate wherein new communication patterns emerge, bottom-up communication changes the organization, and differences in talents, structures, and communication networks come forth and promote high-performance organizations.

CURRENT ISSUES AND TRENDS

Creativity and innovation will be the cornerstone of nurses' participation in the health care system of the future. An IOM report (2011) and the 2015 update (Altman et al., 2015) have noted that nurses should and must take the lead in providing care for patients in a complex, rapidly changing health care system. New roles have emerged, such as the clinical nurse leader, who is a bedside leader and coordinator of complex care. Accountable care organizations (ACOs), which will coordinate primary care for groups of patients, provide many opportunities for nurses to demonstrate the value of their advanced critical-thinking and decision-making skills (Hart, 2012).

The emphasis on quality and safety will be the focus of much of nurse managers' and leaders' planning and resultant decision making. The seminal report *To Err Is Human* (IOM, 1999), pointed out that human error was rampant in the health care system, causing lives lost and increasing health costs. Makary and Daniel (2016) have pointed out that medical errors are the third leading cause of death in the United States. Nurse leaders and managers can foster team decision making in a shared governance environment in order to improve processes of care delivery and mitigate errors. Balanced scorecards will increasingly be a part of the manager's and leader's toolbox (Dunham-Taylor & Pinczk, 2015). Although financial considerations in an organization are important, quality, and safe care that is patient- and family-centered is equally important. The Quality and Safety Education for Nurses (QSEN, 2014) competencies will continue to serve as a guide for clinicians and managers alike as they strive to increase personal and organization performance.

Changing reimbursement patterns as a result of the Patient Protection and Affordable Care Act (2010) and changing reimbursement regulations from the CMS (2015, 2016) will challenge nurse leaders and managers to find creative ways to facilitate the delivery of safe and quality care. More than likely costs will go up, but reimbursements may not keep pace with costs.

Despite the need for creativity, a certain amount of standardization must occur if safe patient care is to occur in complex care environments. This involves evidence-based practice (EBP) using standardized guidelines and evidence-informed decision making (EIDM) (Jansson & Forsberg, 2016). However, many nurse leaders have not fully implemented evidence-based nursing practice in their organizations (Melnyk et al., 2016).

Nurse leaders need to advocate for a preferred future for nursing and evaluate the effectiveness of decision making in practice. Both are aimed at making careful projections about what decisions to make—given uncertainty—to improve organizational and system performance. In times of change, nursing has an opportunity to make decisions that proactively direct the future. Nursing has demonstrated its value to the health care system. Therefore nurse leaders must be a party to all decisions regarding how care is delivered in health care organizations via shared governance arrangements (IOM, 2011).

Many hospitals are applying for Magnet recognition from the American Nurses Credentialing Center (ANCC).

One of the 14 Forces of Magnetism from the old model that is incorporated in the new model of five domains involves management style and another promotes interdisciplinary collaboration. These two elements—a management style that is collaborative and the promotion of interdisciplinary staff input in decision making—are evidence-based "best practices" (ANCC, 2016).

The efficiency, efficacy, and effectiveness of health care decisions will continue to enjoy a strong focus in nursing, with shifts toward outcomes specification. As performance improvement specialists, nurses will be challenged to make decisions that directly affect quality, access, cost, productivity, and the "bottom line." Effective approaches to decision making are needed when care is delivered in a complex system in which multiple stakeholders need to be served, time is constrained, and the amount of information is overwhelming. The decisions that nurse managers and leaders make must be translated from the corporate "lingo" into terms that the clinicians understand if true buy-in is to be achieved (Porter-O'Grady, 2015). Furthermore, all nurses need to have leadership competencies, including the ability to make effective decisions (IOM, 2011). Nurses need to be at the forefront of all decision making in health care, including at the governing board level.

RESEARCH NOTE

Source
Shirey, M.R., Ebright, P.R., & McDaniel, A.M. (2013). Nurse manager cognitive decision-making amid stress and work complexity. *Journal of Nursing Management, 21*, 17–30. doi:10.1111?j.1365-2834.2012.01380.x

Purpose
The aim of this qualitative study is to describe how nurse managers make decisions in a complex and stressful work environment.

Discussion
In this qualitative descriptive study, the authors interviewed 21 nurse managers. The data from their interviews resulted in a cognitive model for decision making. Inputs into the model were:
- Person/resource demands including managerial work experience
- Situation factors including work complexity-ambiguity, overload, uncertainty, interruptions, gaps (presumably gaps in information)
- Environmental resources, which included organizational culture and context

The decision-making processes consisted of: appraisal of threat; cognitive decision making; reflective questions such as who and what; salient factors (similar to the factors in clinical reasoning models) including cues, patterns, tradeoffs, past experiences, data; and further questions such as why and when. The outputs considered how the nurse manager's decisions affect nurse managers, nursing staff, colleagues, patients and families, and organizations.

Application to Practice
Expert managers, like expert clinicians, are more apt to take the context of decision making into their decision-making processes. Novice managers tend to use a step-by-step approach to decision making. Supportive cultures tend to ameliorate the high stress of the decision-making process. In order to support the development of nurse managers' decision-making process, organizations can provide education about the manager role and then help nurse managers balance personal and professional role responsibilities on a day-to-day basis. Just as tired and distracted clinicians are more prone to errors in decision making, so, too, are stressed and distracted nurse managers.

CASE STUDY

Effective decision making relies, in part, on analyzing alternative levels of uncertainty or risk. Staffing and scheduling decisions exemplify this. In addition to making "apples to apples" comparisons through such tools as staffing matrices recommended by professional bodies, daily and monthly patient census data and patient acuity and nursing intensity data can guide unit managers in their analysis, which might precede a request for more staffing. In addition, the nurse manager needs to have an awareness of the environment in which care is delivered in order to make the analysis complete. Fig. 4.4 is an example of a decision tree. A nurse manager from the intensive care unit could use such a decision tree to justify an increase in staffing. The tree has several branches, and, depending on the end point, an increase in needed personnel could be handled in several ways. Diagrams such as decision trees can be invaluable in understanding complicated alternative solutions. These diagrams are useful in assessment and problem definition and in considering the available alternatives for dealing with a problem. Once the alternative is chosen, a plan must be formulated for implementing the approach chosen. The choice implemented must be evaluated. Note, however, that the decision tree in Fig. 4.4 only lists three alternatives. A more complex tree could be constructed that includes more alternatives based on a different combination of tree branches.

New research on knowledge representation has shown that human cognition is more effective through visualization rather than text. Decision trees, fishbone diagrams, problem continuums, and flowcharts are frequently used as visualization tools in problem analysis. To assist in visualization techniques, managers could consider placing a large grease board, dry-erase board, or flip chart in their office to quickly map out various alternatives.

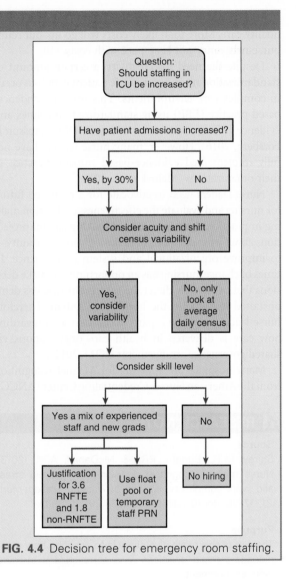

FIG. 4.4 Decision tree for emergency room staffing.

■ CRITICAL THINKING EXERCISE

Alan Field is a nurse who has been working on a surgical floor for about 2 years following his graduation from nursing school. He is caring for a postoperative patient who had posterior neck surgery. The postanesthesia care nurse relayed that the dressing had been changed twice in the past hour due to blood saturation. When Nurse Field went to assess the patient, he found the patient restless and thrashing about. The patient's dressing was again saturated with blood. The patient's dressing had to be changed three more times. Nurse Field notified the physician of his findings and actions. The physician stated bleeding was normal and dressing should be reinforced, not changed. However, during an additional assessment Nurse Field found the patient restless and the patient was soaked with blood from head to the buttocks. Nurse Field tried to calm the patient, but the patient continued to thrash about. Although the surgeon had directed the nurse not to change the dressing, Nurse Field felt he had no choice but to change the dressing. During the dressing change, the nurse had to put pressure on the surgical site in order to stem the bleeding, and he also noticed swelling and hardness at the incision sites. Although the surgeon was not concerned when the first phone call was made, Nurse Field knew in his gut this bleeding was not normal. He continued to put pressure on the incision and asked another nurse to call the physician. The other nurse did so and told the physician that Nurse Field requested that the patient be seen by the physician. Despite his complaints for having to come back to the hospital in the middle of the night, the physician returned and decided to return the patient to surgery. Later Nurse Field heard that the patient recovered in the intensive care unit (ICU), but restlessness continued because the patient had not disclosed his alcohol use and the fact he was on antischizophrenia medication. His restlessness in the ICU after the bleeding had abated was due to withdrawal from alcohol and medication.

Using the SBAR framework identify:
1. What was the situation?
2. What was the background information?
3. What was Nurse Field's assessment?
4. What was Nurse Field's recommendation?

Since Nurse Field did not have the patient's medical history, how could a full history have been obtained before surgery? What specific questions could have been asked to prevent the lack of crucial information needed to care for the patient? As you consider the SBAR scenario, think about how Tanner's (2006) model could assist you in your SBAR communication and decision making, such as by noticing patient cues, interpreting the cues, responding to the cues, and finally reflecting on the outcome of the SBAR process.

5

Managing Time and Stress

Susan R. Lacey, Karen S. Cox, Adrienne Olney

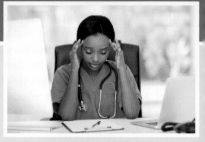

http://evolve.elsevier.com/Huber/leadership

"We find our bootstraps and tug. But we can't come to terms with circumstances whose terms we don't yet know. An uncertain future leaves us stranded in an unhappy present with nothing to do but wait."

Daniel Gilbert, PhD, Professor of Psychology at Harvard University and author of Stumbling on Happiness

Stress can manifest as good stress or negative stress. There are physical, mental, and even professional benefits to *good stress* or *eustress* (Nelson & Simmons, 2004). Good stress provides a feeling of accomplishment, but stressful experiences that are perceived as negative result in a variety of conscious or subconscious responses to regain stability or *homeostasis* (Seyle, 1950). The nature of these responses may be physical, mental, psychological, spiritual, or any combination of these. If these fail, an individual's resources are depleted, which can threaten general well-being.

Stress is not only emotional but also physical. For example, physical insults that stress the body, such as a surgical procedure, serious illness, or traumatic injury, can lead to *stress-induced hyperglycemia* (McCowen et al., 2001). This is caused when blood glucose levels increase as a response to the stressor and need for the body to heal. Fatigue is another physical byproduct of stress. For example, nurses experience high levels of rapid and continuous change. Overwhelming feelings of stress, exhaustion, and burnout are associated with what is called change fatigue (McMillan & Perron, 2013).

Photo used with permission from michaeljung/Getty Images.

The negative consequences of stress for individuals, organizations, society, and the economy are well documented (American Institute of Stress, n.d.). Work-related stress has been called *The 21st Century Black Death* (Lundberg & Cooper, 2011). This phenomenon demands swift and comprehensive action.

Work-related stress affects productivity and effectiveness at work, but it also may negatively affect personal lives and relationships (Rosch, 2001). The converse is also true. Rosabeth Kanter, the leading social scientist in the work–home phenomenon, explained that it is nearly impossible to compartmentalize what happens at work and home so that neither enters the other domain (Kanter, 1977). She called this phenomenon *spillover*.

A recent article in *The Atlantic* provided a window into the impact and consequences of stress in relation to cost and personal health. The effects of stress are estimated to cost $180 billion or 5% to 8% of annual health care expenditures (White, 2015). Stress:

1. Increases the incidence of chronic and costly conditions, such as diabetes, Alzheimer's, and cardiovascular disease
2. Increases addiction and mental health conditions associated with job insecurity, unjust dealings with employees, or poor leadership decisions that influence the work conditions of employees
3. Is linked to over 120,000 deaths per year in the United States from physical and mental health conditions

Governmental and organizational reports about work-related stress most often reference the work of Paul Rosch, MD, FACP, a leader in the field of occupational stress, specifically, his publication "The Quandary of Job Stress Compensation" (Rosch, 2001). Rosch calculated the combined direct and indirect cost of work-related stress to be a staggering $300 billion per year. Although the article is considered dated by scientific standards, it remains the most widely referenced in support of national discourse, research, and large-scale planning in the area of work-related stress.

DEFINITIONS

Stress is defined as a negative emotional experience that is associated with biological changes that trigger the body to make adaptations (Rosenthal, 2002). This means that stress can be a physical, mental, psychological, or spiritual response to a stressor experience that is evaluated by the individual as taxing or exceeding resources and threatening to one's sense of well-being. It was originally conceptualized as a syndrome having a variety of induced changes, including measurable physiological components, such as an increase in heart rate or a rise in blood sugar levels, as well as emotional ones. Chronic stress can lead to acute and chronic health problems. **Job stress** is a tension that arises related to the person-in-environment demands of a person's role or job. Job stress, or "disquieting influences," can accumulate into levels that are too high, reach the point of burnout, and manifest as emotional and/or physical exhaustion and lowered job productivity. Levels of job stress that are either too low or too high decrease individual productivity.

Time management is a deliberative process of identifying and focusing on the activities needed to accomplish tasks and goals. Individuals cannot control time itself; therefore they need to learn to manage the available time more efficiently and effectively. This may be difficult, especially when comfortable habits need to be changed, but time management is a major strategy for managing stress. **Time management** is defined as the accomplishment of specified activities during the time available. It is the process of managing the things an individual does with his or her available time. At its core, time management is self-management.

THE RELATIONSHIP BETWEEN TIME AND STRESS

Situational stress and the need to respond in a timely manner is true for most types of work, and particularly in health care. Clinicians and leaders anticipate and even prepare for stressful situations. Time-sensitive care and decision making may produce mild to severe stress. As if time-sensitivity for single events were not stressful enough, it is typically compounded by multiple stressful events that occur at or near the same time. For example, there are specific times designated for medication administration, tests, and procedures. If a clinician fails to complete the treatments or therapies within a defined window of time, a cascade of events may follow, from submitting an incident or variance report to patient harm. In life-threatening emergencies, response time is even more critical. Ineffective or inaccurate interventions may result in lasting consequences for patients— or even death.

Time management involves a deliberative process of identifying, focusing, and completing activities needed to accomplish specific tasks and achieve goals (Claessens et al., 2007). Since it is impossible to control time, individuals must manage the time they have in the most efficient and effective way. The time an individual has to complete all regular and unexpected responsibilities may vary depending on the type of position held. Nonetheless, the delivery of health care exists in an environment where time is finite. Box 5.1 displays strategies that can be used for time management at work.

Nurses work shifts of time, such as 8- or 12-hour shifts. If time (a shift) is finite, the nurse must make

---

BOX 5.1 Strategies for Time Management

- Block time for daily rounds for both patients, families, and staff; some days will have longer blocks of time.
- Schedule blocks of time to tackle e-mail. Consider this for the end of your day, not the beginning.
- Prioritize e-mails to address people first—staff issues, patients, and family issues.
- Schedule blocks of time for an "open" door to your office; invite staff to visit.
- Post your daily schedule on your office door with beeper number and/or cell.
- Take note cards to meetings where only listening is required; write personal notes to recognize staff for their contributions and recognize birthdays.
- Schedule periodic "lunch with the manager" sessions for both night and day shifts.
- Set realistic follow-up deadlines for staff issues, questions, and concerns.

fairly accurate estimates of the amount of time each patient encounter will consume during that shift based on what needs to be done during that encounter. During real or anticipated budgetary constraints, many organizations seek to reduce labor costs. Because labor expenditures are greatest within nursing, reducing the number of staff nurses on a unit is one strategy to improve the bottom line. However, there is also a need to increase reimbursement for good clinical outcomes and positive patient experiences, and this requires the presence of adequate numbers of nurses to deliver needed care.

The Centers for Medicare and Medicaid Services (CMS), the nation's largest payer, bases 30% of reimbursement on the patient experience and 70% on clinical outcomes (CMS, 2014). If the number of nurses is reduced on a given unit or shift, good outcomes may be compromised, and therefore reimbursement may be compromised. For instance, if normal nurse-to-patient ratios are modified from 1:5 to 1:7 without additional unlicensed assistive support, the time spent on patient encounters will naturally have to be decreased and the availability of nurses will be diminished. Chronic cycles of suboptimal staffing create stress and fatigue.

Evidence has linked higher nurse-to-patient ratios with poorer clinical outcomes (Aiken et al., 2002). Many believe current staffing models are incongruent with professional practice standards, patient needs, and the organization's ability to maximize reimbursement. This perpetual grind makes it difficult for staff nurses to feel good about nursing or encourage others to join the profession. Many nurses have buyer's remorse for choosing nursing as their career, even more so compared with nurse practitioners and physicians (Peckham, 2015).

Leadership decisions are also time sensitive. Adequately staffing units, responding to a community health crisis, deploying rapid-cycle improvement initiatives when benchmarks fall, and addressing unanticipated budget shortfalls are but a few of the challenges requiring a rapid response. When unexpected conditions are added to regular responsibilities, nurses may experience what experts call *Complexity Compression,* which has been linked to burnout, turnover, and other types of work-related stress (Krichbaum et al., 2007). Nurses experience this when they must manage unplanned (complexity) and regular responsibilities simultaneously (compression). A prime example is the issue of constant interruptions in the environment of care or high "churn" of admissions and discharges, which are not factored into tight workloads.

MORAL DISTRESS

Beyond complexity compression and its consequences is what has been described as moral distress. Moral distress can be defined as a psychological, emotional, and physiological experience of suffering that occurs when a person acts in ways that are inconsistent with deeply held ethical values, principles, or moral commitments. It is seen as a two-stage process of initial and reactive moral distress experiences (Sasso et al., 2016). This is a common problem for health care professionals, especially nurses. It is linked to issues related to patient care, including ethical dilemmas that can put professionals in difficulty and give rise to feelings of unease. Organizational constraints or the perception that professional values and health care standards are being compromised may trigger moral distress (Sasso et al., 2016).

Moral distress occurs when an individual knows what ethical action should occur but is prevented from doing so by either internal or external barriers (Rushton, 2006). Internal obstacles include personal characteristics such as fear or lack of confidence. External obstacles include a lack of resources, structures, or processes that prevent taking the desired and right action (McCarthy & Deady, 2008). A nurse may be prevented from acting by organizational constraints, lack of time, lack of management support or power, policies, regulations, or legal considerations. A remedy may lie in the type of education and training that nurses receive about how to analyze and solve ethical dilemmas at work. Nurses can be assisted in building competencies in a range of moral competencies that moral agents have, such as moral sensitivity, moral imagination, moral responsiveness, moral comportment, moral virtues, principled compassion, moral courage, moral knowledge, and moral empathy and resilience (McCarthy & Gastmans, 2015).

Those who work in health care have a fundamental need to establish therapeutic patient and family relationships. The unpredictable nature of health care work, combined with complex and shortening encounters, can create the potential for ethical dilemmas and moral distress beyond expectations for individuals who choose a career in health care. Unrelenting ethical and moral conflicts can lead to high levels of stress. The response may include cognitive dissonance, acute physiological changes, and chronic physical or mental health issues (American Psychological Association, 2013).

RESILIENCE

Countering the negative aspects of workplace stress is the concept of resilience. **Resilience** is defined as an ability to bounce back. Resilient people exhibit personal characteristics of an internal locus of control, prosocial behavior, empathy, positive self-image, a sense of optimism, and an ability to organize daily responsibilities (Pines et al., 2012). Empowered people are thought to be more resilient, and for nurses there is an association between stress resiliency and psychological empowerment. Because the behavioral skills needed to manage interpersonal conflict and its feelings of powerlessness and psychological distress can be taught, nurses can learn to resist stressors, manage conflict, and boost resilience (Pines et al., 2012).

LEADERSHIP AND MANAGEMENT IMPLICATIONS

Creating an Environment to Prevent and Address Work-Related Stress

To prevent and address work-related stress, creation and innovation are needed. A **creation** is something new that did not previously exist in that form and occurs in a multitude of fields, not just the arts (Creation, n.d.). Experts who study creativity may differ on the requisite attributes of creative individuals and exact steps in the creative process. However, most agree that *intention* is the critical first step (Ditkoff, 2010). Without intention, no action is ever taken.

Innovation and innovators in the health care industry are highly sought after. But to innovate is to alter, change, or transform something that exists in a stable system (Marshall, 2013). On the other hand, creativity is less frequently discussed in the industry, and in some cases, is maligned. For example the term *creative accounting* is used to describe illegal or unethical activities and does not convey the positive aspect of creativity, which is to produce something needed or valued. Industry leaders prefer to predict the future based on the past and innovate within the current system as opposed to envisioning the future based on what is desired and creating it (Scott, 2003). The former is thought to use hard data, and the latter, subjective or unknown information, inspiration, and feelings. Creativity does not require one to suspend all intellect. Indeed, creative individuals use all of the senses, as well as abstract and concrete thought. Without concrete and abstract thought, it would have been impossible for Salvador Dalí to have painted *The Persistence of Memory* or for British scientist Sir Tim Berners-Lee to have written code for the first web browser, which became the genesis of the world wide web (World Wide Web Foundation, 2015).

Getting Started

It is challenging to envision creating a health care organization focused not only on addressing work-related stress when it occurs but also on having structures and processes in place to prevent them from happening in the first place. This is particularly hard while in the midst of persistent demands from payers, consumers, regulators, and even the overarching uncertainty of the Affordable Care Act of 2010 (ACA) mandates. It has always been challenging to secure the necessary resources for prevention, even for patient care. However, failure to do so puts employees at risk, which in turn can jeopardize the lives of patients. It is no longer possible to wait for more evidence about the human and financial costs of work-related stress. Waiting for more stability in the industry, which may never come, wastes precious time. Once that is embraced and there is genuine intention, then design and creation can begin in earnest. This intention and corresponding action will call for bold leaders who reject reactionary quick fixes. Based on the evidence this can lead to the interconnected outcomes of employees with greater resilience and performance, improved patient outcomes, and measurable and sustained financial benefits.

Strategies

Stress management. Stress management is important for nurses as they cope with stress at work. This is also true for nursing students and new nurses. Among the many stressors are needing to meet professional and academic demands, fear of failure, the workload of taking care of patients, and insecurity about clinical competence or lack of knowledge. Stress and anxiety are often high during times of education and training when the nurse or student is developing clinical skills. Two low-cost and easily implemented stress-management techniques are mindful meditation and biofeedback. Both were found to decrease anxiety, and mindfulness also significantly lowered stress levels in nursing students (Nowrouzi et al., 2015; Ratanasiripong et al., 2015).

Workplace intervention strategies for stress can be either individual-level stress management and burn-out interventions or organizational-level workplace health-promotion programs. For the individual nurse, mindfulness-based stress reduction has evidence of effectiveness; for mental health, psychosocial interventions decrease burnout (Nowrouzi et al., 2015). The Research Note and Box 5.2 also provide some guidance on stress management.

Organization-directed prevention measures can be directed to management style, incentives and career structures, educational opportunities, salaries, and recruitment and retention practices (Nowrouzi et al., 2015). Research on conflict management styles found that nurses who worked in supportive work environments and who avoided conflict (avoidant style of managing conflict) experienced less work stress (Johansen & Cadmus, 2016). In addition, conflict and communicative stress feed off each other in a cycle that contributes to destructive working conditions. Nurses manage conflict and stress through respectful and caring communication and mismanage it through disrespectful communication. Building relationships can be fostered in organizations by formal and informal social gatherings, mentoring, social

media, and deliberate culture creation (Moreland & Apker, 2016). Perceived supportive work environments are characterized by perceptions that supervisors are supportive, there is fairness, and there is open communication. Stress is reduced when nurses feel that win–win solutions occur in the work environment (Johansen & Cadmus, 2016).

One example is the implementation of new nurse residency programs. In response to the stress and anxiety ("transition shock") that new nurses feel in the transition from nursing education to nursing practice, organizations are instituting nurse residency programs. They may be up to a year long. New nurses are mentored and guided during this residency in order to support their coping, reduce their stress, and augment their time-management capabilities. This is a major recruitment and retention strategy. In addition, it is a visible component of a supportive work environment (Rosenfeld & Glassman, 2016; Rush et al., 2013).

Informal nurse leaders can employ a combination of person-directed stress management techniques (for themselves) and organization-directed stress management techniques (for the sake of the work group). Clearly, a supportive work environment is critical, so any interventions that improve nurses' perceptions of the work environment are helpful. Role modeling and setting a tone of respectful and caring communication aids conflict resolution and stress reduction. Informal leaders can take the initiative to address workplace issues in a proactive and evidence-based manner so that nurses see that their issues are being evaluated fully and fairly for problem resolution.

Wellness programs in the larger context. There are a variety of strategies that individuals and organizations need to employ to prevent and address work-related stress. There is no shortage of research, workshops, websites, and blogs about how to reduce stress. Although sources may emphasize the benefits of one strategy over another, most include similar recommendations. Using these strategies can serve as the inspiration for creating this new, vital environment. Instead of employees trying to find their own way through the maze of strategies, the newly created health care environment would provide on-site (or reimbursement for) work-related stress prevention workshops and retreats. Just as the traditional employee health staff conduct new and ongoing physical health screening for risky behaviors such as smoking or substance use, additional screening for resiliency,

---

BOX 5.2   Personal Strategies to Decrease Stress at the Workplace

- Learn chair exercises and complete them while catching up on e-mails or talking on the phone.
- When possible, take the stairs to reenergize yourself.
- Get a de-stress buddy at work and contact him or her when you need to vent—this is someone you completely trust and ideally someone outside of your unit.
- Have a "getaway" place at work where you can spend a few minutes in silence and thought.
- Get off the unit for at least your lunch break. Do not eat at your desk.
- Schedule lunches with other people outside your unit. This commitment ensures your escape and has the added bonus of putting yourself with another person not associated with your own unit.
- Schedule "think time" appointments at least once a week for a block of time; get out of your office for these times.
- Have a fruit bowl instead of chocolate or candy on your desk
- Bring a water bottle to work and refill as needed to keep hydrated.

coping strategies, and support networks needs to be a part of the work structure. Once screened and a profile developed, the employee can use the information to select from wellness options beyond smoking cessation, hypertension, and diabetes management programs in consultation with a wellness professional.

It is common practice to compensate employees who take advantage of preventive health care services. There are some organizations that pay for alternative health care, such as gym memberships, massage, and acupuncture, but that is not the norm. Given the costs of work-related stress, the health care environment of the future will provide full or partial compensation for a much wider array of prevention services that fit the needs of the individual employee. As personalized medicine forges a pathway to realize the potential of matching therapies to an individual's DNA for disease states, wellness offerings should match the employee's needs for work–life balance and prevention of work-related stress. Examples of wellness initiatives and programs might be offered in multiple formats, but could include self-care, setting boundaries, relaxation, and journaling.

Self-care. One of the most important strategies to mitigate individual stress is self-care. Though everyone needs to spend time on themselves, clinicians often put the needs of others ahead of their own. It is difficult to effectively care for patients and their families or be productive at work if clinicians and leaders do not care for themselves. Self-care is unique to each person, but the following are generally accepted as important self-care activities (Fisher & Keenan, 2010): taking personal time each day, getting enough sleep (7–8 hours), nutritious intake and adequate hydration, some form of exercise, and a strong support network, which includes friends, family, and counseling, if necessary. Box 5.2 displays personal strategies for decreasing stress at the workplace.

Setting boundaries. Setting boundaries is one way of engaging in self-care (Gionta, 2009). Family members and even friends faced with a health care question, concern, or crisis call on nurses and other clinicians to provide advice, and in some cases, direct care. In an effort to respond and be helpful, clinicians may overextend themselves, sacrificing their own needs or those of their direct family members. In some ways, it is flattering. It validates one's knowledge, skills, and expertise. However, when requests exceed a person's capabilities, it is reasonable to refer them to other experts and services.

Boundaries need not be exceedingly rigid and may change over time. For instance, someone who does not have a husband, wife, partner, or children may seem to have the capacity to take on extra work and may need to set more boundaries than those who have these commitments to others. Clearly, boundaries should be set based on individual needs, not gender, stereotypes, or even where someone is on the lifespan. The most important thing is that setting them should not induce more stress on the individual than not having them at all.

Relaxation. Finding ways to relax can also help one avoid and reduce stress. Because stress can produce both emotional and physical responses, it is important to learn to relax the body and mind, even for short periods. There are numerous relaxation techniques and even apps to download to help a person relax. It is not necessary to devote long periods or find a special environment to achieve a state of relaxation. One can relax anywhere and for any amount of time (Seaward, 2013). By calming the mind, physiological responses to stress are also reversed, which allows the individual to think more clearly.

Journaling. Keeping a diary or journal was a part of many individuals' lives when they were younger, but most do not continue the practice into adulthood. There are many benefits in keeping a journal. For those who recognize they are experiencing stress but are not fully cognizant of the specific triggers, experts suggest keeping a journal to identify situations that cause stress, the response or action to the stressor, and whether these actions lowered their stress or not (Ullrich & Lutgendorf, 2002).

The work of clinicians and leaders in health care is time sensitive, and time management is, for all intents and purposes, personal management. Journaling about situations that challenge personal time management will provide clarity. This clarity may shed light on learned behaviors that may be sabotaging one's quest for effective time management. Saunders (2013), an international expert and coach in the area of time management, outlined and described secrets to effective time investment. They are priorities, expectations, and routines. Fully understanding these three things can unlock the potential to manage even the most chaotic situation, regardless of the context, at work or home.

Organizational Recommendations

Clearly, organizations are experiencing financial pressures, which makes adding the necessary work required

BOX 5.3 **Institutional Strategies to Decrease Stress at the Workplace**

- Assess stress levels and stress-management strategies of employees.
- Institute the AACN Standards for Establishing and Sustaining Healthy Work Environments.
- Ensure that management and leadership education includes vital behaviors and competencies.
- Structure evaluations of managers, directors, supervisors, and senior-level management with leadership and management behaviors that provide stress-management strategies.
- Ensure transparency of information and set effective communication patterns.
- Implement a top-down approach to sharing and owning quality improvement and outcomes.

to create a new environment that prevents and addresses work-related stress a challenge. However, either way, employees will experience work-related stress, which will negatively affect the organization in one way or another. Therefore it is a matter of which approach (proactive or reactive) an organization wants to take: up front with prevention and early intervention or after the fact with employee loss of productivity, increased sick days, and/or turnover. If an organization chooses the proactive approach, beginning the work to create this environment does not seem as daunting and is a prudent business decision. Box 5.3 displays a list of institutional strategies to decrease stress in the workplace. They are not an exhaustive list, nor are they intended to be prescriptive. Instead they are meant to generate discussions while this new environment is planned.

Related evidence-based management strategies to address work-related stress include healthy work environment standards and empowerment strategies.

Healthy work environments standards. A healthy work environment (HWE) is one that is safe, empowering, and satisfying. HWE standards are further discussed in Chapter 3. The American Association of Critical-Care Nurses (AACN) has established six standards that support healthy work environments (AACN, 2005). Although developed for nurses, they are applicable for all types of employees. These standards and supporting statements are displayed in Table 5.1.

Empowerment. Employees who are empowered in their jobs are also more engaged and satisfied. Research indicates that structural empowerment leads to higher productivity and satisfaction for the employee, which translates to more satisfied customers. Customer satisfaction stems from the empowered employee's ability to correct a problem at the time it occurs. This leads to better fiscal health for the organization in both direct and indirect labor and benefit costs (Woods, 2005). Empowerment for nurses is manifested in shared governance structures where nurses are engaged and participate in solving clinical practice issues. Shared governance structures are a hallmark of the Magnet Recognition Program®. There is a growing body of evidence that links Magnet hospitals to better clinical and patient level outcomes, as well as to better nursing outcomes (e.g., lower turnover and higher satisfaction), compared with non-Magnet hospitals (Aiken et al., 2008). Improved clinical and organizational outcomes translate to improved financial health.

Clinicians are also empowered by gaining new knowledge and skills beyond required clinical competence. In

TABLE 5.1 **AACN Standards for Establishing and Sustaining Healthy Work Environments**

Standard	Statement
Skilled Communication	Nurses must be as proficient in communication skills as they are in clinical skills.
True Collaboration	Nurses must be relentless in pursuing and fostering true collaboration.
Effective Decision Making	Nurses must be valued and committed partners in making policy, directing and evaluating clinical care, and leading organizational operations.
Appropriate Staffing	Staffing must ensure the effective match between patient needs and nurse competencies.
Meaningful Recognition	Nurses must be recognized and must recognize others for the value each brings to the work of the organization.
Authentic Leadership	Nurse leaders must fully embrace the imperative of a healthy work environment, authentically live it, and engage others in its achievement.

addition, if these new skills also allow them to be a part of developing solutions to clinical and organizational problems, this can lead to even greater engagement and satisfaction. For example, the Clinical Scene Investigator Academy is currently administered by AACN (Lacey et al., 2012). The program teaches staff nurse teams skills in advanced leadership, quality improvement methods, project management, accurate data management, and how to translate nursing care into fiscal terms. To date, the national program has significantly improved nurse-sensitive outcomes, such as pressure ulcers, catheter-associated infections, ventilator-associated pneumonia, and patient satisfaction. In addition, in the first 3 years of the program the improvement projects (N = 42) had an aggregate fiscal impact on the organizations of over $29 million (Lacey et al., 2016). In recognition of the sustained, programmatic impact, the two nurse scientists who developed the original program were named Edge Runners by the American Academy of Nursing in 2015.

Special Considerations for Nurse Managers

With any unit or department, workflow modifications creep into the manager's routines, creating chaos in a well-planned day. The unit manager has one of the most difficult jobs in meeting the challenges of managing and leading employees, as well as meeting priorities that flow from higher management. The challenge of meeting the expectations of the multiple roles of the nurse manager can produce stress that reveals itself as role strain, which is an unpleasant feeling of frustration and an intense labile emotional state (Richmond et al., 2009). This may lead to communication breakdowns, the sense of failing, and intense anxiety about job performance.

There is a scarcity of evidence about how stress affects the nurse manager role. However, Shirey and colleagues (2010) have provided a rich source of qualitative evidence about sources and factors related to stress, outcomes of this stress, and coping strategies used to decrease stress. In the study, nurse manager participants reported key sources of stress to include dealing with people—specifically related to people with negative attitudes or employees with subpar work performance; patient and family complaints; physician interactions; and working within the political nature of the hospital with a lack of transparency and collaboration. Staffing was noted as the most stressful part of their role. High stress is experienced by nurse managers and stems from the challenges of a multifaceted job with myriad sources

of stress (Kath et al., 2012). Although there is a relationship between job satisfaction and intent to quit, when stress is high for nurse managers, other factors show strong relationships with stress (Kath et al., 2012). Having support from others (e.g., supervisors, comanagers, and coworkers) is a factor that decreases stress (Kath et al., 2012; Shirey et al., 2010). The amount of autonomy and predictability in the job mitigates the negative effects of stress as well (Kath et al., 2012).

There is nothing stopping us from creating this new environment that addresses work-related stress, except for the limits (real and imagined) placed on ourselves and organizations. It takes leadership and vision to see the business case for being proactive. Some of the most brilliant minds work in health care. Together nurses can build a preferred future state that results in managed stress and promotion of healthy work environments where all employees flourish.

CURRENT ISSUES AND TRENDS

Health care delivery environments are characterized by chaos, complexity, high risk, and high stress. This is not likely to change. Clinicians and leaders function in environments with increasing unknowns while trying to take appropriate daily actions as well as predict and plan for the future. This is a highly stressful situation. Individuals respond to unknowns in a fairly predictable pattern, which happens rapidly and primarily in one's subconscious. The process includes mentally triaging proven strategies used in similar situations, selecting and modifying the strategy, and evaluating the strategy in real time or as needed.

There is long-standing evidence that fear of the unknown is a normal part of human nature. (Öhman, 2000). It is also known that fear is linked to the feeling of danger. A recently published study found that subjects presented with *certain danger* had significantly lower stress than subjects presented with *potential danger* (de Berker et al., 2016). In this study one group of participants, the *certain danger group,* was told when they picked up a rock a snake would be under it. The other group, *the potential danger group,* was told a snake may or may not be there. The researchers concluded that when participants knew something would occur ahead of time, they were able to mentally and physically prepare. In addition, physiological responses such as heart rate and breathing were significantly higher for participants in the potential danger group than those in the certain danger group.

Scientists in the field of psychology have studied a person's ability to predict or envision the future in normal and uncertain times. Noted psychologist Daniel Gilbert (2007) outlined his thesis in *Stumbling on Happiness,* using scientific evidence coupled with analogies and real-world examples. What he and other social scientists found is that the need to control and predict the future is central to the human condition. It is part of what distinguishes us from other species. In addition, he offers compelling evidence that even those with a great deal of experience, expertise, and cultural wisdom find it difficult to accurately predict the future and make good choices when presented with new and uncertain situations. Specifically, prior experiences coupled with current realities do little to help accurately predict or envision the future, especially when the stakes are high. He extends the logic with additional evidence that in a person's struggle to gain control, make better predictions, and thus make effective plans and choices, individuals fill in details of missing information even if these details are inaccurate. As the brain is *filling in* inaccurate details from memories, perceptions, and emotions, it allows people to reweave the narrative to one they believe or want to be true.

The research supporting Gilbert's logic is applicable to the current health care industry. Clinicians and leaders make efforts to predict the future and make decisions based on their predictions. Unfortunately, just as Gilbert's work has proven, historical evidence supports the reweaving of narratives and undesirable outcomes. Organizations introduce new initiatives or cut services in response to *expert* predictions, only to realize when the future becomes the present, it looks nothing like the prediction, rendering the initiatives and related expenditures relatively useless.

An example of significant scale occurred in the 1980s. In response to payer demands, specifically the introduction of diagnosis-related groups (DRGs), reimbursements declined significantly (Fetter et al., 1980). Hospital leaders and external experts predicted vastly reduced margins, and experts recommended reducing expenditures as the best way to address the negative financial impact of DRGs. On face value, that was prudent and a common business practice given the anticipated loss of revenue. They recommended consolidating organizations, reducing or eliminating services, and closing facilities, primarily within a defined geographical region. Nurse layoffs occurred. These recommendations led to a frenzy of mergers, acquisitions, and closings (Federal Antitrust Policy in the Health Care Marketplace, 1997). Some mergers created complicated partnerships. Many were ill conceived with little or no input from staff, referring physicians, or the communities served. Faith-based and secular hospitals merged, buildings were shuttered, and hybrid names and slogans emerged. Stark philosophical differences, disruption or elimination of services, and disgruntled staff and physicians made sustaining such mergers difficult. To make matters worse, loyal consumers of one hospital or another felt betrayed. It did not take long for many of these hospitals and systems to unmerge, costing even more money, all because experts inaccurately predicted the long-term consequences of this strategy. Some mergers did survive, but rebuilding trust with providers and consumers took many years.

The current example is the odyssey surrounding the fate of the ACA, which has added formidable uncertainties not only for clinicians, leaders, organizations, and systems, but also for the industry's key drivers: payers, consumers, and regulators. The ACA passed along party lines and was signed into law on March 23, 2010 (US Department of Health and Human Services, 2014). Legal challenges were swift and aggressive. The Supreme Court upheld the constitutionality of the law, specifically the individual mandate, on June 28, 2012, after hearing arguments in the *National Federation of Independent Business v. Sebelius* case (Barnes, 2015). Nevertheless, challenges continue. These continued challenges create speculation regarding how decisions about the ACA will influence current external health care drivers and compound stress in the environment.

Even with the compelling evidence that we lack the ability to accurately predict the future, there is no evidence suggesting we cannot *create* our desired future. In fact, this advice is often suggested to nurses.

Predictions and Risk

A prediction is a statement (or thought) about a future event based on past experiences and knowledge (Prediction, n.d.). Everyone makes predictions or forecasts about the future many times a day, most of which are made subconsciously. Some predictions involve low risk. Thus an inaccurate prediction may cause a temporary inconvenience, but not stress. For example, a person driving to work who failed to listen to the current traffic report takes the regular route but is soon stuck for an hour behind an overturned vehicle.

Nurses make predictions in clinical practice based on assessment and clinical judgment. For example, a nurse may predict that following a standardized protocol will result in desired outcomes such as avoidance of catheter-associated urinary tract infections. If the protocol is evidence based, then prediction is low risk.

Other predictions would be considered high risk. If high-risk predictions are inaccurate, the consequences may cause intense stress, anxiety, depression, and even financial loss. Examples of personal situations that require high-risk predictions include choosing or leaving a job, selecting a partner, and buying or selling a large amount of company stock. Nurses are often faced with high-risk predictions in practice, and this is a source of work stress. For example, unstable patients, code

situations, or rapid decompensation may result in the need for instant reactions and/or high-risk predictions about treatment.

One additional important aspect of making predictions is that predictions may affect others in positive or negative ways. When clinicians and leaders in health care initiate actions based on predictions, the actions often affect others in small and large ways. Clinicians make predictions every day based on tacit and empirical knowledge. Most would prefer using the term *prognosis*, not prediction, but they are similar. For example, a nurse predicts that if the patient has difficulty swallowing when provided a sip of water, he may have difficulty eating solid food, and recommendations and actions occur based on this prediction. Likewise, when leaders make predictions and take subsequent actions about real or anticipated changes in demand from key drivers (e.g., payers, consumers, regulations, and the fate of the ACA), many people may be positive or negatively affected.

RESEARCH NOTE

Source
Hoolahan, S.E., Greenhouse, P.K., Hoffmann, R.L., & Lehman, L.A. (2012). Energy capacity model for nurses: The impact of relaxation and restoration. *The Journal of Nursing Administration, 42*(2), 103–109.

Purpose
This study examined the effect of stress management techniques, in particular a restoration room on the unit, on nurses' levels of stress. The investigators also assessed whether the restoration room had an effect on unplanned absences and nursing turnover.

Discussion
A restoration room was created on the study unit, and health coaches taught a 6-week stress-reduction workshop. On average the nurses used the restoration room five times during the study period. Stress levels were

measured using the Nursing Stress Scale both before and after the intervention. This scale showed an overall reduction in stress, but it was not statistically significant. Because of attrition by study participants, not enough nurses completed the study to adequately measure reductions in unplanned time off or turnover. However, anecdotally, the nurses appreciated the restoration room and continued to use it after the study period ended.

Application to Practice
This study considered the importance of stress reduction on a nursing unit. Although the sample size was not large enough to detect statistically significant differences, it did support the idea that a restoration room and a stress-management program were useful in helping nurses to manage their stress. It is important that staff nurses find ways to deal with their daily stress on the unit.

CASE STUDY

Nurse Maria Vasquez is thrilled with the results of creating a new unit council and implementing AACN's Healthy Work Environment (HWE) Standards. A year ago, when she became manager of an inpatient unit, she felt as though everything was crashing in on her. The unit was struggling with many issues, including poor patient outcomes, decreased morale, stressed staff nurses, and a high nurse turnover rate. Nurse Vasquez knew that changes had to be made on the unit, so she decided to establish a unit council to address some of the practice issues.

Continued

CASE STUDY—cont'd

The new unit council and Nurse Vasquez decided to use AACN's HWE Standards. The first standard they wanted to tackle was skilled communication. They first created several workshops to teach this skill and were very pleased with the response. All staff, including physicians and respiratory therapists, attended. Follow-up workshops were then scheduled to be completed every year.

The unit council decided to track whether the workshops had any effect on the nurses' stress and burnout, so they decided to use the Nursing Stress Scale (NSS) to measure the stress levels of the unit nurses both before and after the workshop.

Nurse Vasquez was very pleased to see that not only did patient outcomes improve on the unit, but nurses' stress scores on the NSS significantly improved as well. She was also happy to find that turnover on the unit had also decreased.

CRITICAL THINKING EXERCISE

Nurse Whitney Gould was initially very excited about her new job as nurse manager of a 50-bed regional intensive care nursery. She has experience in both leadership and management, but she is not a clinical expert in this area. The director she reports to *is* an expert in the field, as was the nurse manager of this unit for many years before Nurse Gould. The staff nurses are skeptical about Nurse Gould not having specific practical experience, but do realize her leadership skills are refreshing. However, they continue to go to the director for practice issues.

Nurse Gould has established a unit council as well as "lunch with the manager" sessions for both the day and night shifts. She hopes this will give the staff opportunities to voice their issues, concerns, and vision for the unit.

However, the director and Nurse Gould have significant differences about a leadership versus management focus on the unit. The director wants management tasks completed, whereas Nurse Gould believes that the unit needs a strong focus on leadership, role modeling, coaching, and mentoring in order to empower the nurses to own their own practice.

The director constantly pressures Nurse Gould about being behind on e-mails, human resources issues, and budget variances. Recently, meetings have been held with the director regarding education issues on the unit, but Nurse Gould has not been invited. Nurse Gould experiences a rising stress level.

1. What problem(s) do you see for Nurse Gould in this scenario?
2. Why is it a problem?
3. What sources of stress are present?
4. How might Nurse Gould's stress affect the stress of the nurses on the unit?
5. What should Nurse Gould do first?
6. What factors should Nurse Gould assess and analyze?
7. What strategies could be employed to help control stress and enhance coping?

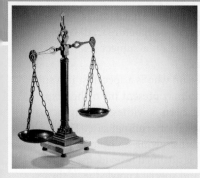

Legal and Ethical Issues

Lynn S. Muller

> *"Law is a framework of authority directed by ethics."*
> **L.S. Muller © 2011**

It takes a special person to consider a career in nursing. Not only is a nurse smart and technically savvy, but there is an essence of caring that simply cannot be taught. Because nursing is known as the profession of caring, society grants nursing autonomy or control over its own practice. The American Nurses Association's (ANA) *Nursing's Social Policy Statement: The Essence of the Profession* (2010, p. 25) indicates "competence is foundational to autonomy," with the profession ensuring nursing competence through professional regulation of nursing practice via standards and ethical codes of practice, legal regulation of nursing practice via state licensure requirements and law pertaining to criminal and civil wrongdoing, and self-regulation in which all nurses retain personal accountability for their own practice (Cooper, 2014).

The practice of nursing is constrained by both legal and ethical boundaries. Law and ethics are two sides of the same coin. Whether a legal mandate or an ethical obligation, the results are the same. Unlike scientific facts, with black and white boundaries, the law provides guidance, mandates, and parameters for lawful practice, and the facts are ever changing. For example, when nurses see a blood culture result, the result can be placed on a finite

range of acceptable norms. However, when examining legal requirements, there may be shades of gray.

No one can practice as a nurse without meeting the legal requirements of the state(s) of licensure. When embarking on a nursing career—or if the nurse has been licensed for some number of years—it is critical that the state board of nursing websites be checked regularly for practice alerts and new laws, as well as legal and regulatory changes for all state(s) in which the nurse practices. A complete list of all state boards of nursing can be found at *https://www.ncsbn.org/contact-bon.htm* through the National Council of State Boards of Nursing (NCSBN, 2016a). Although foundational nursing theory is time honored, it is critical in today's fast-moving digital world that nurses take responsibility for their own knowledge and stay current. The nursing license is a privilege, not a right, which the nurse is given by meeting the licensing requirements throughout his or her career.

Some laws are designed to protect the nurse, and other laws are there to protect the public from errors or wrong practices done by the nurse. As health professionals, nurses have a duty to perform their practice consistent with all relevant laws, scopes of practice, standards of practice, and codes of ethics consistent with the nurse's education and experience. The concept of title protection, which pertains to who can call themselves "nurse," is designed to provide the public with safe, effective nurses who can be relied on to practice to the current standard of care. By establishing minimum mandatory standards, complemented by specialty certifications and mandatory

---

Photo used with permission from Photos.com.

Disclaimer: The information contained in this chapter is for educational purposes only. It is not legal advice, which can be given only by an attorney admitted to practice in the jurisdiction/state(s) in which you practice.

continuing education, the public can depend on nurses regardless of location or facility where practice occurs. It is imperative that nurses acquire and maintain nursing practice skills and competencies. Patient outcomes rely on competent professional practice.

DEFINITIONS

Legal and ethical concepts contain a variety of specific terms requiring definition.

Legal Terms

Cross-examination: The opportunity for the attorney to ask questions in court of a witness who has testified in a trial on behalf of the opposing party. The questions on cross-examination are limited to the subjects covered in the direct examination of the witness, but it is important to note that the attorney may ask leading questions, in which he or she is allowed to suggest answers or put words in the witness's mouth (Hill & Hill, 2016). These questions are usually answered with "yes" or "no."

Damages: The amount of money that a plaintiff (the person suing) may be awarded in a lawsuit. There are many types of damages. Special damages are those that were actually caused by the injury and include medical and hospital bills, ambulance charges, loss of wages, property repair or replacement costs, or loss of money due on a contract. The second basic area of damages is general damages, which are presumed to be a result of the other party's actions but are subjective both in nature and determination of the value of the damages. These include pain and suffering, future problems and crippling effect of an injury, loss of ability to perform various acts, shortening of lifespan, mental anguish, and loss of companionship.

Deposition: The taking and recording of the testimony of a witness under oath before a court reporter in a place away from the courtroom before trial. A deposition is part of permitted pretrial discovery (investigation) set up by an attorney for one of the parties to a lawsuit demanding the sworn testimony of the opposing party (defendant or plaintiff), a witness to an event, or an expert intended to be called at trial by the opposition.

Direct examination: The first questioning of a witness during a trial or deposition (testimony out of court), as distinguished from cross-examination by opposing attorneys and redirect examination when the witness is again questioned by the original attorney. Questions on direct examination cannot be answer with "yes" or "no."

Expert testimony: Opinions stated during trial or deposition (testimony under oath before trial) by a specialist qualified as an expert on a subject relevant to a lawsuit or a criminal case.

Expert witness: A person who is a specialist in a subject, often technical, who may present his or her expert opinion without having been a witness to any occurrence relating to the lawsuit or criminal case. This is an exception to the rule against giving an opinion in trial, provided that the expert is qualified by evidence of his or her expertise, training, and special knowledge. If the expertise is challenged, then the attorney for the party calling the expert must make a showing of the necessary background through questions in court, and the trial judge has discretion to qualify the witness or rule that he or she is not an expert or is an expert on limited subjects.

Fact witness: A lay witness who has firsthand knowledge of certain facts, having made observations, and can testify to material facts.

Lay witness: A witness who is not an expert witness.

Liable: Responsible or obligated. Thus a person or entity may be liable for damages due to negligence.

Material fact: A fact upon which all or part of the outcome of a lawsuit depends.

Malpractice: See professional negligence.

Negligence: Failure to exercise the care toward others that a reasonable or prudent person would do in the circumstances or taking action that such a reasonable person would not.

Profession: Any type of work that needs special training or a particular skill, often one that is respected because it involves a high level of education (Cambridge Dictionaries Online, 2016a).

Professional judgment: "The process of forming an opinion or evaluation (characterized by or conforming to the technical or ethical standards of a calling requiring specialized knowledge and often long and intensive academic preparation) by discerning and comparing" (Busch, 2016, p. 5).

Professional negligence: An act or continuing conduct of a professional that does not meet the standard of professional competence and results in provable damages to his or her client or patient. Such an error or omission may be through negligence, ignorance (when the professional should have known), or intentional wrongdoing. However, malpractice does not include the exercise of professional judgment even when the results are detrimental to the client or patient.

Ethical Terms

The four principles that form the cornerstone of biomedical ethical decision making are (1) autonomy, (2) beneficence, (3) nonmaleficence, and (4) justice.

Autonomy: The client's right of self-determination and freedom of decision making.

Beneficence: Doing good for clients and providing benefit balanced against risk.

Nonmaleficence: Doing no harm to clients.

Justice: The norm of being fair to all and giving equal treatment, including distributing benefits, risks, and costs equally (Cooper, 2014).

Biomedical ethics also recognizes a number of rules that are related to the four fundamental ethical principles and, likewise, provide guidance in dealing with ethical dilemmas. Examples of commonly applied rules are fidelity, veracity, confidentiality, and privacy. *Fidelity* means being loyal and faithful to commitments and accountable for responsibilities. *Veracity* is the norm of telling the truth and not intentionally deceiving or misleading clients. *Confidentiality* prohibits some disclosures of some information gained in certain relationships to some third parties without the consent of the original source of the information. *Privacy* is a right of limited physical or informational inaccessibility (Cooper, 2014).

BACKGROUND

State Law and Nursing: Education and Licensure

Part of the way that a profession improves itself is to review its educational requirements and update as appropriate. More than ever, today's nurse is well educated, because many states and territories are moving toward a minimum educational level of a bachelor's degree in nursing (BSN) for new nurses entering into the profession (NursingLicensure.org, 2013). This trend has been accelerated by *The Future of Nursing,* a report of the Institute of Medicine (IOM, now called the National Academies of Sciences, Engineering, and Medicine, Health and Medicine Division) (IOM, 2011) and its 80% BSN by 2020 challenge. New York was one of the first states to propose "BSN in 10," a concept that would require all nurses with an associate degree in applied sciences/nursing (AAS) or 3-year diploma from a hospital nursing program to obtain a BSN by their 10th year of licensure. Many hospitals, particularly those with the Magnet Recognition Program® designation, have established policies that reflect this

model, even though states have not yet enacted such laws. Although the National Council Licensure Examination (NCLEX) is a national standard, it is also a minimum national standard and may be only one element of the legal requirements for licensure in a particular state or territory (NCLEX, 2016). In addition, advanced practice is another area of state law that defines the requirements, both educationally and clinically, for who may practice with a state-issued certification and/or supplemental license (laws and regulations vary by state), especially for nurse practitioners (APRNs).

> "APRNs include certified registered nurse anesthetists, certified nurse-midwives, clinical nurse specialists and certified nurse practitioners. Each has a unique history and context, but shares the commonality of being APRNs. While education, accreditation, and certification are necessary components of an overall approach to preparing an APRN for practice, the licensing boards—governed by state regulations and statutes—are the final arbiters of whom is recognized to practice within a given state. Currently, there is no uniform model of regulation of APRNs across the states. Each state independently determines the APRN legal scope of practice, the roles that are recognized, the criteria for entry into advanced practice, and the certification examinations accepted for entry-level competence assessment. This has created a significant barrier for APRNs to easily move from state to state and has decreased access to care for patients" (APRN Joint Dialogue Group Report, 2008, p. 5).

In each state, the nurse practice act, administered by the state board of nursing, is the singular authoritative source to identify the educational, clinical, continuing education, fees, and all other requirements to satisfy the state's licensure requirements.

THE LEGAL SYSTEM AND SOURCES OF LAW

Nurses, nurse managers, and health care facilities are all subject to being found **legally liable** (i.e., legally responsible) for harm caused to others by civil wrongs. More specifically, liability is created when the law imposes a civil obligation on a wrongdoer to compensate an injured party for the consequences of a wrongful act. As shown in Fig. 6.1, there are two sources of legal liability—torts and contracts (Cooper, 2014).

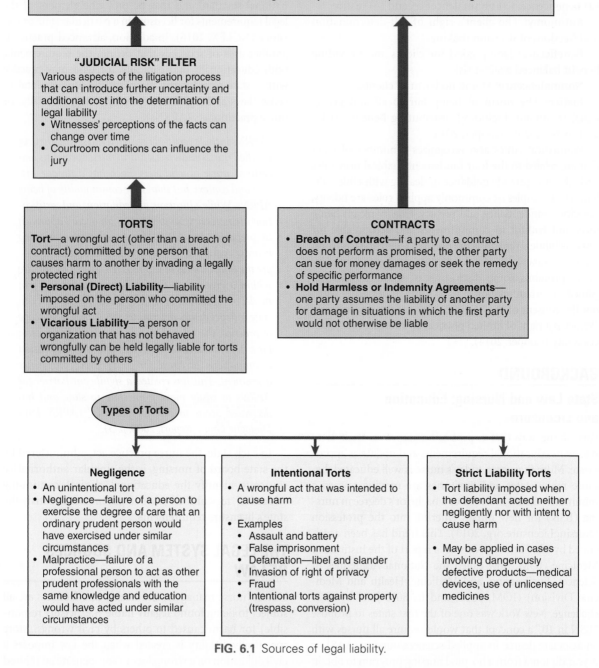

FIG. 6.1 Sources of legal liability.

The most common source of legal liability for nurses and nurse managers is a *tort*. A tort is a wrongful act (other than breach of contract) committed against another person or organization or their property that causes harm and can be remedied by a civil (rather than criminal) lawsuit. Examples of a tort are intentional emotional distress or false imprisonment. Although torts most commonly give rise to *personal* (or *direct*) liability for the person committing the wrongful act, in some cases another person or organization may also be held *vicariously* liable for the same wrongful act they did not commit. For example, when a nurse commits a tort, the nurse may be found to be directly liable and the nurse's employer also may be found to be vicariously liable for the nurse's wrongful action (Cooper, 2014).

As indicated in Fig. 6.1, determination of legal liability as a result of a tort depends on more than just the various technical elements of the tort that must be proved by the injured party (plaintiff), the presentation of various available defenses by the defendant, and the formal rules of the judicial system regarding the litigation process. In the case of torts, the legal outcomes are often influenced also by what may be termed *judicial risk*. This refers to various aspects of the litigation process that can introduce further uncertainty and additional cost into the determination of legal liability. Judicial risk can result in findings with respect to legal liability that are not based solely on the merits of the case nor on the rules of law applicable to the case (Cooper, 2014).

What we refer to as the legal system is a multifaceted structure of federal, state, and local laws. In addition, there are regulations, which are rules that have full force and effect of law. In other words, in addition to statutes, there is a whole structure of rules created through an enabling statute. Such statutes give authority to an agency, such as the state board of nursing. There are two major divisions in the structure of the law: civil law and criminal law.

Civil Law

There are different standards by which defendants are judged in civil litigation: simple or regular negligence and professional negligence or *malpractice*.

Tort

A tort is a civil or personal wrong, compared with a crime, which is a public wrong. The purpose of tort law is to adjust losses by compensating one person because of the actions of another. Therefore the only remedy available in a civil lawsuit based on tort is monetary damages (i.e., money). Each intentional tort represents a direct interference with a person's physical integrity or right to property. Personal freedom is a fundamental right. One does not waive a fundamental right, such as personal integrity, automatically. On the contrary, a person must be aware that he or she possesses a particular right and can intentionally relinquish it. This is the basis for the concept of informed consent.

Informed consent is a good example of a knowing and voluntary waiver of rights in the medical setting. In the absence of such a waiver of rights, a person touching or keeping another in a clinic, hospital, or any place he or she chooses not to be may be liable for assault, battery, or false imprisonment. Informed consent is a statutorily created right given to potential recipients of medical treatment. Most state statutes express that it is the duty of the physician to fully inform the patient as to the risks and benefits of a proposed procedure. The physician must also advise the patient of alternative treatments, if any, as well as the option to refuse any treatment. For the patient to be fully informed, the physician must advise the patient of all the potential risks and benefits of each option, including refusing the proposed treatment. Unless there is a specific statute, such as in the case of some advanced practice registered nurses (APRN), the physician's duty of informed consent is never transferred or delegated to a nurse.

Intentional torts include assault, battery, false imprisonment, and trespassing. These terms are often confused because they also exist within criminal law.

Negligence. For a civil lawsuit to be successful in negligence, there are four required elements. These elements are commonly referred to as duty, breach, cause, and harm. All four of the elements must be proven, and the burden of proof is on the plaintiff (the one who brings the complaint). The plaintiff must prove that there was a well-established duty and an obvious breach of such duty. These proofs are not sufficient without also establishing the causal connection to the harm claimed. Proof of damages (harm) is an essential element to a negligence case. Negligence is sometimes referred to as simple negligence, compared with malpractice or professional negligence. This standard is used in cases such as motor vehicle accidents, personal injury (outside the medical setting), and property damage. The *standard of proof* for a simple or regular negligence case is that of a reasonably prudent person.

The concept of negligence is based on the idea that there can be a generally uniform standard of human behavior. The simplest example of this is that when one drives a car, there is a generally accepted expectation that each person will operate the vehicle in a reasonably prudent and careful manner. Each time there is a motor vehicle accident, it is likely that one or more persons deviated from the reasonably prudent person's standard, and liability may attach. However, state statutes may limit or expand a person's ability to bring a cause of action via a lawsuit (Muller, 2007).

Professional negligence (malpractice). The standard by which a licensed professional nurse (RN) will be judged comes from a governmental standard. The nurse's licensure and scope of practice are derived from the state's nurse practice act. All states, as well as US territories (Puerto Rico and Guam), have a nurse practice act. Links to all state boards of nursing and those states' nurse practice acts can be found on individual state board of nursing websites or through the National Council of State Boards of Nursing (NCSBN, 2016a). Nurse practice acts provide broad statements defining nursing practice, delineating the educational and other requirements for licensure and renewal, giving notice to the public of the sort of behaviors that can be expected from a nurse, and identifying what unacceptable practices might subject a nurse to disciplinary review or sanctions.

Professions develop a standard for themselves through a complex process of discussion and interaction within the profession and with other professions; knowledge dissemination such as peer reviewed professional journals; meetings; development of standards, guidelines, and statements; networking with colleagues; and the development and refining of academic programs both at the undergraduate and graduate levels for the profession. In addition, each profession has an obligation to monitor its members and self-police the behavior of its own.

For more than 14 years, nursing has been recognized by the general public in a Gallup poll as a highly esteemed profession. Nurses have the respect and admiration of the American people and were acknowledged as the most trusted profession (American Nurses Association [ANA], 2015a). Nurses should take great pride in this recognition. However, it also reminds nurses that they are always being watched by the public and are expected to conduct themselves in a professional, ethical, and truthful manner. Such accolades could easily be lost.

Professional Safeguards

Civil law controls those circumstances when an individual, the plaintiff, feels that he or she has been harmed by another. If the other person, known as the defendant, is a professional, the law provides for *professional liability*, also known as *malpractice*. Professionals are provided with many safeguards to avoid them being wrongfully accused of malpractice. Some of these safeguards include:

Statute of Limitations: A statutory time limit (most commonly 2 years) by which a plaintiff must file a lawsuit against a professional or lose that opportunity forever. In many states, there are exceptions to the time limitation for infants (children under a prescribed statutory age at the time of the alleged event) and an extension of time if the plaintiff was unaware of the injury at the time. One example is if a surgical count was incorrect at the completion of a procedure, an instrument or other substance was left in the patient's abdominal cavity in error, and the nurses "signed off" on the count. The patient is discharged, goes home, and does not have any symptoms or problems for 30 months, at which time it is discovered that the item has encapsulated, become infected, and the patient now requires additional surgery and/or suffers some other harm, even death. It is possible that a lawsuit could be filed as late as 2 years after the discovery of the indwelling item. The standard basis to file a professional liability/malpractice lawsuit is the time when the patient knew or should have known.

Affidavit of Merit: Another safeguard to protect the professional is the requirement of an affidavit of merit. An affidavit of merit is a sworn document by a like kind of professional (a doctor for a doctor defendant and a nurse for a nurse defendant) who reviews the injured patient's chart, and, based upon the reviewer's education and experience, makes a statement that the case has merit and should be permitted to go to trial. Their opinion will also include that there is a likelihood of the plaintiff's success at trial.

The person who reviews the record and provides the affidavit may never testify or have any other contact with the case.

Sources of Law: Laws are found in case books, as well as online in official reports and legal research services. A reported case is one that can be found in an official reporter. There are state as well as federal reporters. When entered into a reporter, the case is printed and becomes part of the ever-growing body of case law. It is important to remember that what is heard on the news, no matter the source, is simply news (maybe entertainment) and is not admissible as evidence at trial (Muller, 2007). Official sources of law need to be consulted and used when drawing conclusions.

Under both federal and state rules of evidence, the only way to prove professional negligence is through the use of expert witnesses. Expert witnesses need to be knowledgeable and up to date in their fields and familiar with texts, journals, and the relevant accepted standards of practice. These individuals are often published authors, leaders in the field, or academics.

The Nurse as Witness

There are times when a nurse is called on to testify at a deposition or appear to testify in court. The nurse may have been present in the hospital, clinic, or office setting where he or she made certain observations. This does not mean necessarily that the nurse is a party to the case; the nurse may not be a defendant. There are two general categories of witnesses who testify at trial: the fact witness and the expert witness.

A **fact witness** is someone who can testify from his or her own observations. In other words, the nurse can apply his or her senses to a fact or set of circumstances. (e.g., I saw . . . I heard . . . I smelled). For example, the nurse might have observed a patient fall in a hospital hallway, but it was not his or her patient; the person was with another staff member, but the nurse saw the fall. That nurse could testify as a fact witness (sometimes referred to as an eyewitness) to those events that were seen, heard, or felt. A fact witness may not offer an opinion, but must testify only as to personal knowledge.

An **expert witness** is a person with specialized knowledge who aids the judge and jury (in the case of a jury trial) to understand something that is beyond the scope of the average individual. There are multiple standards in determining whether one can be considered an expert witness. Experts base their opinions and their testimony on their knowledge, education, and experience. State and federal rules of evidence require that a patient claiming that a professional is responsible for his or her injuries and damages use a "like-kind" expert witness to prove his or her case (Federal Rules of Evidence 703,704) (Legal Information Institute, 2015).

A professional liability case cannot be proven without an expert witness who can testify as to actions or inactions of the professional defendant. Simply put, only a nurse can testify as to the standard of care and scope of practice of another nurse. If the nurse works in a specialty area such as professional case management, the operating room, or the emergency department (ED), a like-kind nurse should be the one to testify as an expert for that particular nurse defendant.

There are typically two experts: one for the plaintiff and one for the defendant nurse. An expert witness is only as good as his or her education and experience in two critical ways: first by establishing and maintaining credibility by having expertise in the required field, and second by withstanding cross-examination by the plaintiff's attorney. The fastest way to be excluded as an expert witness is to "step outside your sandbox." Any document, text, or other material that an expert refers to in his or her written report and/or testimony must be available and, in most cases, is admissible into evidence.

It is important to note that if the expert refers to such a document, he or she must be fully familiar with the entire document. It would be appropriate cross-examination for the nurse to be asked about something in the text or other reference that has nothing to do with the present case and that the expert made no reference to; it goes to the expert's credibility. In other words, did the expert simply "cherry pick" a small portion of a reference that related to the facts, or is that expert fully familiar with the foundational materials? In recent years, some states have permitted professionals whose practice area overlaps with the defendant's to testify, although other states interpret the "like-kind" expert strictly. The attorney who seeks a nurse's assistance as an expert should be fully familiar with the criteria in the jurisdiction. However, even those experts who are experienced in courtroom testimony can be enticed to step outside their area of expertise. The next thing that happens is that there is an objection to the witness and his or her testimony in whole or in part, the expert's credibility is ruined, and an otherwise solid case begins to crumble (Muller, 2011).

Criminal Law

Criminal law is based on statutes. Statutes are laws created by the legislature and signed into law by the executive, the governor for state laws and the president of the United States for federal laws.

Crimes are prohibitions against behaviors that are so egregious that they offend society, not just the individual victim. Crimes are punishable with fines and/or jail, depending on the level of the offense and other factors, and these consequences are delineated in the criminal statute. Nurses can be subject to criminal law for such behaviors as stealing or misusing narcotics, practicing without a license, or intentionally causing physical harm to a person in their care. These criminal offenses violate the public trust and safety and carry serious consequences.

LICENSURE, MULTI-STATE, AND DISTANCE PRACTICE

There is no doubt that the world in which nurses practice today has been dramatically and forever affected by advances in technology. Gone are the days when the only interaction between nurse and patient was at arm's length. Today, with the advent of electronic health records (EHR), telephonic, e-mail, text, and video connections, nurses and patients can interact from across town or across the country. Distance communications need to be considered with great caution: Just because we can, does not mean we should. The law is slow to catch up with technical advances. Although there has been much talk about cost-effective interventions through electronic means, the nurse must adhere to the law. As it stands today, nurses must be licensed in each and every state/jurisdiction in which they practice.

"Uniform Licensure Requirements (ULRs) are the essential prerequisites for initial, endorsement, renewal and reinstatement licensure needed across every NCSBN jurisdiction to ensure the safe and competent practice of nursing. ULRs protect the public by setting consistent standards and promoting a health care system that is fluid and accessible by removing barriers to care and maximizing portability for nurses. They also assure the consumer that a nurse in one state has met the requirements of the nurses in every other state. ULRs support the fact that the expectations for the education of a nurse and the responsibilities of a nurse are the same throughout every NCSBN member board jurisdiction in the United States." (NCSBN, 2011)

The Nurse Licensure Compact (NLC) allows nurses to have one multistate license, with the ability to practice in both their home state and other compact states. There are currently 25 states in the NLC (NCSBN, 2016b). In 2015 significant revisions were made to the NLC Model Act, requiring all legislatures to revisit the issue. Revisions were made, in part, in response to objections from some states, and it is hoped that the NLC will grow significantly in the coming years. If a nurse lives or works near another state's border, it is often tempting, and may be requested, that the nurse speak telephonically or go in person to deliver care to persons in the neighboring state. Thus it is imperative that nurses be licensed in each state in which they deliver care; otherwise care can only be legally delivered to patients in the state in which the nurse is licensed.

Distance practice is nothing new, but the tools and technologies available today make distance practice far easier and will become more and more common. Telehealth, telemedicine, and case management practice are examples where distance practice occurs. There is a two-pronged test to determine if a distance communication is permitted, whether by telephonic, e-mail, or other electronic device. The first test is that the nurse must examine the content of the communication, and the second test is whether that communication constitutes the practice of nursing.

Example #1: Nursing process begins with assessment. A "systematic, dynamic process by which the nurse, through interaction with the client, significant others, and health care providers, collects and analyzes data about the client. Assessment is broader than observing and data gathering. It includes the application of processes such as critical thinking and professional judgments used in prioritizing, identifying immediate and anticipated need, analyzing medical and nursing interventions aimed at appropriate outcomes, and providing for holistic continuum of care" (ANA, 2016, p. 1). Assessment can start with a simple telephone call, "Good morning. How are you?"

If the nurse asks that simple question, "How are you?", and the patient responds with symptoms, then the nurse, based on his or her knowledge and experience, uses critical thinking, makes professional judgments, and takes action. That is the practice of nursing. To conduct such a dialogue across state lines, the nurse must be licensed in the state where the patient is located. Therefore in this example the nursing process has been established, and licensure is necessary.

Example #2: The caller contacts the patient and says, "Good morning, I'm calling to follow up and remind you of your appointment with Dr. Smith. I've arranged for transportation; the car will pick you up tomorrow morning. Is that ok? Is there anything else I can do for you?" No assessment occurred, no nursing process was initiated, and no nursing skill, based on education and training, was required to conduct this communication. Anyone with minimal training (such as a high school graduate) could perform this task. Review of Chapter 9 on delegation will be helpful and provide parameters for appropriate task delegation.

LEGAL DOCUMENTS AND THE NURSE

It is important for the nurse to have a working knowledge of certain legal documents that affect practice. It is not uncommon for the nurse to encounter powers of attorney or advance directives for health care (also referred to as living wills or powers of attorney for health care, depending on the jurisdiction). Patients are asked before admission whether they have a living will or similar document, but what happens to that document varies greatly from facility to facility, even in the same state. The most important thing that the nurse must take away from a discussion of legal documents is that the nurse must actually see the document. It is not enough for an individual to say, "I am the health care representative/proxy" or "I'm the power of attorney," which is simply a misuse of the term.

Power of attorney is the document used for the appointment of another person, referred to as the principal, and empowers that person (the attorney-in-fact or agent) to act on behalf of the principal. In other words, by way of a legal document, one person gives authority to another to act and perform certain functions on behalf of that person. The power of attorney is a document, a writing, prescribed by state law, which can grant very limited or very broad powers to the attorney-in-fact

(the agent). It is common to hear people say, "I have power of attorney." That may be a true statement if there is a document that assigns such a power, but it is actually incorrect to say, "I am the power of attorney." Misusing these terms overextends or improperly limits the authority of the attorney-in-fact.

Confusion regarding these terms often stems from those states that permit the use of the term "power of attorney" to extend to health care proxies and directives, commonly called living wills. New York, Michigan, and California are among the states that use a durable power of attorney for health care as the legal document for use as a living will. Other states, like New Jersey, use an advanced directive for health care (The New Jersey Advance Directives for Health Care Act, NJ. Stat. §. 26:2H-53–78). No matter what "power" an individual is asserting, without actually seeing the document (or a facsimile thereof where permitted), the nurse may risk a Health Information Portability and Accountability Act of 1996 (HIPAA) violation or other liability exposure by disclosing information to one who is not entitled to such access (Muller, 2008).

Guardianship

Parents are the guardians of their children until the child reaches the age of majority in the particular state. Typically, this is at 18 years of age, but there are exceptions. Certain states have greatly reduced the age of consent, particularly in the medical setting. It is important to understand the purpose of the rule of law and the requirements in the state(s) in which the nurse practices.

A *guardian* is a person appointed by a court via a judge. In the normal course of events, a parent is the guardian of their child, but all that changes on the child's eighteenth birthday. There are many types of guardians. *A general guardian* is appointed if the court finds that an individual is incapacitated, according to that state's legal definition of incapacity, to govern or manage his or her affairs. The general guardian exercises all rights and powers of the incapacitated person concerning both the rights of the person and his or her financial assets, income, and responsibilities (NJ. Stat. §3B:12—24.1). The nurse must pause when any person represents to the nurse, the hospital, or the agency that they are the guardian of a person or custodian of that person's affairs. They *must* provide you with a copy of the specific court order naming him or her as the guardian over a named person, with any limitations to that guardianship.

A *guardian ad litem* is a temporary appointment of a person by a court to act on behalf of another for a specific purpose. Typically it is an adult who will take legal action on behalf of a minor child or an adult who is unable to handle his or her own affairs, even when represented by an attorney. For example, the guardian ad litem may file a lawsuit for a child who is injured in an automobile accident or by some other means. A *guardian ad litem* may also be appointed following the death of a person in order to file claim against an estate on behalf of a child or incompetent adult (Muller, 2008).

The Problem of the Adult Child

When a child reaches the age of majority—18 years in most jurisdictions—the parent no longer has access to medical records, nor do parents have the right to make medical decisions for their children. It is difficult for a devoted loving parent to simply stop, when yesterday the privilege and burden of making medical decision for their child(ren) fell to them, and then the next day, on the eighteenth birthday, this stopped. The problem is further magnified when the child has a disability and special needs. The nurse is in a unique position to have insight and understanding into the child's (now a young adult) needs. In cases where the young adult is not competent to make his or her own medical decisions, guardianship may be a viable option. In most states, this is a complex procedure requiring an attorney's advice and at least one court appearance.

For a child who is unable to communicate but has the mental capacity to make his or her own choices, the legal documents described in this chapter are useful tools. It is the nurse's legal and ethical duty to protect the adult "child's" autonomy and not simply accept a parent's intervention, without lawful authority, just because it may seem easier at the moment. Along with incredible advances in prosthetics, electronic aids, and assistive devices, children and adults who were once unable to function in schools, universities, and the workforce are now able to. Thus the limits are being tested with regard to individual autonomy.

Confidentiality and Access to Medical Information

Patient confidentiality has been a central theme to medical and nursing practice for generations, but the rules governing access and release of medical records were solidified more than 20 years ago with the advent of HIPAA (Public Law 104–191). Even though HIPAA is federal law and preempts state law, there is great variation from state to state. HIPAA is a minimum mandatory standard. States are permitted to provide additional protections to their residents, but no law can limit or reduce a right provided under federal law. An interactive map is available at *http://www.healthinfolaw.org/comparative-analysis/individual-access-medical-records-50-state-comparison* and provides a state-by-state comparison. Iowa, Alabama, and New Hampshire are examples of states whose law was preempted by HIPAA and provides no additional access or rights. California, Colorado, New York, and Nevada provide greater access and protection; they require release of medical records to those who properly make requests in a specific number of days, even though providers are permitted to charge reasonable fees for accessing and copying records (Milken Institute School of Public Health, 2012). One of the goals of EHRs was to make provision of medical records to patients who request them easier to access, faster and less expensive to copy, and more accessible to patients.

Demonstrating Compliance

Legal compliance is demonstrated by holding and maintaining a professional license in each and every jurisdiction in which the nurse practices, whether in person, telephonically, or through other means of electronic communication. The nurse must maintain up-to-date knowledge through continuing education as mandated by the state(s) of licensure and adhere to all applicable laws and regulations.

Adhering to all applicable federal, state, and local laws, as well as employer policies, is the general principle of necessary compliance, but there is a hierarchy to these duties. Federal law *preempts* state law. Law will always supersede hospital or other employer policies and procedures. Legal compliance is broader than simply following the rules for correct drug dosage, route, and observations of the patient; it starts with patient assessment and goes through full discharge of duties at the standard of care of a reasonable and prudent nurse.

Regulatory Compliance

Regulations are rules that have the same effect as laws. They are created based on a statute, giving authority to an agency or the director of an agency, to create regulations to further the purpose of the enabling statute.

HIPAA has now been a part of health care and health care practice for 20 years. Protecting health information is the core of the law and all the regulations that followed. Nurses need to be familiar with who the privacy officer is in whatever entity they work and use resources to educate and reeducate themselves with the requirements in their state.

The HIPAA Privacy Rule was published on December 28, 2000, with the goal of providing consumers with greater rights for protection of individually identifiable health information, sometimes referred to as personal health information (PHI). In the spring of 2003, there were further modifications to the Final Privacy Rule. The key to HIPAA, and all the changes and improvements over time, is meeting the educational requirement (at minimum, a yearly update) and demonstrating genuine compliance. The Privacy Rule is only part of HIPAA compliance requirements. There are complex regulations controlling the use of electronic communications, including telephone, fax, e-mail, and text messaging, as well as billing and reporting requirements (Muller, 2007).

HIPAA responsibilities come to us as building blocks. The patient privacy rules and access to medical records do not go away when a new responsibility is added. Each new aspect, addition or modification of the law requires that each practitioner have not only a basic understanding of HIPAA (1996), but an ever-enlarging knowledge base regarding HIPAA, the Health Information Technology for Economic and Clinical Health (HITECH) Act, which is a portion of the American Recovery and Reinvestment Act of 2009 (ARRA) 26 USC 1 and the Final Omnibus Rule (2013), and subtle changes that continue to be made. Most recently, in January 2016, the HIPAA restriction on the disclosure of PHI was modified by agency amendment. "The Department of Health and Human Services issued a final rule expressly permitting certain HIPAA covered entities to provide to the [National Instant Criminal Background Check System] NICS limited demographic and other necessary information about these individuals" (Obama, 2016, p. 1). It is important to obtain and update knowledge of all HIPAA and state privacy and confidentiality mandates.

The Personal Representative

The US Department of Health and Human Services (HHS) "recognizes that there may be times when individuals are legally or otherwise incapable of exercising their rights, or simply choose to designate another to act on their behalf with respect to these rights. Under the Rule, a person authorized (under State or other applicable law, e.g., tribal or military law) to act on behalf of the individual in making health care related decisions is the individual's 'personal representative.' Section 164.502(g) provides when, and to what extent, the personal representative must be treated as the individual for purposes of the Rule. In addition to these formal designations of a personal representative, the Rule at 45 CFR 164.510(b) addresses situations in which family members or other persons who are involved in the individual's health care or payment for care may receive protected health information about the individual even if they are not expressly authorized to act on the individual's behalf" (HHS, 2016, p. 1).

ETHICAL COMPONENTS

In addition to potential legal concerns, nurses and nurse managers are often faced with ethical dilemmas in connection with decision making. Ethical dilemmas require that decisions be made about what is right and wrong in situations in which an individual has to make a choice between equally unfavorable alternatives. Like other health care professionals, nurses traditionally have faced ethical dilemmas arising primarily out of clinical practice. These dilemmas have involved conflicts among principles and/or rules attributable to common morality (socially approved norms of human conduct), standards articulated in professional codes of ethics, public policies promulgated by government agencies, and the personal values of the health care professionals themselves. Ethical dilemmas faced by nurses and nurse managers also arise as clashes between the principles, rules, values, and standards of clinical/professional ethics and those of organizational/business ethics.

Although the domain of clinical ethics is the care of clients, the domain of organizational ethics is a facility's business-related activities, including, among others, marketing, admissions, transfer, discharge, billing, and the relationship of the facility and its staff members to other health care providers, educational institutions, and payers. These are activities that also directly affect the care of patients. Organizational ethics reflect a health care facility's basic values that serve as guides for proper and acceptable behavior in decision making. Together, clinical and organizational ethics reflect a health care facility's concern that, whether related to the continuum of care or the continuum of services related to that care, ethical dilemmas should be resolved based on values-centered principles that focus on doing the right thing and taking the right action.

Professional responsibility is something each nurse must deal with every day in his or her practice. If an error occurs, but no one knows, is it any less an error? This is the point where ethics and legal mandates come together. Using the distance practice example, the question is, is it wrong? Or is it wrong only if I get caught? In this author's opinion, it is fundamentally wrong, and accepting responsibility for such errors in judgment and practice are the duty of each and every nurse. "Nurses bear primary responsibility for the nursing care that their patients and clients receive and are accountable for their own practice" (ANA, 2015b, p. 15). Whether nurses are discussing distance practice, medication errors, HIPAA violations, or any other deviation from acceptable nursing practice, it is that accountability that sets nurses apart as the most trusted profession.

Incident Reports

Incident-reporting systems are set up as a way to report errors, especially safety errors. They are used to gather data and information about patient safety occurrences for organizational learning. There are three types of incidents: a harmful incident, a no-harm incident, and a near miss (Hewitt & Chreim, 2015). Incident-reporting systems are part of risk-management efforts and are voluntary but set an expectation for reporting. Their effectiveness has not been substantiated (Stavropoulou et al., 2015). Barriers to reporting include personal reasons such as fear, accountability, and nurse characteristics as well as organizational factors such as culture, the reporting system, and management behavior (Vrbnjak et al., 2016). One study found that hospital personnel frequently encounter safety problems that they themselves can resolve on the spot. Fixing and forgetting, instead of fixing and reporting, was the main choice when handling near misses (seen as unworthy of reporting), solving a patient's safety problem (seen as unique or a one-time event), or encountering recurring problems (seen as inevitable, routine events). Although common, fixing and forgetting does not serve as the best organizational handling of patient safety or its risk-management efforts because it does not make patient safety more preventive. Nurses may incur liability and

risk, with possible ethical implications, if incidents are not properly reported so that investigation and organizational intervention can occur.

Code of Ethics

In addition to these basic moral principles and rules of biomedical ethics, nurses are also provided standards of conduct by professional codes of ethics. For example, the ANA's *Code of Ethics for Nurses With Interpretive Statements* (2015b) provides nonnegotiable standards as to the ethical obligations and duties of those who enter the nursing profession. The ANA indicated that the Code was developed as a guide for carrying out nursing responsibilities to be consistent with quality in nursing care and the ethical obligations of the profession. The focus is not on giving precise answers to specific ethical problems but rather on providing general guidance as to how to act when faced with ethical dilemmas.

LEADERSHIP AND MANAGEMENT IMPLICATIONS

By the very nature of their work, nurses and nurse managers are decision makers who are constantly faced with making choices in personal, clinical, and organizational situations. These decision-making situations are commonly fraught with legal and ethical issues that often become entwined. As members of a profession, nurses and nurse managers are guided by both legal and ethical considerations in making decisions. The legal aspects of nursing management center on decision making and supervision. Because all nurses retain personal accountability for their own acts and the use of knowledge and skills in the provision of care, personal accountability cannot be assumed by another. Nurse managers keep their own personal accountability for their own specific acts, but they are accountable also for their acts of delegation and supervision (Cooper, 2014).

Nurse managers carry the major responsibility for developing and upholding the standards of care for the staff. Nurses and nurse managers carry the accountability for the supervision of others, who are often unlicensed assistive personnel. Supervision includes monitoring the tasks performed, ensuring that functions are performed in an appropriate fashion, and ensuring that assigned tasks and functions do not exceed competency or require a license to perform. Nurse managers use their autonomy to make decisions about practice situations. They are accountable for carrying out supervisory responsibilities; proper notification; assessing the competency of staff; training, orientation, and evaluation of staff; reasonable staffing decisions; and monitoring and maintenance of professional treatment relationships with clients, called *nonabandonment* (Cooper, 2014).

The managers of any health care organization are responsible to the policy-making body of the organization and hold an obligation to comply with the laws of society at local, state, and national levels. Managers are responsible for ensuring that laws are adhered to in the actions of management itself and also in the actions of those employees who assist the managers in carrying out the mission of the organization. Concern for the law involves three general areas: personal negligence in clinical practice, liability for delegation and supervision, and liability of health care organizations (Cooper, 2014).

Personal Negligence in Clinical Practice

Activities of clinical client care involve corresponding legal accountability and risk. Errors do happen, and some lead to injury to a client. At minimum, nurses have an ethical obligation to nonmaleficence, or to do no harm to clients. This duty is discharged in part by remaining competent in knowledge and skills and the standards of practice. Nursing negligence/malpractice occurs when the nurse's actions are unreasonable given the circumstances, fail to meet the standard of care, or when the nurse fails to act and causes harm. In nursing, harm related to clinical practice commonly arises from negligent acts or omissions (unintentional torts) and a variety of intentional acts (intentional torts), such as invasion of privacy or assault and battery. To establish legal liability on the grounds of malpractice (professional negligence), the injured client (plaintiff) must prove these four elements:

1. A duty of care was owed to the injured party.
2. There was a breach of that duty.
3. The breach of the duty caused the injury (causation).
4. Actual harm or damages were suffered by the plaintiff.

Common clinical practice areas that give rise to allegations of malpractice include the general areas of treatment, communication, medication, and the broad category of monitoring/observing/supervising/surveillance. Examples of common negligence allegations in nursing malpractice suits include patient falls, use of restraints, medication errors, burns, equipment injuries, retained foreign objects, failure to monitor, failure to ensure safety, failure to take

appropriate nursing action, failure to confirm accuracy of physicians' orders, improper technique or performance of treatments, failure to respond to a patient, failure to follow hospital procedure, and failure to supervise treatment (Cooper, 2014).

Both nurses and nurse managers have a duty to follow organizational policies and procedures when reasonable. Nurse managers are advised to review policies and procedures carefully, including the language used, in order to adhere to legal and ethical parameters more closely. Clearly, management in nursing practice means that nurses must fulfill obligations and duties both to clients and to the organization. This means using knowledge, skill, and decision-making abilities to reduce the incidence of negligence and malpractice by employees as a way to reduce harm to clients and legal risk to the organization. As the primary coordinators of care, nurses need to manage the environment of care delivery. Ensuring staff competence and reporting incompetent practice are key activities. For example, in nursing, legal and ethical issues arise when a nurse is impaired by substance abuse. The overall consideration is protecting the client from harm. Confronting suspected abuse must be done carefully, but when an incident occurs, the nurse manager has a responsibility to intervene (Cooper, 2014).

Liability of Health Care Organizations

Health care facilities face extensive exposure to legal liability from several sources in addition to the liability faced by nurses and nurse managers arising out of malpractice in clinical practice and negligence in the process of delegating and supervising. These sources include negligence of their employees, negligence of independent contractors, corporate negligence arising out of the facility's responsibilities to hire qualified employees and monitor and supervise their activities, and failure to comply with numerous laws and regulations, especially those related to employment issues. Nurse managers have important roles to play in helping their organizations control facility liability arising from each of these sources (Cooper, 2014).

Nurse managers can help the facility avoid corporate liability by, among other things, ensuring that those who report to them remain competent and qualified and have current licensure. Nurse managers should also report dangerously low staffing levels, incorrect mixes of staff for effectively meeting the health care needs of clients, and report incompetent, illegal, or unethical practices to appropriate authorities. Nurse managers have an important role to play in compliance with human resources (HR) areas of hiring, performance appraisal, management of employees with problems, and termination (Cooper, 2014).

HR management is a major area for organizational liability. Nursing is a labor-intensive occupation. Some organizations are unionized. Labor and employment law includes various laws and regulations that deal with issues related to hiring, firing, employee benefits, compensation, overtime, workplace safety, privacy, drug testing, and preventing discrimination, harassment, and violence. Because of the volume, variety, and complexity of local, state, and federal HR-related laws and regulations, organizations have HR departments whose function is to implement strategies and policies related to employee management.

Mandatory Reporting

Among the many duties under one's professional license to practice nursing is the duty to report. This duty sits firmly on the fence between legal and ethical responsibilities and is a good example of those times when a legal obligation is affected by ethics. This duty to report includes observations of children, elders, disabled, developmentally compromised, and anyone who is at risk or in a vulnerable situation. Licensed professionals have had an affirmative "duty to warn" ever since the 1976 decision of the Supreme Court of California in the case of *Tarasoff v. Regents of the University of California*, 551 P.2d 334 (1976). Since that time, nurses and other health professionals have struggled to identify the triggering point in a patient relationship that rises to the statutory "duty to warn" (Muller & Fink-Samnick, 2015). Initially, the case stood for the concept that if there was a specific threat against an individual, the therapist (in that case) was legally obligated to warn that individual and enable him/her to take steps to protect themselves. In other words, the threat had to be specific to an identifiable individual. Citing previous cases, the court said, "We recognize the difficulty that a therapist encounters in attempting to forecast whether a patient presents a serious danger of violence. Obviously, we do not require that the therapist, in making that determination, render a perfect performance; the therapist need only exercise 'that reasonable degree of skill, knowledge, and care ordinarily possessed and exercised by members of [that professional specialty]

under similar circumstances'" (Tarasoff v. Regents of the University of California, 1976, p. 8).

In 2007, the California legislature codified Tarasoff, along with subsequent cases. The then-new law increased the duty to one that is twofold: (1) the duty to inform the potential victim of the risk and (2) the duty to inform appropriate law enforcement. In the passage of time, states have adopted varying duties for nurses, therapists, social workers, physicians, and other practitioners. It is critical that nurses make inquiry and be fully familiar as to the requirement(s) of the state(s) in which they practice. The National Conference of State Legislatures (NCSL, 2015) lists those states that have laws in place. There are three types of laws: mandatory reporting, permissive reporting, and no reporting requirement at all. The NCSL report focused on mental health professionals, but it is a valuable resource for nurses as well (NCSL, 2015).

Ethical Decisions

Many of the decisions nurses and nurse managers make on a daily basis have an ethical component and may involve conflicts among ethical responsibilities. These conflicts may involve clashes between the following:

- Two ethical duties to the client (e.g., duty to respect autonomy and duty to benefit the client)
- The client's rights and benefits (e.g., withholding or withdrawing treatment in respect for a client's right to die by forgoing treatment at any time and treating or continuing treatment that is expected to produce more good for the client)
- Duties to self and duties to the client (e.g., a nurse's desire to remain on the same shift because of parental responsibilities and the need to advocate for better treatment of the clients by some health care practitioners on that shift)
- Professional ethical provisions and religious ones (e.g., a professional code requiring the recognition of the client's right to self-determination and a nurse's religious beliefs prohibiting abortion).

When ethical dilemmas are encountered in dealing with clinical matters, health care professionals commonly refer to various principles, rules, and standards for guidance in making moral decisions. Principles and rules are normative generalizations that provide guidance in ethical decision making. Although rules are more specific in content and restricted in scope than principles, neither can fully guide action but instead must be complemented by judgment for a decision to be made (Cooper, 2014). Many organizations employ an ethicist and have ethics committees that operate to provide a source of support and guidance for ethical dilemmas faced by nurses in organizations.

CURRENT ISSUES AND TRENDS

Legal Issues and the Changing Family Dynamic

The ideal American family is no longer a "mother, father and 2.5 children" (Carroll, 2007), and even if the number of children remains constant, the makeup of the family has changed. According to one definition, a family is "a social group of parents, children, and sometimes grandparents, uncles, aunts, and others who are related" (Cambridge Dictionaries Online, 2016b). On June 26, 2015, the US Supreme Court issued its decision in *Obergefell et al. v. Hodges, Director, Ohio Department of Health, et al.* The court held that, "The Fourteenth Amendment requires a State to license a marriage between two people of the same sex and to recognize a marriage between two people of the same sex when their marriage was lawfully licensed and performed out-of-State" (Obergefell v. Hodges, 2015, pp. 3–28).

The traditional US concept of a family is clearly undergoing change. Nurses are confronted with families who may be structured in ways that are completely different from their own life experience and beliefs. Although nurses are entitled to their personal beliefs, those beliefs must remain outside the nurse–patient relationship. The duty as a nurse is to obey the law and act toward all patients, their families, and/or family caregiver with respect, providing them with the care and education that the circumstance requires. This issue is also directly related to the issue of consent and who may give consent for treatment on behalf of the patient. Questions in the practice setting should be referred to supervision, administration, or legal counsel within the facility or practice setting.

Staffing

In view of the significant degrees of change and uncertainty associated with the legal and ethical aspects affecting decision making in nursing care management, there are important current issues and trends in this area. A major current and continuing issue is the nurse shortage, which for a number of reasons is expected to continue in the foreseeable future. This issue gives rise to a number of legal and ethical challenges for nurse managers and staff nurses. The nurse shortage has resulted in a major problem called short staffing caused largely by increases in cost-cutting measures and other financial constraints, as well from deterioration of working conditions. Short staffing refers to the use of an insufficient nursing staff on a unit or in a facility for the number of patients requiring care at various acuity levels. Consequences commonly associated with short staffing include:

- Deterioration of patient outcomes in terms of increased mortality and failure-to-rescue rates (Needleman et al., 2011)
- A general decline in the quality of patient care (Buerhaus et al., 2007; Hassmiller & Cozine, 2006)
- Deterioration of nurse outcomes resulting from increased burnout and greater job dissatisfaction (Agency for Healthcare Research and Quality [AHRQ], 2007)
- Increases in organizational costs resulting from increased turnover (American Hospital Association, 2002; Hassmiller & Cozine, 2006; PricewaterhouseCoopers, 2007)
- Legal liability

In an effort to deal with short staffing, nurse managers are often required to do the following: float nurses to areas in which they are not cross trained, an action that also increases the client-to-nurse ratio closer to staffing requirements; use agency (temporary) personnel; and use unlicensed personnel. Staff nurses, nurse managers, and health care facilities all face numerous possibilities of legal liability—as well as dilemmas involving conflicts between clinical and organizational ethics—as a result of short staffing and actions taken in an effort to temporarily solve this problem (Cooper, 2014).

Nurses need to focus on their use of expert judgment in practicing the highest legal and ethical standards in the quest for high-quality care and services. In some instances, they may also be called on to demonstrate moral courage, which is the courage to honor ethical core values in the face of personal risk. Strategies that are available to the nurse leader chiefly focus on the use of multidisciplinary teams because they can provide an expert group approach to addressing moral and ethical issues. Although not providing definitive answers, the use of a group approach increases the knowledge and ideas that can be brought to bear on the situation and increases analysis that helps to shape the best possible decision under difficult circumstances.

RESEARCH NOTE

Source

Ben-Assuli, O. (2015). Electronic health records, adoption, quality of care, legal and privacy issues, and their implementation in emergency departments. *Health Policy*, *(119)* 287–297.

Hill, G., & Hill, K. (2016). Cross examination. In LAW. COM. Retrieved from http://dictionary.law.com/Default.aspx?selected=408

National Conference of State Legislatures. (2015). *Mental Health Professionals' Duty to Warn*. Retrieved from http://www.ncsl.org/research/health/mental-health-professionals-duty-to-warn.aspx

Skehan, J., & Muller, L. (2016b). Reducing disparities in the LGBT community. *Professional Case Management Journal, 21*(3), 156–160.

Purpose

The purpose of this article was to review and analyze proposed and actual uses of electronic health records (EHR) and health information exchanges (HIE) in the emergency department (ED) and the implications and impact of use of these technologies from the clinical and legal standpoint. The focus was on the current body of evidence regarding the status of care quality as Health Information Technology (HIT) implementation becomes more common.

Discussion

The study reviewed use of EHR around the world and found varying degrees of success. One large and successful study was that of the veterans' health system in the United States. This particular study included over 1000 hospitals. Overall, the study found a greater degree of success in non-profit public (government run) hospitals. Training and readiness had a direct impact on the success and compliance with the newly adopted programs. Regulations requiring EHR have a direct impact on compliance and Medicare and Medicaid use, which—although lower at the time of the study—has increased due to regulatory mandates for phased-in implementation. In the ED, ease of use and accessibility of the system may well be a barrier to adoption if the system design does not take into account physicians' busy workflow.

Legal and privacy concerns are significant due to the rapid advancement of technology. Portable devices and security of patient information are paramount in analysis of the costs and benefits of EHR. One concern was that convenience may lead to carelessness, such a "cut and paste." The issue of accidents or mistakes while using these new systems (due to information technology [IT] glitches and bugs) raises new and unanswered questions about potential liability as it relates to professional liability (malpractice). In addition, there is concern that interaction with the IT system may negatively affect the quality of care, thus again exposing medical professionals to liability. Protecting and maintaining patient privacy has always been a nursing responsibility, but with the advent of uploading and sharing of medical information through an electronic system, these burdens take on new concerns.

Application to Practice

Particular concerns were raised with regard to certain practice areas, such as maternity, contraception, and sexual and mental health. Logic would also indicate that other sensitive areas such as drug and alcohol use, HIV/AIDS, sexual orientation, and transgender issues would generate privacy issues. Would patients resist being forthcoming with sensitive information, knowing that their information would be put into "the system"? Nurses need to be sensitive to patient concerns and use interviewing and observational skills to overcome potential gaps in necessary information.

Policies and procedures are critical to framing how nursing will use electronic access, information, and reporting. Safeguards must be established in cooperation with the IT department. Nurses must always be mindful of HIPAA implications and participate whenever possible in the creation and modification of polices affecting patient privacy. Segregating personal information from patient information and protecting patient privacy must never become lax. Compliance with HIPAA and state privacy laws must be at the forefront of practice.

CASE STUDY

Ohio and Kentucky are an example of the complicated practice issues surrounding nurse licensure, state-to-state variations, and Nurse Licensure Compact (NLC) issues. There are 25 states in the NLC, meaning 25 states are not in the NLC. Suppose a nurse practices near the border of Ohio and Kentucky. The southern border of Ohio is contiguous to the border with northern Kentucky. In fact, the airport for the greater Cincinnati area of Ohio is in Kentucky and known as the Cincinnati/Northern Kentucky International Airport. Thus it is quite common for people (patients) to cross state lines without even thinking about it. Nurses must stop, analyze,

CASE STUDY—cont'd

and make a knowing decision. Since 2007, Kentucky has been a member state of the NLC; Ohio is not (NCSBN, 2016b). Therefore a nurse whose primary residence is in Kentucky can practice in 24 other states, but not in Ohio. A nurse residing in Ohio who wishes to practice nursing in Kentucky must apply for and receive a Kentucky nursing license through the process of reciprocity (also known as endorsement). This process includes an application, fees, background checks, license verification in the home state, and review of transcripts. Once licensed, the nurse must then comply with any and all requirements for nurses' licenses in Kentucky, including but not limited to, renewal applications, fees, continuing education, and compliance with the laws of the state of Kentucky.

The one thing the Ohio nurse—now licensed in Kentucky—will *not* have is a Kentucky NLC license. The nurse can now practice nursing in both Ohio and Kentucky but not in the other 24 compact states. The state of residence is controlling and cannot be changed unless the nurse actually and permanently moves to an NLC state (such as the Ohio nurse moving to Kentucky) and makes a new NLC application with proof of residency. If that happened, the former Ohio nurse would still have to maintain his or her Ohio license in addition to the Kentucky license. The lack of national uniformity in state licensure laws makes nursing practice complicated. However, each nurse must still be knowledgeable about all state nurse practice act laws and regulations that apply to his or her practice in order to practice legally and maintain his or her license.

▌ CRITICAL THINKING EXERCISE

You are the nurse manager of the ED. At 2:00 on Sunday morning, a patient presented in the ED with severe pain, was doubled over and sweating, and had nausea and a fever in excess of 103°F. On paper the individual was John Smith, but when asked, she stated that her name was Wanda Smith. Wanda was quite beautiful, wearing a cocktail dress, with impeccable makeup and long, wavy blonde hair. The patient was unable to sit in the waiting area due to her pain, and after a very short wait was escorted to a treatment area.

The ED nurse (RN) on duty began his assessment of the patient. He noted that on the portion filled out by the patient, the boxes for male or female were left blank. After assisting the patient onto an examination table, the RN said, "I really don't like surprises. Am I going to be surprised when I lift the covers to examine you?" Wanda replied, "I'm not a real girl."

Upon examination, the RN discovered open, weeping wounds in the groin and on male genitals. The RN asked the patient the cause of the wounds and added, "Did someone hurt you?" The patient responded by explaining that they were tape burns from her efforts to "mask" the genitals in female clothing, even swimsuits. She further explained that she had tried twice before to

have a doctor examine her but became frightened and walked away. The RN said, "We're here to help you."

1. By what name should the RN call this patient?
   a. John Smith
   b. No name
   c. Wanda Smith
   d. Sir
   e. Ms.

2. Should the RN ask the patient personal questions about his or her anatomy?
   a. No
   b. Yes, to quench his curiosity
   c. Yes, to conduct a full and accurate assessment based on actual anatomy as it relates the patient's health risks and wellness
   d. None of the above

3. When the RN goes on break, he should:
   a. Laugh and joke about the patient where the patient cannot hear him
   b. Say nothing about the patient in a social setting
   c. Tell co-workers that they have a "tranny" on the unit
   d. Inform the nurse manager how to address the patient and any other pertinent information that needs to be shared with other shifts (Skehan & Muller, 2016a)

Communication Leadership

Kathleen A. Vertino

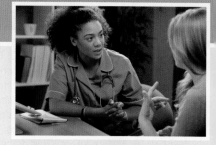

ⓔ http://evolve.elsevier.com/Huber/leadership

Communication is a process by which meaning is assigned to the needs, feelings, perceptions, and interpretation of what is brought to our awareness. There are a number of variables that influence how we assign meaning to our experience and thus affect how we communicate. Successful health care outcomes are dependent on clear communication; therefore all nurses need proficiency in interpersonal skills. Nurse leaders and managers must be mentors, coaches, and role models for effective interpersonal and team communication in order to ensure safe patient outcomes, effective teamwork, and staff satisfaction.

The purpose of this chapter is to enhance nurse leaders' understanding of the pivotal role that communication plays in health care by elucidating the complexities present in human communication, by addressing current key communication issues in health care, and by offering pragmatic strategies using communication models that can be applied to a variety of health care settings.

DEFINITIONS

Communication is based on mutual understanding. Clarity of meaning is derived from a clear definition of terms related to communication. Relevant definitions are as follows:

- **Interpersonal communication:** Communication between two or more individuals involving face-to-face interaction while all parties are aware of the others on an ongoing basis. Each person sends and receives information while continually adapting to the other actors.

- **Non-verbal communication:** Unspoken, this communication is composed of affective or expressive behavior.
- **Persuasion, negotiation, and bargaining:** *Persuasion* is the conscious intent by one individual to modify the thoughts or behaviors of others. *Negotiation* is a dialogical discussion between two or more parties to arrive at an agreement about some issue. To *bargain* is to make a series of offers and counteroffers about what each party will do, give, receive, etc., until an agreement is reached to the satisfaction of all. All three of these involve communication. Persuasion uses argumentation and appeals to logic, whereas negotiation and bargaining may involve some sense of compensation and perhaps coercion, such as bullying or condescending behaviors.
- **Verbal communication:** Includes both written and spoken communication.

BACKGROUND

The literature supports the importance of effective team and interpersonal communication at all levels of an organization. Not only is this key in preventing medical errors, but effective communication and team functioning have also been shown to contribute to patient and staff satisfaction (Nicotera et al., 2014). Despite the focus on patient safety for the past several years, serious issues continue. Specifically, "underreporting of events and near misses, inadequate and unsafe staffing, long work hours, communication lapses, and training and compliance issues" have been reported (Kear & Ulrich, 2015, p.116).

Furthermore, individual, team, and group communication is influenced by organizational climate and culture (see Chapter 3). An organization with a rigid bureaucratic one-way communication network or lack of transparency will impede effective communication among all levels of the organization. A less rigid, more open, transparent structure will encourage creative problem solving and healthy conflict resolution, elements that are needed for healthy organizations. Open communication practices are important because this builds trust. Trust, respect, and empathy are three ingredients that foster positive communication outcomes.

Proficiency in verbal, non-verbal, and written communication is a key leadership quality. Leaders must possess the skills necessary to communicate vision, ensure the mission, and create a culture where this can be achieved. Leaders also need special communication skills in order to implement change.

Interpersonal relationship skills—including the ability to communicate—are as essential to a leader's personal set of leadership skills as psychomotor skills are for a clinical nurse. Leadership ability is predicated on a facility for communication. Human interaction issues are an area where leaders can spend a considerable amount of time. Power and conflict become important focal points of human interaction in organizations that may need managerial intervention or resolution through persuasion or negotiation. Because nurses may frequently be in situations in which they need to persuade others to cooperate, proficiency in managing conflict, bargaining, negotiating, and the art of "crucial conversations" is essential for nurse leaders.

The foregoing skills require practice, experience, assertiveness, and confidence, which are necessary elements in the nurse leader's armamentarium.

Nurses need to be able to feel safe enough to articulate needs, viewpoints, and ideas for improvement of health care and the work environment. Feeling that one has not been heard can be a source of true frustration, anger, and conflict.

Nurse leaders and managers play a crucial role in the management of information and communication for the purpose of effective care coordination and the avoidance of unsafe and error-prone care situations. Clearly providers need high-quality information and access to health care information systems and effective communication models. Nurse leaders are responsible for developing care delivery systems with adequate structure and an effective communication system that enhances care coordination. These systems of communication need to enable patient rescue and safety by coordinating care, preventing information loss, and improving methods of surveillance.

In sum, the crux of the work of successful nurse leaders as communicators depends on their ability to listen and provide empathy to staff needs in order to establish trust and respect and to model behavior and language that sets the tone for a positive and supportive work environment. Equally critical is the development and fostering of similarly effective communication skills in all nurses for peer-to-peer, colleague, and followership interactions.

COMMUNICATION THEORIES AND MODELS

Communication is a process in which information, perception, and understanding are transmitted from person to person. It is important to nurses and is an integral part of any relationship. Nurse leaders and managers can view communication as a tool to accomplish work and meet goals. The significance of communication revolves around its effectiveness and the climate in which communication occurs. Effective communication is enhanced by clear, direct, straightforward, and frequent message transmission. Trust, respect, and empathy are the three ingredients needed to create and foster effective communication.

Much of what was written in the past with respect to communication in health care was about teaching techniques and skills such as interviewing and how to elicit information from patients. These works also included explanations regarding how to reflect, clarify, summarize, provide feedback, use silence, and actively listen. Learning communication techniques is not enough. Communication is more than messages, and human beings are more than senders and receivers. Further, communication models specifically written for nursing are limited, and rigorous studies using randomized controlled trials or systematic reviews to determine the effectiveness of models applicable to nursing practice are not well documented.

Communication is a process that is affected by a number of internal and external variables, takes place on multiple levels of complexity, is difficult to measure, and for which standardized instruments are lacking (Foronda et al., 2015). However, Vertino has developed models to assist in explaining the complexities inherent in human communication (see Figs. 7.1 and 7.2).

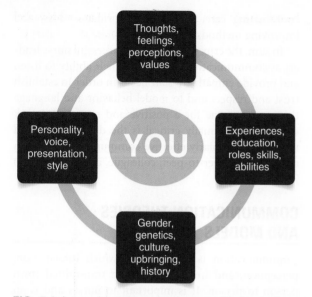

FIG. 7.1 Internal predisposing factors. (Redrawn from Vertino, K.A. [September 30, 2014a]. Effective interpersonal communication: A practical guide to improve your life. *OJIN: The Online Journal of Issues in Nursing, 19*[3], Manuscript 1.)

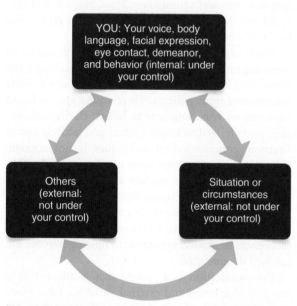

FIG. 7.2 Interaction of internal and external variables. (Redrawn from Vertino, K.A. [September 30, 2014a]. Effective interpersonal communication: A practical guide to improve your life. *OJIN: The Online Journal of Issues in Nursing, 19*[3], Manuscript 1.)

Intrapersonal and Interpersonal Communication

Decades ago, Abraham Maslow developed a model for understanding human needs. He identified that how we respond, react, and behave is based on our needs and whether they are being met. Thus this model is still relevant and is a useful framework for understanding human communication. At the bottom of Maslow's pyramid of human needs are our most basic needs for survival, followed by safety and security, love and belonging, esteem and appreciation, and finally altruistic needs, like fulfillment by helping others and reaching psychological maturity.

Our most basic needs will not be met if we are not able to communicate. Babies cry when they are hungry, tired, uncomfortable, and in need of safety and security. They do not usually speak until about age 1, and then they start to form words, yet their caregivers know what they want and provide for them in their pre-verbal state. This happens because we use body language, facial expressions, and other sounds to communicate. Thus, as a species, we would not survive without communication between and among us, and unmet needs can be a source of conflict, misunderstanding, and anger. There are a number of factors that can influence how we respond. Figs. 7.1 and 7.2—developed by this author and previously published—will help to elucidate this point.

Fig. 7.1 depicts several internal variables that can influence who we are and how we process information—and thus how we respond to the world. However, certain parts of this model are not indelible but dynamic and ever changing. As we grow and mature, our mentors, education, and experiences may influence our thoughts, beliefs, values, and perceptions. Most people grow and evolve with time. Some individuals, however, for a number of reasons, have fixed ideas, perceptions, beliefs, and values that may not change over time. The purpose of the model is to demonstrate that we are complex beings. Therefore it is important to understand that all of these variables exist and can influence how we and others view the world. Having this understanding provides a framework for developing insight into our own behavior, and thus can serve to promote empathy when communicating with others.

With that in mind, Fig. 7.2 depicts how communication may be affected by the interaction of external variables (others, a situation) and internal variables (you).

Similar to Fig. 7.1, this figure is simple, but the possibilities that can exist between and among the variables within the boxes are multitudinous. Further, and more importantly, is that the "internal factors" are the only thing under our own control. We have little or no control over others or the situation, because those are external to us. This point is exceedingly important. When one tries to control other people and situations through various means, communication is likely to be misunderstood, and conflict can be the result. However, when one works on the "you" variables depicted in Fig. 7.2—what you are in control of—a positive outcome will more likely be the result. Why? Because your focus is on your own behavior, facial expression, tone of voice, choice of words, and expressing your feelings and needs. Thus you are communicating in an authentic manner. You are not attempting to force a solution by controlling another person or the situation.

Words and language are powerful tools that can be used to harm or heal (Sears, 2010). Non-verbal communication, such as use of the body and face, can also convey a strong message. To be most direct and straightforward, verbal and non-verbal communication should

be congruent, meaning that our verbal and non-verbal are consistent. Communication problems in interpersonal relationships, whether personal or occupational, can be a source of conflict due to misinterpretation of what was said or meant. Conflict can arise in the work environment when communication is unclear, indirect, or misunderstood.

Unresolved conflict can lead to resentment, backbiting, bullying, and other dysfunctional behaviors. A supportive work environment, positive communication between staff nurses and leadership, and frequent feedback on job performance facilitate nurse job satisfaction. Setting a positive and cooperative tone within a work group is each member's responsibility. Moreover, it is incumbent upon nursing leadership to set the tone of the work environment (such as promoting a healthy work environment) and model impeccable interpersonal communication for the staff.

Helpful Cures for Ineffective Communication

Many times individuals get caught in a situation and are just at a loss for words or cannot come up with the response that feels just right at the time. Table 7.1 displays

TABLE 7.1 Possible Causes, Consequences, and Cures of Ineffective Interpersonal Communication

Possible Causes	Consequences or Possible Interpretations	Possible Cures
1. Social/familial/organizational/cultural taboos regarding "no talk" issues	Frustration; Helplessness; Lack of trust; Substantive issues are ignored	Talk openly about the cultural taboos and how they may have contributed to a climate wherein people are reluctant to share or tackle difficult issues.
2. Poor conflict management skills	Inappropriate and misdirected anger; Finger pointing; Blaming	Learn how to respectfully disagree; Become comfortable with affect (yours and others)
3. Poor negotiation/problem-solving skills	Knee jerk responses; Temporary fixes (Band-Aids); Focus is on "putting out fires" rather than vision	Learn collaboration; Become comfortable with unfinished (long-term) solutions
4. Lack of empathy/understanding of others	Poor team work/spirit; Lack of cooperation; Wasted time and resources	Widen your perceptions and awareness of those around you and the environment
5. Unresolved emotional issues, e.g., history of physical or emotional abuse	Distorted perceptions of the world; Misinterpretation of the motives and messages of others; Distorted responses to communication of others	Resolve your issues and do not focus on other people's issues; to do so means you are avoiding looking at your issues.

Continued

TABLE 7.1   Possible Causes, Consequences, and Cures of Ineffective Interpersonal Communication—cont'd

Possible Causes	Consequences or Possible Interpretations	Possible Cures
6. Poor self-image/self-esteem	Perceived attacks Perceived threats Perceived losses Fear of others or situations	Same as above
7. Negative self-talk (e.g., "I'm a mess.")	Contributes to low self-image and lack of respect from others	Same as above
8. Lack of boundaries	Can be caused by history of abuse	Same as above
9. Lack of insight	Blindness to your faults and flaws robs you of opportunity for personal growth	Be open to input from others Ask for honest feedback Be willing to take constructive criticism
10. Physical or mental illness	Pain, depression, anxiety affects one's ability to focus, listen, and respond	Take care of your health; no one else will do this or should do this for you
11. Hidden agendas, politics, games and tests	Disdain and lack of trust for authority figures Secrets create disempowerment and dependency, which can lead to increased stress, burnout, and lack of creativity and motivation	Do not participate in gossip, rumors, or back-stabbing Demonstrate integrity in all you do Be honest Own your own mistakes
12. Lack of tolerance for change and uncertainty	Playing out scenarios in advance robs you of the opportunity for growth Decreases spontaneity, creativity	Life is not always predictable Change is a part of life Develop a comfort level with it
13. Feigned or planned ignorance, lack of accepting responsibility: "I don't want to know, I don't need to know, it is not my problem."	Disempowers Promotes or maintains unnecessary dependency Allows passing the buck, lack of accountability Promotes immature behavior	As above, communicate clearly and articulately (in writing) who owns what and who has responsibility for what Follow through on your responsibilities Meet deadlines on time
13. Lack of clear plain speech or writing: acronyms, codes, slang, hashtags, accents, culture, apps, jargon	Distancing strategy Power move You can appear uneducated	Never use slang or improper English in professional situations If you lack these skills, learn them
14. Caretaking and enabling behavior	Takes the focus off you and your business Creates unnecessary dependency upon you by other adults who should be caring for themselves	Focus on you and not others Mind your own business Take better care of yourself

From Vertino, K.A. (September 30, 2014a). Effective interpersonal communication: A practical guide to improve your life. *OJIN: The Online Journal of Issues in Nursing, 19*(3), Manuscript 1.

suggested causes, consequences, and possible cures for ineffective communication. This may help to understand how misunderstandings occur and how to avoid (or confront) as needed.

Tools for effective communication and speaking up. Poor communication has consequences for patient safety and can be deadly. Medical errors can be avoided and work environments can become healthier if health care professionals acquire the ability to speak up and discuss emotionally or politically risky topics. Communication breakdowns can be either honest mistakes or undiscussables. Honest mistakes are accidental or unintentional slips and errors such as confusing labels, competing tasks, language barriers, distractions, or gaps during handoffs. Undiscussables occur when someone knows of risks or something being wrong but does not speak up or chooses to ignore or avoid it. A person may back down from the conversation (Maxfield et al., n.d.).

VitalSmarts, the Association of periOperative Registered Nurses, and the American Association of Critical-Care Nurses worked on research to address communication failures and avoidable medical errors. Their 2005 study called *Silence Kills* was followed by the 2010 study *The Silent Treatment,* which confirmed that poor communication is harmful and that despite encountering resistance, nurses need to be enabled to speak up about dangerous shortcuts, incompetence, and disrespect. A safety culture where people speak up when there is a strong suspicion of risk needs to be developed using the communication skills of exceptional nurses and organizational strategies (Maxfield et al., n.d.).

There are some useful tools developed by the Agency for Healthcare Research and Quality's TeamSTEPPS program (AHRQ, 2016) (discussed later in this chapter). With specific scripting, these tools help nurses communicate fully and clearly as well as speaking up when appropriate. For example, AHRQ has developed a pocket guide *(http://www.ahrq.gov/teamstepps/instructor/essentials/pocketguide.html#passbaton)* that presents CUS assertive statements and "I Pass the Baton." The CUS model is a tool to help nurses speak up/speak out in uncomfortable situations. A script is presented, using "I am **c**oncerned," "I am **u**ncomfortable," "this is a **s**afety issue." "Stop the line" is one script used. A constructive approach for managing and resolving conflict is the DESC script: **D**escribe the situation, **e**xpress how the situation makes you feel, **s**uggest other alternatives, and state **c**onsequences in terms of impact on team goals. "I Pass the Baton" is a handoff strategy for the transfer of information during transitions of care. The opportunity to ask questions, clarify information, and confirm the status is established. The script includes introduction, patient identifiers, assessment, situation, safety, background, actions, timing, ownership, and what comes next.

Another helpful tool for effective communication and speaking up is called *crucial conversations,* which gives guidance on providing constructive feedback. Based on a book by Patterson and colleagues (2011), a crucial conversation is defined as a discussion between two or more people where the stakes are high, opinions vary, and emotions run strong. Billed as tools for talking when the stakes are high, the focus is on alleviating failure to communicate. The choices when facing crucial conversations are to avoid them, face them but handle them poorly, or face them and handle them well. Examples of crucial conversations range from ending a relationship to talking to a team member who is not keeping commitments or has a personal hygiene problem to giving an unfavorable peer or performance review. Dialogue skills are learnable. The book and training courses help people learn how to create conditions that make dialogue the path of least resistance; how to use key skills related to talking, listening, and acting together; and how to master tools for talking when the stakes are high. For nurses, this training promotes a culture of safety because team members can then talk about issues and concerns openly even when they touch on areas of silence in health care—such as incompetence, poor team work, and disrespect—or are difficult, risky, or emotionally charged. Some organizations have crucial conversations training for staff to build skills in how to speak and be heard.

Evidence-Based Practice and Communication

Evidence-based practice (EBP) was developed following several reports by the Institute of Medicine (IOM, now called the National Academies of Sciences, Engineering, and Medicine, Health and Medicine Division) that cited staggering numbers of poor patient outcomes related to preventable medical errors. EBP is the preferred model of nursing care for the future. EBP encompasses clinical knowledge coupled with research evidence and patient preference to develop best practices, and it is supported by a number of regulatory organizations. However, despite growing evidence for support of EBP, incorporation of this model into daily clinical practice, "remains inconsistent and presents complex challenges" (Pryse et al., 2014, p. 244). In order for EBP to work in an organization, nurse leaders and those in the work environment must be well informed and supportive of individual nurses who wish to incorporate EBP principles into their nursing care. Pryse and colleagues (2014) developed and tested two psychometric instruments, the *EBP Nursing Leadership Scale* and the *EBP Work Environment Scale,* that can be used by nurse leaders to determine support for EBP within their organization.

One example of EBP that can be readily learned and implemented by nurses is motivational interviewing (MI). MI is an EBP that is supported in the literature as being successfully used by nurses, especially in behavioral health, but it also is expanding into many areas of practice. Briefly, MI is a "collaborative conversation style for strengthening a person's own motivation for change" (Hettema et al., 2014, p. 325). MI uses motivational language to enhance one's ability to make lifestyle changes to promote good health outcomes. Because shared decision making and consideration for patient preference are necessary elements of MI, as the primary caregivers, nurses have the most optimal opportunity to work with patients on behavior change through ongoing communication with them.

Furthermore, MI is a useful tool that can be used by nurse leaders to motivate the workforce and promote change. For example, MI coupled with coaching can enable staff to adopt and integrate EBP into their practice (Hettema et al., 2014). And most importantly, MI principles are a consistent style of communication that is collaborative, respectful, and collegial.

Transformational Leadership and Communication Style

Transformational leadership is a leadership style of communicating that has been well supported in the literature as contributing to nurse satisfaction and retention, decreased medical errors, promotion of a positive work environment, and improved team functioning. It can affect organizational climate and change (Green et al., 2014). The basic goal of transformational leadership is to empower staff to take ownership of their own development (see Chapter 1).

Transformational leadership is designed to inspire, excite, and engage staff to become stakeholders in a shared mission and vision. Reflecting on Maslow's hierarchy of needs, it is obvious that the need for belonging and inclusion in group/family/team is very basic. Nothing feels worse than being shunned or left out, as this can evoke feelings of unworthiness. Effective transformational nurse leaders will engage their staff through role modeling and mentorship of inclusion behaviors such as developing rapport, sharing vision and decision making, providing constructive feedback, and communicating successful outcomes. The communication of transformational leaders is focused on positive interchanges, rather than punishment, and inclusion in decision making versus authoritarianism. Transformational leaders also know

how to share vision and mission and how to motivate the workforce. This is accomplished by communicating the vision with passion and commitment that is contagious. Transformational leaders need to listen more than they talk, be open to all new ideas, and create a culture of safety, transparency, and empathy (Sears, 2010).

ORGANIZATIONAL CULTURE AND CLIMATE

Health care organizations are complex, and role expectations and responsibilities of leadership can change from facility to facility. Some health care organizations are moving away from bureaucratic and hierarchical organizational structures to more facilitative-shared governance models. Some have even adopted the model of servant leadership (see Chapters 1 and 3).

The entire tone of the organization is based mostly on unspoken cultural norms. Because nurses make up the bulk of the health care workforce, having nurse leaders at the helm of the organization can influence the culture and climate of the organization as a whole.

For example, a vision is communicated by means of passion and commitment that needs to be contagious. Leaders need to listen more than they talk, be open to all new ideas, and create a culture of safety, transparency, and empathy (Sears, 2010).

For most of the past century, concern for the manner by which human beings are treated has increased, not only on an international and national level but also in business and industry. The need for humane behavior toward people—especially in communication behavior—is particularly important as health care evolves into a larger and more complex industry. For example, bullying, discriminatory, and hateful language communicates disrespect, inflames passions, and disrupts healthy work environments.

According to workplace specialists, job satisfaction has been found to include much more than salary increases, decreased overtime, and tangible rewards. Appreciation, trust, and respect are not quantifiable but are extremely valuable. These, as well as support for individual growth and a sense of purpose, have been identified as important factors in job satisfaction. Job satisfaction means having a leader who is fair and honest, listens to concerns, and helps the team to develop knowledge, attitudes, and skills to advance their careers. Some have suggested that nurses probably do not leave agencies; they leave dehumanizing nursing leaders. Nurse leaders need to be in touch with the degree to which nursing staff are satisfied. Job satisfaction remains an important issue in the workplace environment, given nurse shortages and high reported levels of burnout. Fackler and colleagues (2015) found that as nurses' perceived power increased, they were more likely to have an "improved perception of their work environment" (p. 267). Communicating trust and respect are central aspects.

Nurse leaders can set the tone and expectations for everyone they come in contact with, not just those who directly report to them. Much has been written about the effectiveness of informal power and that more often than not, those without official title and position have more influence among leaders and peers than those with formal title and position (see Chapter 1). Therefore any nurse can exert influence on the cultural norms and climate of the organization, and nurse leaders should model this empowerment approach for all nurses.

It is proposed that if health care personnel—especially nurses—are regarded in a manner that acknowledges all characteristics of human beings, then these personnel will tend to regard the patients, clients, peers, and professional colleagues in a similar manner. Because registered nurses (RNs) constitute the largest health care occupation in the United States, with 2.7 million jobs of the approximately 4.8 million people employed in hospitals in the United States (US Department of Labor, Bureau of Labor Statistics, 2012), humanizing efforts become important to the fabric of health care.

HOLISTIC AND SPIRITUAL HEALTH CARE

Numerous papers have been published in the health care literature regarding spirituality, but for the most part they have focused on palliative, end-of-life care, and parish nursing. In the past, the responsibility of providing spiritual care for hospitalized patients largely fell to the hospital chaplain. However, The Joint Commission (TJC, 2008) has included requirements regarding spiritual care of hospitalized patients, and there is an expectation for documentation of spiritual assessments. This is necessary because social, spiritual, religious, and cultural values and beliefs may indeed affect individual patients' health care decisions and preferences. Because individuals are bio-psycho-social-spiritual beings, the holistic paradigm is the desired mode of health care

delivery and needs to be reflected in communication and practice. The spiritual component of the holistic paradigm of health care has received the most recent attention; however, because a holistic model of health care encompasses body, mind, and spirit, holistic health care and spiritual care must be discussed concurrently.

Spirituality is in itself complex, unique, and difficult to define and measure because it is a broad general term that is not easily operationalized (Wu et al., 2015). Burkhart and colleagues (2011) defined spirituality as "a dimension of human beings associated with the human expression of meaning, purpose, and transcendence in life" (p. 2463). Spirituality can indeed overlap with religious practices, beliefs, and rituals as well, and the difference between the two is not always clearly understood. Regardless, there is a great need in health care to provide holistic care (body, mind, and spirit) to patients regardless of religious, ethnic, or cultural characteristics, in a humane (nonjudgmental and compassionate) manner. Respect for all persons and their beliefs is an essential component of holistic health care and nursing practice.

Alternative and complementary medicine, homeopathy, Ayurveda, and natural healing such as Reiki have increased in popularity in recent years. Although there has been a recent resurgence in the popularity of energy healing and Reiki, this is not new. Therapeutic touch (TT) was introduced to nursing practice by Dolores Krieger in the 1970s (Krieger, 1979).

Although Reiki, for instance, has been used in hospitals (Rand, n.d.), these modalities of "healing" fall under the auspices of New Age practices and are controversial in their benefits as well as lacking evidence in the scientific literature (Joyce & Herbison, 2015). These modes of delivering care may have gained success and popularity not necessarily because people are looking for more natural cures but because there is a relationship, bond, rapport, or human connection with the practitioner. Whether the provider of care practices traditional or alternative medicine does not matter, what matters is the patient's feeling of connectedness and trust for the health care provider. Within that sacred space of interpersonal trust and understanding lies spiritual communication and care. It is in that space where healing occurs.

Spirituality in Practice

The literature reveals there are many questions about the ways in which spirituality assessments are conducted and whether one assessment tool can prove adequate in measuring the significance of spirituality in the lives of individuals, all of whom may interpret its meaning differently. Simply asking the patient or family if they desire a visit from the chaplain, priest, rabbi, minister, or church elder may provide the patient with an opening to discuss his or her religious preferences and/or spiritual beliefs. Listening in a nonjudgmental manner may be enough to encourage the patient to share. If the patient shares his or her beliefs and asks about the nurse's, this is acceptable reciprocal communication that will serve to build rapport.

Implementing spiritual care in clinical practice within a facility is an example of communication leadership. In order for hospitals to fully integrate spiritual care as part of the organizational mission, a concerted effort is needed by health care leaders both in education and practice to assist staff in discovering personal barriers that may prevent their ability to tend to patient's individual spiritual needs (Battey, 2012). Moreover, leadership needs to become much more familiar and comfortable with the current models that are available and adapt one to meet the needs of their particular organization and staff (Battey, 2012; Wu et al., 2015).

LEADERSHIP AND MANAGEMENT IMPLICATIONS

Extensive documentation in the literature exists regarding the disruptive and distracting communication interactions that occur not only between nurses and between nurses and professional colleagues (e.g., physicians, pharmacists, administrators) but also between nurses and patients. The research, the literature, and common knowledge from media accounts indicate that nursing personnel experience high turnover rates, job dissatisfaction, and burnout; many RNs are leaving the profession. The shortage of nursing personnel in most areas of the United States has had a negative effective on retention of nurses. The work environment is described as hostile to nurses, and patient outcomes of increased severity of illness and mortality have been directly related to poor communication skills of the staff. The clinical ambiance and interpersonal communication received by nurses need to change. Leaders can set realistic goals, model appropriate communication practices, and make a difference where nurses live and work.

With the advent of changes in health care and subsequent shrinkage in resources, new methods of communication have been developed to aid staff in providing high quality care while accounting for patient preference and published evidence. The next section discusses models that can be employed by nurse leaders to address issues in the health care environment resulting from ineffective communication.

Hostile Work Environment

Nurses work in complex, highly interpersonal, relationship-based work environments.

Professional relationships can be problematic. Conflict, poor colleague relationships, decreased job satisfaction, reduced productivity, and quality/safety concerns result. Leaders can help nurses gain insight into their own behavior, how it affects others and the work environment, and how to use strategies to cope, become resilient, and advocate for workplace communication improvements at all levels.

There is support on a national level to promote effective communication and collaboration. It is important that positive interdisciplinary relationships are established and are active in the organizational culture. The workplace does not have to be hostile. Nurse leaders have a responsibility to communicate zero tolerance for bullying and a hostile environment.

The professional nurse traditionally has had the closest and longest interpersonal contact with patients compared with most other health care providers. In this same health care system, technology rules in a labor-intense service industry, as seen in all the buildings, equipment, and sophisticated monitoring machines that need to be operated by human beings. Yet nursing colleagues, as well as other health care professionals, overlook the need to communicate with one another in a holistic and humanizing way.

According to the Workplace Bullying Institute (2016), although many good nurses have been driven out by toxic environments, many other nurses have just accepted those environments. Whatever solutions have been proposed thus far do not seem to be working, as this problem continues to plague the profession *(http://www.workplacebullying.org/)*. Unfortunately, this does not apply only to staff nurses who work in hospitals. This can also occur between junior and senior faculty members and anywhere else where a "pecking order" exists. The phenomenon has been called "eating our young," and solutions that reverse these practices need to be found and implemented.

Nonviolent Communication

Expanding on nonviolent communication (NVC) concepts developed by Dr. Marshall Rosenberg (2004), Melanie Sears (2010) took aim at the health care system in her book *Humanizing Health Care*. In a nutshell, NVC is predicated on the notion that our language, which is based on our culture and experience, is replete with judgment, criticisms, labels, and phraseology that is bound to create defensive reactions in others and is considered violent. Further, and more importantly, she quotes Rosenberg to say, "the labels, analyses and judgments of others are *tragic* expressions of your own unmet needs" (Sears, 2010, p. 56).

Recalling our earlier discussion of Maslow's hierarchy of needs, this makes perfect sense. Unmet needs in the area of belonging—a basic need—can create issues of safety or feelings of insecurity or of feeling threatened. Anger or helplessness are two responses that may be seen in people trying to protect themselves. Also recall the discussion of personal variables and internal predisposing factors discussed in Fig. 7.1 and how these variables shape how individuals view the world. No one is safe in a hostile work environment. Therefore, when one feels threatened or unsafe, one may regress to an earlier stage of development when they felt safe and respond in a childlike manner. This may account for behavior that we may consider to be immature.

Sears proposed a four-part nonviolent communication process grounded in compassion, empathy, and honesty. She stated that "Empathy is one of the simplest yet most potent technologies on the planet. It is a low-cost, high yield solution that everyone can use" (p. 88).

The four parts include making an observation, expressing a feeling, expressing a need, and making a request without demanding. Table 7.2 is an adaptation of these four parts of NVC developed by Rosenberg.

Nurses are by and large caretakers of others and thus may be great at making observations. But they may lack the ability to express their own feelings and needs and lack the ability to make a straightforward request. By becoming proficient at expressing their own feelings and needs and communicating requests in a clear, direct manner, nurses are providing for their own self-care. Only in this way can nurses truly care for others.

TABLE 7.2 Four Parts of Nonviolent Communication (NVC)

Clearly Expressing (Without Blaming or Criticizing)	Empathetically Receiving (Without Hearing Blame or Criticism)
1. Making an observation	1. What you observe
2. Expressing a feeling	2. How you feel based on your observation
3. Stating what you need	3. How you feel based on what you are hearing
4. Making a request (without demanding)	4. Hearing the request for an action to be taken.

From Rosenberg, M.B. (2004). *We can work it out: Resolving conflicts peacefully and powerfully.* Encinitas, CA: Puddledancer Press.

Team/Group Communication: TeamSTEPPS and SBAR

Nurse leaders need to be familiar with group theory because little is accomplished in a health care facility without individual participation in a team, group, or meeting. Participation in groups is a necessary part of the functioning of the larger organization. In principle, the degree to which individual need satisfaction is achieved differentiates effective from ineffective groups; the greater the individual's satisfaction, the higher the probability of group effectiveness (Hersey et al., 2013).

Group theorists have articulated different stages of group development. One of the most popular theories, first postulated by Tuckman in 1965, contains four stages as follows: forming, storming, norming, and performing. In the forming stage the group needs direction in defining tasks, goals, and objectives. Members are unclear regarding their respective roles in the group. This initial period can be chaotic and confusing. The next stage is storming. As the name connotes, there can be conflict, and indeed there must be conflict for the group to sort through issues such as leadership, power, and roles. Usually there is some willingness to accept the group goals and objectives, but there are still differences of opinion, competition for recognition, and attempts to influence the group. During the norming period, there is greater agreement on the task goals as the group develops cohesiveness and adjusts to the group and task. Finally, during the performing period, the members are thinking as one and willingly performing the task. There is camaraderie and team spirit as the group becomes self-managing (Hersey et al., 2013).

Members assume a variety of roles within the process of a group. Most are constructive in nature, contributing to the discussion, solving the problem, and achieving the group goal. These roles may be questioning, suggesting possibilities, taking notes, and summarizing the group's progress. However, some roles are not helpful. The most disruptive periods in group process are with intergroup dissonance and competition. It is at these levels that members may behave in roles that hinder group effectiveness, such as criticizing, attacking, or name-calling. The leader needs to intervene as appropriate with discussions of goals, standards, and feedback on behavior and progress for individuals or the group, depending on the situation. The degree to which roles are not helpful probably influences member satisfaction, and certainly interferes with communication and collaboration (Hersey et al., 2013). For example, using a generic team-based communication model, Matzke and colleagues (2014) analyzed conversations between nurses and physicians. Their findings indicated that although about half of the conversations were considered collegial, communication was status based rather than team based. Status-based communications were described as patterns that allow an individual with more perceived power to be more forceful and directive in his or her communication toward other team members. Unfortunately, this autocratic style of communication does not support team building or promote good working relationships, and this can lead to preventable medical errors.

Research in small task group process has also revealed movement from an initial organization through a period of disorganization or chaos to reorganization at a level that achieves a goal. A group is defined as two or more people, and it exists to meet the needs of each individual in the group so that each will be satisfied. The leader's four major styles of communication used with task groups are similar to those for individuals (telling, selling, participating, and delegating). The process includes moving from defining, clarifying, and involving to empowering according to the leader's assessment of the readiness of the group (Hersey et al., 2013). The relationship styles of defining, clarifying, involving, and empowering suggest the highest probability of success for the manner in which the leader relates to the group.

TeamSTEPPS

The Agency for Healthcare Research and Quality (AHRQ) has collected data regarding patient safety over many years. They discovered that poor communication was the number one cause of preventable medical errors (Kleiner et al., 2014). After discovering the staggering number of preventable medical errors and recognizing that communication problems were cited as the number one contributor, the AHRQ partnered with the Department of Defense (DOD) and developed the TeamSTEPPS program (AHRQ, 2016).

TeamSTEPPS is an evidence-based, comprehensive education and training program designed to improve patient safety by eliminating preventable medical errors related to ineffective team communication. TeamSTEPPS stands for **T**eam **S**trategies and **T**ools to **E**nhance **P**erformance and **P**atient **S**afety. TeamSTEPPS has been adapted and implemented effectively in a number of health care settings and across numerous specialty areas. Much support exists in the literature documenting the utility and effectiveness of TeamSTEPPS. The program consists of five key principles: team structure, leadership, situation monitoring, mutual support, and communication. Fig. 7.3 is a visual depiction of the five key principles of the TeamSTEPPS program. Extensive education and training programs are available on the AHRQ website.

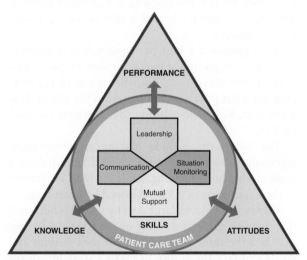

FIG. 7.3 Model of TeamSTEPPS key principles of teamwork. (From Agency for Healthcare Research and Quality. [2016]. *TeamSTEPPS: Strategies and tools to enhance performance and patient safety.* Rockville, MD: Author. Retrieved from http://www.ahrq.gov/professionals/education/curriculum-tools/teamstepps/index.html)

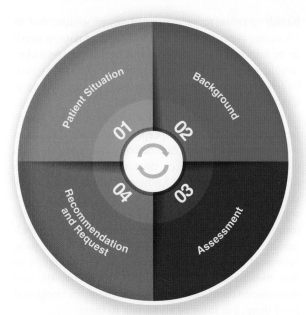

FIG. 7.4 Four steps in the SBAR process.

SBAR and Handoff Communication

To address the "communication arm" of the TeamSTEPPS model pictured at the left side of Fig. 7.4, strategies such as SBAR have been created to enhance teamwork communication. One of the strategies that has been well documented and is familiar to nurses is SBAR, which stands for: Situation, Background, Assessment, and Recommendation.

Compton and colleagues (2012) implemented SBAR education across a large multihospital health system and found that SBAR was generally well understood, but it was inconsistently used across facilities and was sometimes inaccurately viewed as a "document rather than a verbal technique" (p. 261). In addition, Anderson and colleagues (2014) conducted a review of 45 papers discussing bedside handoff tools. They found that utilization of a specific method or model for a clinical handoff is documented in the literature, and although no single tool was consistently successful, a customized approach was well supported. Fig. 7.4 demonstrates the four steps involved in SBAR.

Although originally developed to facilitate communication between nurses and providers in urgent care situations (Compton et al., 2012), SBAR has demonstrated utility in other situations. SBAR promotes nurse-to-nurse reporting of focused, timely, prioritized information during shift and round reporting (Cornell et al., 2014) (see Chapter 4 for more on SBAR).

TeamSTEPPS huddles—another strategy for development of team cohesiveness and used for handoff communication—have been found to create a "shared mental model" within the team and promote employee satisfaction (Glymph, et al., 2015, p. 185; Plonien & Williams, 2015). HUDDLE stands for Healthcare Utilizing Deliberate Discussion Linking Events. The purpose of the huddle is to exchange information and brief team members on potential patient safety concerns proactively. Huddles can be briefings at the beginning of the day or can be called at any time throughout the day if a team member has a concern. Debriefing, another type of huddle implemented in the TeamSTEPPS model, is a review process after an event. In order for this model to be fully successful it is imperative that leadership supports, educates, mentors, and models these important patient safety team processes (Glymph et al., 2015). Units use huddles at the top of each shift or change-over as a standardized and real-time way to address critical communication needs and to make sure that information is consistently communicated.

COMMUNICATION TO FACILITATE CHANGE: KOTTER

In alignment with the goals of the Institute of Medicine's (IOM, 2011) report on *The Future of Nursing*, nurses are called upon to "lead change to advance health," yet the report acknowledges that several barriers exist that prevent nurses from responding to this call and participating fully in the rapidly changing health care environment. Kotter (1996) proposed a model in business for making change in organizations. This framework underscores that all change is made by communication, and the effectiveness and *sustainability* of the change is based on the skilled communication of the leadership and stakeholders endorsing the change process.

Kotter (1996) suggested the following are needed to empower people to make change: communicate the vision to employees, make structures compatible with the vision, provide the training employees need, align information and personnel systems, and confront supervisors who undercut needed change. Further, he suggested that structures, skills, systems, and supervisors are generally the four barriers to any transformational process. Before implementing change, the nurse leader is well advised to first analyze the communication pattern currently in place at the macro and micro level and to be cognizant of

BOX 7.1   Kotter's Eight-Stage Process of Creating Major Change

1. Establishing a Sense of Urgency
2. Creating the Guiding Coalition
3. Developing a Vision and a Strategy
4. Communicating The Change Vision
5. Empowering Broad-Based Action
6. Generating Short-Term Wins
7. Consolidating Gains and Producing More Change
8. Anchoring New Approaches in the Culture

From Kotter, J. (1996). *Leading change* (p. 21). Boston, MA: Harvard Business School Press.

the organization's general culture, climate, and politics. Box 7.1 outlines the points of Kotter's change process.

Leadership must be part of the guiding coalition in all of these stages to be supportive and communicate needed change. Kotter stated that the barriers that can interfere with change are: "inwardly focused cultures, paralyzing bureaucracy, parochial politics, a low level of trust, lack of teamwork, arrogant attitudes, a lack of leadership in middle management, and general human fear of the unknown" (p. 20). He also stated that organizations that are more manager versus leader oriented will not produce needed change that is sustainable, because managers "plan, organize and control," whereas leaders "establish direction, align people, and motivate and inspire," qualities that are needed to "produce extremely useful change" (p. 26).

CURRENT ISSUES AND TRENDS

Diversity in Patient Population and Health Care Workforce

Global health care is a current reality. Moderate to large cities in the United States contain university-based medical centers that provide education to health care personnel from all over the world. In the same vein, the patients to whom nurses provide care have emigrated from many countries of the world. Patients and health care personnel come from every religion, culture, race, and ethnicity. Because of this diversity, nurses need to be aware of—and have respect for—individual cultural differences that may affect health care delivery.

For example, a female patient may wish to have a female provider, particularly if her religious beliefs prohibit her from disrobing in front of a male who is not her husband. Nurses need to find her a female provider. Also, a Catholic nurse or doctor may recuse himself or

herself or refuse to participate in any procedure that, in his or her view, does not respect life. That request needs to be honored. Both patients and health care providers should be allowed to be comfortable with their own beliefs without judgment, criticism, or repercussions. Communications need to reflect this.

Leaders and managers must set the tone for acceptance of diversity and be prepared to make allowances when necessary so that care delivery can continue in an efficient manner. Further, nurses are not expected as health care providers to know everything about every culture, but they are expected to respect all human persons. Nursing is a profession in which nurses become intimate with patients on many levels. People are vulnerable when they are sick. They may cry out in pain, scream at us, laugh with us, and disclose things to us that they have not shared with anyone else. We feed them, bathe them, dress them, walk them, and poke and prod them, but most of all we talk to them.

It is quite acceptable to admit that you know nothing about their particular native country, ethnicity, habits, food, and/or religious practices. Most people are happy to share this with you. Food is usually a great place to start because nurses need to know their patient's dietary restrictions. This may also arise when dining with co-workers who abstain from consuming certain food items. The key point is to respect patients' and colleagues' beliefs, values, morals, and manner of dressing, washing, praying, eating or fasting—and never judge another because his or her manner of living differs from your own.

COMMUNICATION ISSUES

Teaching Communication

There are many approaches to teaching communication skills to nursing students. Most approaches are based on procedures, techniques, and/or rubrics that provide an agenda of topics for specific case situations. Communication seems to be such a broad topic that it is unclear what to include. In addition, teaching communication skills is particularly challenging in culturally diverse situations. What is needed is a general communication theory specifically for nursing that will provide a framework from which to teach communication skills to nursing students.

The NVC model is applicable to all situations in nursing practice, and thus it can serve as a benchmark theory. This nursing theory can be used with other nursing theories to provide a unique perspective on the communication dimension of interpersonal interactions. NVC is a simple model with relatively few steps. It provides examples of how to choose words and language. This—coupled with the author's models depicted in Figs. 7.1 and 7.2 regarding how our own shaping can influence us—provides the nurse with insight and serves to provide possibilities to change negative, unhelpful communication patterns. It provides direction to change relationships into empathetic interaction patterns and attitudes.

Another model with similar underpinnings is the VERA framework. The VERA (validation, emotion, reassurance, activity) framework for communication was developed to meet a need for nursing students who were at a loss to communicate with persons with communication difficulties (Hawkes et al., 2015). Because the focus is on compassion, expression of emotion, and providing validation via support, it very much resembles the principles of NVC.

There is a need to determine a theoretically based and research evidence–supported approach to teaching communication. It is important that this approach be most effective in developing interpersonal communication skills in nursing students to ensure that they have the highest probability of responding in an empathetic manner with patients in critical life situations.

Patient Privacy

A related concern for the management of information and communication is how to prevent breaches of patient confidentiality. The Health Insurance Portability and Accountability Act (HIPAA) provisions have heightened awareness about and presented strategies to protect patients' privacy and data security in health care transactions. For example, fax transmissions need to be secure, and security measures need to be taken to protect computerized databases and electronic transmissions. End-user encryption is commonly used for data security. Health care providers' actions that disseminate confidential information can harm patients. For example, some nurses are uncomfortable performing handover reporting at the patient's bedside because of the risks of sharing patient information where other persons may be within earshot. Discretion and sensitivity are best used in these situations. Systems, processes, and structures can be altered to protect patient privacy.

Communication in Emergencies

Communication effectiveness becomes crucial in times of emergency or disaster. In fact, often one of the key outcomes of disaster drills is to identify breaks in the communication system so they can be fixed before a real-time event occurs. As discussed earlier, TeamSTEPPS was initially developed to address communication issues between nurses and providers during critical patient events. Communication at these times must be impeccable. The AHRQ offers a plethora of team communication tools on their website for teams to practice and role-play so that they can be prepared to address issues efficiently during emergency situations.

One leadership situation occurs when a nurse presents a proposal to a committee who must be convinced to release the money for a project that is vital to the care of clients. Strategic planning and a written business plan are used to determine how to maximize the message delivery. This may include knowing how to structure the communication non-verbally as well as verbally so that a positive impression is created to set the stage for a full and impartial hearing.

Written Communication

The entire health care system relies on reliable, efficient tools and methods to produce timely and accurate patient documentation. The nursing profession, at the hub of the health care system, is called upon to produce the lion's share of the day-in, day-out documentation that exists in health care facilities. Proficiency and professionalism are imperative in all written documentation. One must have a command of the English language in order to produce written information that is useful and readable. Patient documentation is only one form of written communication needed by nursing staff. Promotions and awards in the profession are usually based on written documentation of performance and outcomes endorsing an individual staff member. Grants and funds for projects are based upon extensive written proposals that address specific criteria. Quality improvement initiatives within a hospital can be awarded based on both written proposals and oral presentations, such as those making a business case for a clinically based initiative. Sharing information with colleagues is nurses' professional responsibility, such as by authoring textbooks and journals and providing expertise as peer reviewers and subject matter experts.

Electronic Communication and Social Media

With the advent of e-mail and explosion of social media and cell phones, the avenues of communication have changed. Health care systems have kept pace by developing extensive internal information technology (IT) departments that have engineered electronic medical records, secured e-mail servers for communication between patients and their providers, and developed numerous health care "apps." Electronic communication has assisted us to be better informed regarding our patients. However, within the professional health care realm, there is a tendency to rely on these modes of communication when other methods would be preferable and more appropriate. For instance, there are definite times when a face-to-face conversation is preferred to an e-mail. Warrell (2012) noted that there are four times you should *never* use e-mail: (1) when you are mad, (2) when rebuking or criticizing, (3) if there is any chance your words could be misunderstood, or (4) when you are canceling or apologizing. In our busy professional lives, it is easier to send off a quick e-mail than to pick up the phone or walk down the hall; however, e-mail distances us from others and is really only the preferred means of communication when information is simply being conveyed. It is not appropriate for a back-and-forth dialogue where feelings need to be expressed and opinions heard.

Similarly, texting, social media, Facebook, Twitter, and hashtags (#) can be overused, making face-to-face conversations a thing of the past. Video chatting provides a nice way to have a conversation and actually see the person. There are several very good health care apps that have been produced for downloading on smartphones for free or at a fairly minimal cost. Some of these apps are very useful; some are a waste of time and money. The important thing to remember is to maintain professionalism and appropriate boundaries when using social media and to be judicious in what information is shared about yourself and others publicly. Many organizations have formal social media policies to help nurses navigate around what is appropriate for sharing on social media. Patient privacy, potential HIPAA violations, perceived bullying, and damage to reputations are major concerns.

RESEARCH NOTE

Source

Vertino, K.A. (2014b). Evaluation of a TeamSTEPPS initiative on staff attitudes toward teamwork. *Journal of Nursing Administration, 44*(2), 97–102.

Purpose

It is well documented that poor team communication is the number one contributor to preventable medical errors. Poor team communication can also lead to low morale, high nurse turnover, and a hostile work environment. The purpose of this study was to determine whether a customized TeamSTEPPS training program conducted with nursing staff on an inpatient hospital unit would lead to changed attitudes toward teamwork.

Discussion

The study had two research questions: (1) Does TeamSTEPPS implementation with nursing staff on an inpatient unit result in improved attitudes toward teamwork?, and (2) Are there differences among occupational groups (RNs, LPNs, NAs) and years of clinical experience on attitudes toward teamwork? The theoretical framework for the study was based on Kotter's Change Model. A pre-experimental (pre-test/post-test) repeated measures design was used, and 26 staff were provided with a 4-hour classroom training session in TeamSTEPPS. This was followed by site visits, coaching, and mentoring to provide support and follow up, coupled with periodic phone and e-mail communications. Of the original 26 staff who completed the pre-test and received the training, 18 were eligible to take the post-test. The instrument used for testing was the TeamSTEPPS Teamwork Attitude Questionnaire (T-TAQ) a 30-item attitude assessment questionnaire. Descriptive statistics as well as a repeated measures analysis of covariance (ANCOVA) with two within (pre/post) and one between (occupational group) factors with three levels (RN, LPN, NA) were used. Covariates were years of experience and baseline (pre-test) T-TAQ scores. Results indicated that there was statistical significance at $p \leq 0.001$ across all five teamwork constructs tested by the T-TAQ. Neither occupational group nor years of experience moderated any of the T-TAQ scores or subscales, which indicated that they had no effect. Two exit questions were posed to the staff, asking (1) if they felt teamwork had improved, and (2) if they felt there was a culture change on the unit as a result of the training. These responses were analyzed using Chi-square. 82% thought there was an improvement in teamwork on their unit ($p = 0.008$) but only 61% thought there was a culture change ($p = 0.467$, ns). Results indicated that TeamSTEPPS training did result in improved attitudes toward teamwork.

Application to Practice

This study could not have been conducted without support from nursing leadership. Four-hour training classes had to be provided to all eligible full- and part-time staff on all three shifts, which took considerable planning between the project director and the nurse manager of the unit. Upper level nursing management needed to be engaged as Kotter's "guiding coalition" as well. Despite challenges in implementation of the training sessions and limitations of the study, the results support that a tailored, short-term unit-based intervention can result in changed attitudes toward teamwork of nursing staff.

CASE STUDY

Nurse Olivia Smith works as a charge nurse on a busy inpatient unit. The unit was somewhat chaotic because they had seen three nurse managers come and go in the past 18 months. Responsibility for the floor frequently fell to the charge nurses. Nurse Smith generally spent her days on duty feeling somewhat frustrated because she seemed to be responsible for so many patient care problems as well as staffing issues. Short staffing has resulted in mandatory overtime and frequent call-ins. Staff are complaining of burnout and feeling powerless to change anything on their units. Further, when there were staffing concerns on other units, Nurse Smith might be pulled from her regular duties to fill in elsewhere, only to return to the floor to find other patient care and staff issues awaiting her, or providers approaching her with unsolved problems that had arisen when she was away.

Staff and leadership frequently asked for support from Nurse Smith because she was efficient, organized, and trustworthy. She heard about the TeamSTEPPS program from another nurse and decided to read about it. She went to the AHRQ website and found all the material. This convinced her to attend a training session. She discussed this with her nurse manager and promised that upon returning from the training program she would provide training for the nurses on the unit. Nurse Smith learned about the importance of daily huddles, briefs and debriefs, and wrote a short proposal to leadership to train the nurses. She implemented these on her unit. After just a few short weeks, staff began to work more together as a team, felt more supported by one another, and the morale on the unit was improving despite the fact that the workload had not changed.

CRITICAL THINKING EXERCISE

You are the charge nurse for the weekend inpatient psychiatric unit. A newly admitted patient is known to you and the other staff. The patient has multiple psychiatric and medical comorbidities. His care is generally very complex, involving both medical and psychiatric providers due to his documented diagnoses of bipolar disorder, alcohol dependence, and diabetes. He is frequently hospitalized due to exacerbations in his medical and psychiatric conditions and due to non-adherence to medications and outpatient follow up-appointments. On admission to the floor, he is initially loud, demanding, and exhibiting manic behavior. He is disheveled, his face is flushed, his speech is pressured, and his mood is very labile. When he sees you he begins crying, stating he is in terrible pain from his diabetic neuropathy; he complains his hands and feet are burning and tingling. Because you have a rapport with him, he allows you to check his blood sugar. It is 537.

1. What are your priorities in caring for this patient?
2. Who do you call first and why? What do you say?
3. Using the SBAR tool, succinctly describe what you would report when making a call to the provider(s).

Team Building and Working With Effective Groups

Anne Gallagher Peach

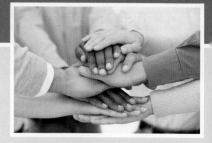

http://evolve.elsevier.com/Huber/leadership

Nurse leaders in today's health care organizations must be skilled communicators, collaborators, and facilitators with an exquisite ability to lead the collective work of individuals. At times they will serve as a leader for a team or group, and at other times they will serve as a member. Being capable of both leading and following are essential skills for nurses. A significant percentage of work completed in organizations today is done through the collaborative efforts of different types of teams or work groups. There is an even greater emphasis on shared leadership in nursing as well as working with other health care professionals as part of an interdisciplinary or multidisciplinary team. Understanding the characteristics of teams, groups, and the basic principles for attaining successful outcomes increases the leader's effectiveness.

Health care leaders recognize that an interdisciplinary, team-based approach is essential for high-quality, patient-centered, coordinated, and effective health care. Teamwork allows for greater exchange of information, ideas, and problem solving to address the complex issues of health care. Engaging teams in this process allows for diverse points of view, creativity, innovation, and an enhanced ability to adapt to continuous or sudden change. The health care environment continues to evolve at an unprecedented rate with new specialized knowledge, scientific and technological advances, and redesign of care processes. A high degree of specialization exists, even within a particular profession. The nursing profession, for example, includes individuals with a variety of different roles, including direct care registered nurses, licensed practical nurses, nurse practitioners, clinical nurse specialists, nurse educators, nurse midwives, and nurse anesthetists. Establishing effective teamwork across various specialties within and across professions is key to interdisciplinary collaboration to address and adapt to the constant state of change in health care.

The ability to collaborate is essential for optimal patient outcomes. The focus of health care organizations today is to achieve the Institute of Health Care Improvement's (IHI, 2016) Triple Aim. The goal is "simultaneously improving the health of the population, enhancing the experience and outcomes of the patient, and reducing per capita cost of care for the benefit of communities." The shift in payment methodologies from fee-for-service to value-based purchasing and accountable care has created incentives and penalties for organizations to improve quality, efficiency, and the overall value of health care. The expectation for health care leaders is to continuously improve while delivering safe, high-quality patient care. Changing reimbursement methodologies, increasing governmental regulation, and managing care across the continuum require a high level of engagement between clinical disciplines, non-clinical staff, and senior management. Just as in other industries, rapid information dissemination and the shift to a knowledge worker–based service society are some of the social and economic forces operative in health care. These forces converge to create the tumultuous change currently underway in health care delivery. Teamwork is the solution.

Employees who work in a collaborative manner with others and who are able to work effectively within a team

---

Photo used with permission from Photos.com.

context can provide the strength, structure, and resiliency to deal with work complexities and changes. Today's health care organizations are considered *learning organizations* (see Chapter 2), and there is a renewed emphasis on the role of teams. Just as interdisciplinary teams play an important role in delivering mental health, home care, rehabilitation, hospice, and other community-based services, hospitals and large health care systems engage teams as an essential element of their core processes and structure. This is the general way now that business gets done in all health care settings. The Institute of Medicine (IOM, now called the National Academies of Sciences, Engineering, and Medicine, Health and Medicine Division) suggests that working as part of an interdisciplinary team is an essential core competency of health care professionals and suggested that professionals cooperate, collaborate, communicate, and integrate care in teams to be sure that care is continuous and reliable (Grenier & Knebel, 2003).

Because health care professionals are specialists, it is incumbent on leaders to bring people together in groups and teams to build on their knowledge and strengths and ultimately to ensure safe, effective care. Leaders have an ever-increasing role to ensure that teams are effective, efficient, and productive. In their book *The Wisdom of Teams: Creating the High-Performance Organization,* Katzenbach and Smith (2015) claimed that teams should be the basic unit of organization for most businesses as a way to reach the highest levels of performance.

The IOM's (2001) six aims for improvement are: safety, effectiveness, patient centeredness, timeliness, efficiency, and equity. To achieve these goals teams must work together collaboratively and cooperatively, eliminating silos and tearing down institutional barriers. Team building is a strategy for designing, implementing, developing, and nurturing work teams in organizations. These work teams are a specialized subset of the many types of groups that form or are formed in organizations.

In nursing, group process theory relates to both how to be therapeutic with clients and how to work as an employee within an organization that is often large and complex. Nursing has an integral role as a member of the health care team. As a caregiver, the nurse serves a key role as a patient advocate and frequently serves as the coordinator of care with other members of the team (see Chapter 16). The nurse tracks whether different interventions have been effective or whether alternative pain strategies might be needed. As a care provider spending significant time with the patient, often a nurse will see fine, distinct changes in a patient's condition before other members of the health care team. Nurses oversee the plan of care in home health, long-term care, hospice, and many other settings. The nurse is involved more intimately and more proximately than any of the other health care providers in managing the total health care of the patient. Therefore understanding and developing skills in group process and group dynamics is essential within the context of leadership and management in nursing because of the group functioning and coordinative aspects of nursing practice. Equally important is the nurse's role in coordinating multidisciplinary and interdisciplinary teams. They often rise to the occasion and lead these teams. Because care is complex and involves the expertise of many disciplines, nurses need strong group process and interaction skills to communicate clearly and collaborate effectively with a variety of colleagues.

DEFINITIONS

A **group** is defined as any collection of interconnected individuals working together for some purpose. Groups are important in organizations, not only because of informal network dynamics, but also because of the multitude of formal committees, task forces, councils, and teams in the contemporary organization. A **committee** is a relatively stable and formally composed group. Committees are a specific type of group in that they are stable, meet periodically, and have an identified purpose that is part of the organizational structure. There is a mechanism for maintaining and selecting members. Typically, committees have official status and sanction within an organization. For example, there are policy and procedure committees, quality and patient safety committees, and ethics committees.

A **task force** is a temporary group of individuals formed to carry out a specific mission or project. Task forces may solve a problem that requires a multidisciplinary approach. A **council** is an advisory group of individuals who may be elected or appointed and that has a defined charter or purpose and meets regularly. In a nursing shared governance model, the councilor structure is commonplace. Councils promote collegiality and engagement. Nursing may have unit practice councils, a hospital practice council, and a leadership council, as well as specific areas of focus, such as a nursing research council or education council.

Collaboration a complex phenomenon that brings together two or more individuals, often from different professional disciplines, who work to achieve shared aims and objectives such as working together toward a common goal for the patient (Fewster-Thuente & Velsor-Friedrich, 2008).

Communication is the style and extent of interactions both among members and between members and those outside the team. It also refers to the way conflict, decision making, and day-to-day interactions occur (Wellins et al., 1991) (see Chapter 7).

Team building is defined as the process of deliberately creating and unifying a group into a functioning team. A **team** was defined by Katzenbach and Smith (1993, p. 45) as "a small number of people with complementary skills who are committed to a common purpose, performance goals, and approach for which they hold themselves mutually accountable." Teams are interdependent, with shared responsibility to achieve the goals and their successes or failures. Teams have the authority to coordinate activities and tasks; team members may have defined roles, duties, or responsibilities.

The distinction between a work group and a true team is crucial. Health care leaders may mistakenly assume that simply calling a group a *team* actually makes it a team. As Katzenbach and Smith (1993, 2015) emphasized, the group becomes a true team only by doing its collective work. The team goes through a developmental process that takes time and the investment of energy to materialize. Many collective entities in today's organizations are called *teams* yet clearly function more as work groups than true teams.

A **work group** is a collection of individuals who are charged with completing a specific activity or mission. Work groups come together to share information and ideas, and they may make some decisions mutually. However, the members of the work group have individual work products for which they are responsible, and these consume their major focus and effort. For example, in a patient care unit, the unit secretary has certain responsibilities, as do the charge nurse, direct care nurse, and nurse manager. The boundaries remain fairly clearly separated when the collective entity is a work group. Each person may view his or her role as being individually accountable, but there is little to no collective accountability.

This is in contrast with a true team, which is a collective entity where the leadership rotates and is shared by various members of the team, depending on appropriateness and fit of skills and abilities. In a true team, there are collective work products, for example, the provision of quality patient care to all of the patients housed in the department or seen in the clinic. There is group as well as individual accountability. If one member of the team is having a problem, it is not just that individual's problem; instead it becomes a team problem for all members of the team to pull together to resolve. An example of team thinking is "No one sits down until we can all sit down" or "No one goes home until we all go home." If quality outcomes are difficult for one team member, all team members are affected by this and become engaged in helping the affected team member meet expectations. In the management book *The Goal* (Goldratt & Cox, 2016), the author tells a parable about taking a Boy Scout troop on a hike. When it was discovered that Scout Herbie was slowing the whole group down, the weight in his backpack was redistributed, and the troop sped up. This is how a high-performing team works.

BACKGROUND

Group interactions are a pervasive element of the health care environment in which nurses work. A basic understanding of groups helps nurses function more effectively. These principles apply to any group, whether an actual team, a committee, task force, council, or an informal group effort. Group interactions are composed of the following elements (Book & Galvin, 1975):

- The *process* that the group undergoes to reach outcomes. This relates to the unique way the group interrelates and begins to work together. The leader can assess group process through observation. What is the process that occurs while the group is accomplishing its task?
- The *standards* that regulate the group's behavior. This relates to the specific values and norms (ground rules) that are chosen for meetings, group processing, and group interaction. Which ones are chosen and which are discarded?
- The process of *problem solving* or *decision making* that the group adopts. Does the group solve problems?

How are decisions made? Are group decisions made by consensus, or are decisions made by an individual with group input (as occurs when the group participates but the decision is made by a leader or manager)? Do members of the group support decisions once they are made?

- The *communication* that occurs among group members. What are the internal patterns and styles of communication used by group members? To whom does the group communicate? Do they report as a subcommittee to a full committee? If a team, does the team have frequent communication with external team leaders? What are the internal and external modes of communication for group input and output? What are the communication gaps within the group?
- The *roles* played by each member. Members will adopt a variety of group roles within the group, but roles are fluid. Members may take on different roles in different situations. It is important to remember when assessing group interactions that roles in the group may be formal roles, clearly established by the leader or the group. However, there are additional roles that each group member moves in and out of that best suit him or her (such as clarifier, harmonizer, or devil's advocate). Clarity in the more formal roles, such as team leader, facilitator, recorder, and timekeeper, is important to avoid confusion and avoidable conflict.

Groups tend to go through a series of stages in their work and development. Farley and Stoner (1989) originally identified these as (1) orientation, (2) adaptation, (3) emergence, and (4) working. The first stage, *orientation,* occurs when the group first forms and the members begin to relate to one another and the task. The group needs to develop trust and define boundaries in order to establish involvement and identification. The second stage, *adaptation,* occurs as the group begins to develop a collective identity and differentiate roles. The group needs a facilitative structure and climate to maximize its processing and to work through the establishment of roles, rules, norms, and a common language. The third stage, *emergence,* occurs as control issues arise. Disputes, disagreements, confrontations, alliances, and power struggles mark this stage of determining control over the group in order to emerge with a more consolidated identity. The final stage, *working,* occurs when conflict and dissention dissipate and the group achieves greater cohesion through negotiation.

The group is now focused primarily on decision making and productivity. The stages may overlap and are not necessarily sequential. The group leader pays attention to the stage of the group as a way of monitoring the group's development and progress. For example, in the orientation stage, the leader may need to be more alert to the need to intervene personally than would be the case in the working stage when the group has achieved a higher level of maturity.

WHY GROUPS ARE FORMED

In nursing, the formation of groups occurs primarily for one of two reasons: (1) to provide a personal or professional socialization and exchange forum, or (2) to provide a mechanism for interdependent work accomplishment. Groups can be social, professional, or organizational in purpose. The following are some reasons why groups would be established in organizations:

- Group activities can create a sense of status and esteem, allowing an individual to be part of something bigger than him or herself
- Groups allow an individual to test and establish reality.
- Groups allow engagement of individuals with leaders to share responsibility, decision making, and accountability for outcomes.
- Groups function as a mechanism for individuals to work collectively and cooperatively to get a job done.
- Groups address complex problems or tasks by a diverse group of individuals with specialized knowledge and/or skill.
- Groups can maximize leaders' strengths and minimize their weaknesses.

A major part of the working environment of nurses is the accomplishment of work through group activity. The work group provides an institutional and professional identity for an individual nurse, and work groups become a focus for interpersonal relationships, support, and social integration. Job satisfaction, positive relational leadership, and positive quality outcomes are linked (Wong et al., 2013). Factors related to job satisfaction include working conditions, job stress, role conflict and ambiguity, role perception, role content, and organizational and professional commitment (Lu et al., 2012). In addition, being part of a healthy group or team is related to the level of organizational commitment by the team member. Individuals with an emotional connection to their work group have lower levels of turnover and higher levels of engagement (DiMeglio et al., 2005; Manion, 2004, 2009).

Work groups can be disrupted by factors such as downsizing, reorganization, absenteeism, loss of leadership, bullying, and turnover. Work group disruption has been linked to negative outcomes (Kalisch & Begeny, 2005; Kalisch & Lee, 2010). In a study of four hospitals, interpersonal relations were found to be an important part of nurses' job satisfaction. Interpersonal relationships are integral to work group functioning. Things get done because of relationships among people; nurses need to build successful collaborative relationships among multiple levels of colleagues, key people, organizations, and patients (Laramee, 1999). The level of nursing teamwork has been found to be directly linked to missed nursing care (Kalisch & Lee, 2010).

One vulnerable group of nurses are new graduates. There has been extensive research suggesting that workplace bullying occurs particularly with new graduates. Read and Laschinger (2013) found the sense of community and similarity between the ideals and beliefs of the nurses within a work unit affected the perception of bullying. Some of the job characteristics related to workplace bullying include workload, job control, reward, and recognition. Budin and colleagues (2013) found that support from their leader or a mentor had an impact on the likelihood of a new graduate being a victim of bullying. Bullying may affect the trust, communication, and cohesiveness of a group. Furthermore, informal work group norms exert a strong influence on nurses' behavior and functioning within a group. See Chapter 5 for more on nurse residency programs for new graduate nurses as an antidote.

Work group relationships can reinforce behaviors and rationalization, thus leading to deviant behaviors such as workarounds that become passively or actively accepted. Debono and colleagues (2013) conducted an extensive literature search of studies concerning nurse workaround behaviors. There were several themes related to teamwork. First, workarounds may be individual or supported by a group who share the belief that rules are "flexible." When that is the case, there is also an understanding of who will and will not perform a workaround. Second, nurses may justify working around policies and procedures as necessary to benefit the patient. Finally, the acceptance or proliferation of workarounds can be affected by a variety of factors, including group norms, leadership, professional structures, personal relationships, and organizational culture.

Clearly, there is a strong relationship between work groups, interpersonal relationships, leadership, and outcomes such as nurses' behaviors and perceptions. Work group relationships are a powerful mechanism influencing both good and bad outcomes in nursing practice.

ADVANTAGES OF GROUPS

Groups have the potential for being a driving force for change in an organization. Ronco (2005) identified the potential positive impact groups can have on an organization:

1. *Synergy:* Groups have the potential to perform at higher levels than an individual would on his or her own.
2. *Positive individual impacts:* Groups have the potential to improve every member of the group or at least help each one reach his or her highest potential.
3. *Motivation:* Groups have the potential to motivate their individual members and provide encouragement, constructive criticism, and praise.
4. *Diverse thinking:* Groups have the potential to engage in diverse thinking, thereby identifying problems that might otherwise go unnoticed or ignored and exploring solutions.
5. *Linkage to the larger organization:* Groups have the potential to make individuals feel more connected to the larger organization.

Veninga (1982) identified the following five major advantages of group problem solving over individual problem solving:

1. *Greater knowledge and information:* Obtaining a broader and wider range of knowledge and experiences creates a higher-quality input into group problem solving. The insights of one member can stimulate the thinking of other group members. This is especially true with today's highly specialized health care workers.
2. *Increased acceptance of solutions:* If there is a decision to be made in an organization, people can get together in a group to talk about it so that the people themselves are more committed to the decision. When individuals who are going to be affected by a decision are part of the decision-making process, they do not have to be convinced of the rightness of the decision and are more likely to be committed to implementing it.
3. *More approaches to a problem:* Complex problems are typically more manageable when a number of

perspectives are mixed together to address the problem. The advantages include blending and complementing individual learning and problem-solving styles to capitalize on strength through diversity.

4. *Individual expression:* Groups allow for individual expression, and in organizations specifically, there may be few mechanisms for expression of individual perspectives. Sharing information and getting input are best done in groups. Sometimes groups allow people to express themselves, for example, if they are anxious about a change or if morale is low.

5. *Lower costs:* If the group is functioning in a positive and constructive manner, the use of a group can be less expensive than the use of individual effort to accomplish a task. Group decision making is cost effective if it saves time. For example, when a group meets for one session as opposed to the leader meeting multiple times with multiple individuals, the leader and possibly the group members save time.

Groups are one vehicle for creative problem solving, stimulating innovation, and building consensus. To be successful, the leader must be skilled at facilitation, ensuring the meetings have a clear purpose and are organized, focused, and productive, with balanced participation by team members. An effective meeting will start and finish on time and result in a balanced discussion of pros and cons on a particular topic or issue and required next steps, actions, follow up, and specific member assignments and accountabilities. These practices demonstrate the leader's organizational skills and respect for the contributions by all team members and their time. It is imperative that there is a clearly defined purpose for a group, particularly when the group is part of a larger organization. Ideally this is an early discussion by the group and is determined with the input of all members. The purpose and value of the group should be evaluated periodically as well as whether the team is meeting its goals. Is it functional? Is it accomplishing the task to which it was assigned or committed? If not, should the group be disbanded or reorganized?

When the work output of any group is analyzed, meetings can be financially costly endeavors. For example, when the number of hours spent by all committee members is multiplied by their individual hourly salary and fringe benefit cost and added together to compute a committee total, the sum of costs for the group may be astounding. This is one reason for paying attention to how well the group is functioning. Just as

important is assessing whether the group adds value to the organization and the individuals involved. If team members are not actively contributing to the group's charge, their role and time on the team may be wasted energy and may drain the enthusiasm and effectiveness of the group. The cost of group work can be balanced by calculating its value in increased productivity or risk/cost avoidance.

A highly functioning group may have a profound impact on an organization. Such groups often identify and solve complex problems. Participation and involvement in a group decision typically results in individuals being more engaged and committed to a decision, even if there is disagreement. Disagreement and conflict are important elements for the leader to guide teams through and are often very productive factors in solving problems. In this way, leaders of teams can demonstrate effective means of resolving differences, which are commonplace in health care.

DISADVANTAGES OF GROUPS

Ronco (2005) identified the six potential negative impacts groups can have on an organization, including negativity, passivity, individual focus, groupthink, vocal minority, and the ethical dark side. Veninga (1982) also suggested a seventh: disruptive conflicts.

1. *Negativity:* Research suggests that people working in groups tend to be more negative than if they work individually.

2. *Passivity:* People may become passive participants in a group versus being active participants. Unbalanced participation may lead to feelings of resentment, jealousy, and disillusionment. Some may "slide by" on the work effort of others.

3. *Individual focus and individual domination:* Individuals may have difficulty thinking globally and objectively. Instead, they may focus on how a discussion affects them as an individual. They may also dominate the group, compromising the group process. Their strong opinions may stifle discussion, creativity, and innovation. As a result, the group or leader may need to divert its energy and productivity into working out interpersonal dynamics rather than moving forward on the group's task.

4. *Groupthink:* Groups may reach quick agreement and be unwilling to challenge or debate. Sometimes decisions result from pressure—by the group, leader, or external

deadlines—to complete the work. Groups may influence individual members when the majority of the group feels a certain way about an issue or task. The minority members of the group who may disagree experience an element of pressure because of psychological dynamics related to subtle pressure for group acceptance and conformity. Creative and innovate ideas may be lost if a group reaches decisions too quickly.

5. *Vocal minority:* Groups have a tendency to allow the most vocal members of a group represent the overall views of the group even when they are the minority of members. It may be difficult to be a devil's advocate or to adopt the role of bringing alternative critique points to the group for consideration because of a concern about not being personally socially accepted or fear of conflict. For example, derision and humiliation can occur if members react with strong negative opinions.

6. *Ethical dark side:* Groups have the potential, based on the power of the group, to not support ethically positive choices.

7. *Disruptive conflicts:* If people perceive an adverse effect on a group member or members or if they feel threatened, conflicts usually emerge. Conflicts can accelerate in a competitive environment when members vest in their own position and are not willing to consider a different point of view. Conflicts that are about substantive issues actually help the group become more effective in their decision making. However, when conflicts occur over differences in personality, opinion, or clashes of values, these conflicts can become destructive. Although it may seem contradictory, conflicts can serve as a control mechanism in a group and may actually result in far superior outcomes. When group members are comfortable respectfully disagreeing with each other, a premature acceptance of decisions can be avoided because opposing viewpoints are considered.

GROUP DECISION MAKING

Group work can be—and typically is—a slow process. It takes more time for a group to arrive at a decision than for one person to make the decision.

In addition, a continuum of decision-making power may be vested in a group (Fig. 8.1). A group or committee has certain powers, tasks, and functions, as well as certain parameters or latitude in terms of how far to go in making a decision. Decision power is a matter of degree, with four distinct points on the continuum of authority for decision making: authoritative, consultative, joint, and delegated.

On one end of the continuum is *authoritative decision making,* where the leader makes the decision. In this process there is input, perhaps, but not necessarily a vote. One example of this is in some medical emergencies, such as cardiac arrest, where there is no time for discussion, and the leader needs to take control and direct the team. This style is generally ineffective in nonemergencies because it can generate increased cynicism and employee disengagement.

Consultative decision making occurs when decisions involve employee participation, but the leader still makes the final decision alone. Group members may make certain recommendations, but these must then go to the leader, chairperson, or head of the group, who makes the final decision. There is more participation with this type of procedure, but the ultimate decision is not under the control of the group members. This type of decision making is used in nursing with task forces, quality committees, and shared governance councils.

Some decision procedures result in *joint decision making.* In this approach, the entire group decides, whether by a two-thirds vote, simple majority, consensus, or some other process. In a joint decision procedure, the team members have as much influence as the leader. The leader has one voice, one vote. The leader

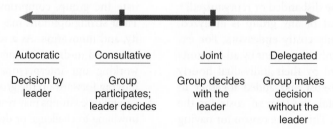

FIG. 8.1 Range of decision powers.

can use persuasion, but when it comes to the final vote, the leader's vote is equivalent to that of any other member of the group. This is fundamentally different from the leader making the decision with group input. This is the type of decision making used in a multidisciplinary team. Every voice is heard and valued equally. In nursing, individual unit and hospital councils may have the authority to implement certain decisions related to clinical practice.

Finally, at the other end of the decision continuum is the *delegated decision procedure*. This occurs when the committee chair or leader allows participants to make the final decision. For example, the establishment of a self-directed work team for the purpose of self-scheduling involves decision delegation. The leader may set up the basic parameters to follow, such as ensuring an appropriate number of staff by role and experience for a particular shift for the entire schedule before it is released. In nursing, many leaders assign self-scheduling as a way to engage the team and allow for flexibility in scheduling. The true test of delegation decision making is whether the leader overrides the followers' decision. Technically, the leader would not have the authority to veto or override unless he or she determined the decision made would compromise safety or the organization's well-being. For example, new legal mandates supersede group decision making. If it is truly a delegation situation, the leader would go forward with the approach that the decision is the choice of the group. The group then becomes accountable for the outcome and is responsible for fixing any resulting issues. Hersey and colleagues (2013) labeled these same four procedures as *authoritative, consultative, facilitative,* and *delegative* decision-making styles.

It is advisable for the followers in any group to determine who has the authority to make decisions. Knowledge about what type of group it is and what delegation or decision making can be anticipated is critical to participation. A leadership or conflict moment may occur when a group assumes that they have the authority to make decisions but the leader has a different idea. Clarity before beginning work on an issue prevents unnecessary conflict and augments productivity. However, group members and leaders need to become skilled and comfortable in handling interpersonal dynamics.

Group decision making may be time consuming. Therefore the leader needs to be skilled at allowing the appropriate amount of discussion to occur, particularly ensuring that varying opinions are presented before a decision is made. It can be derailed if the leader is not skilled at facilitation, does not have a clear purpose for meeting, or is disorganized, unfocused, or allows unbalanced participation or discussion. Meetings that do not start and finish on time show a lack of respect toward the participants. When there is limited discussion of the pros and cons of a particular topic or issue, members of the group may feel disenfranchised and limit their attendance or participation. Leaders need to be skilled at ensuring there is equal participation and that ideas and suggestions by all members of the group are taken into account. Group members and leaders need to become skilled and comfortable in handling interpersonal dynamics, including conflict.

WORKING WITH TEAMS

In health care, multidisciplinary and interdisciplinary care teams are necessary for survival. Teamwork affects clinical performance, and team training is an effective strategy for improving patient safety. Implementation strategies and organizational conditions matter (Salas & Rosen, 2013). Organizational design principles and management approaches that strive to prevent patient injury and improve quality include the use of high-reliability theory. High-reliability health care organizations are characterized by an organizational commitment to safety, back-up steps built into processes, safety measures, and an organizational culture for continuous learning (Riley et al., 2010). These organizations provide safe care and use deliberate design to minimize errors. Applied to nursing, the concept is *high-reliability teams.* Using reliability principles, multidisciplinary and interdisciplinary teams can focus on reducing flaws in care processes, increase the consistency of appropriateness of care delivery, and improve patient outcomes. Team training and system design are the key hallmarks of high-reliability patient care units. Members of high-reliability teams have four key behaviors: situational awareness, use of standardized communication, closed-loop communication, and a shared mental model, which can be enhanced with interdisciplinary team training (Riley et al., 2010). High-performance teams are essential to an organization's efficiency and effectiveness because high-quality work outcomes and cost control are impossible without communication, collaboration, and teamwork.

Nurse leaders need to learn how to create, lead, and manage teams; all nurses need to know how to be effective team players as well. Skilled leaders listen, invite, and encourage participation by members of the team. They understand the individual strengths and weakness of each member. The formation of a well-functioning group or team is never the work of just the leader. Members, as followers, give input, participate in decision making, share responsibility, and hold themselves and each other accountable for the outcomes of the group. A highly skilled and effective professional is not necessarily a highly skilled and effective group member. There are distinct skill sets involved, and all are beneficial for nurses. Leaders and staff members alike should be able to function both independently and interdependently with others. They should have the judgment to know when and which form of functioning is more appropriate. Regardless of their role as leader or member of a group, the vision and goals of the group must be embraced by everyone to be effective.

Types of Teams

Three types of teams found in health care are (1) primary work teams, (2) leadership teams, and (3) ad hoc teams (Manion, 2011). Primary work teams include all forms of operational teams, including patient care teams such as a medical intensive care team and teams organized by a focused area, such as the rapid response team or a quality improvement team. In the operating room, teams are often based on the specialty (e.g., a cardiovascular or an orthopedic team). The senior executive team is an example of an executive or management leadership team. At the hospital department level there may be a leadership team that is composed of the nurse manager, charge nurses, and perhaps an educator. Project teams and problem-solving teams are examples of ad hoc teams found across settings and sites. Specific problem-solving teams in departments are other examples of ad hoc teams, frequently referred to as task forces. The chief characteristic of these teams is that they are created to perform a very specific piece of work. When that work is completed, the team dissolves. Designing, building, and implementing effective work teams requires a specific methodology and process. A primary work team fails if it behaves like a collection of individuals operating from narrowly defined jobs; if it is composed of the wrong mix of members, size, structure, responsibility, or expertise, or if it cannot fluidly shift activities and adapt to changes. Teams need to be designed based on the work responsibilities and the skills and competencies required by the work of the team. After the team design is determined, the next step is to build the team by incorporating the essential elements needed to function. These include a common purpose, agreed-on performance goals or results-driven structure, competent members, a common approach for the work, complementary skills, collaborative relationships, mutual accountability, standards of excellence, external support, and principled leadership (Manion et al., 1996). The complementary skills that are needed in the right mix to do the team's task fall into at least three categories: technical or functional expertise, problem-solving and decision-making skills, and interpersonal skills. There are defined characteristics of *highly effective teams* (Wynia, 2012, pp. 1327–1328) (Table 8.1).

Managing this development process is a key leadership function. This means that the leader guides the team in the development of its purpose. Team members are more likely to coalesce into a strong team if they have been given the time and opportunity to carefully reflect on their purpose and agree on what they do and for whom they do it. This leads to a unified commitment. The team becomes a true team by doing its work. Specific performance goals give it direction and also provide evaluative criteria by which the team's success can be measured. Although it is simplistic to say that the team has common working approaches, unnecessary conflict occurs in this area if the leader and team members have not established these key processes. Agreement is needed about how things are going to be done and by whom. This ranges from the establishment of team behavioral norms to agreement on procedural issues. This step usually requires a significant amount of time and will continue to be addressed throughout the lifetime of the team. When foundations are laid carefully, effective teams can emerge (Manion, 2011).

Team Dynamics

The dynamics of interdisciplinary teams create some unique challenges. When teams are comprised of professionals who have been educated, socialized, and are used to a unique vocabulary, professional values, and standards and practices, then it may become challenging for them to work across disciplines. Regrouping people into multidisciplinary groups increases the diversity of the team and is essential to ensure high-quality, coordinated, reliable care. Yet, many professionals are more comfortable functioning independently instead of as part of a team. Lencioni (2006) promoted the idea that to overcome the common turf

TABLE 8.1	Values and Principles of High-Functioning Health Care Teams	
Share Values Among Team Members	**Principles to Guide Team-Based Care**
Honesty	*Clear roles*
Put a high value on open communication within the team, including transparency about aims, decisions, uncertainty, and mistakes.	Have clear expectations for each member's functions, responsibilities, and accountabilities.
Discipline	*Mutual trust*
Carry out roles and responsibilities even when inconvenient, and seek out and share information to improve even when it is uncomfortable.	Earn each other's trust, creating strong norms for reciprocity and greater opportunities for shared achievement.
Creativity	*Effective communication*
Be excited by the possibility of tackling new or emerging problems, seeing errors and unanticipated bad outcomes as potential opportunities to learn and improve.	Prioritize and continuously refine communication skills using consistent channels for candid and complete communication.
Humility	*Shared goals*
Recognize differences in training but do not believe that one type of training perspective is uniformly superior; recognize that team members are human and will make mistakes.	Work to establish shared goals that reflect patient and family priorities and that can be clearly articulated, understood, and supported by all members.
Curiosity	*Measurable processes and outcomes*
Delight in seeking out and reflecting on lessons learned and using those insights for continuous improvement.	Agree on and implement reliable and timely feedback on successes and failures in both the overall functioning of the team and achievement of specific goals.

Data from Wynia, M.K., Von Kohorn, I., & Mitchell, P.H. (2012). Challenges at the intersection of team-based and patient-centered health care: Insights from an IOM working group. *Journal of the American Medical Association, 308*(13), 1327–1328.

battles and the tendency team members have to function in their own narrow scope (silo thinking), the team needs to have a pressing, time-constricted goal upon which to focus.

Other perils and pitfalls can occur when teams are assigned—not designed—including (Manion et al., 1996):
- There is confusion about the team's work.
- The team lacks real authority.
- Structural team building is not done.
- Dysfunctional behavior occurs and team members don't know how to constructively deal with it.
- Team-based outcome measures and coaching are lacking.

Trust and communication are critical elements of building effective work teams. It is not enough to simply structure the team. Team members need to learn to work collaboratively and interdependently. Team performance and effectiveness are important managerial concerns. Dysfunctional team behaviors can occur. Lencioni (2002) identified five key dysfunctions of a team as absence of trust, fear of conflict, lack of commitment, avoidance of accountability, and inattention to results.

Teams form, grow through stages, and mature. Team dynamics change throughout this process. Teams benefit from team building and developmental training. Articulating and negotiating expectations for healthy interpersonal behavior benefits team development. A key characteristic of an emotionally intelligent team is one that has established norms that guide team member behaviors (Cherniss & Goleman, 2001).

Team norms are best established when the team initially forms. They are continually revisited, modified, and expanded throughout the life span of the team. The process for developing norms is usually leader initiated and begins with a conversation within the team about how members expect each other to behave and contribute. The norms are usually developed during a group meeting in which ideas are shared, refined, and finally negotiated with all team members. Appropriate topics for behavioral norms include, but are not limited to, expectations around communication, both at the individual and group levels; how team members treat each other; how support is to be demonstrated; decision-making processes; and how conflict is to be handled. For example, one team developed the following expectations of each other:

I expect you to:

- Communicate in an open, honest, and direct manner with me
- Give me feedback when my behavior creates a difficult or uncomfortable situation for you
- Persist and work with me on difficult issues until we reach a mutually agreeable resolution
- Pitch in gladly, provide help when asked, and look for ways to help each other out
- Respect confidences and not share sensitive information we discuss with others without my knowledge or permission
- Be trustworthy as evidenced by honoring and meeting commitments made, including being on time and staying engaged (being present) throughout the meeting
- Refrain from using technology and "multitasking" during meetings
- Be loyal to absent team members, and present them in the best light to others

Often these norms are referred to as the *team operating agreement,* the *code of conduct,* ground rules, or *articulated expectations.* Once the norms are identified, in many teams the members sign them, indicating agreement, and the norms often are posted in sight in the workplace. These norms are more than just a paper exercise. They signify that the team member agrees to live by the expectations and address other team members who do not. As new members join the team, it is important to share team members' expectations. It is also beneficial to revisit the defined expectations on a regular basis.

Team effectiveness is dependent not only on how individual members of the team perform and adhere to norms, but also on the degree of communication, cooperation, and the emotional intelligence of the individual members and the leader of the team. The ability to manage conflict and have self-awareness is essential for a team to reach peak performance. The greater the performance of a team, the greater is the advantage to the group members, their customers, and the organization.

COMMITTEES

An essential part of any nurse's role is to be involved in committee and group work. Work is accomplished through people, and the quality of care is furthered through committee actions. It is also important to nurses' job satisfaction and autonomy to have an avenue of involvement and participation in which to actively solve problems and retain autonomy over nursing care. Shared governance models incorporate staff nurse participation in groups and committees as a core element of how work gets accomplished.

Some people prefer not to participate in committees because they dislike the time involved or because they are frustrated with the psychodynamics of group process and decision making. However, committees are a mainstay of organizations and can be an important way to make changes in clinical practice. Lencioni (2004) believed there is no substitute for a good meeting—one in which there is passionate, dynamic, and focused engagement—to gather the collective wisdom of the group. Understanding committee workings facilitates the process of being a more effective nurse.

Committee structures are preferable in the following two kinds of situations:

1. *Situations in which each member's input is needed to attain a certain goal.* For example, a committee may be set up to review patient safety issues in a department, such as patient falls. If the work cannot be done alone or if there is a need to have everyone's agreement or support, then a committee is probably appropriate.

2. *Situations in which diverse representation facilitates implementation of proposed activities.* To have a diverse group of people provide input in order to get the job done, a committee should be created. For example, a multidisciplinary products committee could be established to develop a process in which existing and new products would be reviewed before large purchases are made. This approach allows nurses to evaluate new products and look at value to patient care, including safety, efficacy, and cost. It also provides a disciplined approach to product review, with an aim of preventing duplication of products and promoting good stewardship of precious funds.

Types of Committees

Several types of committees are found in organizations. One kind is the *standing* committee, which, as the name implies, is a constant, ongoing part of the organizational mission, performing critical and essential functions. For example, policy committees are standing committees because there always are policies to write and review. The same is true for a patient safety committee because these functions and activities are ongoing and continuous.

Contrasted with a standing committee is the task force, also called a *project team* or *ad hoc committee*. This is a committee that is developed in response to some emergent or immediate need. A need arises, and a group is formed. A task force is not part of the organizational core mission. It is formed in response to a specific circumstance that arises or to study a specific problem. The committee is expected to disband when the issue is resolved. Examples are a search committee to replace an advanced practice nurse or a problem-solving group dealing with patient throughput in the emergency department and bed availability within the hospital.

Some groups or committees are structured to gather together members *based on organizational position or job position.* For example, all the nurse managers may belong to a group of nurse managers, or staff nurses may belong to a staff nurse council. By holding the position of nurse manager, the person belongs to that committee. This provides an opportunity for peer interaction, support, and problem solving.

There are multidisciplinary interdivisional committees. A *multidisciplinary* committee includes participants from several divisions, locations, or specialties. The participants may all be from within the institution or from both inside and outside the organization. These committees are often used to coordinate and eliminate boundary conflicts. Some examples are a products committee, a risk management committee, or a patient safety committee in which nurses, physicians, and allied health colleagues work together to improve patient care and reduce interprofessional conflicts. In some cases, multidisciplinary teams are formed using a committee structure (e.g., to develop a critical pathway such as sepsis screening). Other committees may be cross-functional (e.g., nurses meeting with members from the information technology or facilities management department to discuss and resolve issues).

Within organizations, committees perform a central role in the implementation of the strategic plan. A committee is a group that can assume responsibility and be held accountable for planning, implementing, and evaluating the outcomes of a strategic goal translated to the operational level. Committees accomplish some departmental activities and provide a mechanism for increasing staff participation in decision making. In an environment characterized by complex work, committees become a major vehicle for resolving issues related to the organization's mission. Two elements promote efficient and effective committee decision making: appropriate representation (by including people affected by changes) and delegation of an appropriate level of authority to the committee (Manion, 2011).

Committees evolve over time. To remain vital, committees need to be evaluated regularly for congruence with organizational mission and contribution to outcomes. The committee's goals and outcomes should be reviewed annually, with membership reevaluated and changed as necessary. If asked to be on a committee as a department representative, it is advisable for the nurse to explore the nature and characteristics of the committee. The nurse needs to determine the authority level delegated to this particular committee, remembering that this delegation may be formal or informal. Another factor involves assessing the personal level of interest in the work of the committee. Other factors include whether the people on the committee are highly motivated, whether they are task- or relationship-oriented people, and what committee politics exist. The feedback mechanisms and the committee's productivity are key characteristics. The track record of the committee is reflected in its output. These characteristics are important for the nurse to understand before deciding whether to participate. Preparation for followership enhances both personal and committee productivity. It is also helpful to clarify any expectations for the committee role being considered. For example, is the nurse there to share individual opinions or to represent others in the department? This role requires more active solicitation of colleagues' opinions and ideas.

EFFECTIVE MEETINGS

Meetings are common occurrences in health care organizations. Whether a meeting involves a group, a committee, or a team, the leader's role is to maximize the benefits of the meeting. Structuring a meeting for effectiveness requires preparation and effort. To manage effective meetings, the leader should consider the purpose of the meeting. Some of the most common reasons meetings are ineffective are that the purpose of the meeting is not clear or there are too many competing issues on the agenda for a single meeting (Lencioni, 2004). For example, a brief team huddle would become ineffective if it turned into a decision-making group about a key department issue.

Probably the most common type of meeting is held for *information dissemination or sharing.* For example, the designated leadership person calls the group together to let the members review the organization's performance scorecard. That may include the organization's and the individual department's performance in financial management, patient experience scores, quality scores, and employee measures such as turnover. A meeting is called to disseminate information about what is happening and to provide time for questions and answers. Perhaps there has been an organizational change, such as the decision that one unit is going to be consolidating with another unit or that a new building, department relocation, or new service is being planned.

One familiar form of information sharing is the end-of-shift report. Pertinent, important information about patients is reviewed and discussed by staff members from the outgoing and incoming shift. The shift hand-off report is a very common form of this type of meeting. This is a very short meeting at the beginning of the shift with all team members to review the upcoming shift or any short topics that need to be communicated.

Second, there are meetings held for the purpose of *opinion seeking.* The goal of these meetings is open dialogue to solicit group and individual opinions and ideas on specific topics or issues. This purpose does not imply that decision making is the prerogative of the group. Seeking opinions is an input strategy and may be used for only gathering data or testing group reactions. For example, an opinion-seeking meeting may be called to invite input on equipment purchases for budget requests.

The third type of meeting is held for the purpose of *problem solving and/or decision making.* The meeting is structured to solicit help in clarifying, analyzing, and solving a specific problem. This type of meeting is more action oriented. Group participation in decision making is encouraged. For example, group problem solving or unit meetings may be called to discuss ways to solve problems related to patient safety issues or complex and challenging patients or family members. Meetings for the purpose of problem solving must follow a methodical structure; otherwise they are likely either to deteriorate into a complaint session or to result in ineffective or unacceptable recommendations. Effectively leading these groups requires strong facilitation skills and knowledge in problem-solving techniques.

Yet another type of meeting is a *strategy* meeting. These meetings are less frequent—perhaps quarterly or annually—and focus on reviewing the organization's vision and strategic goals, developing future goals and strategies for the department or work group, or tackling one issue in great depth, such as implementing a shared governance model or a new model of care delivery. This may be called by executive nursing leaders as a "summit," a "retreat," or "town hall meeting."

Preparing for Meetings

In the most effective groups, all members are clear about the purpose of the meeting they are attending, are prepared, and help the group stay focused on the purpose. When the group becomes distracted by other issues (for example, getting side-tracked by operational issues during a strategy meeting), focus is lost and the meeting time is wasted. This is a sign that the meeting structure may need to be evaluated.

In preparing for a meeting, a leader should make certain that the committee's process stays true to the purpose of the meeting. In other words, there should not be a mix of items in the same meeting. For example, basic information dissemination is not appropriate at a quarterly strategic meeting. This does not mean that any of these items are less important, but introducing them in the wrong venue or with the wrong timing will reduce the effectiveness of the meeting.

A timed agenda may be a helpful way to facilitate the group's process. This involved identifying on the agenda, next to each item, the anticipated amount of time allotted for discussion. It might be beneficial to review the proposed time with committee members before the meeting to ensure the estimates are realistic. It should serve as a guideline rather than a rigid parameter. It is important not to cut off discussion prematurely or force a decision when a particular discussion is productive but takes longer than anticipated. One effective strategy is to do a time check with the members and adjust accordingly. This may require an adjustment in the agenda. Many leaders organize the agenda items according to priority topics. Some leaders have a brief agenda and add to it to cover any pressing issues or topics based on the team's input. This can be done at the beginning of the meeting or after planned agenda items are covered. Meetings can rapidly become disorganized without an agenda or a carefully facilitated discussion. The leader must be mindful of the time allotted for the meeting.

Leader Duties

The leader of the group can facilitate meeting effectiveness by preparing and dealing with both the task and the people involved. The leader should listen carefully, process the interactions, control the flow, and keep the meeting directed toward accomplishing the objectives. The ideal size of a group depends on the work to be accomplished. If group interaction and getting everyone's input is important, the size of the ideal group is small, perhaps 4 to 7 people, with 12 being the upper limit. Members should be carefully selected for providing best input, being representative, and having potential contribution to the work.

The leader needs to start on time and be alert to seating positions. Some leaders assign seating to maximize group participation and prevent disruption. The leader can facilitate effectiveness ensuring that all members of the team have an ability to actively participate. The leader may need to control compulsive talkers, drawing out silent members, protecting junior members, encouraging the clash of ideas, discouraging the clash of personalities, preventing the squashing of creative ideas, and closing on a note of achievement (Jay, 1982). The leader also needs to attend to careful meeting wrap-up. Summarizing the group's accomplishments after the meeting and verifying task assignments going forward are important leader responsibilities. Box 8.1 presents a checklist for leading effective meetings.

Without thought and preparation, people may go into a meeting focused on their own issues, biases, and perspectives; they may not be tuned in to how to be productive within the meeting. However, even in a negative situation, individuals may choose to participate in a way that assists or enhances the process by making constructive suggestions about how things could be done better. This is an ideal situation, one to be encouraged, structured, and facilitated by the leader.

The duties of the chairperson include preparation of the physical environment. Comfort and convenience engineering is part of the leader's responsibility in terms of preparing an environment that is conducive to people being satisfied, productive, positive, and working together. The worst-case situation occurs if the meeting room is uncomfortable, including being too cold, too hot, too noisy, too small, or too large. Another challenge is when technology does not work. The chairperson should ensure the meeting room, including the technology, is set up appropriately. Consider how to facilitate group work through hosting functions related to breaks,

---

BOX 8.1 Effective Meetings Checklist for Leaders

- Identify the purpose of the meeting
  - Information dissemination
  - Opinion seeking
  - Problem solving
- Prepare an agenda and related materials
  - Identify time needed for each item on the agenda
- Identify the category of each agenda item
  - For information
  - For development
  - For implementation
  - For change in the system
- Set the size of the group and identify type of members needed
- Carefully select members (based on skill and expertise)
- Distribute agenda and related materials such as previous minutes well in advance of meeting with instructions for assignments due and materials to be reviewed before the meeting
- Start on time and finish on time
- Listen carefully and summarize discussion and assignments at the end of the meeting
- Ensure balanced dialogue by all members
- Process the interactions
- Control the flow of interactions
- Keep the meeting directed toward accomplishing objectives

Data modified from Jay, A. (1982). How to run a meeting. *Journal of Nursing Administration, 12*(1), 22–28.

---

food, and beverages. It is human nature for members to be more relaxed and productive in comfortable surroundings. With the reliance on technology versus the need for people to "be present" during a meeting, many leaders have added technology breaks.

As all nurses are pressured to do more with less under severe time and travel constraints, conducting meetings assisted by technology has become a major strategy. The prevalence and ease of technology, such as video conference calls, webinars, Internet-based meeting technology, real-time (synchronous) discussion boards, and related audio or video technology strategies are commonly employed. These become useful ways to save time by eliminating travel to an in-person site. However, specific problems may occur, such as technology incompatibility, speed of transmission, connection failures, or other delays in transmission that result in people talking over one another or hesitancy in speaking, a lack of interpersonal modulation due to absence of body language, or a tendency to forget about people who are not actually in the room. Ensuring that the agenda, minutes, assignments, and presentations are sent in advance might mitigate some of the technology difficulties. Despite these known issues, nurses will increasingly experience meetings assisted by technology.

Positive meeting dynamics are a shared responsibility between the leader and group members. A leader has a responsibility to prepare in advance for the meetings and provide participants support in their preparation. The participants' responsibility is to read and be prepared, show up on time, participate openly and positively, share responsibility for managing the group's dynamics, and attend to the task at hand. Depending on the meeting, the leader needs to prepare an agenda with handouts and background materials and distribute them to the members to give them time to review. Most materials can be sent electronically to members. The better prepared members are, the more they can participate, positively affect the quality of decisions, and feel gratified by their participation.

If the leader's preparation activities include generating an agenda or reviewing the status of agenda topics, questions to ask when organizing and preparing include the following:

- Where are we/what is the current status?
- What else needs to be done?
- What supporting materials might help the committee members?
- Who should be invited?
- Are there other experts or people from other departments that can contribute to this committee's process?

A leader who does not distribute materials in advance may limit the effectiveness of the meeting because members will not be prepared.

CONSTRUCTIVE GROUP ROLES AND BEHAVIORS

Savvy group leaders and members understand that people in groups assume a variety of roles. In a now-classic work, Lancaster (1981) identified both group building roles and group maintenance roles as being a part of group interactions. Group building roles include *initiator, encourager, opinion giver, clarifier, listener,* and *summarizer.* Group maintenance roles include *tension reliever, compromiser, gatekeeper,* and *harmonizer.* The

group building roles concentrate more on relationship functions than on task functions; the group maintenance roles focus more on task functions than on relationship functions. Effective groups need a balance of members and roles.

Beyond the more general group roles are specific, structured roles that can help increase the effectiveness of the group. For example, one positive way to handle meetings is to identify a facilitator. This is often the formal group leader or individual in a position of authority, but it does not have to be. If this is a true team, the role of facilitator may rotate among team members. In a committee, the facilitator is probably the committee chairperson. A facilitator conducts the meeting, ensuring that everyone has the opportunity to speak, maintains the focus of the meeting, and ensures that group dynamics remain positive.

A group recorder is also needed. The task of taking minutes or summarizing discussion and decisions may need to be delegated to a clerical support person (if possible) if group members are averse to taking on the task of recording outcomes. However, a recorder who is a group member technically can do far more than just take minutes. This person should be in tune with the group processing and with the inputs and roles of group members and help keep the group on time. The recorder can provide feedback to the facilitator in terms of how to improve the process. One key tip is to construct a standardized meeting agenda and a record (or minutes) to facilitate the process. It is helpful to decide in advance the level of detail required in the minutes to avoid lengthy minutes and potentially unnecessary effort.

One useful way to expedite group work is to use a laptop computer to directly enter draft minutes. It is also valuable to summarize actions and assignments at the end of the meeting. Some leaders choose to allow the recorder to summarize discussion on a topic versus composing detailed minutes on each topic. Sending out minutes and talking points or a summary of items discussed and decisions made shortly after the meeting can support continued engagement and communication of the group.

Finally, group members who believe that they can be active participants—each with equal status in the meeting—are generally more engaged and feel empowered. The three components of facilitator, recorder, and group members contribute to the design of a positive working group. All can share in the basic group role functions. As with teams, leaders should establish ground rules for members of the group to facilitate maximum engagement. Some common rules may include:

- Meetings begin and end on time
- Members need to be on time, prepared, and stay for the entire meeting
- No cell phone or computer use during the meeting except on scheduled breaks
- One person speaks at a time
- No sidebar conversations

DISRUPTIVE ROLES AND BEHAVIORS

Another role that the group leader assumes is that of process facilitator. The leader must observe group members' actions and be prepared to control or redirect disruptive behaviors. It is important to focus on the behavior that needs to be adjusted and not label an individual in a group. Although the leader has a responsibility to deal with these nonproductive behaviors, in a mature team or highly effective group this is also a responsibility of other group members. If the issue is not addressed by a fellow group member, then the leader needs to be prepared to address the behavior. However, it is very hierarchical thinking to leave this responsibility solely to the leader, and doing so reinforces the formal hierarchy in the group. It is also important that the leader, facilitator, or group member avoids embarrassing a member of a group publicly because the impact on the group will be equally disruptive. Many times individuals do not have insight concerning their own behavior or its impact on the group. It can be a "teachable moment" to enhance an individual professionally by diplomatically redirecting to positive behavior. In the following sections are some types of disruptive group members that are encountered (Jacobs & Rosenthal, 1984), with strategies for the leader to use in managing the behavior of the group member. See also Chapter 7 for further information such as crucial conversations.

Compulsive Talkers

A common disruptive behavior is seen in individuals who are compulsive talkers. Often their behavior can be modified. One suggestion is to thank them for their input and then ask to hear from others on that same topic before they are given the opportunity to speak again, as a way of guiding and opening up the meeting to be more effective. If this behavior continues to affect the group negatively and the individual is not receptive to this subtle feedback, meeting with the person after the group work and giving direct, constructive feedback about the negative impact of the behavior may be necessary. There are techniques that can be shared with them to assist them in future meetings, such as asking them to keep track of the number of times they have spoken on a particular subject. In a mature team, it would be expected that this issue could be brought up and dealt with by any team member.

Nontalkers

The nontalkers are the quiet ones. They may not be comfortable speaking in front of a group or may process information more slowly than other members of the group. It is important to create a safe environment where their ideas are considered. Some approaches include offering them the option of submitting their ideas in writing or directly asking them to share their thoughts on the matter at hand. Anyone in the group can specifically ask them questions to draw them out, thereby opening up a broader range of group input. Preparing members in advance by distributing the agenda or letting them know where their input will be crucial is also a way to include the nontalkers. Sometimes these individuals need time to think through their thoughts before they engage in a conversation, unlike their more spontaneous and verbal peers. It is most important to understand their communication style and not embarrass them in front of a group if they are not engaged in discussion.

Interrupters

The interrupter must be addressed because this person is demonstrating a lack of awareness or self-control. The interrupter can be a problem in groups because the person can stifle conversation. Individuals who are interrupted may feel violated and wonder why they are not given the courtesy of finishing a thought and having their full input considered. Anyone in the group can halt the interruption, control, and redirect the interrupter. This can easily be accomplished by saying, "Let's allow Joan to finish what she was saying." If the group does not intervene, it is the responsibility of the facilitator. One consideration when developing ground rules for the group is to list no interruptions as an expectation. Interrupters may be individuals who process information quickly. It might be beneficial to meet with them privately to give them some examples. They might not have insight concerning their behavior and actions needed to support communication within the group.

Squashers

Squashers try to squash an idea before it is even developed. Suggestions about processes or procedures that have not been proven or even tried are much easier to criticize than are facts or opinions. Persons who are averse to change may have a litany of reasons why a potential solution would never work or why this proposed project simply cannot or should not happen. Often these are people who do not want to take a personal risk or undergo the personal effort of making a change, so it is easier to squash everything and maintain the status quo. Especially during brainstorming sessions, the leader must be alert to and have a method for containing the squasher. An easy way to influence this is to set the expectation at the beginning of the session by saying, for example, "For this exercise, please do not engage in analyzing or saying anything negative about the ideas thrown out until we have them all identified." There will be time later that allows dissecting and critiquing a new idea. Negative remarks adversely affect the level of creativity in any group, but an individual may have a wealth of experience and knowledge such that they discern pitfalls and barriers more quickly than others. Careful team discussion guidance is needed.

Distracted or Unreliable Members

Unreliable members really may not be committed to the group's work. They may be distracted, which they exhibit in a variety of ways, including arriving late, leaving early, answering phone calls, texting, or reading e-mails during the meeting. They may not be prepared for the meeting. Ultimately, they are not contributing to the ongoing group work or the task at hand nor are they invested in the group's goals. The leader needs to address this issue with them. One possible solution is to meet with them privately and discuss whether they are interested and able to be part of the group. There are times when individuals overcommit and, as a result, do not fulfill their obligations to the group or others. Sharing the observed group behavior and expectations is essential should they wish to be part of the group. If they do, it might be beneficial to give them a specific assignment with accountability. If this does not work, they may need to be released from the group or placed in an advisory role.

MANAGING DISRUPTIVE BEHAVIOR IN GROUPS

The most useful way to have an impact on negative behaviors is to lead the group through the clarification of their working expectations. When group members have clearly identified what they need from each other to work together productively in a group setting, they have established the norms for acceptable and non-acceptable behavior.

The nurse leader can take an active role in structuring group work for positive processing and effective outcomes. It is important to control the flow to modulate disruptive group members without embarrassing them. Another way is to structure positive and constructive group roles among members. Peer pressure is a powerful group behavior modification tactic, especially for group members for whom approval of the rest of the group is important. The leader's vision, enthusiasm, interpersonal relationship skills, and empowerment of followers all facilitate group effectiveness.

LEADERSHIP AND MANAGEMENT IMPLICATIONS

Leaders play a significant role in the success of an organization and, specifically, patient safety, quality, and joy at work. The ability to work with a committed collaborative group, team, or committee is essential for an organization to continue to grow and improve as well as retain top talent. It is well documented in the literature that nursing job satisfaction and burnout correlate with the degree of teamwork, the work environment, professional practice, and degree of professional and collaborative working relationships with both the nursing team and medical staff. For example, new nurses in nurse residency programs report difficulty in working on project and patient care teams if they have not had prior exposure or background. Because of the growing use of interdisciplinary teams, leaders and managers can structure in mentored experiences so that new nurses specifically can grow in knowledge and skill in teamwork. See Chapter 7 for more on communication leadership for teams and groups. Health care organizations that have managers with an effective management style that allows a degree of autonomy, promotes interdisciplinary relationships, and promotes professional development have a lower turnover among the nursing staff.

The leadership and management role is essential in ensuring that groups, teams, and committees are effective. With limited resources the leader should consider the work to be accomplished, determine the structure most suited to do the work, put the structure in place, and facilitate the work process. This requires a leader who understands the basic differences among work groups and teams, committees, and informal groups. The leader also needs to be able to think carefully about the work to be accomplished and determine whether it is primarily collective or individual work.

The leader's role includes selecting the right members, inspiring them to participate, preparing critical questions, developing agendas and background materials, summarizing the minutes and developing talking points, continually coaching the group for effective functioning, and guiding the long-range strategy. This is a planning, coordinative, and tracking function. Leaders and managers address questions such as:

- What is the task?
- What is the best way for this task to be accomplished?
- Is collective work involved?
- Do we need a team, or will a good work group or committee suffice?
- How many meetings will it take?
- How much effort is required?
- How can the tasks be divided?
- How can they be delegated?

In planning for meetings, a good leader puts in the time and effort to provide preliminary information and documents so that all members are prepared when they come to the meeting, they know what the issues are, and they are familiar with the background of the task to be accomplished. The leader facilitates the group coming to some agreement about norms for decision making, length of discussion, when to vote or use consensus, and the process through which the task is completed efficiently and effectively. This is done as a deliberate agenda item that the leader initiates, opens for discussion, and brings to closure. Sometimes an off-site retreat is used to employ high-relationship and group-forming strategies. Nurses may find that the group leader role challenges them to plan, organize, coordinate, and evaluate the work of the group.

An effective leader understands that a process is involved in creating effective, engaged work teams, highly functioning groups, and committees. The process requires facilitation and a significant amount of coaching

from the leader. The leader's style must fit the development stage of the group, with the leader providing more extensive structure and direction in early stages and minimal structure and direction in later stages. The leader must support the work and at times coach the team or group. Skill, capability, and readiness of the group must be assessed. Ensuring they have appropriate resources is imperative. Finally, celebrating the success of the group, team, or committee is essential, with the understanding that recognition is personal. Although some individuals enjoy public recognition, others prefer private recognition such as a note or private comment about a job well done.

CURRENT ISSUES AND TRENDS

Creating Healthy Workplaces

The creation of a positive and healthy work environment is a key issue in health care. Organizations continue to struggle with attracting and retaining highly qualified nurses and other members of the health care team and with motivating employees who are highly engaged and experience joy in their work. There is much evidence that confirms that an unhealthy work environment contributes to unsafe conditions that result in medical errors, poorly coordinated and ineffective care, as well as conflict and stress among members of the health care team (Roth et al., 2015). In 2005 the American Association of Critical-Care Nurses (AACN, 2005) released *AACN Standards for Establishing and Sustaining Healthy Work Environments: A Journey to Excellence.* The six standards are as follows: skilled communication, true collaboration, effective decision making, appropriate staffing, meaningful recognition, and authentic leadership. These are recognized in nursing as the gold standard for health care organizations (see also Chapters 3 and 4).

A healthy work environment assumes that the relationships one has with colleagues and co-workers are positive and respectful. Leadership plays an important role in supporting the nursing team. Ensuring adequate staff, an appropriate workload, and mutual respect among not only the nursing team but also with other disciplines is critical to creating and sustaining a healthy work environment. Another aspect of a positive workplace related to groups is nurses' need to see problems solved and difficult aspects of work resolved so that conditions improve over time. Effective problem-solving groups are a crucial aspect of making this happen.

TeamSTEPPS

In the early 2000s, the Agency for Healthcare Research and Quality (AHRQ), in partnership with the Department of Defense, began working on a patient safety initiative that was directed at improving teamwork in health care settings. TeamSTEPPS was the result (AHRQ, 2016). The acronym stands for **T**eam **S**trategies and **T**ools to **E**nhance **P**erformance and **P**atient **S**afety. The premise is quite simple. Anyone who touches a patient (nurse, physician, pharmacist, technician) must work together to ensure the delivery of safe and high-quality care. It is aimed at helping health care professionals work together more effectively as a team. TeamSTEPPS teaches professionals to understand each other's roles and collaborate to improve the quality of the care they deliver (see Chapter 7). The aim is to foster a culture where any member of the team has the freedom to respectfully question authority when there is a question that an error may be occurring. It teaches the team that questioning authority need not be threatening. In the airline industry, there is similar training known as crew resource management.

One example is a structured process for communication to ensure information is clearly exchanged between members of the team. There is a specific training curriculum used to integrate teamwork principles. This program is much like a boot camp in teamwork and interdependent relationships. It offers a host of innovations such as team huddles, patient handoff briefings, time-outs before commencement of a surgical procedure, and the SBAR (situation, background, assessment, and recommendation) technique for communicating information in a concise manner. The website *http://www.ahrq.gov/teamstepps/index.html* offers an impressive number of resources (see Chapter 7 for more on SBAR).

Innovation Centers

Fostering innovation is essential as health care continues to transform with targeted focus on continuous improvement and breakthrough novel ideas and approaches to patient care (see Chapter 2). Health care organizations today are being measured on quality results, the patient experience, and the cost of care. Innovation groups and committees are engaged in total quality management (TQM) initiatives, continuous quality improvement (CQI) methods using techniques such as Lean, Six Sigma, and rapid response teams (see Chapter 18).

A common way of thinking about problems is to look for an individual to blame. The result of systems thinking is to capture the energy of teams to tackle systems problems. An overall focus on quality has led to adoption of business management concepts such as Lean and Six Sigma. These are customer-focused and data-driven approaches to deriving best practices. The focus is on reducing process variation and then on improving process capability. Lean focuses on process speed and reduction of waste and inefficiencies; Six Sigma focuses on process quality toward fewer defects.

Many organizations have created innovation centers as a means to discover new ways to address health care challenges. New health care products and services are being tested—and in some cases commercialized—through collaboration with clinicians, scientists, entrepreneurs, and business partners. Innovation centers are focused on disruptive innovation as a way to expedite change. This may involve developing new techniques and approaches to operational efficiency including testing new workflows, patient care redesign, standardization, and teamwork through simulation and hands-on experiential learning.

Leaders are cautioned that creativity and innovation at a team level require diversity in membership and perspective. Diverse teams have the freedom to challenge the status quo and engage in creative problem solving. Nursing leaders play a crucial role integrating with other disciplines in making a commitment to ensure that teams feel supported and have the freedom to creatively identify new ways to address clinical processes and care redesign. Leaders who understand and use these techniques and the process of innovation can be very effective in disseminating and implementing novel approaches to patient care.

Multidisciplinary Quality Improvement Teams

Whether continuous quality improvement (CQI), total quality management (TQM), Lean, Six Sigma, or some related quality improvement program, direct care nurses are expected to participate more actively in multidisciplinary quality improvement teams. In an organization that looks at problems as systems problems, the next step is to acknowledge that anyone involved in that part of the system needs to be engaged in solving the problem. Therefore coordinating patient care and solving problems through interdisciplinary committees and groups with people of equal status is the strategy best suited to solving systems problems.

The basic strategy behind each of these systems-based approaches is to bring together interdisciplinary collaborative groups. This means that if there is a problem in patient care, the physicians, nurses, ancillary staff, and any other direct caregivers work together to identify issues and possible solutions. Solutions that are identified can be tested and evaluated through collaboration. The facilitator does not have to be a content expert or the person with the most expertise in that problem area. In fact, having the most expertise in a

problem area can actually be problematic when functioning as a facilitator because it becomes too tempting to take over the process. The individual's facilitation skills are crucially important.

Establishing equality among peers regardless of status and using expertise and responsibility result in a different way of looking at work, which has implications in terms of how nursing practice may change. It also means nurses are going to continue to be involved more substantially in groups, committees, and teams. Multidisciplinary teams are not just for problem solving and process improvement. The current pace and complexity of the world today also demands that new approaches to care delivery be considered by teams.

RESEARCH NOTE

Source
Lancaster, G., Kolakowsky-Hayner, S., Kovacich, J., & Greer-Williams, N. (2015). Interdisciplinary communication and collaboration among physicians, nurses, and unlicensed assistive personnel. *Journal of Nursing Scholarship, 47*(3), 275–284.

Purpose
To explore the potential for hospital-based interdisciplinary care provided by physicians, nurses, and unlicensed assistive personnel (UAPs).

Discussion
The authors conducted qualitative, semistructured, face-to-face individual interviews with physicians, nurses, and UAPs involved in direct care in a large metropolitan hospital. The interviews included 10 questions, and participants from throughout the organization were invited to participate. The information gathered from the interviews was transcribed and coded, identifying emergent patterns and themes.

The study suggested that physicians, nurses, and UAPs generally function as separate health care providers with little discussion among them. The study also identified that although there is still a hierarchal relationship between physicians and nurses and nurses and UAPs, relationships are changing. Although physicians and nurses have a tendency to work together more closely, UAPs are usually excluded from any type of meaningful discussion or dialogue involving patient care. There is a lack of understanding of the potential value each member of the team could offer the team.

Application to Practice
The findings of this study shed important light on the opportunity that still exists to create and support the ongoing development of effective teams both within nursing and across disciplines. Inter-professional collaboration and engagement by the team will improve patient safety and quality outcomes. Houser and colleagues (2012) found that hospital nursing units where there is a high level of participation in had better patient outcomes, including fewer infections and pressure ulcers. Harter and colleagues (2010) identified that employee perception of their work environment affects employee retention, customer loyalty, and the financial performance of the organization. Continuity and quality of care are more likely to occur when there are collegial relationships among nursing and other disciplines. Other research (Adams & Bond, 2000) found that interpersonal relationships, cohesion as a team, and collaboration with the medical staff affected nurses' job satisfaction.

The major premise behind developing a high-functioning team in this study is that it is essential for patient safety and high-quality outcomes. A secondary impact is on employee retention and customer loyalty. Perhaps it is no surprise that although improvements have been made in teamwork, there is still more work to do. Leaders play an important role in fostering an environment where there is clarity in roles and responsibility, mutual trust, effective communication, and accountability. Coaching members of the team to reach their full potential and work across disciplines is vital.

CASE STUDY

A Patient Care Leadership Team

A patient care leadership team was created in a midsize community hospital. The members were the directors of the various nursing divisions, the clinical laboratory, medical imaging, respiratory therapy, pharmacy, and perioperative services. This team established its purpose statement, identified its values, and developed a code of conduct that outlined its membership behavioral expectations. Although these individuals had long worked together, this approach with a shared leadership responsibility for the clinical services was new to them.

Michelle, the director of the pharmacy, agreed to be the team's first formal leader. One of the biggest challenges facing the team was the need to dramatically and quickly improve the patient experience scores throughout the organization. This was the underlying primary reason for the formation of the team. In the past, this would have been identified as a responsibility of the individual directors and managers, primarily those in nursing. However, there was serious concern about the quality of care that these low patient experience scores represented, and as a result this team was assigned the leadership responsibility for intervening in a positive way to raise the scores. Although the work of the team is only briefly presented here, their approach demonstrates the concept of collective leadership and joint or mutual accountability.

One of the strategies these leaders developed was related to mentoring the inpatient care units where the scores were most problematic. They decided that each team member would accept responsibility for mentoring the staff of a specific inpatient area. For example, as the director of the pharmacy, Michelle agreed to mentor one particularly challenging patient care unit that had recently appointed a new manager. Patient satisfaction scores had been inconsistent from month to month. Michelle began making rounds in the department, helping the nursing staff troubleshoot patient and family issues and coaching them in service recovery when there were problems. She also had the opportunity to interact with staff to understand the ways the pharmacy and nursing team could work better together to improve service and care. They jointly worked together to address issues she was not aware of, including issues related to medication reconciliation, medication delivery times, and errors being made in deliveries from the pharmacy to the nursing unit. There was a real commitment to improving care as a team. The results were surprisingly impressive. Not only did the patient satisfaction scores rise, but so did employee morale, collaboration, and teamwork between the nursing and the pharmacy department. The new manager had the support of a seasoned and respected manager.

Michelle and the pharmacy team benefited as well. Her leadership capacity deepened significantly, and she became recognized and sought after for attributes that had not been apparent in her work as pharmacy director. It was quite remarkable to see the results when these team members accepted joint accountability for something that in the past had been the accountability of individuals. It was also striking that Michelle was so well accepted by the nursing staff when previously a silo mentality would have prevented the formation of this type of coaching relationship between members of two different disciplines. The pharmacy team was very appreciative of the efforts to improve communication with the nursing staff.

It takes skilled team leadership and followership to capitalize on team strengths to create an effective, efficient, and highly productive team that endures over time.

Involving members in change and solving shared problems helps both members and management. Members benefit because they are involved in what affects their work. Management benefits because involvement tends to reduce resistance and increase ownership of the change or solution. The health care delivery system benefits as high-performing teams tackle and solve systems problems, improve collaboration, and promote quality and safe patient care.

CRITICAL THINKING EXERCISE

Organize into a small group, then select a leader. Take a few minutes to do this, and then select or appoint a process recorder. Here is your assignment:

The leader is a nurse manager at Valencia Community Hospital. She has been asked to lead a task force to evaluate the effectiveness of the nursing department's committee structure. The task force has been asked to create a methodology for conducting the evaluation and then making recommendations for streamlining the current structure, consolidating committees that overlap, and improving the effectiveness of the committees. The leader must now lead your group to develop a plan while preserving a sense of teamwork. The process recorder is to prepare a summary of the group's work and report as requested.

1. Observe the process the group uses to select its own leader. Did anyone try to avoid selection? Was someone an enthusiastic volunteer? How long did the process take? Were the selection criteria discussed? What were the selection criteria?

2. What method was used to select/appoint a process recorder? What power strategy was used to make this decision?

3. What is the problem identified in the task?

4. What did the group leader do to handle the situation?

5. What should the group leader do to handle the situation?

6. How did group members respond to the task?

7. What leadership and management strategies might be effective?

8. What could the leader and followers consider changing in the situation?

9. How did group members feel about what happened?

Follow up this exercise with one that tackles a similar problem: this time the leader has just been informed of a serious morale issue in the department. A few very vocal, negative staff members are intimidating and using bullying tactics to coerce their co-workers in uncomfortable ways. No one wants to speak up, and everyone thinks it is the manager's responsibility to fix the problem. This group needs to work together to develop a plan for dealing with this negative behavior.

9

Delegation in Nursing

Jayne Josephsen

http://evolve.elsevier.com/Huber/leadership

Although the roles and responsibilities of delegation have transformed over time, the foundational need for nurses to delegate is not a new concept. Florence Nightingale herself identified the need for the nurse to delegate tasks to others (Saccomano & Pinto-Zipp, 2014). The necessity for delegation has evolved and expanded as health care has developed and transitioned into a variety of community and acute care settings (Hasson et al., 2013). Delegation competencies are present throughout a variety of foundational aspects of nursing practice, such as state licensure descriptions, the national licensure examination for nurses, and in the American Association of Colleges of Nursing's baccalaureate essentials (American Association of Colleges of Nursing, 2008). The skill and process of delegation is paramount in the current era of health care reform and will only increase in application and function as the role of the nurse broadens.

Professional roles are often developed and defined when "task-shifting" occurs. The origin of delegation in health care can be traced back to physicians delegating some of their responsibilities to nurses. For example, at one time it was the physician who took vital signs or administered injections. But in present day health care these tasks are often performed by unlicensed assistive personnel (UAP) (Henderwood, 2015). As health care has become more specialized and disease processes more complex, the call for the creation of a team of health care professionals emerged to meet the multitude of patient needs. The health care team today includes a variety of therapists (respiratory, physical, speech), social workers,

chaplains, pharmacists, phlebotomists, and UAP. This task-shifting, or role transformation, is still occurring today, as nurses are required to expand their roles significantly in the contemporary health care environment and work to their full scope of practice (Altschuler et al., 2012; Brady et al., 2015; True et al., 2014).

Ensuring that the nurse's skills and experience are being used optimally is a key strategy to produce positive patient outcomes, manage resources, and improve quality of care while containing costs (American Association of Critical-Care Nurses [AACN], 2004; Brady et al., 2015). To meet these organizational and patient outcome goals, a new vision of the health care workforce is required—one that is team based, interdisciplinary, and in which the ability for the nurse to delegate is essential (Pittman & Forrest, 2015). This team-based approach to patient care necessitates training and education concerning delegation to members of the team as well as a change in approach and practice for nurses (Altschuler et al., 2012). It is crucial for the nurse to take on a leadership role concerning delegation. Nurses will be required to delegate appropriately and coach and teach UAP and other members of the team delegation skills and concepts. Moreover, nurses will be obliged to contribute to the development of organizational processes that enhance the use of effective delegation (Hansten, 2014).

The nurse as leader has a vital role in the workplace concerning patient outcomes, job satisfaction, teamwork, and patient safety. Appropriate delegation is central to all of these outcomes; therefore the nurse is required to master the art and skill of delegation (Bryant, 2015; Kaernested & Bragadottir, 2012). Nurses, whether novice or expert, are expected to perform delegation-related activities along the

Photo used with permission from laflor/Getty Images.

continuum of health care. Awareness of the necessity for effective delegation is vital for positive patient outcomes and a culture of patient-centered care. Open communication concerning delegation in the workplace can lead to discussions and education that permits the connection of delegation concepts to organizational and nursing practice (Hansten, 2014).

Delegation is at the heart of patient-centered care, as it is based on individualizing and customizing health care. With the nurse as coordinator of care, a team-based approach to patient care is used to ensure quality care and to meet the patient's unique needs. A mutual understanding and shared sense of purpose or vision between the nurse and the delegatee (the one who is delegated a nursing responsibility) is necessary for effective delegation (True et al., 2014). Research has shown that missed cares or unmet patient needs that are caused by ineffective delegation can lead to negative patient outcomes and decreased patient and employee satisfaction (Hasson et al., 2013; Papastavrou et al., 2014).

Currently a health care system change is underway as the focus of health care is transitioning from acute care to preventive and community/population-focused services (Bryant, 2015). This system change requires a redesign of the workforce and the likely increasing use and transferring of tasks to a UAP (Craftman et al., 2012; Day et al., 2014; Kaernested & Bragadottier, 2012; Pittman & Forrest, 2015). Ultimately, nurse leaders and other health care providers will need to plan for the best mix of staff to meet patient needs while maximizing members of the team practicing to their full scope of practice (Hansten, 2014). It is clear that delegation is a skill that nurses have an obligation to exercise and refine, as it is at the center of patient-centered care, quality outcomes, cost containment, and resource management in today's health care environment.

DEFINITIONS

An important aspect of effective delegation is communication. The language of delegation possesses a distinct conceptual framework. In order for a shared vision of delegation and care to develop, both the nurse and the UAP or other delegatee must have a mutual understanding of the context and meaning of common terms.

Accountability: The position of retaining responsibility for a delegated task, including supervision. Nurses answer to patients, their employers, their state board of nursing, and a criminal court if there are allegations of inappropriate or unprofessional nursing conduct or actions (American Nurses Association [ANA], 2009). The nurse is accountable to assess the situation, for the decision to delegate, and the appropriateness and supervision of the delegated task. The UAP accepting delegation also has accountability for accepting the delegated task and for the actions carried out performing that task. The National Council of State Boards of Nursing (NCSBN, 2016) defined accountability as being answerable to oneself and others for one's own choices, decisions, and actions as measured against a standard.

Assignment: The transferring of a task to UAP that is within their own level of practice. The task needs to be within the parameters of the UAP's role (such as the client care activity of oral care). Delegation is patient specific (the decision to delegate is made after the nurse's assessment of the patient), the nurse determines whether the UAP has the needed knowledge and skill to perform the task, and the nurse is responsible for supervision and assessment of the outcome of the performed task (College of Registered Nurses of British Columbia, 2013).

Authority: This refers to the legal authority to perform a task. The nurse has the power and control to make decisions concerning the nursing process and delegation of nursing tasks (ANA, 2009; NCSBN, 2005a).

Client Care Activities: Client care activities include tasks and activities necessary to care for clients and produce nursing and health outcomes. Examples include hygiene activities such as dressing and bathing, vital sign measurement, and assisting with ambulation.

Delegation: In their *Joint Statement on Delegation* (NCSBN, 2005b), the ANA and the NCSBN defined delegation in nursing as "the process for a nurse to direct another person to perform nursing tasks and activities" (p. 1). A goal of delegation is workload distribution as well as using all team members in the most resourceful way possible to meet quality patient outcomes.

Delegatee: The delegatee is the person receiving and accepting the delegation. The delegatee must be competent to perform the task and supervised by the delegator.

Delegator: The delegator is the nurse or other health care provider who is delegating the task or responsibility.

Nursing Activities: These involve actions, tasks, and direct client contact, as well as the full scope of the nursing process. The act of delegating certain activities that are performed by the nurse, but not limited to the nurse, does not create a situation in which nursing itself—and the responsibility for it—are delegated away.

Scope of Practice: This is the actions, procedures, and processes that are permitted within the terms of the professional license. It is limited to that which the law allows for specific education, experience, and competency. The UAP scope of practice varies by state due to state-specific licensure laws. In order for the nurse to delegate effectively, the nurse needs to know the state-specific practice guidelines for the UAP.

Supervision: Supervision is the provision of guidance or monitoring of a delegated nursing task. It may occur in a variety of ways, including written and verbal communication (such as giving or receiving reports), observation of the performance of the delegated task, or assessing the patient for evidence that the delegated task has been completed successfully.

Unlicensed Assistive Personnel (UAP): This includes a number of health care disciplines, such as nursing assistants, medical assistants, nurse apprentices, and personal care attendants. The NCSBN (2016) defined UAP as any unlicensed personnel trained to function in a supportive role and to whom a nursing responsibility can be delegated.

THE PROCESS OF DELEGATION

The NCSBN has developed a number of tools relating to delegation and the roles of licensed nurses and assistive personnel that have been collected in the document *Working With Others: A Position Paper* (NCSBN, 2005a). This position paper presented key delegation concepts and the delegation decision-making process. There are two helpful decision trees (visual flow charts): delegation to nursing assistive personnel (pp. 11–12) and accepting assignment to supervise unlicensed assistive personnel (pp. 16–17). Also included in the position paper is a state-by-state review of statues and rules, a summary of multiple organizations' position statements, definitions, and a literature/case law review. These tools are useful and are grounded in the nursing process of assessment, diagnosis, planning, implementation, and evaluation. In addition, the ANA and the NCSBN published a joint statement on delegation (2005) that included background material, a decision tree for delegation to UAP, and communication, supervision, and evaluation guidance and questions. These are valuable guides and classic works, yet they have not been updated. However, in 2016 the NCSBN published *National Guidelines for Nursing Delegation,* which used current research and literature to facilitate and standardize the nursing delegation process. This document

contains a delegation model composed of employer, licensed nurse, and delegatee responsibilities; key definitions, and guidelines for delegation.

The nursing process is organized around the ability for the nurse to integrate practical, theoretical, and intuitive knowledge, skills, and experience (Heath, 2012). This process does not end when the nurse delegates a task. Delegation is a decision-making process that requires skillful nurse judgment. The decision to delegate a task should be based on an individualized patient assessment and evaluation and sound clinical decision making (Bryant, 2015). Before delegating a task the nurse should assess the patient, consider the patient condition, diagnoses, physical and emotional stability, and family issues (Trossman, 2012).

When considering whether to delegate a task, the nurse needs to assess the patient and determine whether the action delegated is complex or if the plan of care of the patient could change rapidly (Catalano, 2015). In this case it is not appropriate to delegate, as the UAP should not be put in a position in which he or she is compelled to make clinical judgments concerning patient care (Bryant, 2015; Hand, 2016). Additionally, if the UAP does not have a sufficient understanding of the patient's condition or the desired outcomes, he or she may not perform the delegated task in a way that supports optimal patient care (Hansten, 2014). In this instance, if the task is still to be delegated, then the nurse is responsible for providing the UAP education about how the task is to be completed and require a return demonstration from the UAP or provide detailed education on the task, which includes outcomes, potential complications, and when to notify the nurse (Catalano, 2015). The nurse can delegate tasks or certain aspects of care but never the nursing process, including assessment and evaluation (Trossman, 2012).

In making a decision to delegate a nursing task, the following five factors should be assessed:
1. Potential for harm: The nurse must determine how much risk the activity carries for an individual patient.
2. Complexity of the task: The more complex the activity, the less desirable it is to delegate.
3. Amount of problem solving and innovation required: If an uncomplicated task requires special attention, adaptation, or an innovative approach, it should not be delegated.
4. Unpredictability of outcome: When a patient's response to the activity is unknown or unpredictable it is not advisable to delegate that activity.

5. Level of patient interaction: It is not advisable to delegate so many tasks that the amount of time the nurse spends with the patient is decreased to the point that a therapeutic relationship cannot be established between the nurse and the patient. (AACN, 2004, p.10)

The delegation process, as outlined by the ANA/NCSBN joint statement (2005) and the NCSBN national guidelines (2016), begins with the preparation/assessment phase and then goes on to outline a five-step process. These steps are (1) the right task, (2) under the right circumstance, (3) to the right person, (4) with the right directions and communication, (5) under the right supervision and evaluation.

When determining the *right task* to delegate, the nurse must determine whether the task falls within the guidelines of established organizational policies, the ANA code of ethics, and legal practice regulations. For example, in some situations the UAP may be allowed to assist with the use of an incentive spirometer, but it is not appropriate for the UAP to assess the effectiveness of the intervention.

The *right circumstance* to perform the task indicates the delegatee has the available resources, equipment, safe environment, and supervision to complete the task correctly. For example, it may be allowed for the UAP to monitor vital signs, but if the patient is having an acute episode of hypertension, then that would require a nurse as opposed to the UAP to monitor the vital signs.

The *right person* is the one who has the education and competency to perform the element of care. The delegatee, then, is legally acceptable to complete the task. For example, some states may allow a UAP to assist a patient in taking their oral medications, but in other states this may not be allowed.

The *right direction/communication* of delegated tasks must be a clear, concise description of the task, including its objective, limits, and expectations. For example, the direction to "Get the patient up in room 1101" is somewhat vague. Rather, the nurse could say "When you get the patient in room 1101 up today, remember he is on hip precautions so he will need assistance getting out of bed and ensuring he is sitting correctly when up in the chair." The difference in these two directions is immense. The first directive is ambiguous and may cause the UAP to miss specific positioning that is necessary for a positive patient outcome.

The *right supervision* of a task includes appropriate monitoring, intervention, evaluation, and feedback as deemed necessary. In most cases, it is recommended that the nurse delegator and delegatee agree on the task, circumstances, and time frame and arrange for feedback in which the delegatee reports or the delegator evaluates progress toward completion of the task. In no instance should the UAP be required to make independent clinical judgments concerning the patient because the nurse is unavailable or unwilling to provide supervision (Bryant, 2015). One way to ensure that both the delegator and delegatee understand what the task is and how to complete it effectively is to follow up a verbal directive with written instructions so that each person can refer to them later.

The UAP has a further role in delegation by being prepared to receive delegation, participate in the communication and information exchange, and ultimately accept the delegated task. The UAP should seek clarification and request additional training/supervision if needed and confirm to the nurse the expectations and plan of action in case an issue arises. Lastly, the UAP is required to accept or deny the delegated task. If the task is accepted, the UAP has also accepted accountability for his or her role in the delegated task (NCSBN, 2005b). Fig. 9.1 highlights areas of accountability for the delegator and delegatee.

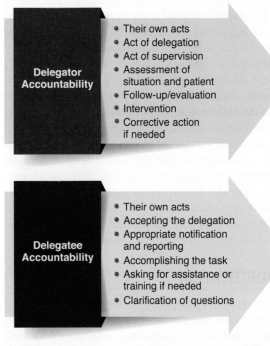

Delegator Accountability
- Their own acts
- Act of delegation
- Act of supervision
- Assessment of situation and patient
- Follow-up/evaluation
- Intervention
- Corrective action if needed

Delegatee Accountability
- Their own acts
- Accepting the delegation
- Appropriate notification and reporting
- Accomplishing the task
- Asking for assistance or training if needed
- Clarification of questions

FIG. 9.1 Delegator and delegatee accountability.

At the core of the five rights of delegation and the roles of the UAP and nurse are three organizational principles that are present in many health care settings today. These principles include organizational and legal guidelines and policies, patient safety and accountability, and knowledge and education (Craftman et al., 2012). These principles can be applied to delegation in very concrete ways. Resistance to change, role and scope of practice confusion, lack of training and education, and poor leadership structures can bring a multitude of difficulties in meeting these organizational principles related to delegation (Pittman & Forrest, 2015).

In the end, delegation is necessary, as the nurse cannot do everything for the patient and meet all of their needs. A team-based environment, using effective delegation, is required for positive patient outcomes (Bryant, 2015). However, appropriate delegation cannot occur if the nurse is unaware of the organizational systems in place to establish competency requirements for the UAP or what the state practice acts legally allow the UAP to perform. Additionally, to meet patient safety and professional accountability guidelines, the nurse must communicate mindfully and respectfully with the UAP concerning the delegated task. Effective communication demands situational awareness and presence in the conversation. Without these items, the information will be relayed in unproductive manner, which will hinder the delegation process and inevitably lead to poor outcomes and ineffective delegation.

Effective delegation is real to the delegatee and to the patient. Delegators permit delegatees to perform the delegated tasks on their own, but only after instilling in them the highest standards of performance and adherence to a shared vision, which is created through a relationship based on mutual respect and a dynamic information exchange. See Fig. 9.2 for a model of dynamic information exchange in delegation. Effective delegation allows the UAP to participate in tasks that offer learning opportunities and professional growth, and it also provides support throughout the process of the task if needed (Finkelman & Kenner, 2013).

PRIORITIZATION

Nurses recognize that priority-setting skills are essential to survival as a direct care ("bedside") nurse, but nursing students and novice nurses often need assistance with developing skills and confidence in prioritization. Time

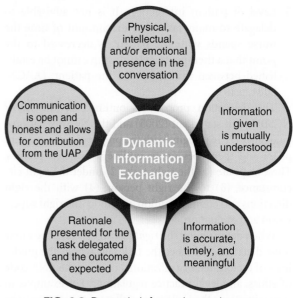

FIG. 9.2 Dynamic information exchange.

management; familiarity with an organization's policies, procedures, and supply locations; the development of efficient routines; and the tension between safety and speed are factors. Newly graduated nurses may struggle with delegation and communication within the nursing care team, all contributing to stress from the urgency and constant changes. Yet it is imperative that they learn how to prioritize the many competing tasks so that patients are best served, the team is respected, and they themselves maintain energy and focus (Nelson, 2010).

Nurses use discretionary judgment and ongoing assessment to prioritize a patient's need for care throughout the caregiving time and as patient situations unfold. Effective nursing prioritization is an advanced skill of nursing practice. It relies on discretionary judgment and ongoing assessment to manage complex and uncertain dynamic situations. Lake and colleagues (2009) found that nursing prioritization of patients' needs for care is a non-sequential decision-making process that is ongoing throughout unfolding patient situations.

Patterson and colleagues (2011) found that there are seven levels to a prioritization hierarchy of nursing activities (high to low): (1) addressing imminent clinical concerns, (2) high uncertainty activities, (3) significant, core clinical caregiving and managing pain, (4) relationship management, (5) documenting, helping others, and patient support, (6) system improvement and cleaning/preparing supplies, and (7) personal breaks and social interactions. This hierarchy can be used to help teach prioritization skills and evaluate the design of health care environments for improvement. As there appears to be no accepted standard for how to prioritize nursing tasks, this framework can be used to evaluate missed nursing care especially in the categories of patient support and documenting activities for quality and outcomes improvement (Patterson et al., 2011). Nurses can improve prioritization skills through knowledge about priority setting; seeing the whole picture; use of the assessment process; time management strategies such as time for planning, completing the highest priority task, and then reprioritizing; acuity ranking; grouping activities; and breaking down activities into smaller steps. Delegation is then an option to extend the nurses' ability to complete the needed patient care duties.

BARRIERS TO DELEGATION

Although delegation is in everyone's best interest for a variety of reasons, the process may be undermined from within the health care setting itself. There may be organizational issues such as time and paperwork pressures interfering with the nurse being able to effectively delegate. Or the organization may not provide support or education concerning delegation or expected outcomes of delegation. These organizational deficits can lead to the nurse being unable to delegate appropriately or effectively and potentially lead to negative patient outcomes (Keogh, 2014).

There may also be issues such as status, risk, or lack of time that can lead to a number of problems. The health care hierarchy often has the nurse as leader or coordinator of patient care delegating to a UAP. This institutional hierarchy may contribute to an ingrained status versus lack of status issue that can be a barrier to effective delegation. Nurses also find delegation time consuming and believe it is easier to do the tasks themselves (Kaernested & Bragadottier, 2012). Or they may believe that if they do it themselves they do not have to worry about the UAP making a mistake, therefore minimizing risk (Trossman, 2012). These are often the beliefs of novice or insecure nurses who have not mastered the art of delegation or internalized the value and contribution of a patient-centered, team-based, health care environment to positive patient outcomes.

Furthermore, when called on to delegate something important, the nurse may discover that he or she has a lack of trust in the UAP (Kaernested & Bragadottier, 2012; Lee et al., 2015). The nurse may fear that there will be a problematic outcome or the patient may be affected negatively if the task is delegated (AACN, 2004). This is a real dilemma, because how can a relationship of mutual trust be developed between the delegator and delegatee if the nurse chooses not to delegate due to an absence of trust? The emotion of fear is often driving this lack of trust and could be a delegation barrier.

Delegation inevitably involves some risk, and this can create an emotional response on the part of the nurse and the delegatee. This risk can be mitigated through effective communication and dynamic information processing. Poor teamwork and communication skills can lead to confusion and anxiety among the team members (Graham et al., 2014; Kaernested & Bragadottier, 2012). This may lead to hard feelings, grudges, or passive aggressive actions of refusing to perform tasks delegated (Hansten, 2014). Moreover, not all members of the team may interpret delegation the same way, or the organization may have institutional barriers in place that discourage collaborative practice among the nurse and the UAP, which can lead to care being omitted. Research has shown that the types of care most often omitted include oral care, hygiene, ambulation, and turning, all of which can lead to significantly poor patient outcomes. This is where delegation and clear communication regarding accountability between the team members is beneficial for the functioning of the organization as well as patient care (Hansten, 2014).

The use of delegation may also be threatening to a nurse's self-esteem or seen by the nurse as their failure to personally accomplish work. This is a genuine issue for novice or younger nurses, as these nurses state that they often feel insecure in their ability to delegate or uncomfortable delegating tasks to older and/or more experienced staff members (Kaernested & Bragadottier, 2012; Saccomano & Pinto-Zipp, 2014). The novice nurse may believe that if he or she delegates then he or she will be perceived as lazy or bossy or create resentment among the UAP (Magnusson, 2013; Trossman, 2012). Nurses may also feel the need to be "indispensible" and believe that if they want the task done right they have to perform the task themselves.

Furthermore, the nurse may not truly understand delegation concepts and may actually be using assignment of tasks rather than delegation as a way to distribute the workload. This type of delegation may be done without consideration of the delegatee and whether the task is appropriate for that UAP or if they would benefit from being assigned the task (Patton et al., 2013). This lack of understanding can cause detrimental patient outcomes, resentment, and mistrust on the part of the UAP, and promote a continuation of poor delegation processes and outcomes.

Likewise, the nurse's type of delegation or leadership style may be a significant barrier to effective delegation (Keogh, 2014). Fig. 9.3 contains descriptions of various delegator leadership styles. Many nurses fall into the "invincible" nurse style; they prefer to do everything themselves so as not to risk delegating to the UAP or transfer some control to someone else. This nurse often stays late after the shift completing documentation and may miss some cares that should have been completed due to trying to do everything him- or herself. This can lead to a nurse/UAP team that is not used to its maximum effectiveness and lead to resentment among the staff as well as issues with nursing management due to excessive overtime or missed cares.

Nurses using the "rationalizer" leadership style are uncomfortable with the act of delegation, and in an effort to appear cognizant of the UAP's time and effort, they will go to great lengths to rationalize to the UAP and others why something was delegated. They are fearful of appearing lazy, but the very act of always rationalizing delegation may create division between the nurse/UAP team. The "pal" is the nurse who wants to be everyone's friend. These nurses do not want to be viewed as pushy or demanding. This type of delegator may come across as a pushover to the UAP, and this can cause trust and lack of respect issues in the nurse/UAP team.

The "shining example" nurse believes that he or she should delegate through example. These nurses feel that if they give a good example of patient care, then the UAP will automatically start doing what is role modeled. Unfortunately, because this type of delegation relies on observation and not communication, it is fraught with a variety of poor communication issues within the nurse/UAP team. Lastly, the "watchdog" nurse views delegation as a real risk and is constantly monitoring

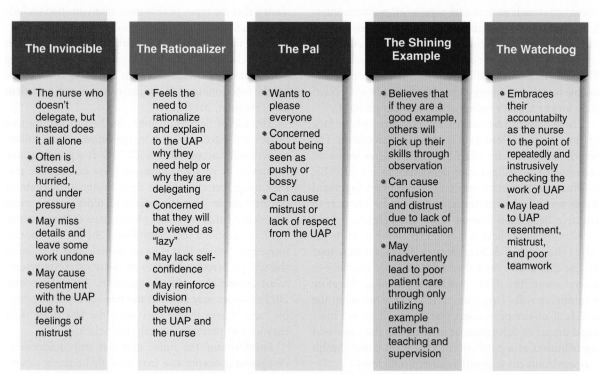

FIG. 9.3 Types of nurse delegators. (Data from Keogh, K. [2014]. Lecturer says delegation should be a part of preregistration courses. *Nursing Standard, 29*[1], 9. doi:10.7748/ns.29.1.9.s7)

and micromanaging the UAP to the point that resentment may enter the nurse/UAP team and lead to poor teamwork and outcomes.

At times the delegatee is a barrier to the delegation process by avoiding delegation. The delegatee may fear criticism regarding mistakes because they lack confidence in their own abilities or may feel that they already have enough workload. The delegated task can be part of the UAP's workload anyhow, and this may be a way for the delegatee to avoid work. If lacking confidence is the issue for the UAP, the nurse can remind the delegatee that he or she does have the necessary experience, skills, knowledge, and ability to perform the task and work with them on any issues.

Solutions to these barriers of delegation are straightforward: mutual respect, feedback, supervision, and communication. Detailed and specific activities need to be communicated through dynamic information exchange to the delegatee. It is essential that the nurse recognizes the importance of the process of supervision and its implications for educational opportunities that focus on delegation competencies. In short, by effectively delegating, the nurse and the UAP are empowered to provide the best quality patient-centered care possible while working to their full scope of practice.

ETHICAL AND LEGAL ISSUES CONCERNING DELEGATION

No review of delegation would be complete without discussing common legal issues surrounding delegation. As with all aspects of nursing there are ethical and legal parameters to be followed. Ethical and legal issues invariably occur when there is a lack of congruency between the nurse's state nurse practice act and organizational policies. Some state nurse practice acts clearly define scope of practice concerning delegable activities, and others are more unclear. Furthermore, some nurse practice acts have not been updated to account for the current prevalence of home and community-based health care delivery, which can cause role blurring and confusion of delegable tasks (Wilt & Foley, 2016). Ultimately, although certain discrete tasks may be delegated in any health care setting, the nursing process consisting of assessment, clinical judgment, and evaluation of outcomes may not be delegated (NCSBN, 2005b; 2016). This foundational fact should direct the nurse's response concerning delegation no matter whether there is a scope-of-practice or organizational issue.

Scope of Practice

Legal guidelines and parameters direct and define nursing and UAP practice. The nurse as delegator is required to know his or her state's nurse practice act and the organization's policies, procedures, and competencies outlined for health care team members (Trossman, 2012). The ANA and each state's nurse practice act speak for the profession of nursing to guide the professional practice of nursing through definitions, standards of practice, and statements about delegation and supervision. Additionally, the state's nurse practice act outlines and defines the activities that only the nurse can perform because harm may occur if they are performed by someone without the necessary skills, knowledge, and abilities. Identification of which tasks are appropriate to nursing and which tasks can be delegated—and to whom—is imperative. It is critical that the nurse is knowledgeable concerning these standards of practice, as he or she must be diligent in monitoring what is being delegated for encroachment or working outside the defined scope of practice (AACN, 2004).

Organizational Issues

The nurse is never permitted under law to passively observe substandard care. The most common situation is of a fellow nurse or other health care provider demonstrably or clearly failing to provide the appropriate care to clients. Substandard care may also come about when a health care agency fails to exercise its corporate duty in providing sufficient numbers of nurses with appropriate delegation and supervision skills to ensure quality care. In the event that the health care agency is compromising care, the nurse will need to initiate an assessment of how much client safety is being compromised. If there is clear actual or potential harm, the nurse must act directly. If the situation in ambiguous, such as an ethical issue, then the nurse must take some action appropriate to the circumstance. For example, this may be reported to the immediate supervisor or the nurse may refuse to participate if that is appropriate. Ethical concerns may also be referred to the organization's ethics committee.

Cost Containment

Legal and ethical issues surround the tensions and trade-offs between quality and cost. For example, what constitutes an unsafe level of nurse staffing is not clear. Nurse leaders face uncomfortable situations when deciding between labor budget pressures and staffing for client care needs. Nevertheless, nurses are held accountable for the quality of their patient care, and inadequate staffing may not provide a legal defense for inappropriate delegation (Owsley, 2013). The increasing use of UAP inherently brings to focus the issues with delegation related to staffing mix and resource management.

Nursing Licensure

Another confusing legal issue is that of the delegated task being connected to the nurse's license. This is often a fear that nurses have concerning delegation of care to UAP. There is the belief that if a task is delegated then all of the liability concerning that task falls only to the nurse. This belief is based on an incomplete understanding of the delegation process. A key aspect of delegation is the UAP accepting the task—and thus some responsibility connected to the task (Catalano, 2015). This does not mean that once a task is delegated the nurse is not accountable for the delegation process. The nurse still needs to ensure the competency of the UAP to complete the task and provide for feedback and supervision. Accountability in delegation means being obligated to answer for one's actions, including the act of supervision. The nurse is ultimately accountable for the appropriateness and supervision of the delegated task. Thus the nurse may be found liable if found negligent in the process of delegating and supervising. The delegatee is accountable for accepting the delegation and for the actions in carrying out the delegated task. Therefore both the delegator and delegate share accountability for the task.

Direct Versus Indirect Delegation

The often puzzling issue of delegation versus assignment can also be a legal issue. Direct delegation is just that, the nurse directly delegating a task to a UAP. Indirect delegation is the organizationally produced list of tasks that the UAP can perform, such as taking vital signs (Catalano, 2015). Although organizations may suggest which acts are delegatable, the nurse is still responsible for the assessment of the patient and the UAP to determine whether it is in the patient's best interests to have the UAP complete a patient care task (NCSBN, 2005b; Wilt & Foley, 2016). Just because the task is on the list of things the facility deems appropriate for the UAP to perform does not mean it is an appropriate task for the UAP to perform in a specific patient situation.

The nurse must be diligent in making a sound clinical judgment as well. For example, it may be organizationally supported for the UAP in a school setting to administer student medications because there may not be a nurse on site. But the school nurse still would need to make a decision as to whether a specific UAP is appropriate to administer medications to students in the nurse's absence (Wilt & Foley, 2016). Ultimately, as coordinator of the patient's care, the nurse is accountable for safe and appropriate completion of tasks concerning his or her assigned patients.

Communication

The skill and quality of delegation can be learned and improved, but the nurse must be aware of his or her own personal barriers, biases, and assumptions that may prevent effective delegation. A basic foundation of delegation is clear communication. The nurse should be available to the delegatee and give and request feedback. The nurse needs to give the delegatee the freedom to perform the task independently if possible, as this will build trust. But the nurse should never delegate tasks that cannot be evaluated or supervised because they do not know how to do the task themselves (AACN, 2004; Trossman, 2012).

Delegation requires skillful written and verbal communication to avoid liability. Clear documentation of assignments and additional clarification of the delegated tasks or training for each health care team member are required when delegating. The organization is responsible for informing nurses of all changes in policy concerning UAP practice and expectations through e-mail, memos, in-services, or staff meetings. The nurse's responsibility is to keep current with updates in the literature and guideline changes in the standards of care concerning delegation as well as to be an advocate for the development and implementation of safe and appropriate delegation standards of care. It is essential that nurses are involved in organizational and legislative processes and policy development so that safe standards of practice are initiated and maintained (Wilt & Foley, 2016).

What to Do When in Doubt

Clearly, client safety and obligation to do no harm are fundamental starting points for any questionable situation regarding delegation (Wilt & Foley, 2016). The nurse has accountability to society at large, as well as to his or her patients and employer. Nurses are held to a standard of patient care in which they use their expertise, knowledge, and skill in decision making (Wilkinson, 2016). When considering a questionable situation, the standards of "reasonable," "prudent," and "good faith" form the foundations for legal and ethical decision making. The nurse can analyze the situation and decide on a strategy. A framework for ethical analysis can be chosen to help clarify values and ethical choices. A legal analysis can be done to assess whether the elements of a malpractice claim appear to be in evidence: duty, breach of duty, proximate cause, and damages (see Chapter 6). Other assessments can be done by consulting organizational policies and standards, the state's nurse practice act, and administrative rulings from the board of nursing. Through reasoned investigation and situation analysis, the nurse then can decide whether to act immediately, document, report, or analyze the situation for future decision making. Ultimately the nurse has an ethical responsibility to advocate for patients if a problematic condition exists (Airth-Kindree & Kirkhorn, 2016).

LEADERSHIP AND MANAGEMENT IMPLICATIONS

The nurse as leader is a core aspect to effective delegation. Key leadership and management skills that the nurse leader is required to use are effective communication, mentoring and coaching, and advocacy for the patient and staff members. Leadership behaviors for delegation and supervision include being available and helping the delegatee through the task actions and decisions. Although there may be a power differential between the nurse and the UAP, how this is perceived by the UAP and the quality of the communication among the nurse/UAP team will have positive or negative implications for patient care. Authoritative attitudes, poor information exchange, and lack of collaboration can lead to negative patient outcomes. Interacting collaboratively and dynamically sharing information is needed for the health of the patient (Amer, 2013).

The nurse as leader is also required to provide coaching regarding delegation. When nurses coach another person they are supporting that person in the development of a professional skill. Providing guidance and leadership in the development of the nurse's ability to delegate is an important aspect of skill building. If the workplace environment is such that delegation is not supported or there are no avenues for a nurse to learn and expand his or her delegation skills, then this can undermine patient outcomes and create an atmosphere of resentment (Amer, 2013).

Invariably there will be potential problems as the use of delegation expands in health care. The nurse leader will need to be aware of techniques to address these potential problems. One such method is the TeamSTEPPS 2.0 (**T**eam **S**trategies and **T**ools to **E**nhance **P**erformance and **P**atient **S**afety) program. The framework followed is based on a foundation of team competencies including knowledge, attitudes, and performance. The principles the program abides by include team structure and the teachable principles of communication, leadership, situation monitoring, and mutual support. Because the team engages in the principles and competencies together, there is an interaction between the outcomes desired and the skill mix of the team itself. This interaction is the basis of providing safe, effective, and quality patient care as well as offering a framework for organizational quality improvement. In TeamSTEPPS 2.0 the task of delegation would fall into a multi-team approach that would provide mutual support through provision of knowledge related to roles and responsibilities, assessment of situational variables, awareness of team functioning, clear and accurate exchange of information, and provision of needed resources. This set of teamwork-based tools provides an "evidence-based framework to optimize team performance across the health care delivery system" (Agency for Healthcare Research and Quality [AHRQ], 2013, p. 4) (see Chapter 7).

Organizational leadership in building the skills related to delegation enhances individuals and builds high-performing teams, as well as enhancing team member awareness of roles and responsibilities and their individual capabilities and limitations (Lanfranchi, 2013). If used effectively, delegation can help team members build skills, confidence, and a shared vision, which can translate into positive outcomes and greater job satisfaction. This causes the organization itself to be accountable for the delegation processes in place and for upholding values of safe patient care and staff development.

CURRENT ISSUES AND TRENDS

Mastering delegation is essential because the current health care system is full of complex patients with chronic illnesses receiving health care in various settings. To meet these patient and industry needs, the nurse will be required to employ his or her full scope of practice. As the role of the nurse expands, it will be imperative that the nurse use delegation appropriately and work collaboratively with the health care team to meet patient outcomes and provide for efficient resource utilization (Josephsen & Butt, 2014). Exercising best practices for delegation and supervision and implementing sound organizational policies surrounding delegation will be crucial for positive patient outcomes.

The act of task delegation is a patient-centered nursing skill that relies on the nurse's use of knowledge, expertise, and abilities. A new vision of how to apply the nursing process to delegation—including assessment and evaluation—in a multitude of settings will be required. Nurses will be challenged to address appropriate delegation in the numerous community settings in which patients receive their care. Nurses will need to master effective communication, embrace the teamwork model of care, and be a patient advocate.

No longer can the nurse ignore organizational policies or legislative actions, because these have a direct impact on patient care and the act of delegation. Nurses as leaders have a unique duty to participate in the development of legislative and organizational policies that support the use of effective delegation guidelines and appropriate scopes of practice—and that address the current health care shift to a multi-team and provider approach to patient care. Delegation is here to stay in health care; it will only grow in application and function. The expanding use of UAP for nursing tasks creates an essential need for the nurse to possess quality delegation and supervision skills, as well as actively engage in patient advocacy and policy development.

One issue that is creating the increasing need for nurses to be skilled at delegation is the transition to community-based and ambulatory care versus the acute care setting (Haughton & Stang, 2012). Currently, many health care interventions are offered in outpatient settings, such as wound clinics, dialysis centers, and anticoagulation clinics. Coordination of care has become a real need in today's health care environment as patients receive care in these various settings from a multitude of health care professionals. Care coordination has developed in an effort to decrease poor patient outcomes and to assist the patient in navigating these diverse providers and settings (Kovner & Knickman, 2011). The Patient Protection and Affordable Care Act (HR 3590) has encouraged a redesign of the health care system to focus on preventive care and wellness and integration of payment for services through a medical home or bundled payment model in which care coordination is at the core (Haughton, & Stang, 2012). This has led to the implementation and expansion of the patient-centered medical home (PCMH) model, based upon the premise of accessible, patient-centered, and coordinated care (Kovner & Knickman, 2011; Lamb, 2013).

Care-coordination models are at the foundation of the PCMH, as patient populations age and tend to have one or more chronic diseases affecting their health. The need for a central person to coordinate their health care services is required. In fact, the National Quality Strategy has identified care coordination as a priority in today's health care (Lamb, 2013). Unfortunately, not all primary care providers or clinics are skilled in care coordination or have the time needed to provide this service in their practice. Therefore more primary care offices are creating leadership positions for nurse care managers related to care coordination to support disease and medication management, patient education, transitional care, and coordination of care with other health care providers (Kovner & Knickman, 2011). In this role it is essential that the nurse is skillful in a variety of leadership abilities (Johnson et al., 2015). It is crucial that the nurse care manager be able to work in a team-based collaborative environment and be able to skillfully delegate. The PCMH is a team-based care milieu, and the nurse may be working with medical assistants, medication technicians, certified nursing assistants, home health clinicians and therapists, administrative staff at the patient's place of residence such as an assisted living or skilled nursing facility, and hired caregivers or informal caregivers such as family or friends. It is believed that teamwork will promote more effective delivery of primary care services, with care coordination being one of them (Lichtenstein et al.; 2015; McDonald et al., 2010; O'Malley et al., 2014).

Delegation is vital to using a health care team effectively. The nurse as care manager cannot perform all needed tasks and interventions; he or she must be able to identify the appropriate team member, assess the team member's abilities, and provide a plan of task implementation that fits in the patient's "big picture" of care. The nurse care manager must then provide for supervision and evaluation of outcomes so that the patient's needs are met across disciplines and various health care and residential sites (Lamb, 2013).

RESEARCH NOTE

Source
Brady, A., Fealy, G., Casey, M., Hegarty, J., Kennedy, C., McNamara, M., et al. (2015). Am I covered?: An analysis of a national enquiry database on scope of practice. *Journal of Advanced Nursing, 71*(10), 2402–2412. doi:10.1111/jan.12711

Purpose
The purpose of the study was to determine how nursing roles are changing or expanding in the current health care reform era.

Discussion
In the modern health care setting, there is a demand for policy makers to develop more flexible roles for nurses. Organizational foci on cost containment, impact of patient outcomes, and review of skill mixes in the health care setting has led to an unprecedented drive for expansion of the nursing role. Evidence has shown that there are benefits to nursing role expansion, such as reduced morbidity and greater use of evidence-based guidelines and protocols. Even so, there are some who question the use of flexible role boundaries and the potential erosion of long-standing nursing values.

This study conducted a thematic analysis via a database of telephone surveys concerning scope of practice for nurses and midwives. A mixed-methods study design was used to include national survey data as well as individual interviews. A total of 9818 telephone inquiries were made available to review. The data review focused on queries related to scope of practice, with identifiers such as "competence, accountability, autonomy, continuous professional development, support, delegation and emergency situations" (p. 2404). Using this as a framework for data cleaning, half of the potential inquiries were deleted. The remaining inquiries were reviewed using a keyword analysis, leaving a total of 978 relevant inquiries to be reviewed for the study.

Nurses from general health care settings, psychiatric, and public/community health settings were represented in the remaining 978 inquiries. Over one-third of the resulting inquires concerned medication management (n = 352), with the majority of these respondent nurses working in community settings. Concerns identified included lack of knowledge of medication administration principles, being asked to perform unfamiliar medication tasks (such as titration), and lack of certainty of scope of practice in certain instances (such as non-nurse medication administration). Questions concerning accountability and delegation in the autonomous community health care environment were also apparent. These concerns related to questions on scope of practice, role boundaries, training, and supervision of unlicensed assistive personnel (UAP). Throughout the data analyzed, nurses expressed concern due to the lack of an organizational structure or policy that verified what activities were in the nurses' and the UAP's scope of practice. Examples included patient assessment being done via the phone, which is a nursing task that normally had been performed in the acute care setting and was now being performed by nurses in the community setting. Nurses expressed that they sometimes found themselves operating beyond what they felt were their professional roles and felt their professional boundaries blurring.

Application to Practice
The shift from acute care to community-based nursing care has forced a redefinition of the nurse's role. There is pressure for organizations to maximize the available staff mix. This may challenge the nurse to navigate uncertain waters. With the emphasis of cost containment, resource management, and coordination of care in the community, nurses will be asked to extend their professional boundaries to meet patients' needs. Yet there is also the need for state licensure agencies and discipline-based organizations to provide definitive guidelines for nurses so that they are reassured they are functioning within their scope of practice. With the increasing use of non-clinical staff to deliver patient care, nurses have the obligation to advocate for clear policy and legislative development to guide issues concerning appropriate delegation, training of non-clinical staff, and supervision. In order for the nurse to adhere to best practice standards there must be formalized policies and practice development support. Role expansion maximizes the use of nurses to their full scope of practice, but initiatives and policies are needed to protect the nurse, the UAP, and the patient, and to promote use of evidence-based guidelines and support the greatest amount of professional development for all team members.

CASE STUDY

It is the beginning of your shift. You have a patient assignment of three patients. One patient, Mr. Jones, is scheduled for an interventional radiology procedure in 1 hour, and he needs to sign his consent before heading to the procedure. Your second patient, Mrs. Blake, is scheduled for discharge to a skilled nursing facility with a pickup time an hour and half from now. The other patient is a new admit that the night nurse has admitted. When going over report with the night nurse it is noted that the new admit, Mr. Marsh, had a spinal fusion. The night nurse reports that she gave him his pain medication at 6:30 AM and that the patient is on mobility restrictions. His call light is on

Continued

CASE STUDY—cont'd

currently. After report ends, you ask the UAP to go take care of Mr. Marsh's call light while you go get the consent signed for Mr. Jones. You also ask the UAP to get Mrs. Black dressed and bathed once Mr. Marsh is taken care of.

As you are getting Mr. Jones ready for his procedure, you get a call from the UAP, who states that Mr. Marsh was up to the bathroom and was now eating breakfast up in the chair but that assistance is needed in Mrs. Black's room. Once in Mrs. Black's room the UAP tells you that every time she touches the patient, the patient grimaces and moans in pain,

so she has not been able to get her bathed or dressed. You review the chart and realize Mrs. Black has melanoma with metastases to her bones. Just then you get a call from Dr. Pike, who is very upset that Mr. Marsh has been up out of bed without his brace and wants to know about his pain level.

How could these seemingly simple delegable tasks have turned into patient pain and discomfort and a doctor's displeasure? What should you do next as the nurse? What part of the delegation process was skipped/missed/or ineffective? (Bowles, 2015; Day et al., 2014).

■ CRITICAL THINKING EXERCISE

Situation: The hospital patient care unit is full and busy with high-acuity patients. The shift is short staffed, but Lindsay, an unlicensed assistive person (UAP), has been floated in to help the RNs. Although you have worked with Lindsay before, you do not know her well. You begin to plan for your delegation. First, you make a list of needed tasks. Then you review your state's nurse practice act to determine whether the task is delegable by going to the computer and going to *https://www.ncsbn.org/contact-bon.htm*. You then search for your state board of nursing's site.

Next, you look at Table 9.1 and mark whether the action is expressly allowed (EA), expressly prohibited (EP), or delegable (D) to a licensed practical or vocational nurse or a UAP or both. Add any comments you may have to the comments column.

TABLE 9.1   Delegable Task Evaluation

	Licensed Practical/ Vocational Nurse	Unlicensed Assistive Personnel	Comments
Administer intravenous antibiotics			
Administer intravenous medications			
Administer heparin			
Access a central line			
Administer dialysis therapy			
Administer a feeding through a percutaneous gastric tube			
Administer one touch glucose monitoring			
Collect a clean urine sample			
Provide simple wound care			
Use a Doppler for pulse checks			
Cleanse healed percutaneous gastric tube site			
Reinforce nurse–patient teaching			
Open sterile pack			
Apply over-the-counter creams or ointments			
Apply heat pads and/or ice packs			
Provide incentive spirometry			
Perform intake/output measurements			
Initiate or change oxygen flow rates			
Participate in patient care plan development			

EA, Expressly allowed; *EP*, expressly prohibited; *D*, delegable (the RN is allowed to assess the UAP or LPN/LVN competency and delegate the task).
Adapted from O'Keefe, C. (2014). The authority for certain clinical tasks performed by unlicensed patient care technicians and LPNs/LVNs in the hemodialysis setting: A review. *Nephrology Nursing Journal, 41*(3), 247–255.

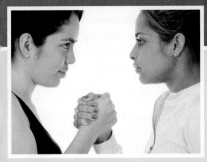

Power and Conflict

Kathleen B. Cox

http://evolve.elsevier.com/Huber/leadership

POWER

Powerless nurses are ineffective nurses, and the consequences of nurses' lack of power have come to light (Manojlovich, 2007). Powerless nurses are less satisfied with their jobs and more susceptible to burnout and depersonalization. Lack of nursing power may also contribute to poorer patient outcomes (Manojlovich, 2007). As the largest health care profession, nursing must use power and influence as a legitimate tool to facilitate change in health care organizations and the health care system. Manojlovich (2007) noted that power is necessary for nurses to influence patients, physicians, other health care professionals, and one another. Nurse leaders recognize that understanding and acknowledging power and learning to seek and wield it appropriately are critical if nurses' efforts to shape their own practice and the broader health care environment are to be successful (Tomajan, 2012).

There are many reasons why power is important to nurses. Despite the fact that some nurses are averse to focusing on power or just never think about it, power and empowerment help nurses, the patients they serve, and the nursing profession. One example is positioning the profession nationally so that nurses can work at the top of their license. Private foundations and prestigious agencies have partnered to leverage their prestige to empower nurses within the health care delivery system. In 2014 the Robert Wood Johnson Foundation asked the Institute of Medicine (IOM, now called the National

Academies of Sciences, Engineering, and Medicine, Health and Medicine Division) to convene a committee to assess progress made on implementing the recommendations of *The Future of Nursing* (IOM, 2010) and identify areas that should be emphasized over the next 5 years. This report outlines specific areas to accelerate implementation of the IOM recommendations for nurses: (1) removing barriers to practice and care, (2) transforming education, (3) collaborating and leading, (4) promoting diversity, and (5) improving data.

Nurses need to understand and use power because they need to have access to the resources needed to accomplish nursing care. Staffing and scheduling are an example of scarce and competing organizational resources. Nurses also need access to information because they coordinate care. Opportunities to learn and grow—and be embedded in a supportive environment—require power to ensure that, although scarce, they are provided fairly and consistently.

DEFINITIONS

Although power connotes strength and ability, the term *power* has different meanings. It can mean the ability to compel obedience, control, or dominate; or it can be a delegated right or privilege as occurs in the power to enact the staff nurse role. **Power** can be defined as the capability of acting or producing some sort of an effect, usually associated with the ability to influence the allocation of scarce resources. Other definitions identify power as the potential capacity to exert influence, characteristically backed by a means to coerce compliance. A key element of power is its aspect of being potential as well as actual.

Photo used with permission from Photos.com.

Classic theory identifies three formal dimensions of power: relational, dependence, and sanctioning. The **relational aspect of power** suggests that power is a property of a social relationship. Many classic definitions indicate that power has to do with relationships between two or more actors in which the behavior of one is affected by the other. Organizational theorists have addressed the concept of power for a very long time. Weber (1947, p. 52) defined power as "the probability that one actor within a social relationship will be in a position to carry out his own will, despite resistance, and regardless of the basis on which this probability rests." Dahl (1957, pp. 202–203) also defined power as an interactive process and stated that "A has power over B to the extent that he can get B to do something B would not otherwise do."

The second formal aspect, the **dependency aspect of power,** was addressed by Emerson (1957), who suggested that power resides implicitly in the other's dependency. Dependency is particularly evident in organizations that require interdependence of personnel and subunits. Daft (2013) defined *interdependence* as the extent to which departments depend on each other for resources or materials to accomplish their task. The highest level of interdependence is reciprocal interdependence. Reciprocal interdependence exists when the output of operation A is the input to operation B, and the output of operation B is the input back again to operation A. Daft noted that hospitals are excellent examples of reciprocal interdependence because they provide coordinated services to patients. Bender and Feldman (2015) addressed the interdependency of nursing practice and the environment, highlighting awareness of the critical role nurses play in shaping environments of care through their practice. Nurses not only focus on patients' care, but they also create beneficial environments of care that optimize health and well-being.

The third formal aspect, the **sanctioning aspect of power,** is the active component of the power relationship, referring to the direct manipulations of the other's outcomes. Sanctions can consist of manipulations of rewards, punishments, or both. Sanctions are a significant part of the process through which parties actually affect one another.

In summary, power is a property of a social relationship between two or more actors in which one is dependent on the other. Sanctions are applied in the form of rewards, punishments, or both. It has been said that, at the core, there are really only two techniques of power: persuasion and coercion. Because nurses are more effective when fostering interpersonal relationships, it is important for nurses to hone skills in motivation, persuasion, and relationship building.

Empowerment

Empowerment is a corollary concept to power in groups and organizations. Through an integrative literature review and concept analysis, Rao (2012) provided insight into the attributes, antecedents, and consequences of empowerment. Nurse empowerment was defined as a state in which an individual nurse has assumed control over his or her practice, enabling him or her to successfully fulfill professional nursing responsibilities within an organization. Empowerment exists simultaneously at the individual, organizational, and psychological levels. Rao (2012, p. 399) noted that "each of these levels of empowerment interact to create the individual nurse's perceived sense of empowerment." Organizational antecedents to nurse empowerment include the "opportunities for mobility and growth and access to resources, support, and information provided within the nurse's work environment" (p. 400). These organizational antecedents (for example, sufficient resources such as staffing) result in individual antecedents that include a nurse's intrinsic motivation, such as the nurse's sense of meaning, competence, self-determination, and impact; educational preparation; and position within the organization. The organizational and individual antecedents lead to psychological empowerment, including a nurse's sense of meaning as expressed in values and work role; competence, which is a nurse's belief that he or she possesses the skills necessary to fulfill the work role; self-determination, which is a sense of control and autonomy over work; and impact, which is a nurse's perception that his or her work has influenced work outcomes.

Rao (2012) summarized the consequences or outcomes of nurse empowerment as (1) the potential for improved nurse and patient outcomes, (2) decreased burnout, (3) decreased job strain, (4) increased trust in the workplace, and (5) increased job satisfaction and work effectiveness. Finally, nurse empowerment can also enable nurses to identify the power that inherently exists in their roles as caring professionals. Rao pointed out that these consequences have been demonstrated in the management literature by researchers who have studied frontline employees and middle managers from a variety of industries.

Organizations set up an organizational structure to get work done. How these structures are set up in health care organizations affects nurses as they deliver nursing care. Structures can empower nurses' work if nurses then have access to opportunities, which in a just culture include needed information, a supportive environment, and resources to do the job. Cziraki and Laschinger (2015) studied the effects of leader behaviors, structural empowerment, nurses' work environment, and staff engagement. Correlations have been found. Nurses who believe they have access to structures such as opportunity, information, support, and resources are empowered. Nurse leaders who acknowledge the importance of nurses' work, engage staff in participative decision making, enable goal attainment, and promote an environment free from constraints foster structural empowerment. Work engagement rises when nurses have access to sources of structural empowerment that enable goal attainment and delivery of quality patient care.

AUTHORITY AND INFLUENCE

Authority and influence are two major content dimensions of power identified in classic theory. There have been three conceptualizations of authority and influence: (1) some authors equate these terms, (2) others tend to equate power with influence and assert that authority is a special case of power, and (3) still others view authority and influence as distinctly different dimensions of power. Several points of contrast are summarized in Table 10.1.

Influence Tactics

Managers operate at the nexus between the nurse and central decision authority levels. Thus they influence the flow and implementation of resources and support. Kipnis and colleagues (1980) were among the first to investigate the influence behavior of managers. Content analysis led to the identification of 370 different forms of influence behavior, which were condensed into 14 categories. Subsequently, factor analysis brought about the following eight forms of *influence behavior:*

1. *Assertiveness* means expressing one's own position to another without inhibiting the rights of others.
2. *Ingratiation* means trying to make the other person feel important, giving praise or sympathizing. Ingratiation is attempting to advance oneself by trying to make another person feel important.

TABLE 10.1 Authority and Influence Contrasted

Authority	Influence
Authority is the static, structural aspect of power in organizations.	Influence is the dynamic, tactical element.
Authority is the formal aspect of power.	Influence is the informal aspect.
Authority refers to the formally sanctioned right to make decisions.	Influence is not sanctioned by the organization and is therefore not a matter of organizational rights.
Authority implies involuntary submission by subordinates.	Influence implies voluntary submission and does not necessarily entail a superior–subordinate relationship.
Authority flows downward, and it is unidirectional.	Influence is multidirectional and can flow upward, downward, or horizontally.
The source of authority is solely structural.	The source of influence may be personal characteristics, expertise, or opportunity.
Authority is circumscribed.	The domain, scope, and legitimacy of influence are typically ambiguous.

3. *Rationality* means using logical and rational arguments, providing pertinent information, presenting reasons, and laying out an idea in a logical, structured way.
4. *Sanctions* are threats. Positive sanctions, or rewards, are addressed within motivation mechanisms.
5. *Exchange* means that to persuade, an exchange is offered; this is sometimes called "scratching each other's back."
6. *Upward appeal* means going to a higher authority. It is the childhood threat of "if you don't play by my rules, I am going to go tell Mom." Upward appeal simply means taking the appeal to a higher authority to arbitrate.
7. *Blocking* means deliberately keeping others from getting their way, threatening to stop working with them, ignoring them, not being friendly, or simply attempting to make sure others cannot accomplish their aims. This may take the form of bullying.
8. *Coalitions* are the result of a group of people getting together to speak or negotiate as one voice.

Influence behaviors translate into power strategies. In their three-nation study of managerial influence styles, Kipnis and colleagues (1984) identified the most to least popular strategies (Table 10.2). Yukl and Falbe (1991) continued the work of Kipnis and colleagues (1980). They developed the Influence Behavior Questionnaire (IBQ), an instrument to measure the influence behavior of managers. In later studies, the IBQ was developed further, and psychometric tests were performed (Yukl et al., 1992, 1993, 2008). The resulting 11 tactics cover a wide range of influence behavior relevant for managerial effectiveness or, in a broader sense, for getting things done in an organization. Influence tactics are identified in Table 10.3.

TABLE 10.2 Most to Least Managerial Influence Strategies Used in All Countries

Strategy's Popularity	Managers Influencing Superiors	Managers Influencing Subordinates
Most popular	Reason	Reason
	Coalition	Assertiveness
	Friendliness	Friendliness
	Bargaining	Evaluation
	Assertiveness	Bargaining
	Higher authority	Higher authority
Least popular	Sanction	

Modified from Kipnis, D., Schmidt, S.M., Swaffin-Smith, C., & Wilkinson, I. (1984). Patterns of managerial influence: Shotgun managers, tacticians, and bystanders. *Organizational Dynamics, 12*(3), 58–67.

SOURCES OF POWER

Individual Sources of Power

Although multiple mechanisms of power have been identified, the most widely accepted power base classification is French and Raven's classic (1959) five sources of power. Their original conceptualization identified the following five power sources (Box 10.1): (1) reward, (2) coercive, (3) expert, (4) referent, and (5) legitimate.

When reward power is used, people comply because doing so produces positive benefits. Coercive power depends on fear. An individual reacts to the fear of the

TABLE 10.3 Definitions of Influence Tactics

Tactic	Definition
Rational persuasion	The agent uses logical arguments and factual evidence to show that a proposal or request is feasible and relevant for important task objectives.
Inspiration appeals	The agent appeals to the target's values and ideals or seeks to arouse the target's emotions to gain commitment for a request or proposal.
Consultation	The agent asks the target to suggest improvements or help plan an activity or change for which the target's support is desired.
Ingratiation	The agent uses praise and flattery before or during an attempt to influence the target to carry out a request or support a proposal.
Personal appeals	The agent asks the target to carry out a request or support a proposal out of friendship or asks for a personal favor.
Exchange	The agent offers something the target person wants, or offers to reciprocate at a later time if the target complies with the request.
Coalition tactics	The agent enlists the aid of, or uses the support of, others as a way to influence the target to do something.
Legitimating tactics	The agent seeks to establish the legitimacy of a request or verify that he or she has the authority to make it.
Pressure	The agent uses demands, threats, frequent checking, or persistent reminders to influence the target to do something.
Collaboration	The agent offers to provide assistance or necessary resources if the target will carry out a request or approve a proposed change.
Apprising	The agent explains how carrying out a request or supporting a proposal will benefit the target personally or help to advance the target's career.

From Yukl, G., Seifert, C.F., & Chavez, C. (2008). Validation of the extended Influence Behavior Questionnaire. *The Leadership Quarterly, 19*(5), 609–621.

BOX 10.1 French and Raven's Five Sources of Power

1. **Reward power** is giving something of value. For example, in nursing, rewards may be a pay raise, praise, a promotion, or a job on the day shift. Reward power is based on the ability to deliver desired rewards.

2. **Coercive power** is force against the will. For example, in nursing, coercive power can be the threat of firing, of disciplinary action, or other negative consequences. Coercive power is the power derived from an ability to threaten punishment and deliver penalties. It is a source of power used to apply pressure so that others will meet what is demanded.

3. **Expert power** means the use of expertise. It is knowledge, competence, communication, and personal power all combined in a reservoir of knowledge and experience. Expert power is a source of power held by those with some special knowledge, skill, or competence in a particular area. For example, the nurse with the greatest expertise in wound dressings will be sought out by other people in the work environment for this expertise. Expertise is an artful combination of skill and knowledge. It may be founded on depth of knowledge and/or psychomotor skill. There is power in the use of knowledge and skill (i.e., because people need you or can benefit from your expertise, power exists). Therefore the use of expertise can be structured to accomplish or influence movement or action toward certain goals.

4. **Referent power** is a little more difficult to understand because it is subtle. It is the use of charisma to influence others. The followers of someone with referent power respond positively to the interpersonal communication and image of the charismatic person. In organizations, this translates into an informal leadership based on liking, charisma, or personal power. Referent power comes from the affinity other people have for someone. They admire the personal qualities, the problem-solving ability, the style, or the dedication the person brings to the work. Referent power can be viewed as an inspirational power because people's admiration for someone allows that person to influence without having to offer rewards or threaten punishments. For example, in the political arena, occasionally there are charismatic political figures or orators. Their influence comes from their followers' liking or identification with them. An example in nursing is Florence Nightingale, who became a symbol of professional nursing. An emotional upsweep is felt by associating with a charismatic person. Referent power is a personal liking and identification experienced by others. Followers attribute referent power to a leader on the basis of the leader's personal characteristics and interpersonal appeal. Physical attractiveness may contribute to referent power.

5. **Legitimate power** means positional power. It is the right to command within the organizational structure based on the hierarchical position held. The president of the United States has power because of holding the position. Legitimate power is the most common source of power. It is what most often is called *authority*. The authority of position gives the person the right to act, order, and direct others. However, leadership and influence need not be confined to those with authority. Every person possesses the ability to tap different sources of power to use in a variety of situations.

Data from French, J., & Raven, B. (1959). The bases of social power. In D. Cartwright (Ed.), *Studies in social power* (pp. 150–167). Ann Arbor, MI: University of Michigan, Institute for Social Research.

negative consequences that might occur for failure to comply. Referent power is based on admiration for a person who has desirable resources or personal traits. Legitimate power represents the power a person receives as a result of his or her position in the formal organizational hierarchy. Expert power results from expertise, special skill, or knowledge. The problem with the French and Raven typology is that the list is not exhaustive, and it ignores organizational sources of power.

Other Sources of Power

Raven and Kruglanski (1975) and Hersey and colleagues (1979) identified two additional sources of power: connection power and information power. A third type of power has also been identified: group decision-making power (Liberatore et al., 1989). These three other sources of power are related to groups and organizations specifically, as opposed to French and Raven's (1959) original five sources of power, which relate more to an individual. These classic ideas provide fruitful areas for nurses to develop expanded sources of power.

Within organizations, the power of connections comes from networking or knowing people and from being able to go across lines laterally to gather information. For example, this occurs when a nurse knows a colleague in another facility with whom he or she can exchange information. For a nurse to know what effective nursing interventions are being used by other institutions helps the institution to be competitive and current. *Connection power* is one strategy to get information accurately and reliably. It may also be manifested as power based on having connections with powerful others. Connection power is based on another's perception that the influencer has access to powerful persons or groups.

Information is power. If information is given away, its power may be lost. This is especially true in situations that require negotiation. If information is used strategically, its possession can be a strong source of power. *Information power* is a source of power that can stem from any person in the organization. Kanter's (1993) classic research suggested that control of resources, especially information, is a major organizational power source. Information power is based on another's perception that the influencer either possesses or has access to information that is valuable to another.

Another source of power is derived from *group decision making.* This means that a creative synergy and force is created when a group comes together, makes decisions, and acts as a united front. For example, some professional groups have formed strong lobbies to influence state and national legislation. With 2.9 million licensed registered nurses (RNs) in the United States (Bureau of Health Professions [BHPr], 2014), group decision making with resultant unity of action could be a powerful strategy for nurses to use to advance nursing's goals or policy agenda. At the unit and organizational level, nurses leverage their group power by using the evidence base and shared governance structure to effect change using data and evidence to persuade.

Persuasive power is an additional source of power identified by later researchers investigating French and Ravens' (1959) taxonomy. *Persuasive power* refers to skill in making rational appeals (Yukl & Falbe, 1991). Yukl and Falbe (1991) differentiated between position power and personal power. Position power consists of legitimate, reward, coercive, and information power. Personal power consists of expert, referent, persuasive power. For nurses, clinical competence (expert power) is a considerable source of power because peers will follow a nurse who is perceived to be clinically competent. This personal expertise power is one way that a nurse becomes an informal leader (Mannix et al., 2013). Another example is in teaching hospitals where new medical residents rotating through a unit may rely on expert clinical nurses as they are learning.

In her structural theory of organizational behavior, Kanter (1993) asserted that those with sufficient power are able to accomplish the tasks required to achieve organizational goals. Conditions in the work environment influence how much productive power is available to employees. According to Kanter, formal and informal systemic structures are the sources of workplace empowerment. Job discretion, recognition, and relevance to organizational goals are important dimensions of formal power. High levels of job discretion ensure that work is non-routinized and permit flexibility, adaptation, and creativity. Recognition reflects visibility of an employee's accomplishments among peers and supervisors. For example, an innovative staff development director or nurse manager whose techniques are reported in a respected nursing journal will enhance his or her influence in the hospital. Finally, relevance of job responsibilities and accomplishments to the organization's strategic plan or current problems is also important. This refers to being a part of the core services or activities of the organization. For example, programs that do not meet the core mission or strategic plan can be vulnerable to elimination during an economic downturn.

Another key systemic structure is informal power, which comes from the employee's network of interpersonal alliances or relationships within and outside an organization. Relationships with people at higher hierarchical levels confer approval, prestige, and backing, whereas peer networks provide reputation and "grapevine" information (Kanter, 1993). Kanter's theory has been tested extensively in nursing populations, and the findings lend support to Kanter's theory.

Kotter (1979) maintained that the basic methods for acquiring and maintaining power are gaining control over tangible resources, obtaining information and control of information channels, and establishing favorable relationships. Basically, acquiring and maintaining power is an exercise in developing credibility by getting people to feel obligated in some way, building a good professional reputation through visible achievement, encouraging identification by trying to look and behave in ways that others respect, and finally, creating perceived dependence either for help or security. Control of information and resources and development of support systems are common elements in both Kanter's and Kotter's theories.

THE POWER OF THE SUBUNIT

Subunit or horizontal power pertains to relationships across departments. Daft (2013) noted that although each department makes a unique contribution to organizational success, some contributions are greater than others. Pfeffer (1981) identified the following structural determinants of power within organizations:

- *Power is derived from dependence.* Simply stated, power comes from having something that someone else wants or needs and being in control of the performance or resources so that there are few, if any, alternative sources for obtaining what is desired.
- *Power is derived from providing resources.* Organizations require a continuing provision of resources such as personnel, money, customers, and technology in order to continue to function. Those subunits or individuals within the organization that can provide the most critical and difficult-to-obtain resources come to have power in organizations. Their power is derived from their ability to furnish those resources on which the organization most depends.
- *Power is derived from coping with uncertainty.* Coping with uncertainty is a critical resource in the organization because it ensures organizational survival and adaptation to external constraints.
- *Power is derived from being irreplaceable.* Members must not only provide a critical resource for the organization but also prevent themselves from being readily replaced in that function. The degree of substitutability is not a fixed thing, however, so it might be expected that various strategies will be employed by individuals and subunits who are interested in enhancing their power within the organization. Some of these might involve the availability of documentation, use of specialized language, centralization of knowledge, and maintenance of externally based sources of expertise.
- *Power is derived from the ability to affect the decision process.* Because decisions are made in a sequential process, it is possible for an individual to acquire power because of his or her ability to affect the premises of basic values or objectives used in making any decision. A person can gain power by influencing the information about the alternatives being considered in the decision process.
- *Power is derived if there is a shared consensus within the organizational subunit.* If individuals within a subunit share a common perspective, set of values, or definition of the situation, they are likely to act and speak in a consistent manner and present to the larger organization an easily articulated and understood position and perspective. Such a consensus can serve to enhance the power of the subunit among other organizational members.

POWER THEORIES

Principles of centrality, uncertainty, and unsubstitutability from the Strategic Contingencies Theory (Hickson et al., 1971) may be used to assist nursing to establish its power base. The Strategic Contingency Theory posits that power among organizational departments can be defined as a dependent variable connected to three contributing variables, or sources of power: (1) coping with uncertainty, (2) non-substitutability, and (3) centrality. Hickson and colleagues defined *uncertainty* as an information deficit pertaining to possible outcomes of future events. *Substitutability* is the degree to which there are available alternatives for completing the activities of a particular subunit, and *centrality* is the degree to which a unit's activities are connected with other units within the organization.

Application of this theory to nursing would mean that nurses must demonstrate that they can handle organizational problems and uncertainties through prevention and information and create conditions within organizations that make them difficult to replace. A high degree of centrality already exists in hospitals because of the nature of nurses' work, which coordinates with all other departments in the hospital. However, centrality can be leveraged to effect organizational improvements. For example, training on and subsequent use of crucial conversations (see Chapter 7) by nurses can be used as a strategy to improve safety and interprofessional relationships.

The Theory of Group Power within organizations (Sieloff, 2003) was developed from a synthesis and reformulation of King's (1981) interacting systems framework and the Strategic Contingencies Theory of power (Hickson et al., 1971). Variables of the Strategic Contingencies Theory of power relate to controlling the effects of environmental forces, position, resources, and role. For example, coping with uncertainty is equivalent to controlling the effects of environmental forces in Sieloff's theory; and centrality and role are comparable to position. Sieloff (2003) noted that although nursing groups are proposed to have a power capacity resulting from controlling the effects of environment forces, position, resources, and role, not all nursing groups have acted powerfully. Therefore four additional concepts were added to the theory as variables that intervened between a nursing group's power capacity and the important element of its ability to actualize that power capacity. These concepts are communication competency, goal/outcome competency, nurse leader's power competency, and power perspective. Every nursing group has a power capacity. The group has the potential to achieve its goals and become a more visible contributor to the progress of the organization. The value of the Strategic Contingency Theory and the Theory of Group Power is that they provide nurse leaders at all levels with strategies that could be implemented to improve a nursing group's actualized power.

LEADERSHIP AND MANAGEMENT IMPLICATIONS

According to Robbins and Judge (2016), leadership and power are two different concepts and need to be defined separately. Leadership is focused on goal achievement in conjunction with followers. Power is used as a way to accomplish the goal, and often followers contribute to accomplishing the goal. Leaders focus on using their leadership downward or laterally to influence others to help them achieve their tasks. On the other hand, power is deployed to influence and to gain something upward or laterally.

Power and Leadership

Power and leadership are closely connected and highly intertwined concepts. This is because power is one of the vehicles by which a leader influences followers to take action. Nurses may be inclined to ignore or avoid an acknowledgment or analysis of power. However, to

lead and manage, nurses need to acquire, possess, and use power. This begins with understanding it.

Hersey and colleagues (2013) described the relationships among concepts of style of leadership, readiness level of followers, and power base use. They indicated that the readiness of followers dictates which leadership style is likely to be successful and which power base would most successfully influence followers' behavior. Combining these concepts maximizes the leader's probability of success. Thus nurses should be able to use Situational Leadership® theory to assess and predict style choice and power source use based on the situation and readiness of followers.

Readiness is the ability and willingness of individuals or groups to take responsibility for directing their own behavior in a situation. There appears to be a direct relationship between the level of readiness in individuals and groups and the power base type that has a high probability of effectiveness (Fig. 10.1). Readiness is a task-specific concept. At the lowest level of readiness, coercive power is most appropriate. As people move to higher readiness levels, connection power, then reward, then legitimate, then referent, then information, and finally, expert power affect the behavior of people. At the highest level, the followers have competence and confidence, and they are most responsive to expert power (Hersey et al., 2013).

If power is the basic energy needed to initiate and sustain action, then power is a quality without which a leader cannot lead. Power is fundamental to leadership in that leadership may be the wise use of power. This is

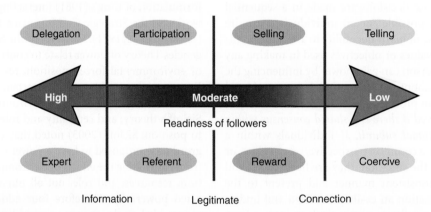

FIG. 10.1 Power related to leadership. (Data from Hersey, P.H., Blanchard, K.H., & Johnson, D.E. [2013]. *Management of organizational behavior: Leading human resources* [10th ed.]. Upper Saddle River, NJ: Pearson.)

especially true for transformative leadership (Bennis & Nanus, 1985). Power need is highly desirable in leaders and managers because power is necessary in influencing others. Assertiveness and self-confidence are associated with power and leadership. Leadership may be characterized as power in the service of others (Kouzes & Posner, 2012), which is also the basis of servant leadership principles. For nurses, this may mean that they need to view power as an integral part of their professional roles in care management and client advocacy. Nursing leadership requires a willingness and ability to take on a power role and to expand the use of power bases.

Centrality and Substitutability

Professional nurses have a high degree of centrality within health care organizations. They are critical to the operation of most health care organizations, and without nurses, many health care facilities would not be able to offer services. Nursing maintains power by being central to the actual delivery of health care services, which is the core business function. Strong chief nurse executives with strong formal power are needed to create conditions within the organization and the health care system that address the IOM's call for nurses to practice at the highest level of preparation. Fortunately, research has demonstrated the relationship between RN staffing and important patient outcomes.

There is strong evidence of the need specifically for registered nurses. For example, the Agency for Healthcare Research and Quality (AHRQ) published a systematic review of the literature on workforce characteristics (Kane et al., 2007). The AHRQ review identified 97 observational studies published between 1990 and 2006 and included 94 of these reports in a meta-analysis. This meta-analysis found strong and consistent evidence that higher RN hours were related to lower patient mortality rates, lower rates of failure to rescue, and lower rates of hospital-acquired pneumonia. Results of the meta-analysis indicated that there was evidence that higher direct-care RN hours were related to shorter lengths of stay. Higher total nursing hours were also found to result in lower hospital mortality and failure-to-rescue rates and in shorter lengths of stay. Based on fewer studies, the review found evidence that the prevalence of baccalaureate-prepared RNs was related to lower hospital mortality rates, that higher RN job satisfaction and satisfaction with workplace autonomy were related to lower hospital mortality rates, and that higher rates of nurse turnover were

related to higher rates of patient falls. The conclusion of the meta-analysis was that higher nurse staffing was associated with better patient outcomes but that the association was not necessarily causal. These findings are confirmed by the extensive research of Aiken and colleagues (e.g., Aiken et al., 2014) and confirmed as global in international studies such as Aiken and colleagues' (2016) European study. This is powerful evidence for nurses' centrality and a strong argument for baccalaureate preparation for nurses.

CONFLICT

The same turbulent health care environment that demands the use of power also creates the conditions that breed conflict. Health care in the United States has gone through dramatic changes, and change has become the norm. Change increases conflict in organizations. Lyon (2012) pointed out the cost of mismanaged conflict:

- *Management time:* The typical workplace manager spends 25% of his or her time dealing with workplace conflict.
- *Presenteeism:* Presenteeism refers to employees who go to work while they are ill and therefore do not perform to their full potential. Unfortunately, presenteeism can be more expensive than absenteeism (Chavez, 2016). The phenomenon can be the consequence of a negative work environment, and many of the health problems that employees experience are the result of the negative psychological effects of an unhealthy workplace.
- *Absenteeism:* Absenteeism is increased due to stress-related illness and the desire to avoid conflict. Companies lose roughly $3600 per year for each hourly worker and $2650 each year for salaried workers for absenteeism (Richards, 2016).
- *Turnover:* Turnover is another cost associated with conflict. According a project funded by the Robert Wood Johnson Foundation (Kovner et al., 2014), the national rate of nurse turnover is that 17.5% of new nurses leave their first job within 1 year, and one in three (33.5%) leaves within 2 years. The rate leveled off somewhat in 2015, and it is at 17.1% (NSI Nursing Solutions Inc., 2016). Further, the average cost of turnover for a bedside RN ranges from $37,700 to $58,400, resulting in the average hospital losing $5.2 to $8.1 million (NSI Nursing Solutions Inc., 2016).
- *Litigation:* Finally, there is the cost of litigation and dealing with grievances. De La Roche (2015) indicated

that months were spent calculating the actual total cost of litigation. To calculate the total cost of litigation in the United States, the average of an attorney's fee ($350 per hour) was multiplied by the time spent in litigation yearly. The time spent in litigation was estimated as an average of 2 hours per day dealing with a single case and 2.5 years to reach a solution. In other words, 1050 working hours are spent in litigation yearly. Thus the cost of the entire litigation process is about $367,500. Given the enormous costs of conflict, the need for conflict management cannot be overstated, and it is essential to focus on the conflict as soon as it arises.

DEFINITIONS

There is no universally accepted definition of conflict (Patton, 2014). Conflict has been studied for a very long time. **Conflict** is defined here as a clash or struggle that occurs when a real or perceived threat or difference exists in the desires, thoughts, attitudes, feelings, or behaviors of two or more parties (Deutsch, 1973). It exists as a tension or struggle arising from mutually exclusive or opposing actions, thoughts, opinions, or feelings. Conflict can be internal or external to an individual or group. It can be positive as well as negative.

Organizational conflict is defined as the struggle over scarce organizational resources. Values, goals, roles, money, or structural elements may be the specific locus of the struggle for scarce organizational resources. For example, two parties may be in opposition because of perceived differences in goals, a struggle over budget allocations, or interference in goal attainment. This opposition prevents cooperation (Deutsch, 1973). **Job conflict** is defined as a perceived opposition or antagonistic process at the individual–organization interface (Gardner, 1992). Conflict levels have an effect on productivity, morale, and teamwork in organizations.

A review of the classic literature revealed several definitions and views of conflict. Social conflict is a struggle between opponents over values and claims to scarce status, power, and resources. According to Deutsch (1973), a conflict exists whenever incompatible activities occur or when one party is interfering, disrupting, obstructing, or in some other way making another party's actions less effective. The factors underlying conflict are threefold: (1) interdependence, (2) differences in goals, and (3) differences in perceptions.

Conrad (1990) indicated that conflicts are communicative interactions among people who are interdependent and who perceive that their interests are incompatible, inconsistent, or in tension. Conflict is thus the interaction of interdependent people who perceive incompatible goals and interference from each other in achieving those goals. Walton (1966) defined conflict as opposition processes in any of several forms (e.g., hostility, decreased communication, distrust, sabotage, verbal abuse, coercive tactics). Interpersonal conflict is a dynamic process that occurs between interdependent parties as they experience negative emotional reactions to perceived disagreements and interference with the attainment of their goals (Barki & Hartwick, 2001).

VIEWS OF CONFLICT

Robbins and Judge (2016) noted that it is entirely appropriate to say there has been conflict over the role of conflict in groups and organizations. Some differing views are:

Traditionalist: In the traditionalist view, conflict is destructive, and all conflict should be eliminated by managers.

Interactionist: The interactionist view is that some conflict is absolutely necessary because peaceful groups can become complacent and unresponsive to the need for change and innovation. According to the interactionist view, conflict can be functional or dysfunctional. Functional conflict supports the goals of the group and improves its performance, whereas dysfunctional conflict hinders group performance.

Resolution-focused: A contemporary perspective on conflict is that conflict is inevitable; therefore conflict must be managed so that the disruptive influence of conflict can be minimized. The negative effects of conflict can be minimized by preparing people for conflicts, developing resolution strategies, and facilitating open discussion. Thus the pendulum has swung from the belief that all conflict must be eliminated to the belief that some conflict is necessary for optimal group functioning, and finally, to the belief that conflict is inevitable and must be well managed.

Conflict can be competitive or disruptive. **Competitive conflict** is similar to games and sports in which rules are followed and the goal is to win or beat an opponent. A **disruptive conflict** is some activity designed to attack, defeat, or eliminate an opponent. It is not based on rules jointly agreed to, and its objective is not focused on winning but rather on disrupting the opponent. The feelings and actions generated by competitive conflict focus on the positive; for disruptive conflict, feelings and actions focus on the negative (Filley, 1975).

Conflict is functional or constructive when it improves the quality of decisions, stimulates creativity and innovation, encourages interest and curiosity, provides a medium through which problems can be aired and tensions released, and fosters an environment of self-evaluation and change (Box 10.2). In contrast, dysfunctional or destructive outcomes include a degrading of communication, reduction in group cohesiveness, and subordination of group goals to the primacy of infighting among members. Extremely high or low levels of conflict hinder performance. An optimal level is high enough to prevent stagnation and stimulates creativity, releases tension, and initiates change. However, it is not so high as to be disruptive or counterproductive (Brown, 1983) (Fig. 10.2).

TYPES OF CONFLICT

Thomas (1992) identified two broad types of conflict. The first refers to incompatible response tendencies within an individual, which Rahim and Bonoma (1979) referred to as *intrapersonal conflict* (Fig. 10.3). *Intrapersonal conflict* means discord, tension, or stress inside—or internal to—an individual that results from unmet needs, expectations, or goals. Intrapersonal conflict is conflict that generates from within an individual (Rahim, 1983a, b, c). It is often manifested as a conflict over two competing roles. For example, a parent with a sick child who has to go to work faces a conflict: the need to take care of the sick child against the need to make a living. A nursing example occurs when the nurse determines that a patient needs teaching or counseling, but the organization's assignment system is set up in a way that does not provide

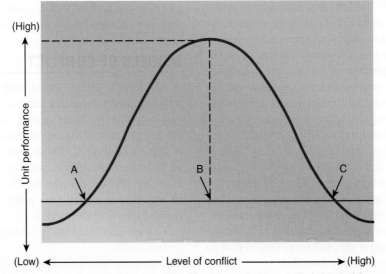

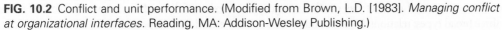

FIG. 10.2 Conflict and unit performance. (Modified from Brown, L.D. [1983]. *Managing conflict at organizational interfaces.* Reading, MA: Addison-Wesley Publishing.)

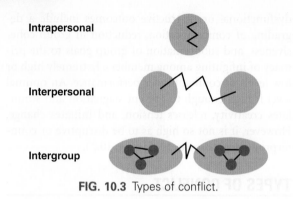

Intrapersonal

Interpersonal

Intergroup

FIG. 10.3 Types of conflict.

an adequate amount of time. When other priorities compete, an internal or intrapersonal conflict of roles exists.

The second use refers to conflicts that occur between different individuals, groups, organizations, or other social units. Rahim and Bonoma (1979) identified these as interpersonal conflict, a category that includes intragroup conflict, intergroup conflict, and interorganizational conflict. *Interpersonal* means conflict emerging between two or more people, such as between two nurses, a doctor and a nurse, or a nurse manager and a staff nurse. In this case, two people have a disagreement, conflict, or clash. Either their values or styles do not match or there is a misunderstanding or miscommunication between them. Interpersonal conflict can be viewed as happening between two individuals or among individuals within a group. When it specifically involves multiple individuals within a group, interpersonal conflict is called *intragroup conflict,* which refers to disagreements or differences among the members of a group or its subgroups with regard to goals, functions, or activities of the group.

Intergroup conflict refers to disagreements or differences between the members of two or more groups or their representatives over authority, territory, and resources. Interorganizational conflict occurs across organizations (Rahim, 1983b; Rahim & Bonoma, 1979). It is conflict occurring between two distinct groups of people. For example, physicians and nurses may disagree about role functions and activities, or lay midwives may seek to perform home deliveries without being prepared as licensed nurse midwives. Sometimes the conflict arises between departments or units as groups. For example, hospital nurses might find themselves in conflict with central purchasing if supplies are provided that do not meet nursing's needs or are defective.

Another view of types of conflict has conflict categorized into three broad types: relationship, task, and process.

Relationship conflict, an awareness of interpersonal incompatibilities, includes affective components such as feeling tension and friction (Rahim & Bonoma, 1979). Relationship conflict involves personal issues such as dislike among group members and feelings such as annoyance, frustration, and irritation. This definition is consistent with past categorizations of conflict that distinguish between affective and cognitive conflict (Amason, 1996), with implications for organizational outcomes. Results of a meta-analysis revealed strong negative correlations between relationship conflict and team performance and also strong negative correlations between relationship conflict and team member satisfaction (DeDreu & Weingart, 2003).

Task conflict is an awareness of differences in viewpoints and opinions about a group task. Similar to cognitive conflict, it pertains to conflict about ideas and differences of opinion about the task (Amason & Sapienza, 1997). Task conflicts may coincide with animated discussions and personal excitement, but by definition are void of the intense interpersonal negative emotions that are more commonly associated with relationship conflict.

Other studies have identified a third distinct type of conflict, labeled *process conflict* (Jehn, 1997; Jehn et al., 1999). It is defined as an awareness of controversies about aspects of how task accomplishment will proceed. More specifically, process conflict pertains to issues of duty and resource delegation, such as who should do what and how much responsibility different people should have. For example, when group members disagree about who is responsible for completing a specific duty, such as during delegation by the RN, then they are experiencing process conflict.

MODELS OF CONFLICT

Pondy (1967), Filley (1975), and Thomas (1976) described conflict dynamics across a temporal sequence of stages or phases. These models provide significant insight into understanding the nature of conflict phenomena (Table 10.4). These models are similar in that all indicate that conflict follows a predictable course. However, they differ in the number of identifiable stages or elements in a particular pattern. The following elements exist in all the models:

- Causes, identified as conditions, that occur before the conflict
- Core processes, including the perception that conflict exists, followed by some kind of affective state or emotional response

Pondy (1967)	Filley (1975)	Thomas (1976)	Robbins & Judge (2016)
1. Latent (antecedent conditions)	1. Antecedent conditions	1. Frustration	1. Potential opposition
2. Perception and feeling	2. Perceived conflict	2. Conceptualization	2. Cognition and personalization
3. Behavior manifestation (manifest)	3. Felt conflict	3. Behavior	3. Intentions
4. Aftermath	4. Manifest behavior	4. Others' reactions (interaction)	4. Behavior
	5. Resolution or suppression	5. Outcome	5. Functional or dysfunctional outcomes
	6. Conflict aftermath		

TABLE 10.4 Comparison of Four Process Models of Conflict

- Conflict behaviors, including a variety of behaviors from very subtle to violent
- Effect that includes outcomes such as resolution or aftermath consequences

Cause, Core Process, Effect

Wall and Callister (1995) described a generic model of conflict. As with any social process, there are causes and a core process that have effects. These effects in turn have an impact on the original cause. This conflict cycle takes place within a context (environment), and the cycle flows through numerous iterations. Wall and Callister (1995) indicated that the model is a general one that displays how the major pieces in the conflict puzzle fit

together. The value of this model is that concepts from all other models may be subsumed under the major concepts of this generic model. In addition, the simplicity of the model facilitates the discussion of conflict according to cause, core process, and effect. Fig. 10.4 uses Wall and Callister's model as a beginning and incorporates the work of Boynton (2012), Patton (2014), and Robbins and Judge (2016).

Causes of Conflict

According to Wall and Callister (1995), conditions that occur before conflict is identified are causes. Patton (2014) identified the causes of conflict as personality differences, value differences, blurred job boundaries,

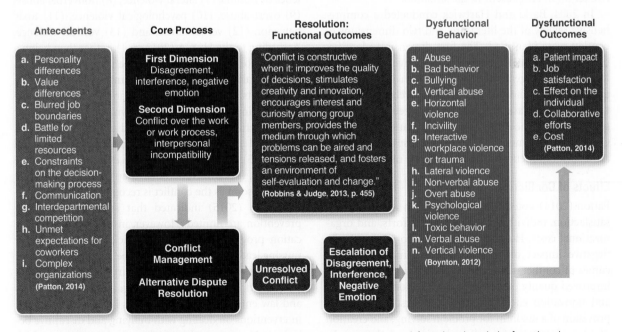

FIG. 10.4 Conceptual framework: antecedents, core process, and functional and dysfunctional outcomes of intragroup conflict.

battle for limited resources, constraints on the decision-making process, communication, departmental competition, unmet expectations for co-workers, and the complexity of organizations.

The Core Process of Conflict

Although conflict has been defined in many different ways, disagreement, interference, and negative emotion are thought to underlie conflict situations (Barki & Hartwick, 2001). Disagreement, interference, and negative emotion can be viewed as reflecting cognitive, behavioral, and affective manifestations of interpersonal conflict. Disagreement is the most commonly discussed and assessed cognition in the literature. Although a number of different behaviors have been associated with and may be typical of conflict, they do not always indicate the existence of conflict. Conflict exists when the behavior of one party interferes with or opposes another party's attainment of its own interests, objectives, or goals. A number of affective states have been associated with conflict. However, it is the negative emotions such as fear, anger, anxiety, and frustration that have been used to characterize conflict. Barki and Hartwick (2001) proposed that interpersonal conflict exists only when disagreement, interference, and negative emotion are present in the situation.

In 2004, Barki and Hartwick conducted a comprehensive review of the literature, and two dimensions of conflict were identified. The first dimension identifies disagreement, interference, and negative emotion as three properties generally associated with a conflict situation. The second dimension identifies relationship and task content or task process as two targets of interpersonal conflict encountered in organizational settings. Conflict management and alternative dispute resolution are also components of the core process of conflict.

Effects of Conflict

Patton (2014) noted that conflict has an impact on job satisfaction, individuals, collaborative efforts, and organizational costs. However, the most serious effect is the negative impact on patients. Positive functional outcomes of conflict include increased group performance, improved quality of decisions, stimulation of creativity and innovation, encouragement of interest and curiosity, provision of a medium for problem solving, and creation of an environment for self-evaluation and changes. In contrast, dysfunctional outcomes include development

of discontent, reduced group effectiveness, disrupted communication, reduced group cohesiveness, and infighting among group members, which then overrides the focus on group goals (Robbins & Judge, 2016).

BULLYING AND DISRUPTIVE BEHAVIOR

Interestingly, many authors addressed the negative impact of unresolved conflict, but few have addressed the escalation of conflict to dysfunctional behavior. There is evidence in the literature that conflict leads to disruptive behavior, which is defined as "personal conduct (words, actions, or inactions) beyond that normally accepted as respectful interpersonal behavior, which disturbs the work environment and/or potentially poses a risk to delivery of safe and quality healthcare" (Health Quality Council of Alberta [HQCA], 2013, p. 3).

Disruptive behavior is the term used by the medical profession to describe this phenomenon, and the nursing profession is also concerned with disruptive behavior (HQCA, 2013). Boynton (2012) explained that overlapping terms are used to describe disruptive behavior in the workplace. Disruptive behaviors include (1) abuse, (2) bad behavior/bullying, (3) covert abuse, (4) horizontal violence, (5) incivility, (6) interactive workplace violence or trauma, (7) lateral violence, (8) nonverbal abuse, (9) overt abuse, (10) psychological violence, (11) toxic behavior, (12) verbal abuse, and (13) vertical violence. According to the HQCA (2013, p. 4), rather than being a one-time occurrence, "disruptive behavior is usually ongoing, escalates over time, and is cumulative in the effect on patients, the staff, and the organization." Disruptive behavior in the workplace is shown to have significant negative effects on individuals and on patient care and safety, and it can undermine the organization itself (Small et al., 2015). Given that conflict can escalate to disruptive behaviors, it is imperative that management of conflict occurs as soon as the conflict is recognized.

Skehan (2015) indicated that studies on bullying prevention are limited. However, institution-based education programs with active participation from senior nursing leaders and managers can be adopted from other disciplines. For example, the Department of Education (*https://safesupportivelearning.ed.gov/index.php?id=01*) and law enforcement communities have evidence-based interventions on dealing with bullying and disruptive behaviors. Nursing can benefit from such programs, which have demonstrated a decrease in disruptive behaviors. For example, for early intervention, crucial conversations training can help.

CONFLICT SCALES

Three conflict inventories are available to measure conflict. The Rahim Organizational Conflict Inventory-I (Rahim, 1983b, c) is designed to measure three dimensions of conflict: intrapersonal, intragroup, and intergroup. The Perceived Conflict Scale (Gardner, 1992) contains four subscales of conflict: intrapersonal, interpersonal, intergroup/other departments, and intergroup/support services. This scale is designed to measure conflict in nursing. Cox (2014) developed a new intragroup conflict scale based on Barki and Hartwick's two dimensions. The scale consists of six subscales: (1) interference over the task, (2) negative emotion over the task, (3) negative emotion and interference related to interpersonal incompatibilities, (4) disagreement over the task process, (5) disagreement over the task, and (6) disagreement related to interpersonal incompatibilities.

CONFLICT MANAGEMENT AND ALTERNATIVE DISPUTE RESOLUTION

Although conflict management and conflict resolution are often used interchangeably, there are differences in the terms (Rahim, 2010). Conflict management involves the control, but not resolution, of a long-term or deep-rooted conflict. In contrast, conflict resolution involves eliminating all forms of conflict. Negotiation, mediation, and arbitration are often referred to in discussions of conflict resolution. These terms are also included under the umbrella of *alternative dispute resolution* (ADR). ADR consists of several forms of conflict resolution that are used to avoid going to court (Brubaker et al., 2014).

Conflict Management Styles

Although other labels have been used for conflict management styles, those identified by Thomas in 1976 are the most frequently cited. The author labeled the five conflict management styles as accommodating, avoiding, collaborating, competing, and compromising.

- *Accommodating* results when one party seeks to appease an opponent; that party is willing to be self-sacrificing.
- *Avoiding* emerges when a person recognizes that a conflict exists and wants to withdraw from it or suppress it.

- *Collaborating* ensues when the parties to conflict each desire to fully satisfy the concerns of all parties. The intention is to solve the problem by clarifying differences rather than by accommodating.
- Competing occurs when one person seeks to satisfy his or her own interests regardless of the impact on the other parties to the conflict.
- *Compromising* may develop when each party to the conflict seeks to give up something and sharing occurs, with the result of a compromised outcome. There is no clear winner or loser, and the solution provides incomplete satisfaction of both parties' concerns (Robbins & Judge, 2016).

Shargh and colleagues (2013) indicated that each of the conflict management styles can be used for different situations. The challenge is for nurses to know when to use each style. Thomas (1976) identified situations for the appropriate use of each conflict management style (see Table 10.5).

Carefronting

Sometimes conflict between two individuals can be managed by carefronting, which is defined as "a method of communication that entails caring enough about one's self, one's goals, and others to confront courageously in a self-asserting, responsible manner" (Kuperschmidt, 2008, p. 12). The term *carefronting* was coined by David Augsburger, a family therapist, in 1973. Issues are the focus of the interaction. Individuals speak for themselves but in a way that decreases defensiveness and allows another person to hear the message. "I" messages are used; "you" messages are avoided.

In her carefronting model, Briles (2007, p. 53) provided a script for carefronting. She suggested that the wording and sequence provided here will help keep the conversation in control. The specifics of a particular conflict situation can be incorporated in the blanks.

1. When you _____, (Describe the perpetrator's action.)
2. I felt _____ (Describe your reaction to the perpetrator's action.)
3. because it _____. (Describe what the perpetrator's actions looked, felt, sounded, or seemed like to you.)
4. Was it your intent to _____? (Describe your interpretation of his or her actions—then stay absolutely silent until he or she responds. Silence is

TABLE 10.5	Use of Conflict Management Styles According to Situation
Conflict Management Style	**Situation**
Collaborating	When both sets of concerns are too important to be compromised
	When objective is to learn
	To merge insights from people with different perspectives
	To gain commitment by incorporating concerns into a consensus
	To work through feelings that have interfered with a relationship
Accommodating	To allow a better position to be heard and to show reasonableness
	When issues are more important to others than yourself
	To build social credit for later issues
	To minimize loss when you are outmatched and losing
	When harmony and stability are especially important
	To allow subordinates to develop by learning from mistakes
Competing	When quick, decisive action is vital
	On important issues where unpopular actions need implementing
	On issues vital to organization and when you know you are right
	Against people who take advantage of non-competitive behavior
Avoiding	When an issue is trivial, or more important issues are pressing
	When you see no chance of satisfying your concerns
	To let people "cool down" and regain perspective
	Gathering information supersedes the immediate decision
	When others can resolve the conflict more effectively
Compromising	When goals are important but not worth potential disruption of more assertive modes
	When equal power opponents are committed to mutually exclusive goals
	To find temporary settlements of complex issues
	To arrive at expedient solutions under time pressure

Adapted from Thomas, K.W. (1977). Toward multidimensional values in teaching: The example of conflict behaviors. *Academy of Management Review, 2*(3), p 487.

uncomfortable for most people; if you stand your ground, chances are he or she will answer.)

5. In the future, I'd like you to _____. (Describe how you would like him or her to behave from now on.)

6. Are you committed to doing that? (Again, stay absolutely silent until he or she responds.)

7. If you continue to behave the way you did, I will _____. (Describe how you intend to respond if he or she behaves the same way in the future.)

The carefronting script is great for nurses to have in their repertoire of tools for managing conflict.

Studies of Conflict Management in Nursing

Older studies in nursing found that avoiding and compromising were the most frequently used conflict handling intentions in nursing. For example, Sportsman and Hamilton (2007) conducted a study to determine prevalent conflict management styles chosen by students in nursing and to contrast these styles with those chosen by students in allied health professions. The associations among the level of professional health care education and the style chosen were also determined. A convenience sample of 126 university students completed the Thomas-Kilmann Conflict Mode Instrument (TKI). The difference was not significant between the prevalent conflict management styles chosen by graduate and undergraduate nursing students and those in allied health. Some of the students were already licensed in their discipline; others had not yet taken a licensing examination. Licensure and educational level were not associated with choice of styles. Women and men had similar preferences. The prevalent style for nursing students was compromise, followed by avoidance. The prevalent style for allied health students was avoidance, followed by compromise and accommodation. Compared with the TKI norms, slightly more than one-half of all participants chose two or more conflict management styles—commonly avoidance and accommodation—at the 75th percentile or above. Only 9.8% of the participants chose collaboration at that level.

CONFLICT RESOLUTION

Conflict resolution involves eliminating all forms of conflict. Negotiation, mediation, and arbitration are often referred to in discussions of conflict resolution. These terms are also included under the umbrella of alternative dispute resolution (ADR). According to Knickle and colleagues (2012) the resolution continuum includes negotiation, mediation, arbitration, and litigation as a spectrum of third-party dispute resolution.

Negotiation: Negotiation can be used by individuals to come to an agreement or in third-party negotiations such as ADR. Negotiation is the major process used in any ADR technique. It is the process whereby two or more parties come to an agreement. There are no official rules for the negotiation process. Robbins and Judge (2016) described negotiation as a five-step process: (1) preparation and planning, (2) definition of ground rules, (3) clarification and justification, (4) bargaining and problem solving, and (5) closure and implementation.

Principled Negotiation: Principled negotiation is an approach proposed by Fisher and colleagues (1992), who urged negotiators to use the following five fundamental principles to negotiate effectively with each other instead of against each other:
1. Separate the people from the problem.
2. Focus on interests, not positions.
3. Invent options for mutual gain.
4. Insist on using objective criteria.
5. Know your BATNA (**B**est **A**lternative **t**o **N**egotiated **A**greement).

The authors were also the first to coin the acronym BATNA. This term essentially describes the need to conceive of creating and developing backup plans when all else fails. Invariably, not even the best intentions to find agreement will necessarily come to fruition.

Conciliation: A conciliator is like a third friend who might attempt to intercede in an argument between two other friends. Conciliators attempt to diffuse the negative emotions that are often involved in the conflict, and they strive to establish more effective communications between the parties. They attempt to understand each party's point of view as a basis for common ground. The conciliator might also meet with managers and co-workers who are involved in order to have greater insight into the conflict situation (Brubaker et al., 2014).

Mediation: Mediation is often used when the parties have tried to negotiate on their own, but the negotiation has not been successful. The mediator is a process expert and acts as a neutral third party. Although the mediator controls the process, the parties control the outcome. The mediator's job is to listen to the evidence, assist the parties to understand each other's viewpoint regarding the controversy, and then facilitate the negotiation of a voluntary resolution to the conflict situation (Brubaker et al., 2014).

Arbitration: Arbitration also involves the use of a neutral third party, which may be an individual or panel. The arbitrator(s) make the decision for the parties in conflict. Arbitration may be binding or non-binding (Brubaker et al., 2014).

There are a number of advantages of ADR. It is usually faster and less costly than litigation. Each individual in the conflict situation has the opportunity to explain their perceptions of the situation. ADR is more flexible and responsive to the individual needs of the people involved, and it is less formal than litigation. Because of the parties' involvement in the process, greater commitment results, and the parties may be more compliant. Confidentiality is maintained as well as the relationship, which is especially important if the relationship will continue.

Face Negotiation Theory

Face negotiation is the focus of a theory developed by Ting-Toomey to describe and explain differences in responses to conflict on the basis of cultural backgrounds (Ting-Toomey, 1988; Ting-Toomey & Kurogi, 1998). This theory draws on the idea that *face* is a metaphor for our public identity, or self-image, and is an important element of social situations throughout the world. Specifically, face is "a projected image of one's self in a relational situation" (Ting-Toomey, 1988, p. 215). In the theory, *facework* refers to specific verbal and non-verbal messages that help maintain and restore face loss and uphold and honor face gain. All individuals want others to see them in a certain way, even though they may not be consciously aware of this desire.

Ting-Toomey (1988) originally considered face negotiation theory as a way to explain differences in conflict communication styles stemming from cultural preferences for individualism versus collectivism. She proposed that those in cultures best described as *collectivistic* would be more likely to seek to uphold "other-face," whereas those in *individualistic* cultures would more likely seek to uphold "self-face."

Face negotiation theory builds on the five-style dual-concern framework developed by Rahim (1983a) and is based on the degree to which a person is concerned with self-interest, as well as with the interests of others. The five styles are problem solving (also called *integrating, collaborating,* or *cooperating*), forcing (also called *competing* or *dominating*), avoiding (also called *suppressing* or *withdrawing*), yielding (also called *obliging, accommodating,* or *smoothing*), and compromising (Putnam & Poole, 1987; Rahim, 2010). The theory posits that collectivistic cultures favor the avoiding, yielding, and compromising styles; in contrast, individualistic cultures reputedly favor forcing and problem-solving styles (Ting-Toomey, 1988).

In 1998, the face negotiation theory was revised, and the dimension of self-construal (self-image) was discussed in terms of the independent and interdependent self, or the degree to which people conceive of themselves as relatively autonomous from or connected to others (Ting-Toomey & Kurogi, 1998). The revised theory posits that the degree to which people see themselves as autonomous (independent; self-face) or connected to others (interdependent; other-face) is a better predictor of conflict interaction than their cultural or ethnic background. Ting-Toomey and Kurogi (1998) also added the concept of power to the theory to explain communicative differences based on the cultural dimension of power distance. In low power-distance cultures, differences in treatment based on status are less accepted. On the other hand, in high power-distance cultures, differences in treatment based on status are more accepted. The authors proposed that individuals of different status levels in low power-distance cultures are more likely to use the forcing style to resolve conflict, whereas in high power-distance cultures, those in lower status roles may use styles such as yielding.

Two cross-cultural empirical tests of the revised face negotiation theory supported much of the theory (Oetzel & Ting-Toomey, 2003; Oetzel et al., 2001). The 2001 study involved a cross-cultural comparison of four national cultures (Oetzel et al., 2001). In the 2003 study of face negotiation theory, Oetzel and Ting-Toomey tested the underlying assumption that face mediates the relationship between cultural or individual-level variables and conflict styles. The findings provide supportive evidence of the face negotiation theory, especially that face concerns provide a mediating link between cultural values and conflict behavior. The authors also suggested that these findings are particularly significant given the relatively large sample size across four national cultures.

Results of the studies indicated that nursing administrators need to be more attuned to face issues in the conflict dialogue process. The findings of Oetzel and Ting-Toomey (2003) demonstrated that display of other-face concern, which is maintaining the poise or pride of the other person and being sensitive to the other person's self-worth, can lead to a collaborative, win–win integrative approach or an avoiding approach. In contrast, individuals who are more concerned with maintaining self-pride or self-image during a conflict episode would devote effort to defending their conflict position to the neglect of other-face validation issue. Face negotiation theory has been applied to physician communication in the operating room (Kirschbaum, 2012).

Conflict Resolution Outcomes

Whatever the conflict resolution style used, the individual must be aware of the outcome that results from the strategy selected. The outcomes of conflict are what actually happens as a result of the conflict management process. The three ways in which conflicts resolve are (1) win–lose, (2) lose–lose, and (3) win–win (Filley, 1975) (Box 10.3).

Filley (1975) described the win–win resolution as the optimum conflict management. Win–lose and lose–lose resolutions also occur, but effective managers should seek win–win resolutions. Win–win strategies focus on problem solving.

BOX 10.3 Conflict Resolution Outcomes

Win–Lose
One party exerts dominance.

Lose–Lose
Neither side wins.

Win–Win
An attempt is made to meet the needs of both parties simultaneously.

Data from Filley, A.C. (1975). *Interpersonal conflict resolution.* Glenview, IL: Scott, Foresman; Filley, A., House, R., & Kerr, S. (1976). *Managerial process and organizational behavior.* Glenview, IL: Scott, Foresman.

Conflict Resolution Inventories

Several instruments have been developed to measure conflict handling styles. In the Organizational Conflict Inventory-II, Rahim (1983b, c) divided the handling of interpersonal conflict into the two dimensions of concern for self and concern for others—both in high and low degrees—to form a grid. Rahim then adapted Blake and Mouton's (1964) five types of handling interpersonal conflict (forcing, withdrawing, smoothing, compromising, and problem solving) into five styles of handling interpersonal conflict (avoiding, obliging, compromising, integrating, and dominating). The inventory measures the five identified styles.

Thomas and Kilmann (1974) also developed a style assessment and diagnosis inventory, called the Thomas-Kilmann Conflict Mode Instrument (TKI). Their grid uses dimensions of assertiveness and cooperativeness on high to low degrees. The five styles are avoiding, accommodating, compromising, competing, and collaborating. This model blends a description of an individual's behavior on assertiveness and cooperativeness dimensions in situations in which the concerns of two people appear to be incompatible. The behaviors of individuals are thought to be a function of both personal predispositions and situational contingencies. Avoiding is low on both assertiveness and cooperativeness; collaborating is high on both aspects. Competing is high on assertiveness and low on cooperativeness; accommodating is low on assertiveness and high on cooperativeness. Compromising is in the middle.

LEADERSHIP AND MANAGEMENT IMPLICATIONS

Organizational Conflict

Thomas (1976) identified a "big picture" structural model of conflict that examines four factors that seem to influence the way conflict is handled in organizations: behavioral predispositions of individuals, social pressure in the environment, the organization's incentive structure, and rules and procedures. Different levels of power exist as a result of bureaucratic hierarchy and the resultant position power.

Organizational conflict is a form of interpersonal conflict that is generated from aspects of the institution, such as the style of management, rules, procedures, and communication channels. Conflicts that arise when an individual's needs and goals cannot be met within the system are generally organizational. Conflict may be necessary to groups and organizations. Conflict serves to unify and bind together a group by setting boundaries and strengthening a group's identity. Conflict may help stabilize a group by serving as a test of opposing interests within the group. Conflict may help integrate a group by distributing power. Thus conflict may be necessary for the growth of a group and its members and serves to stimulate creativity, innovation, and change.

Organizational leadership sets a tone for conflict and conflict management. This occurs because leaders and managers model behaviors of positive or negative conflict management and choose when and how to intervene in conflict situations. Choice of intervention style and timing of conflict management are functions of the individuals' behavioral predispositions and environmental pressure coupled with the organization's reward structure and coordination and control methods.

Specifically related to organizational conflict and the focus on groups in organizations, Pondy (1967) identified three strategies to use when attempting to resolve organizational conflicts by using bargaining; rules, procedures, and administrative control; and a systems integrator. Bargaining might be useful when a conflict exists over scarce monetary resources. The administrative control approach might be helpful when clarification of role boundaries is needed, such as disagreements over delegation by RNs. The systems integrator approach might be appropriate in a matrix structure or where there is a need to coordinate personnel in vertical and horizontal organizational structures.

Johansen (2012) identified strategies for nurse managers to use to resolve conflict. The strategies are also useful for all nurses:

- *Recognize conflict early.* Recognizing the early warning signs of conflict is the first step toward resolution. Pay attention to body language and be cognizant of the moods of the staff.
- *Be proactive.* Address the issue of concern at an early stage. Avoiding the conflict may cause frustration and escalate the problem.
- *Actively listen.* Focus attention on the speaker. Try to understand, interpret, and evaluate what is being said. The ability to listen actively can improve interpersonal relationships, reduce conflicts, foster understanding, and improve cooperation.
- *Remain calm.* Keep responses under control and emotions in check. Do not react to volatile comments. Calmness will help set the tone for the parties involved.

- *Define the problem.* Clearly identify and define the problem. A clear understanding of the issues will help minimize miscommunication and facilitate resolution.
- *Seek a solution.* Manage the conflict in a way that successfully meets the goal of reaching an acceptable solution for both parties.

The goal of conflict resolution is to create a win–win situation for all. Although it is not realistic to think that every conflict can be resolved in such an ideal fashion, win–win solutions are a worthy goal requiring hard work, creativity, and sound strategy.

CURRENT ISSUES AND TRENDS

There are numerous trends and issues in the continually changing health care environment that have an impact on nursing and health care organizations related to power and conflict. The Strategic Contingencies Theory (Hickson et al., 1971) may provide insight into strategies based on principles of uncertainty, centrality, and non-substitutability that nursing can use to address the issues and trends and thus establish a power base in health care organizations. One of the most significant trends in the health care environment is technology. Nurses are already using information technology in the workplace, but advancements in health care technology move at a rapid pace. This contributes to nurses' change fatigue. However, nurses need to stay at the forefront of the advances, embrace these advances in technology, and develop expertise in their use to leverage power.

Perhaps the most important reason for nurses to stay at the forefront of technological advances is that medical errors are the third leading cause of death in the United States (Makary & Daniel, 2016). Medical errors are defined by the IOM (1999) as the failure of a planned action to be completed as intended or the use of a wrong plan to achieve an aim. James (2013) referred to medical errors as preventable adverse events and separated the errors into these categories: (1) errors of commission, (2) errors of omission, (3) errors of communication, (4) errors of context, and (5) diagnostic errors. Ehteshami and colleagues (2013) indicated that a variety of technologies reduce medical errors, especially medication errors, and prevent them in the health care system. Nurses are at the forefront of implementing information technology and use their expertise power throughout the process.

Electronic health records (EHR) are an example of technology that increases the effectiveness of health care

and reduces medical errors through reminders, alerts, and internal intelligent capabilities. This can help intragroup and intergroup conflict and litigation. It has the potential for increasing communication effectiveness. Given the extent of medical errors, the Strategic Contingencies Theory may provide insight into strategies that can be used to establish a power base in health care organizations. Nurses already have a high degree of centrality in health care organizations because of their coordinating functions. Use of technology to prevent medical errors is a place for nursing to demonstrate the ability to cope with this uncertainty and also demonstrate that nurses are non-substitutable.

Participation in High-Level Decision Making

Nurses need to participate in high-level decision making in order to influence patient care and the nursing profession. Power needs to be leveraged and conflict managed. The Robert Wood Johnson Foundation's (RWJF, 2015) Future of Nursing Campaign for Action advocated for a nurse in every boardroom. Thew (2016) suggested that if nurses are interested in entering the boardroom, they need to (1) find an organization in which they are interested, (2) know their own strengths, (3) express interest, and (4) not allow time constraints to interfere with participation in the boardroom.

Arms and Stalter (2016) described six competencies needed by nurses who are serving on boards and/or policy committees so that they can contribute in a productive manner. These competencies include a professional commitment to serving on a governing board; knowledge about board types, bylaws, and job descriptions; an understanding of standard business protocols, board member roles, and voting processes; a willingness to use principles for managing and leading effective and efficient board meetings; an appreciation for the ethical and legal processes for conducting meetings; and the ability to employ strategies for maintaining control during intense/uncivil situations.

Building a Personal Power Base

Huston (2008) emphasized the importance of building a personal power base and proposed 11 strategies that can be used by both nurse managers and staff to establish a personal power base. These are demonstrating expertise possibly through certification, identifying positive role models and seeking mentoring relationships, networking and coalition building, maintaining freedom of maneuverability, being aware of self, staying focused on goals, choosing battles carefully, demonstrating willingness to take risks, giving up some ego, working hard and being a team player, and finally, taking care of oneself. The author concluded that building a personal power base will take time, but the outcome is the ability to achieve personal and professional goals and is therefore well worth the effort.

Political Action

With 2.9 million registered nurses in the nation, the nursing profession should be a tremendous force in political and public policy debates. Nurses have great potential to contribute to the development of health policy through political action, and their involvement in health policy development ensures that health care is safe, of a high quality, accessible and affordable. Knowledge, skills, and abilities in understanding, using, and managing power and conflict are crucial to nursing in both personal and professional arenas.

RESEARCH NOTE

Source

Hart, C. (2015). The elephant in the room: Nursing and nursing power on an inter-professional team. *The Journal of Continuing Education in Nursing, 46*(8), 349–355.

Purpose

This qualitative study was intended to examine the way in which perceptions of power (professional agency and self-determination in decision making), voice (the ability to both speak out and be heard in decision making), and status influenced how various professions experienced and performed their roles within an inter-professional team.

Discussion

The study was framed methodologically by a modified grounded theory approach, which drew on elements of Charmaz's (1990) social constructionist grounded theory and the theoretical perspective of structural interactionism. This study was conducted with a well-established inter-professional team in a large, urban Canadian mental health institution. The team included representation from nursing (staff nurses and advanced practice nurses), medicine, social work, psychology, occupational therapy, and behavioral therapy, as well as administrative, nonprofessional staff. Purposive sampling was done to recruit 15 to 20 participants from across the inter-professional team. Although initial efforts easily recruited non-nurses and administrative staff, the recruiting of staff nurses required additional approaches. Open-ended interviews of approximately 1 hour each were conducted with 15 participants,

only three of whom were nurses. Grounded theory techniques of concurrent data collection and analysis, constant comparison, and theoretical sensitivity (Glaser, 1978; Glaser & Strauss, 1967) guided the analysis. There was a clear discrepancy between the nurses' description of their role and the description of their role by other members of the team. Other professionals described how the nurses had considerable power but often did not use their power. The nurses felt that their voices were not heard in the inter-professional team and other team members did not appreciate the complexity of roles played by nurses. Unwanted tasks were often delegated to the nurses. The lack of recognition made nurses resist by using behaviors such as ignoring or altering other team members' care plans or withdrawing from discussion in team meetings. The space in which the nurses worked also contributed to the nurses feeling undervalued. Nurses could not participate in team meetings because their work did not allow them to leave their patients. Also, other professionals were able to withdraw from emotional situations by going to their offices or taking a short break, but nurses were not able to do so.

Application to Practice

Findings support a need to go beyond the current focus on competencies and competency development to a deeper understanding of how professional groups experience and then respond to issues of power within an inter-professional context. Addressing systemic factors that lead to nurses feeling undervalued in inter-professional teams is imperative.

CASE STUDY

The new nurse manager of the medical unit at City Hospital wants to implement a new nursing delivery model. A functional nursing model had been in place on the unit for a number of years. In the functional nursing method of patient care delivery, staff members are assigned to complete certain tasks for a group of patients rather than care for specific patients. For example, the RN performs all assessments and administers all intravenous medications, the licensed practical or vocational nurse gives all oral medications, and the assistant performs hygiene tasks and takes vital signs. A charge nurse makes the assignments and coordinates the care.

Continued

CASE STUDY—cont'd

The nurse manager is considering a modular nursing model, which is a modification of team nursing and focuses on the patient's geographic location for staff assignments. The patient unit is divided into modules or districts, and the same team of caregivers is assigned consistently to the same geographic location. The concept of modular nursing calls for a smaller group of staff providing care for a smaller group of patients. The nurse manager believes that the new model would meet the needs of both patients and staff. The assistant nurse manager opposes the implementation of the modular nursing model. She has been employed on the unit for 20 years and firmly believes that the functional nursing model has worked well. She sees no reason to change. The two have had many heated discussions on this issue. During a staff meeting, the nurse manager presented information on the modular nursing model in the hopes of stimulating discussion and gaining staff support. During the presentation, the assistant nurse manager yelled, "I will never support a modular nursing system, and if you continue to attempt to make this change, I will make every effort to make sure that it is not successful."

1. What are the dimensions of power and conflict evident in this case study?
2. How is it possible to turn the situation around?
3. How can a win–win situation be created?
4. What power and conflict resolution strategies might be helpful?
5. Which communication techniques would be most constructive?
6. What are the disagreements, interference, and negative emotions involved in this situation?

▎CRITICAL THINKING EXERCISE

Mary is a registered nurse who graduated 2 years ago from a BSN program. She moved from Cincinnati to a small town in Indiana and now works at the local community hospital. This is her second job since graduating. Mary has been having issues with her co-worker Jean, who is a licensed vocational nurse. Jean often makes snide remarks about Colleen being "a big city girl with little experience" and belittles her when she speaks up at staff meetings. Several times over the past month, Mary has asked for assistance from Jean and was told she needed to "learn to set priorities better." Another time when Mary asked for information about a patient, Jean rolled her eyes and stated, "You can find the information in the electronic health record." On another occasion, Mary asked Jean for assistance with a 300-pound patient. Jean ignored her and walked away. Mary recognized she was being bullied and needed to take steps to stop it.

1. What are the dimensions of power and conflict evident in this case study?
2. How is it possible to turn the situation around?
3. How can a win–win situation be created?
4. What power and conflict management strategies might be helpful?
5. Which communication techniques would be most constructive?
6. What are the disagreements, interference, and negative emotions involved in this situation?

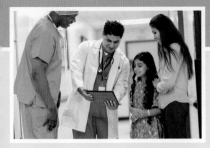

Workplace Diversity

Michael Soon Lee

http://evolve.elsevier.com/Huber/leadership

One of the biggest issues affecting health care today is that of cultural diversity. Differences in the workplace can offer opportunities and create challenges, depending on how they are perceived and handled by the parties involved. As a professional group, nurses are far from representative of the populations that they serve. According to a 2015 survey by MinorityNurse.com (2015), 9.9% of registered nurses (RNs) were Black or African American (non-Hispanic) while African Americans amounted to 13.2% of the population; 8.3% of RNs were Asian while Asian Americans amounted to 6.3% of the population; 4.8% of RNs were Hispanic or Latino while Latino Americans amounted to 17.4% of the population; and 0.4% of RNs were American Indian or Alaskan Native while these groups amounted to 2% of the population.

Culture and diversity affect how people behave and are what are known as "cultural tendencies." For example, many Americans tend to be in a hurry and are known for talking and even walking fast. In fact, there is a common saying in the United States that "time is money." However, this does not mean that every American is in a rush, so it is important to treat every person as an individual with unique needs and wants. Although cultural tendencies can give clues about why and how someone may behave or what they may believe about health care, it is important not to stereotype persons by assuming that everyone from the same culture will act the same way.

Photo used with permission from asiseeit/Getty Images.

DEFINITIONS

The Merriam-Webster Dictionary ("Diversity," n.d.) defined **diversity** as "the state of having people who are different races or who have different cultures in a group or organization." This definition includes race, gender, physical ability, religion, age, sexual orientation, and many more differences. **Cultural diversity** is defined by the Oxford Dictionary ("Cultural diversity," 2016) as, "The existence of a variety of cultural or ethnic groups within a society."

Everyone views the world through their own unique set of lenses, which are colored by their past experiences and those of people around them. This forms their culture. Merriam-Webster ("Culture," n.d.) defined **culture** as "the beliefs, customs, arts, etc., of a particular society, group, place, or time; a particular society that has its own beliefs, ways of life, art, etc. and a way of thinking, behaving, or working that exists in a place or organization (such as a business)." The Office of Minority Health (OMH, 2013, p. 10) defined culture as ". . . the integrated pattern of thoughts, communications, actions, customs, beliefs, values, and institutions associated, wholly or partially, with racial, ethnic, or linguistic groups, as well as with religious, spiritual, biological, geographical, or sociological characteristics. Culture is dynamic in nature, and individuals may identify with multiple cultures over the course of their lifetimes." There is a complex nature to culture, which has been defined and studied across many disciplines.

BACKGROUND

The United States is the most ethnically diverse country in the world, with over 100 racial, ethnic, and cultural groups. The US Census Bureau (2014) estimates that minorities (anyone who is not a single-race non-Hispanic White) will be the majority in America by 2044 as a result of both immigration and growth rate. The nation's racial and ethnic minority groups, especially Hispanics, are growing more rapidly than the non-Hispanic White population, fueled by both immigration and births. This trend has been taking place for decades, and the Census Bureau has announced that minorities now account for a majority of births in the United States (Frey, 2014). Results from the 2010 census show that racial and ethnic minorities accounted for 91.7% of the nation's growth since 2000. Most of that increase, from 2000 to 2010 (56%), was due to Hispanics. Non-Hispanic Whites, although still a majority of the nation's population, accounted for only 8.3% of its growth over the decade.

Another important part of the explanation for changing birth patterns is that on average minority populations are younger than Whites and thus are more likely to be having and raising children. There are notable differences by race and ethnic group in median age, which is the age at which half a group is younger and half older. The national median age in the United States in 2011 was 37.3. Non-Hispanic Whites have the oldest median age at 42.3 years, and Hispanics are the youngest at 27.6 years old. Non-Hispanic Blacks and non-Hispanic Asians are also younger than Whites at 32.9 and 35.9 years, respectively (US Census Bureau, 2014).

Social change, not just demographic change, is also driving recent birth rate trends. A rising number of multiracial babies are being born to couples that include one White parent (US Census Bureau, 2014). The Census Bureau has individuals respond to the race question based on self-identification. For the first time, in the 2000 census, people had the option to self-identify with more than one race.

Statistics show that the racial/ethnic profile of nurses—predominantly White and female—does not reflect the general population. There are many benefits to having a staff that reflects the population of the patients being served. First, patients will be more comfortable being around nurses who speak their language and understand their culture, which can often result in more positive medical outcomes and compliance. Second, a diversity of backgrounds can provide a greater number of solutions to daily challenges because of differing experiences, ideas, and ways of thinking that can be used to solve problems. Third, having a culturally diverse staff can make it much easier to hire more minority nurses.

When nurses and patients are from different backgrounds, it can make communications more challenging than when the participants are from the same culture. This can be frustrating for everyone involved, but in the health care field, miscommunications can be fatal.

To reduce cross-cultural miscommunications and improve patient satisfaction, the multicultural competence of health care practitioners needs to be improved. The first step toward multicultural competence is to recognize one's own prejudices and learn about other people's differences. The problem is that many Americans are afraid to ask people about their culture because of the idea that "we don't want to offend anyone." The challenge with this thinking is that if nurses do not ask about people's differences, then the only option is to make assumptions. It is far more likely that others will be offended by people making assumptions than asking them directly about differences in their behavior or beliefs. In fact, asking other people directly about their culture can often help build rapport and a much deeper working relationship than simply talking about the weather or current events. To do this, ask "Where are your ancestors from?"

It is okay to take a sincere interest in a co-worker's or a patient's culture. Exploring and assessing the individual's preferences can bring to light the impact of culture on health care needs. Their culture could have an impact on their views about health issues such as health care, diet, and lifestyle. In reality, when people do not ask others about their cultural differences, those unasked questions can create a kind of "cultural static" that can keep the nurse from hearing a co-worker or patient clearly. This is a part of patient assessment and is also important for fostering co-worker relationships. The nurse could miss an important fact that would enlighten care delivery and healthy work environments.

THE IMPACT OF CULTURE

Nurse managers who supervise multicultural teams need to become aware of how culture can affect their interaction with one another and with patients. Just some of the factors that can hinder effective cross-cultural communications include:

- **Comfort with the familiar.** We all tend to be attracted to people who are more like us than different from us. In fact, those who are unlike us can often make us uncomfortable and even anxious. Effective leaders tend to seek a diversity of people and ideas in order to have a wide selection of options from which to choose in order to solve problems. Yet fostering comfort with the unfamiliar is needed.
- **Assumed similarity.** We tend to assume that others are like us in our beliefs, behaviors, and communication style. For example, Americans tend to be very direct in communications, believing we should "say what we mean," whereas Asians tend to be more indirect and leave more unsaid than expressed. This can lead to the belief on the part of Americans that Asians are reluctant to be forthcoming about health care concerns, medications they are taking, or other related issues. Fostering an open, inclusive, and healthy work environment with respectful communication is needed.

Health Equity

According to the World Health Organization (2016), "Equity is the absence of avoidable or remediable differences among groups of people, whether those groups are defined socially, economically, demographically or geographically." Currently, individuals across the United States from various cultural backgrounds are unable to attain their highest level of health for several reasons, including the social determinants of health, or those conditions in which individuals are born, grow, live, work, and age, such as socioeconomic status, education level, and the availability of health services. Health inequities are directly related to the existence of historical and current discrimination and social injustice, and one of the most modifiable factors is the lack of culturally and linguistically appropriate services, broadly defined as care and services that are respectful of and responsive to the cultural and linguistic needs of all individuals.

Health inequities result in disparities that directly affect the quality of life for all individuals. Health disparities adversely affect neighborhoods, communities, and the broader society, thus making the issue not only an individual concern but also a public health concern. In the United States, it has been estimated that racial health disparities are associated with substantial annual economic losses nationally, including an estimated $35 billion in excess health care expenditures, $10 billion in illness-related lost productivity, and nearly $200 billion in premature deaths (Ayanian, 2015). It is believed that concerted efforts to reduce health disparities could thus have immense economic and social value.

According to the 2014 National Healthcare Quality and Disparities Report (Agency for Healthcare Research and Quality [AHRQ], 2015), "Historically, Americans have experienced variable access to care based on race, ethnicity, socioeconomic status, age, sex, disability status, sexual orientation, and residence location." This study found that Blacks had worse access to health care than Whites for about half of measures of access, Hispanics had worse access to care than Whites for two-thirds of access measures, and Asians and American Indians and Alaska Natives had worse access to care than Whites for about one-third of access measures.

Leaders in health care, government, and business must address the persistent disparities at the national, state, and local levels, as both an ethical and an economic imperative. In fact, eliminating racial disparities in health care is vital to pushing the entire health care system toward improving quality while containing costs—so-called value-based care. Since 2003, Congress has mandated that the federal government produce the annual National Healthcare Disparities Report as part of the effort to monitor national progress in this domain.

Ayanian (2015) outlined five principles for eliminating racial disparities as part of health care reform:

1. Provide insurance coverage and access to high-quality care for all Americans.
2. Promote a diverse health care workforce.
3. Deliver patient-centered care.
4. Maintain accurate, complete race and ethnicity data to monitor disparities in care.
5. Set measurable goals for improving quality of care and ensure that goals are achieved equitably for all racial and ethnic groups.

The term **health disparities** is often defined as "a difference in which disadvantaged social groups such as the poor, racial/ethnic minorities, women and other groups who have persistently experienced social disadvantage or discrimination systematically experience worse health or greater health risks than more advantaged social groups" (Virginia.gov, 2016). When this term is applied to certain ethnic and racial social groups, it describes the increased presence and severity of certain diseases, poorer health outcomes, and greater difficulty in obtaining health care services for these races and ethnicities. When systemic barriers to good health are avoidable yet still remain, they are often referred to as "health inequities" (Virginia.gov, 2016).

In addition, even with expanded insurance coverage, racial minorities are less likely to receive needed behavioral health services comparable to that received by non-Latino Whites (Alegria et al., 2012). Health disparities exist beyond racial and ethnic groups; for example, individuals with lower incomes are more likely to experience preventable hospitalizations compared with individuals with higher incomes. In addition, lesbian women are less likely to receive preventive cancer screenings than their heterosexual counterparts, and men who have sex with men are less likely to have access to health and behavioral health care than the general population of men (McKirnan et al., 2013).

Without effective health provider and patient communication in a language both can understand, there is an increased risk of misdiagnosis, misunderstanding about the proper course of treatment, and poorer adherence to medication and discharge instructions (The California Endowment, 2003). These factors have a direct impact on desired health outcomes.

Improving Quality of Services and Care

A 2012 study by the Kaiser Family Foundation found that 26% of Native American/Alaska Natives, 18% of African Americans, 16% of persons of Asian descent, and 12% of native Hawaiian/Pacific Islanders lacked health insurance. In a 2013 study of the non-elderly uninsured, 32% of all Hispanics, 14% of all African Americans, and 6% of all Americans of Asian/Pacific Islander descent reported they lacked health insurance. The same study looked at all non-elderly, uninsured Americans and found that 71% of this population had one or more full-time workers in the family yet were uninsured (Kaiser Family Foundation, 2015).

According to census figures published in 2012, 50.4% of all children in the United States (31.8 million children) are identified as belonging to a racial or ethnic minority (US Census Bureau, 2012). The 2013 census found that around 11% to 12% of persons under age 19 with household incomes less than $50,000 per annum were without health insurance. Some 27% of non-native born persons under 19 were without health insurance in

2013. At the same time, 12% of Hispanics under the age of 19, 7% of African Americans under the same age, and 8% of persons under the age of 19 of Asian descent lacked health insurance (Smith & Medalia, 2014).

Although it is commonly believed that health disparities occur simply because of a lack of health insurance and access to health care, disparities exist even after access to the health care system has been improved. New studies have shown, for instance, that there are stark differences in health outcomes of African-American and Caucasian patients with the same conditions even when they are treated by the same doctor. Studies have also shown that diagnoses, treatments, and quality of care can vary greatly depending on a number of factors that affect minority communities, including language barriers, lack of insurance coverage, and differential treatments based on the population group. This is important because racial and ethnic minorities are among the fastest growing of all communities in the United States and comprised approximately 39% of the total US population in 2013 (US Census Bureau, n.d.).

THE NATIONAL CLAS STANDARDS

The National Standards for Culturally and Linguistically Appropriate Services in Health and Health Care (the National CLAS Standards) were originally developed in 2000 by the Health and Human Services Office of Minority Health (OMH) and then enhanced in 2010 (OMH, 2013). They were intended to advance health equity, improve quality, and help eliminate health care disparities by providing a blueprint for individuals and health and health care organizations to implement culturally and linguistically appropriate services. The original National CLAS Standards provided guidance on cultural and linguistic competency, with the ultimate goal of reducing racial and ethnic health care disparities. Adoption of these standards was designed to advance better health and health care in the United States. Since 2000, the original National CLAS Standards have served as catalyst and conduit for efforts to improve the quality of care and achieve health equity.

The HHS Office of Minority Health undertook the National CLAS Standards Enhancement Initiative from 2010 to 2012 to recognize the nation's increasing diversity, reflect the tremendous growth in the fields of cultural and linguistic competency over the past decade, and ensure relevance with new national policies and legislation, such as the Affordable Care Act. A decade after the publication of the original National CLAS Standards, there was still much work to be done. Racial and ethnic disparities in health and health care remained a significant public health issue, despite advances in health care technology and delivery, even when factors such as insurance coverage, income, and educational attainment are taken into account.

The enhanced National CLAS Standards are built on the groundwork laid by the original National CLAS Standards and are composed of 15 standards that provide individuals and organizations with a blueprint for successfully implementing and maintaining culturally and linguistically appropriate services (see Office of Minority Health at https://www.thinkculturalhealth. hhs.gov/pdfs/EnhancedCLASStandardsBlueprint.pdf). Culturally and linguistically appropriate health care and services—broadly defined as care and services that are respectful of and responsive to the cultural and linguistic needs of all individuals—are increasingly seen as essential to reducing disparities and improving health care quality.

Cultural and linguistic competency strives to improve the quality of care received and to reduce disparities experienced by racial and ethnic minorities and other underserved populations. Through the National CLAS Standards Enhancement Initiative, a new benchmark was established for culturally and linguistically appropriate services to improve the health of all individuals.

State Legislation: Mandating Cultural and Linguistic Competency Training

In the years since the launch of the original National CLAS Standards, a number of states have implemented legislation pertaining to culturally and linguistically appropriate services (OMH, n.d.). For many health professionals and organizations, the original National CLAS Standards served as a driver or model for what the legislation could include. Training has been legislated or proposed, and at least six states have moved to mandate some form of CLAS competency for elements of the health care workforce.

Federal Legislation: Affordable Care Act of 2010

The Affordable Care Act of 2010 laid an important foundation for advancing health equity and improving the quality of services to diverse communities. There are numerous provisions in the health care law related to cultural and linguistic competency, and the enhanced National CLAS Standards serve as a resource, at all levels, in these areas.

Legislative, Regulatory, and Accreditation Mandates

Culturally and linguistically appropriate services are increasingly included in or referenced by local and national legislative, regulatory, and accreditation mandates. For example, the Patient Protection and Affordable Care Act (the Affordable Care Act), Pub. L. No. 111 to 148 (2010), as amended by the Health Care and Education Reconciliation Act of 2012, Pub. L. No. 111 to 152 (2012)—referred to collectively as the Affordable Care Act—contains several provisions related to culturally and linguistically appropriate services.

Diversity: The Americans With Disabilities Act and Inclusive Excellence

Workplace diversity focuses on inclusiveness beyond race and gender. It also applies to being inclusive of persons with hearing, vision, mobility, and other challenges. The Americans with Disabilities Act (ADA) provides workplace protection for persons with disabilities:

> *Barriers to employment, transportation, public accommodations, public services, and telecommunications have imposed staggering economic and social costs on American society and have undermined our well-intentioned efforts to educate, rehabilitate, and employ individuals with disabilities. By breaking down these barriers, the Americans with Disabilities Act (ADA) will enable society to benefit from the skills and talents of individuals with disabilities, will allow us all to gain from their increased purchasing power and ability to use it, and will lead to fuller, more productive lives for all Americans. The Americans with Disabilities Act gives civil rights protections to individuals with disabilities similar to those provided to individuals on the basis of race, color, sex, national origin, age, and religion. It guarantees equal opportunity for individuals with disabilities in public accommodations, employment, transportation, State and local government services, and telecommunications (US Equal Employment Opportunity Commission, 2002).*

Under the ADA, employment discrimination is prohibited against qualified individuals with disabilities. This applies to persons who have impairments; these must substantially limit major life activities such as seeing, hearing, speaking, walking, breathing, performing manual tasks, learning, caring for oneself, and working. An individual with epilepsy, paralysis, HIV infection, AIDS, a substantial hearing or visual impairment, mental retardation, cancer, mental illness, or a specific learning disability is covered; but an individual with a minor, nonchronic condition of short duration, such as a sprain, broken limb, or the flu, generally would not be covered (US Equal Employment Opportunity Commission, 2002).

The Association of American Colleges and Universities (Williams et al., 2005) used the term *Inclusive Excellence* for its initiative to help higher education organizations integrate diversity and quality efforts, place this work at the core of institutional functioning, and realize the educational benefits available to students and the institution when this integration is done well and sustained over time. They saw diversity and inclusion efforts as multilayered processes designed to achieve excellence in learning, research and teaching, student development, local and global community engagement, and workforce development. Three papers were commissioned. A comprehensive framework for organizational change was offered to help campus leaders move to an environment that systematically leverages diversity for student learning and institutional excellence.

GAINING A COMPETITIVE EDGE IN THE MARKETPLACE

Another strong argument for the implementation of workplace diversity and cultural competency in health care is that there are tangible, broad benefits of doing so, including to business operations. Becoming culturally competent has social, health, and business benefits for health care organizations, according to a report from the Equity of Care initiative and the American Hospital Association's Health Research & Educational Trust and Hospitals in Pursuit of Excellence. *Becoming a Culturally Competent Health Care Organization* (Health Research & Educational Trust, 2013) outlined 16 benefits of organizations' ability to meet the health care needs of patients with diverse backgrounds, grouped into three broad categories of social, health, and business benefits:

1. Social benefits
   - Increases mutual respect and understanding between patient and organization
   - Increases trust
   - Promotes inclusion of all community members
   - Increases community participation and involvement in health issues
   - Assists patients and families in their care
   - Promotes patient and family responsibilities for health
2. Health benefits
   - Improves patient data collection
   - Increases preventive care by patients
   - Reduces care disparities in the patient population
   - Increases cost savings from a reduction in medical errors, number of treatments, and legal costs
   - Reduces the number of missed medical visits
3. Business benefits
   - Incorporates different perspectives, ideas, and strategies into the decision-making process
   - Decreases barriers that slow progress
   - Moves toward meeting legal and regulatory guidelines
   - Improves efficiency of care services
   - Increases the market share of the organization

DECREASING THE RISK OF LIABILITY

The literature illustrates the vital role communication plays in avoiding cases of malpractice due to diagnostic and treatment errors. When communicating with culturally and linguistically diverse populations, the opportunity for miscommunication and misunderstanding increases, which subsequently increases the likelihood of errors. These errors, in turn, can cost millions of dollars in liability or malpractice claims. Culturally and linguistically appropriate services can reduce the possibility of such errors.

The National Center for Cultural Competence (n.d.a) noted that health professionals who lack cultural and linguistic competency can be found liable under tort principles in several areas such as treatment in the absence of informed consent. In addition, providers may be presumed negligent if an individual is unable to follow guidelines because they conflict with his or her beliefs and the provider neglected to identify and try to accommodate the beliefs. Additionally, if a provider proceeds with treatment or an intervention based on miscommunication due to poor quality language assistance, he or she and his or her organization may face increased civil liability exposure. Thus culturally and linguistically appropriate communication is essential to minimize the likelihood of liability and malpractice claims (Goode et al., 2006).

COMMUNICATION

Effective communication among nursing supervisors and their subordinates and between nurses with their patients can have a significant impact on the effectiveness of patient care. Failure to communicate effectively could result from language barriers and cultural differences. Cultural competence can help to overcome some of these challenges.

Each patient or staff member is likely to hold varying degrees of allegiance to his or her culture depending on their level of acculturation and what generation they are from. The first generation are new arrivals to the country who may have difficulty speaking English and who hold most tightly to the cultural behaviors of their country of origin. The second generation are the first in their family to be born in America and are usually bilingual, having learned their family's native language from their parents and English in school. They may have some of the beliefs of their parents but may also be greatly influenced by the American culture. The third generation are likely to be very Americanized in their language, ways of thinking, and practices but can still be influenced by the culture of their ancestors. Culture can run very deep, and it is hard to know when it does not affect one's beliefs and actions.

There are numerous resources available on the Internet to assess and improve cultural competence. For example, there is the Self-Assessment Checklist for Personnel Providing Primary Health Care Services, which is provided by the National Center for Cultural Competence at Georgetown University (National Center for Cultural Competence, n.d.b). This checklist asks users to rate themselves on items such as "I understand and accept that family is defined differently by different cultures"; "I accept individuals and families as the ultimate decision makers for services and supports impacting their lives"; and "I accept that religion and other beliefs may influence how individuals and families respond to illnesses, disease, and death."

Another example is the SHARE Approach, a 1-day training program developed by the Agency for Healthcare Research and Quality (AHRQ, 2014) to help health care professionals work with patients to make the best possible health care decisions. It supports shared decision making through the use of patient-centered outcomes research (PCOR). The website lists resources for health care providers and has a fact sheet to provide guidance to health care providers about how to consider cultural differences as they build effective relationships with patients and promote shared decision making.

GENERATIONAL DIVERSITY

A growing challenge in nursing leadership for both nurses in practice and for nurse managers is the management of generational workforce diversity. Sociologists categorize generational groups into cohorts. These cohorts are members of a generation who are linked through shared life experiences in their formative years. As each new cohort matures, it is influenced by what sociologists call *generational markers*. Individuals are all products of their environment. Generational markers are events that affect all members of the generation in one way or another. Thus being aware of generational differences is essential for every organization's leadership in managing a multiage workforce. Each generation possesses unique characteristics and often deems the values and behaviors of another cohort as character flaws instead of cultural differences.

Baby Boomers

The baby boomers, born between 1946 and 1964, are currently occupying the leadership chairs of many executive suites, including those in health care organizations. Boomers present a striking contrast to members of the previous generation, those born between 1925 and 1945, often referred to as the *Mature Generation* or the *Silent Generation*.

Boomers, historically the second largest generation in the workforce, have dominated US society for many years because of their large number. Boomer preferences in every facet of American life are affected by their sheer numbers alone. The boomer phenomenon has been known, tracked by the US Census Bureau, and predicted for many years. As of 2012, the boomers were turning 65, retiring, and entering the Medicare system. They were also beginning to acquire chronic conditions. The implications for health care delivery and financing are enormous. Boomers grew up in a period of unprecedented economic growth during which the United States had virtually no strong economic competitors.

They grew up thinking they were special and that they could ignore or break rules and still be successful. Financial security will remain a central issue for many. Consequently, many boomers will work past the age of retirement. They have questioned traditional authority structures, blurred gender roles, and made vigorous attempts to push systems toward their ideas of perfection. During the Vietnam War, the civil rights confrontations, and Watergate, baby boomers saw clearly the vulnerability of authority; they have been reluctant to accept formal authority since. Their preference is for a more participative and less authoritarian workplace (Hendricks & Cope, 2013).

Generation X

Support for such a workplace environment also comes from members of Generation X (X'ers), born between 1965 and 1980, who share with boomers an aversion to authority but with a decided preference for a balanced life. X'ers are the first generation of latchkey kids; as such, they found the need to be resourceful at an early age. Their childhood years have been marked with economic uncertainty, and thus they are skeptical of traditional practices and beliefs. In their view, employment contracts are agreements that either side can cancel at will, which means that placing their future in the hands of employers makes them extremely uneasy and is thus highly unlikely to occur. The length of time spent with an organization is less relevant to X'ers than how to protect themselves from the capriciousness of business challenges. This creates unique challenges in the workplace for recruitment and especially retention of nurses who are X'ers (Hendricks & Cope, 2013).

Millennials

Both the youngest group in the workplace and the largest group in US history are the millennial workers, those born between 1981 and 1999. This group is known by several other monikers, including *Generation Y, Generation Why?, Nexters,* and the *Internet Generation.* The common marker of their developmental years is technology. This group is the most demographically diverse generation in this country's history. These workers have astonishing multitasking skills. They also tend to have a positive outlook and a desire to improve the world.

Many believe that millennials are shallow on basic skills; but because they grew up with computers, they can create solutions that other generations could not

have imagined. Technology guides their every move. They are problem solvers who grew up in a flourishing economy. Millennials matured in a world in which shortcuts, manipulation of rules, and situational ethics seem to have reigned. They got the message somehow that the final word is not the final word. They do not live to work; they work to live. Thus they have a different set of expectations about the world of work. Most enjoy the liberty of working on their own in a style that favors their work ethic. Millennials have learned that their presence is in demand. To thrive, they need clear definitions of outcomes, resources to do what needs to be done, and a deadline (Hendricks & Cope, 2013).

LEADERSHIP AND MANAGEMENT IMPLICATIONS

Diversity leads to stronger teams with members whose skills complement one another and a broader range of solutions to difficult challenges. However, successfully leading culturally diverse teams requires the ability to consider viewpoints that may conflict with one's own (as well as the majority), to overcome cross-cultural communications challenges, to help the team embrace differences, and beyond. According to the OMH (2013, p. 12), "The enhanced National CLAS Standards emphasize the importance of CLAS being integrated throughout an organization. This requires a bottom-up and a top-down approach to advancing and sustaining CLAS."

Organizational governance and leadership are key to ensuring the successful implementation and maintenance of CLAS. Along with organizational governance, authentic leadership is also need to foster workplace inclusion and a climate that promotes and rewards diversity and inclusion (Boekhorst, 2015). Organization-wide change is needed to leverage the efforts of authentic leaders, organizational reward systems, work group composition, group size, and cooperative goal structures to effect workplace inclusion. Internal processes such as leadership actions are instrumental in managing diversity through engaging resistance to inclusion initiatives instead of silencing them. This supports a vision of an inclusive workplace (Boekhorst, 2015). Strong communication systems and processes need to be in place.

Research shows that there are three major issues in cross-cultural communication: ambiguity, inflexible attitude, and ethnocentrism.

Ambiguity

Cultures provide people with ways of thinking: ways of seeing, hearing, and interpreting the world. Thus the same words can mean different things to people from different cultures, even when they speak the "same" language. When the languages are different, and translation has to be used to communicate, the potential for misunderstandings increases. Each culture has its unique context, value system, and communication style. Ambiguity enters the communication process when the context of the individual's culture and the culture of the listener is not fully comprehended. For example, when people from different cultures come together, they tend to assume certain things (unaware of difference in the communication styles and cultural values) and do not take cognizance of the value system of the other culture. This leads to a situation where the listener not only loses part of the message but also develops an incorrect perspective about the delivered information.

Inflexible Attitude

When they enter a different cultural context, some people tend to avoid exposure or experience of the host culture. This results in introvert behavior and a closed mindset, leading to an impression that the visitor is not accepting the host culture. This leads to missing out on new experiences to learn and adapt to the new culture. Such a behavior, whether conscious or unconscious, dampens the team spirit and deteriorates business relationships.

Ethnocentrism

Ethnocentrism is the assumption that the culture of one's own group is right, moral, and rational—and that other cultures are inferior. Because ethnocentrism is often an unconscious behavior, it is understandably difficult to prevent in advance. When confronted with a different culture, individuals judge it with reference to their own standards and make no attempt to evaluate the new culture from the other culture's point of view. Such a behavior is also characterized by selective listening and value judgments, severely affecting the quality of the communication (Malik, 2015).

Individuals from Western cultures such as the United States tend to prefer direct forms of communication like asking questions, freely providing their opinion, and making direct eye contact. They may consider those who do not act this way to be indecisive, less capable, and possibly even dishonest. In contrast, people from indirect cultures may consider asking questions of those in authority to be disrespectful, withhold their viewpoint especially if it differs from the majority for fear of disrupting group harmony, and avoid direct eye contact, which can be considered aggressive or even disrespectful. They might consider those who do not behave in this manner to be disrespectful, aggressive, and maybe not team players.

Accents and fluency can also create problems in the workplace. Obviously, managers should try not to let an accent or level of English fluency affect their determination of a nurse's intelligence or competence. Unfortunately, research shows that many people make judgments about socioeconomic level, intelligence, or even competence depending on the strength and even the country of origin of an accent. Some in the United States may automatically consider people with British accents to be more intelligent than average, whereas those with Middle Eastern or Latin accents are perceived to be less intelligent (Nelson et al., 2016).

Differing attitudes toward hierarchy and authority can create challenges in the workplace. Geert Hofstede, a Dutch social psychologist, developed a cultural dimensions theory as a framework for cross-cultural communication (Clearly Cultural, 2004–2016a). His dimension for this is known as *power distance* and expresses the degree to which a society handles inequalities among people. People in societies exhibiting a large degree of power distance accept a hierarchical order in which everybody has a place and that needs no further justification. In societies with low power distance, people strive to equalize the distribution of power and demand justification for inequalities of power. For the United States, Hofstede ranked the power distance relatively low at 40, leading to a situation where nurses may commonly call doctors by their first names, whereas in the Philippines the power distance is 94 and nurses may automatically respect doctors and their opinions without question (Clearly Cultural, 2004–2016a).

Decision making can be culturally influenced through Hofstede's dimension known as Individualism versus Collectivism (Clearly Cultural, 2004–2016b). The high side of this dimension, called *individualism,* can be defined as a preference for a loosely knit social framework in which people are expected primarily to take care of themselves and their immediate families. Nurses from these cultures tend to take responsibility for their actions and act more individually than those from collectivist cultures. Hofstede ranks Americans among the highest individualist cultures at 91, with Asian Indians in the middle at 48.

Collectivism is a tightly knit societal framework where people are integrated into cohesive and strong in-groups, often extended families, to look after them in exchange for unquestioning loyalty. Nurses from collectivist cultures tend to look to the team before taking action. The most collectivist culture on Hofstede's scale is Guatemala at 6, China is 20, and the Philippines is 32. It's not unusual with patients from collectivist cultures to have large groups of relatives and friends visit at the same time, which can create challenges for nursing staff to accommodate, especially in crowded shared rooms.

Decision making in collectivist cultures can also be confusing for nurses, because determining who is actually making a medical decision may not be immediately apparent. The patients may look to parents, siblings, grandparents, or others for guidance. The only way to really know who makes the decision is to ask a question such as, "When would you like me to come back?" and carefully watch to see who the group looks to for the answer. This person will likely be the real decision maker (Clearly Cultural, 2004–2016b).

High Context and Low Context

Some people develop a communication style based on socially-influenced ideas about the value of maintaining relationships and thus transfer information by means of shared understandings and context to preserve harmony and save face. Known as high content, this also influences communication orientation and the reluctance to speak up at work (Ward et al., 2016). The assumptions of high context and low context are a part of the health care context, which is always dynamic. The context dictates "where one is coming from" and how information or knowledge is communicated in human transactions or relationships; it is culturally based.

From a global perspective, the cultural context of the Western world is low context. In places such as North America and Western Europe, the explicit verbal or written message carries the meaning. Low-context cultures require extensive detailed explanations, information, and contracts because they are making up for the context that may be missing in a given situation. Decisions are focused around tasks and activities that need to be accomplished. Rules are very clear and tend to be followed precisely.

In high-context cultures such as Asia, South America, Africa, and most of the Middle East, verbal communication is less explicit than in low-context cultures. That which is written or stated rarely carries the meaning. The meaning of the message is understood by reading between the lines for what is not written or stated. In high-context cultures, most of the meaning is assumed to exist by the nature of the situation (i.e., the context). Decisions and activities primarily occur via personal, face-to-face communication, often around a central, authoritative figure. Most nuclear families are high context, relying on high interpersonal interaction and subtle messages. Leaders from a low-context culture may have the power to define the rules of work and to determine what will be rewarded, who gets promoted, what benefits will be offered, and what values will define the organization. In high-context cultures, decisions are made more with face-to-face conversations rather than in formal meetings. Rules tend to be more of a suggestion than an absolute dictum (ToughNickel, 2016). Placing someone from a high-context workplace culture into a setting dominated by leaders from a low-context culture increases the likelihood of perceptions of inequity and workplace conflicts.

CURRENT ISSUES AND TRENDS

Despite targeted efforts, challenges surrounding issues of workplace diversity persist. The most urgent issue is the lack of cultural diversity in the nursing workforce, as seen in the US Census Bureau data. Other issues are hiring nurses from diverse cultures, negotiating postures, and use of interpreters. Various suggestions are offered to address these current issues.

Hiring Nurses From Diverse Cultures

The important issues of recruitment into the profession should specifically include efforts to recruit minorities and individuals from other cultures. The challenge is that managers tend to hire people who are like themselves rather than seek out those with complementary skills to others on their team. Suggestions for hiring more minority nurses are to:

- Increase recruiting efforts from historically minority colleges and universities.
- Watch out for screening procedures that may automatically exclude minority candidates, such as oral interviews, which can put people who are not traditionally verbal at a disadvantage compared with those from high-context cultures.
- Make a concerted and measurable effort to recruit, hire, and retain minority nurses and provide cultural sensitivity training and expectations clarity.
- Ask current staff for referrals and recommendations.
- Develop a hiring committee that is diverse and sensitive to the need to hire minorities.

- Be flexible in reviewing resumes. Recognize that applicants from collectivist cultures may not include or may minimize their accomplishments, as opposed to those from individualist cultures who have a high acceptance of bragging and personal promotion.

Negotiating

There are two types of countries in the world: negotiating and non-negotiating. The United States, Canada, Western Europe, and a few other countries only negotiate the most expensive purchases like cars and houses, whereas they will pay exactly what is asked on almost everything else. In the majority of countries, such as Mexico, Asia, India, South America, and the Philippines, negotiation is expected over everything in daily life (Lewis, 2017). Patients and co-workers from these countries are likely to be much better at haggling than Americans for prescriptions, extra care, and other aspects of health care services. Suggestions for managing negotiations are to:

- Provide education to staff about cultural differences.
- Have trained business office staff or patient representatives available to assist with negotiation initiations.

- Accept negotiation initiations as normal; have scripted responses for those uncomfortable with negotiation.

Interpreters

Patients who are limited English proficient (LEP) are likely to require the services of an interpreter. If at all possible, this person should be a neutral outsider instead of a family member—especially a bilingual child of the client—except in extreme emergencies. Policies and procedures guide health care personnel in the use of interpreter services, which need to be robust and readily available. Knowledge about the major ethnic and cultural groups in the patient population is a key aspect of success. Some suggestions for using interpreters (Refugee Health Technical Assistance Center, 2011) are trained bilingual staff, on-staff interpreters, contract interpreters, telephone interpreters, and trained volunteers can serve as health care interpreters. Some people, however, should not serve as health care interpreters: patients' family and friends, children under 18 years old, health care personnel not involved in direct care, other patients or visitors, and untrained volunteers.

RESEARCH NOTE

Source
Boekhorst, J.A. (2015). The role of authentic leadership in fostering workplace inclusion: A social information processing perspective. *Human Resource Management*, *54*(2), 241–264.

Purpose
The purpose of this article is to present and discuss a conceptual model for an organization-wide approach to developing a climate for inclusion. It explains why authentic leaders are a key source of social information, which then is a major factor influencing the formation of a climate of inclusion.

Discussion
With an ever-increasing trend of workplace diversity, there is the corresponding need to understand and better manage this phenomenon. To advance the knowledge base and literature on workplace diversity, the author explored how a climate for inclusion can foster greater feelings of comfort in the workplace, which in turn encourages the application of diversity/differences directly to work processes, tasks, and strategies—and thereby

better outcomes. Using organizational climate and culture, social information processing, social learning, and authentic leadership theories, the author highlighted the central tenet of ethicality in authentic leadership (authentic leaders tend to engage in ethical behaviors driven by their values and beliefs). A conceptual model was developed, and eight propositions were presented and discussed. An organization-wide change effort to create an inclusive work climate was examined. Key organizational and group structures, processes, and strategies influencing the formation of a climate for inclusion are organizational reward systems, workgroup composition, group size, and goal interdependence.

Application to Practice
Future research is needed for greater understanding of the key determinants and linkages to outcomes. The conceptual model needs empirical testing. The author discusses practical implications for managers and human resources personnel, such as in the recruitment and selection process of leaders, socialization initiatives for new hires, work group design, and organizational reward systems design and management.

CASE STUDY

In a large hospital, many of the nurses had a habit of talking to one another in public in their native languages, which included Filipino, Chinese, Thai, and Hindi. This not only made patients feel uncomfortable but other staff members as well because it was felt that they might be talking about them behind their backs. To make matters worse, these conversations were often punctuated by loud giggling or laughing. The nurse manager has been asked by her boss to get them to only speak English.

1. What are the issues in this vignette?
2. What are the issues from the perspective of the nurses and the manager?

3. Why are people uncomfortable being in an environment where foreign languages are spoken by others?
4. How does this vignette relate to your experience or to the experience of someone you know?
5. What difficulties might the manager encounter in enforcing an English-only policy?
6. How could an English-only policy affect the nurses?
7. Brainstorm strategies to constructively address this situation.

▌CRITICAL THINKING EXERCISE

In a diabetes clinic, there were a large percentage of Filipino nurses. A new nurse manager was unaware that it is customary for many Filipinos to travel back to the Philippines for a month around Christmas to visit their families and celebrate the holidays. This obviously created a tremendous staffing problem as the nurse manager scrambled to fill the vacancies and bring temporary hires up to speed in a short amount of time.

1. What is the problem in this case?
2. Whose problem is it?
3. What should the health professional do?
4. How can the health professionals be culturally competent in this situation?

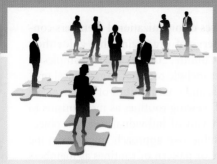

Organizational Structure

Carol A. Wong

@http://evolve.elsevier.com/Huber/leadership

Organizations are essentially social structures that rely on human activity. An organization meaningfully coordinates group activity toward a shared goal because collective efforts are often necessary to manage large-scale work processes and outcomes efficiently and effectively. Many types of organizations are necessary in order to deliver nursing and health care services to diverse populations across sectors and geography. In health care, obvious organizational goals might be safety and quality of care, cost reduction, and increased efficiency. Understanding organizational structure helps nurses be more effective and efficient in their work lives.

Whether as employees or as independent practitioners, nurses work for or interact with organizations. How nurses' roles interface with the structure of the organization influences the accomplishment of organizational goals. Research examples throughout this chapter highlight associations between the organizational structures in which nurses work and clinical, nurse, and organizational outcomes.

DEFINITIONS

Structure refers to the arrangement of the parts within a larger whole. In Donabedian's (1980) classic quality framework of structure, process, and outcomes, structure affects process, which affects outcomes. **Organizations** are entities that contain groupings that consolidate smaller elements into a larger, systematized whole. **Organizational social structure** is defined as the ways in which

Photo used with permission from Kamaga/Getty Images.

work is divided and coordinated among members and the resulting network of relationships, roles, and work groups (e.g., units, departments). The social structure of an organization influences the flow of information, resources, and power among its members.

ORGANIZATION THEORY

Organizations are complex and dynamic. Yet for nurses to function as effective health care workers, an understanding of organizations is essential. There are many ways to understand organizations, and each understanding reflects different assumptions and tensions regarding the nature and dynamics of organizations. The history of organization theory has been shaped by multiple disciplines, including management, engineering, psychology, sociology, and anthropology, and by study over a long period of time. Although this has created a rich and varied understanding of organizations, the field of organization theory contains a variety of approaches to and assumptions about the phenomenon of "organization." Objectivism, subjectivism, and postmodernism reflect three broad perspectives regarding the nature of reality and the nature of knowledge with respect to the concept of "organization" (Hatch & Cunliffe, 2013). These perspectives are reviewed briefly with attention to the meanings of social structure, management, and power.

Objective Perspective

The objective (also called modern) perspective centers interest on causal explanation that entails describing the antecedents and results of a particular phenomenon (Hatch & Cunliffe, 2013). When approached as an objective entity, an organization exists as an external reality, independent of its social actors. Organizations are viewed as logical and predictable objects with identifiable and scientifically measurable characteristics (e.g., size) that can be predicted, observed, or manipulated (Hatch & Cunliffe, 2013). The purpose is to uncover laws that enhance the generalizability of knowledge. Organizational structure is a consequence of both the division of and the coordination of labor, which results in a formal set of interrelated and interdependent roles and work groups. Management determines the *formal* relationships and standardizes the behaviors of individuals and groups in order to align organizational functioning with internal demands (e.g., technology) and external demands (e.g., market conditions, regulatory standards) (Reed, 1992). Typically, power is conceptualized as a resource to be allocated among roles and groups. Modernist theories related to bureaucracy and systems—as well as the schools of scientific management and human relations—have focused on improvements to efficiency, motivation, and performance in the achievement of collective goals (Reed, 1992). These theoretical approaches, which focus on the *formal* aspects of organizations, are examined in detail in this chapter.

Subjective Perspective

In contrast to objectivism, a symbolic or subjective approach to the phenomenon of organization asserts that an organization cannot exist independent of its social actors. The organization is a social reality that can be known only through human experience, relationships, and shared meanings and symbols (Hatch & Cunliffe, 2013). Because knowledge is considered to be relative, open to interpretation, and context dependent, the purpose of inquiries is to uncover collective meanings and understandings that resonate with the experiences of those involved (Hatch & Cunliffe, 2013). Social structure therefore arises from and is continuously transformed through social interaction, which is played out against a backdrop of formal rules and material resources directed by management (Reed, 1992). Power is reflected in the struggle between social actors who proactively and self-consciously shape organizational arrangements and secure scarce resources to serve their interests (Hatch & Cunliffe, 2013; Reed, 1992).

The subjective perspective focuses on the *informal* aspects of organization and on the freedom of individuals to make choices and to influence organizational life. Symbolic–interpretive theorists are interested in "how

the everyday practices of organizational members construct the very patterns of organizing that guide their actions" (Hatch & Cunliffe, 2013, p. 113). Examples of daily social practices include routines (e.g., clinical protocols), interactions, and communities of practice. For example, instead of viewing routines as mechanisms to standardize the behavior of individuals (i.e., an objective approach), a subjective approach might examine the changing nature or pattern of routines as members selectively modify, adapt, and retain practices in response to varying conditions and evidence-based practice. In a community of practice, learning occurs through voluntary social interaction whereby clinicians who are committed to a common interest self-organize informally to build ongoing relationships, partake in joint activities, and share resources (Wenger, 2008). An example in nursing would be an informal group of staff nurses who routinely have lunch together and who come to rely on this activity as a source of knowledge related to patient care in terms of problem solving, information exchange, and networking.

Postmodern Perspective

Departing from the polarization between objectivism (or modernism) and subjectivism (symbolism), the postmodern view offers critique and appreciation by challenging the meanings and interpretations associated with the concept of organization. The basic premise is that the world is known through language. Because language is continually reconstructed and context dependent, knowledge is essentially a power play (Hatch & Cunliffe, 2013). Notions of order and structure are the subject of scrutiny, and organizations may be thought of as chaotic entities characterized by conflicts and misunderstandings (Reed, 1992). Managerial practices and structures within organizations are seen to legitimize the interests of those in power. Even classic organization theorists such as Weber (1978) cautioned that bureaucracies were essentially domination structures that shape the form and purpose of social action through a system of rational rules and norms. Those who control bureaucracies therefore exert significant power over social action. For example, occurrences of sexual harassment can be either ignored or aggressively sanctioned as consistent with organizational values and norms. Thus the postmodern organization is understood both as an arena in which power struggles between dominant and subordinate groups play out and as a text to be rewritten to free its members from exploitative and controlling influences (Hatch & Cunliffe, 2013; Reed, 1992).

Postmodernists challenge the assumption that social structure results from the division and coordination of work among roles and groups. Clegg (1990) suggested that excessive fragmentation of work results in a disjointed and confusing experience for workers who become dependent on more powerful members in the hierarchy to make sense of workflow and goals. To counter this excess control over member actions, he proposed the idea of **differentiation,** whereby people self-manage and coordinate their own activities. Other examples of postmodern approaches to organization include feminist critiques of bureaucracies (e.g., Eisenstein, 1995) and anti-administration theory (Farmer, 1997). Each perspective contributes to stretching the thinking about how organizations are structured and function.

KEY THEORIES OF ORGANIZATIONS AS SOCIAL SYSTEMS

In the field of organizational design, the organization is most commonly approached as a social system from the objective perspective. Different theories within this tradition have contributed to understanding organizational social structure over an extensive period of study. However, these theories have also been critiqued for rationalizing social action, for favoring efficiency and productivity over other values (e.g., equity, justice), and for adopting an elitist view of management (e.g., O'Connor, 1999).

Bureaucratic Theory

Although often criticized for its oppressive qualities and administrative burden, the concept of bureaucracy may be better understood when placed within a historical context. Theorist Max Weber (1864–1920) was a German lawyer, professor, and political activist who noted the push of industrialism toward mass production and technical efficiency (Prins, 2000). Weber sought to explain from a historical perspective how the bureaucratic structure of large organizations differed from and improved on other forms of societal functioning (e.g., feudalism). He viewed bureaucracy as a social leveling mechanism founded on impartial and merit-based selection (i.e., legal authority), rather than a social ordering determined by kinship (i.e., traditional authority) or personality (i.e., charismatic authority) (Weber, 1978).

However, Weber warned of the potential dehumanizing effects of bureaucracies that emphasized purely economic results (i.e., formal rationality) at the expense of other important social values such as social justice and equality (i.e., substantive rationality) (Weber, 1978). Weber's descriptions of authority and rationality are foundational concepts in the study of organizations. His interpretation of hierarchy and its relevance to health care organizations are explored later in the chapter.

Scientific Management School

Arising from the experiences and ideas of business leaders and engineers in manufacturing industries, the scientific management school sought to determine the single best way to structure an organization. A well-known theorist in this field is Frederick W. Taylor (1856–1915), an engineer who authored *The Principles of Scientific Management* in 1914 (Prins, 2000). Along with colleagues, Taylor's vision was to improve labor relations and the low industrial standards that plagued the American manufacturing industry by the application of technical solutions (e.g., time and motion studies) (Prins, 2000). The goal was to enhance organizational performance in a milieu of improved cooperation between management and labor by matching the work performed with the worker's skills and with economic incentives. However, the experiments and engineering techniques associated with this approach were ultimately criticized for reducing the worker to a mere input in the production process (Prins, 2000). The application of scientific principles to improve the task performance and productivity of workers reflected a bottom-up approach to organizational design (Scott, 1992). In nursing, efforts to redesign nursing jobs, such as by using nurse practitioners, or to measure nursing workload often rely on this tradition.

Classical Management Theory

In contrast, classical theorists such as Fayol, Urwick, and Gulick evolved a top-down approach to organizational design. Based on experience as company executives, they identified principles of administration and management functions that could be applied in the design of organizations. Key concepts such as differentiation, coordination, the scalar principle, centralization, formalization, specialization, and span of control became central to the study of organizational structure. These concepts, which describe the *formal* aspects of an organization's social structure and their application to health care organizations, are examined in relation to nursing later in the chapter.

Human Relations School

Theorists in the human relations school emphasized the *informal,* rather than *formal,* aspects of organization social structure. The disciplines of industrial psychology and industrial relations founded this approach, which now persists as the field of organizational behavior (O'Connor, 1999). The social and psychological needs and relationships of workers and groups were thought to be important to work productivity. Improved cooperation between management and workers was proposed to enhance performance and reduce industrial strife (O'Connor, 1999). The famous Hawthorne experiments were influential in this school of thought. Initial interpretations of the Hawthorne experiments suggested that psychological factors influenced worker motivation because improved worker productivity was observed when researchers gave special attention to workers, regardless of changes to physical surroundings (Scott, 1992). Concepts such as job enlargement and job rotation were promoted to offset the alienation workers experienced because of excessive **formalization** and division of work processes (Scott, 1992). Formalization is the extent to which the organization uses explicit rules, procedures, job descriptions, and communications to prescribe roles and role interactions, govern activities, and standardize behaviors (Hatch & Cunliffe, 2013).

Streams of study included leadership behavior, small group dynamics, participative decision making, morale, motivation, and other worker characteristics and behaviors (Scott, 1992). In nursing, this school of thought is reflected in efforts to meet the professional development needs of nurses, enhance nurse autonomy and empowerment, and involve nurses in decision-making processes to improve organizational functioning.

Open System Theory

Open system theory emphasizes the dynamic interaction and interdependence of the organization with its external environment and its internal subsystems. Meyer and colleagues (2010) conceptualized the health care organization as an open system characterized by energy transformation, a dynamic steady state, negative entropy, event

cycles, negative feedback, differentiation, integration and coordination, and equifinality. *Inputs* (i.e., characteristics of care recipients, nurses, resources), *throughputs* (the delivery of nursing services arising from the nature of the work, structures, and work conditions), and *outputs* (i.e., clinical, human resource, and organizational outcomes) were theorized to interact dynamically to influence the global work demands placed on nursing work groups at the point of care in production subsystems.

Contingency theory is a subset of open system theory positing that there is no single right way to structure an organization. Effective organizational performance depends on the fit between the structure and multiple contingency factors such as technology, size, and strategy. Mark and colleagues (1996) applied contingency theory to the evaluation of nursing care delivery system outcomes. The basic premise was that to perform effectively and produce quality outcomes, an organization must structure and adapt its nursing units to complement the environment and technology.

Technology is a core concept in contingency theory and refers to the work performed. Technology can be examined in terms of task uncertainty (i.e., repetitive nature of the task), diversity (i.e., number of different components), and interdependence (i.e., degree to which work processes are interrelated) (Scott, 1992). Highly repetitive and distinct tasks are amenable to mass production technologies (e.g., manufacturing industry). In contrast, highly uncertain and interdependent tasks require discretion, improvisation, and more intense coordination structures across team-driven networks. The work performed by health care professionals such as nurses is often considered to be highly uncertain, diverse, interdependent, and reliant on group coordination. For example, in a study of hospital care for persons with joint replacements, the use of teams with high levels of shared knowledge and goals and mutual respect positively influenced patient-assessed quality of care despite shortened lengths of stay (Gittell, 2004). In this study, task uncertainty was intensified by time constraints (i.e., shorter lengths of stay), task diversity was reflected by the multidisciplinary roles, task interdependence resulted as multidisciplinary work was performed concurrently, and the coordination device was teamwork.

Newer Organizational Theories

In this section, two newer organizational theories that have been applied in health care—including **complexity** theory (see Chapter 1), which suggests that organizations are complex adaptive systems, and **network theory**—are briefly reviewed. Complexity science arose out of the field of physical sciences in the latter half of the twentieth century. It has also provided new perspectives to reconsider both natural and human systems. The theory carries specific assumptions about systems characterized by nonlinearity and feedback loops (Hatch & Cunliffe, 2013; McDaniel et al., 2013). Complexity science is concerned with complex systems and problems that are constantly changing, multidimensional, and unpredictable, comprising interconnected diverse elements and relationships. Concepts such as chaos, self-organization, and complex adaptive systems have been used to understand both irregular aspects of nature and provide frameworks to explore regularities that arise in complex systems. A hallmark of these ideas is the existence of nonlinearities in systems, which means that the behavior of the system is more than the sum of the behaviors of individual components (McDaniel et al., 2013).

The notion that organizations, and specifically health care systems, can be viewed as complex adaptive systems (CAS) has been proposed by organizational researchers (Hatch & Cunliffe, 2013; McDaniel et al., 2013). This perspective has been applied to current issues in today's health care organizations with the goal of finding new ways to understand the roles of individuals and groups (*agents*) and their effects on health care delivery processes. For example, CAS are *nonlinear and dynamic* and do not essentially reach stable equilibrium states. As a result, system behaviors may appear to be unplanned or chaotic (Rouse, 2008). As agents operate in the system, gain experience, or learn and change their behaviors, the overall system behavior naturally changes over time. This change or adaptation and learning tend to result in *self-organization* and these organizational behavior patterns can be viewed as evolving rather than being planned or constructed into the system. However, these emergent behaviors may range from valuable advances to unfortunate errors. In CAS, there is *no single point(s) of control* and, as a result, the behaviors of CAS can usually be more easily influenced than controlled. That is, hierarchy plays a less significant role as knowledge, expertise, and decision making are more distributed across organizational members than invested in authorities at the top of the organization. Leaders using the principles of complexity theory engage in influencing, collaborating,

and relational activities rather than aiming for control of others and the future (McDaniel et al. 2013).

Theories of networks are also applied to organizational structure. Social network analysis, which builds on a systems view of organizations, examines and interprets the structures and patterns of the formal and informal relationships among members of the organization (Tichy et al., 1979). In nursing, for instance, social network analysis has been used to explore the social and geographical ties of senior nurse executives and physicians in the United Kingdom in relation to profession, gender, age, rank, location, and frequency of contact (West & Barron, 2005). **Social capital** is another concept that has been identified in studies using social network theory and refers to resources produced by and rooted in social relationships. The concept is founded on the idea that the relationships among people in the workplace are resources that in turn can provide access to other resources through social exchange (Hatch & Cunliffe, 2013). The concept has been identified by health care leaders as an important resource that is instrumental to the success of health care organizations (Read, 2014). It is receiving current attention in nursing research because greater knowledge about nurses' relationships at work may provide new insights into the creation of healthier work environments that promote positive outcomes for nurses, patients, and health care organizations.

KEY ORGANIZATIONAL DESIGN CONCEPTS

The structure of an organization can be described as the overall way work is divided into tasks and roles, grouped into subunits, and coordinated across an organization. Leaders need to address key elements when they design an organizational structure: division of labor (specialization), departmentalization, differentiation, hierarchy (chain of command), span of control, coordination (integration), centralization and decentralization, standardization, and formalization. In Table 12.1 each of these elements is presented, with definitions and examples, and the following sections describe them.

Division and Coordination of Labor

A formal organization that employs people to achieve predetermined goals divides the work among its members by assigning tasks and delegating responsibilities to

TABLE 12.1	Dimensions of Organizational Design	
Dimension	**Definition or Measure**	**Examples in Health Care and Nursing**
Centralization and Decentralization	The degree to which decision making is concentrated at a single point in the organization versus the degree to which decisions are made by lower-level employees	Centralized or tall organization with several layers of management above the direct care unit level (e.g., unit coordinator, manager, director, vice president, CEO) versus flat organization with one layer (vice president) between unit manager and CEO
Coordination or Integration	The coordination of activities through accountability, rules, and procedures, liaison roles, committees, task forces, cross-functional teams, or direct communication	Bed management specialist role who links across hospital units to manage access and efficient use of available beds, or a quality improvement team that works across patient care programs to improve a particular aspect of patient care such as infection rates, or interprofessional rounds on patient care units
Departmentalization	The basis by which jobs are grouped	Jobs may be grouped by function (e.g., the human resources department) or by product or service/program (e.g., cardiac surgery, palliative care)
Differentiation	The process of dividing the work in an organization *Vertical* differentiation is shown in the number of levels in the hierarchy, and *horizontal* differentiation is shown in the number of departments or divisions across an entire organization	*Vertical* includes several levels from care units to departments or programs/service lines to divisions, and *horizontal* refers to number of units or departments at the same level across the organization
Division of Labor (or Specialization)	The degree to which work activities/tasks in an organization are divided into separate jobs	Large acute care hospitals with several levels of nursing care roles, such as patient care assistants, registered nurses, specialty nurses, advanced practice nurses, etc.
Formalization	The degree to which jobs within the organization are standardized and employee behavior is guided by rules and procedures	Formal job descriptions, certification and educational requirements for each role, standards of practice, clinical protocols, care guidelines, written procedures for various treatments, union contractual agreements
Hierarchy (or Chain of Command)	The structure of authority in an organization The chain of command is an unbroken line of authority that extends from the top of the organization to the lowest level and clarifies who reports to whom	Chief executive officer (CEO) at the top has several vice presidents (e.g., patient care divisions, human resources, finance, etc.) who in turn have directors who in turn have unit managers who may have staff nurses and other professionals reporting to them
Size	Number of employees in the organization	Health system of multiple organizations with 2000 employees versus small rural hospital with 100 employees
Span of Control	The number of subordinates a manager can efficiently and effectively direct	A nurse manager of an intensive care unit with 100 direct reports of nurses and charge nurses versus a manager of a small outpatient clinic with 20 direct reports of nurses plus support personnel
Standardization	The extent to which standard procedures govern the organization's functions and activities rather than using individual judgment	Mission and vision statements, organizational policies and procedures, clearly defined communication channels, or supervisory roles and functions

Adapted from: Hatch, M.J., & Cunliffe, A.L. (2013). *Organization theory: Modern, symbolic, and postmodern perspectives* (3rd ed.), p. 95. Oxford, UK: Oxford University Press.

positions and work units. Structure is a byproduct of the basic need to divide the labor into the specific tasks to be performed and a consequent need to coordinate these tasks to accomplish the activity or goal. The division (or differentiation) of work by occupation or by function is a form of **specialization.** As occupations and functions multiply in number, an organization increases in complexity and **size.** Size is a quantitative measure of personnel, physical capacity, volume of inputs or outputs, or discretionary resources of an organization.

The advantages of specialization include improved work performance and a critical mass of experts (Charnes & Tewksbury, 1993). In health care, specialist roles have emerged to address the increasing complexities of care and technology. Within nursing, specialist roles have also evolved to address particular areas of nursing practice and include advanced practice roles such as clinical nurse educators, nurse practitioners, and nurse anesthetists.

Organizations may also **differentiate** work units by function (also called **departmentalization**) to serve distinct client populations. For instance, rather than a single, general intensive care unit, an organization may establish several intensive care units by medical specialty (e.g., cardiovascular, neurosurgical, neonatal) or grouped into a "service line," such as palliative care or cardiac care programs. At the work group level, nursing care delivery models (e.g., team, primary, or total nursing care models) reflect different ways of dividing and coordinating the work among a team of nurses caring for clients.

Subdividing work may create breaks or fragmentation in work flow, which can be addressed in organizations by integrating work processes across roles and subunits using coordination devices (Hatch & Cunliffe, 2013). At the work group level, coordination may involve specific roles, standardization (programming), groups, or feedback devices. For example, handoff communication and techniques such as Situation, Background, Assessment, and Recommendation (SBAR) are used to coordinate between units or providers in the delivery of care.

In health care, common programming devices used to control work processes are the following:

- Standardization of worker skills coordinates work indirectly by stipulating the kind of training or education required to perform the work. In nursing, the standardization of worker skills might occur if specific degrees or certifications are required for certain roles such as nurse practitioners or critical care nurses.
- Standardization of work processes coordinates work by pre-specifying or programming content before the work is undertaken, such as nurses being required to use clinical protocols or evidence-based best practice guidelines in practice.
- Standardization of work outputs coordinates work through the specification of the results, product, or performance desired or expected and includes the specification of outcome targets such as reduction of nosocomial infection rates.
- Standardization of communication methods coordinates work by providing a uniform structure for information delivery and flow in order to facilitate exchange among those involved in common work processes. In nursing, this might be achieved through electronic health records and relational databases with alerts that allow nurses and other care providers to have direct and simultaneous access to client information in a consistent format.

In addition, feedback mechanisms are used in the transfer of information in an adaptive and reciprocal manner to foster the exchange of information (Gittell, 2002):

- Mutual adjustment coordinates work by using simple informal communication and may occur when one nurse consults another nurse about practice issues, such as how to interpret a policy, or when nurses, physicians, and allied health professionals participate in clinical rounds.
- Direct supervision coordinates work through the use of a supervisor taking responsibility for the instruction and monitoring of the work of others, such as when a nurse supervises the work of assistive personnel.
- Boundary spanning roles coordinate work by managing relationships as well as the bidirectional flow of information and materials across functional divisions. For example, case managers exemplify boundary spanning because these roles manage relationships, exchange information, and negotiate resources with internal and external parties to facilitate care across occupations, services, sectors, funding agencies, and locations.

The types of **coordination** that are used may depend on the degree of stability and predictability of the work situation and the size of the work unit. For instance, acute health care settings are typically characterized as highly uncertain and interdependent work situations in which patient health needs, acuity, and care trajectories are often highly variable and unpredictable. To ensure comprehensive care, nurses coordinate patient care activities with the work of others in a reciprocal manner because the work performed is highly interdependent. As conditions become increasingly uncertain and variable, as in health care, coordination by feedback or specific liaison roles may be used. Improved health care team performance has been associated with both programming and feedback devices because standardized routines may enhance, rather than replace, the interactions among health care providers, particularly in situations of increasing uncertainty (Gittell, 2002). Recent research has shown that improved provider ratings of coordination in inpatient medicine units were linked with an organization's alignment and commitment to high-quality patient care, adequate staffing, resources that support health care professionals to do their jobs, and approaches that promote interactions and communication between nurses and physicians, such as regular multidisciplinary rounding (McIntosh et al., 2014).

At the organizational level, the coordination and division of labor influence the size and degree of organizational centralization and formalization. As organizations grow in size, work units are increasingly subdivided to ensure tasks are accomplished. However, this process slows as organizations become very large, because the gains achieved by subdividing work occur at the expense of the coordination mechanisms necessary to unify system functioning across subunits. In centralized structures, top leaders make all the decisions, and lower-level managers and staff have little decision-making discretion. In a highly formalized job, the individual has minimal discretion over what to do and when and how to do it. Organizational coordination is often measured by the degree of centralization and formalization. Health care organizations tend toward being decentralized and less formalized because professionals are employed to manage highly uncertain work. However, as organizations grow and the work becomes increasingly complex, specialized, and interdependent, there is a pull toward greater centralization and formalization (Hatch & Cunliffe, 2013).

Hierarchy

Hierarchy is the structure of authority in an organization. Authority is equated with the enforcement of regulations, which creates a governing order among the formal social relationships of organizational members (Weber, 1978). Authority is vested in positions, rather than in persons, and creates an impartial mechanism whereby the supraordinate position directs the actions and the norms expected of subordinate positions. Centralization is a multidimensional concept frequently associated with authority and hierarchy and describes the extent to which decision-making authority is concentrated in the top level of the hierarchy (i.e., centralized) versus spread down through the hierarchy (i.e., decentralized). In nursing, shared governance structures signify decentralization. **Hierarchical centralization** can vary according to the decision type.

Corporate strategy is likely to be decided by top executives, whereas procedural work decisions may be decentralized to work units or employees. For instance, a nurse executive could be required to centralize some budgetary decisions, whereas others could be decided at lower levels in the hierarchy. A specific example would be the need to centralize a component of professional development expenditures required by union contracts (e.g., organization-wide funding for nursing certification) in contrast to decisions at the work unit level to possibly fund nurses to attend their specialty conferences (some units do, some do not). Participation is an alternate dimension of centralization that refers to the scope of involvement and influence of organizational members in decision making. Findings from a study of Belgian hospitals showed that nurses who perceived that their work decisions were tightly controlled by a supervisor (i.e., high hierarchical centralization) and they had little influence on program decisions (i.e., low participative centralization) reported lower job satisfaction (Willem et al., 2007).

In addition, hierarchy creates a reporting structure whereby formal lines of communication, in conjunction with role descriptions, delineate the responsibilities and accountability of each position for work processes and outcomes. Organizational positions are traditionally described in terms of staff and line positions (Hatch & Cunliffe, 2013). Staff positions are outside the direct hierarchical authority chain. These positions provide expertise and knowledge to support the line positions in meeting the organization's goals. The clinical nurse specialist (CNS) who is hired for knowledge development and expert consultation for selected patient groups is an example of a staff position. Line positions are in the direct line of hierarchical authority from top to bottom in an organization and are central to controlling or generating the product or service of the organization. Line positions include vice presidents, directors, managers, and frontline nurses because these positions are authorized either to supervise production processes or to produce the organization's output. In nursing, although frontline nurses are commonly referred to as "staff" nurses, these nurses hold line positions that deliver services to care recipients.

Hierarchy also enables organizations to assign responsibilities based on the complexity and skill requirements of the work and to ensure individual accountability. Responsibility is the obligation to take on and accomplish work and to secure the desired results. A manager assigns or delegates responsibility to a subordinate, and thus responsibility flows down the organizational chain. In accepting the obligation of an assigned task, the staff person is accepting responsibility to accomplish the task, whereas accountability is the liability for task performance and is determined in a retrospective analysis of what occurred. The assignment of responsibility and the granting of authority create accountability. Accountability flows upward or outward, from staff to manager or from provider to client. Reporting relationships are important for creating channels of appeal (Weber, 1978), to ensure employees are held accountable for the work assigned, and to invest managers with the necessary authority to ensure the completion of work. The manager represents the organization at the point of contact with staff, and thus the

reporting relationship is also a mechanism by which staff can access organizational resources to identify and solve complex problems. Ideally, managers also apply their leadership skills to reporting relationships to release the energy and talents of people in ways that add value to the work performed. Examples of "value-added" outcomes include improved employee productivity, organizational commitment, and organizational citizenship behaviors.

Organizational Forms

The division and coordination of labor lead to varied organizational forms. As illustrated by the sloping triangles in Fig. 12.1, organizational forms reflect a trade-off between differentiation by function and integration by program. **Differentiation by function** refers to the division of work by occupation. **Integration by program** means the coordination of work around the delivery of particular products or services. Five basic organizational forms can be situated along a differentiation–integration continuum (Charnes & Tewksbury, 1993). Functional and program forms represent extreme examples of differentiation and integration. The matrix form represents the most balanced form. In reality, organizations are not usually found in these pure forms but instead reflect hybrids of the forms described next.

Functional Form

At the extreme left end of the continuum, dividing the work by occupation leads to a functional organization whereby health professions and nonprofessional services

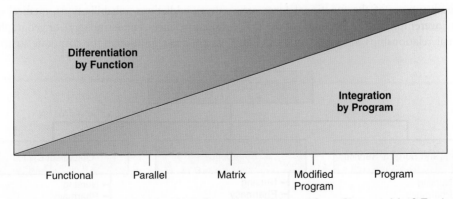

FIG. 12.1 Continuum of organizational configurations. (Adapted from Charnes, M., & Tewksbury, L. [1993]. *Collaborative management in health care: Implementing the integrative organization* [p. 28, Fig. 2.1]. San Francisco, CA: Jossey-Bass. This material is used by permission of John Wiley & Sons.)

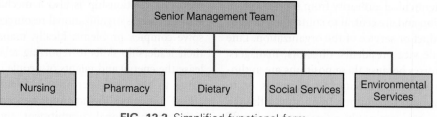

FIG. 12.2 Simplified functional form.

are arranged according to the type of work performed. The emphasis is on the human resources inputs to the organization (Fig. 12.2). Examples are nursing, respiratory therapy, admitting, and environmental services. Within each functional department, management develops specific structures, policies, procedures, and human resource practices. In this type of organizational form, professionals report directly to a discipline-specific supervisor (e.g., nurses would report to a nurse manager). Members of a functional group (e.g., nursing) are likely to interact more frequently, develop social relationships, receive supervision and evaluations from within the group, and conform to professional standards (Charnes & Tewksbury, 1993).

By dividing personnel according to the type of work performed, organizations can capitalize on the expertise, experience, efficiency, and professional standards that each discipline offers (Charnes & Tewksbury, 1993). Other benefits include cost reduction through shared resources; enhanced monitoring of cost, performance, and quality; and promotion of professional development, identity, autonomy, advocacy, and career advancement. Disadvantages of the functional form are its potential to overemphasize professional silos, discourage informal relationships across disciplines, and

fragment care delivery (Charnes & Tewksbury, 1993). Coordination of activities becomes challenging because group members have functionally based differences in work goals, cognitive patterns, and status (Gittell, 2004). Because the work of nursing is highly interdependent with other professional and nonprofessional work, nurse leaders in functional forms may use coordination mechanisms and leadership behaviors to span the boundaries between disciplines and facilitate the flow and exchange of information, resources, and work activities. Although prevalent in health care in the 1980s, functional forms have gradually been replaced by program or matrix forms to enhance patient centeredness.

Program Form

At the extreme right end of the continuum, program organizations emphasize integration of the work by consumer, service, or geography (Charnes & Tewksbury, 1993). The emphasis is on the outputs of the organization (Fig. 12.3). In health care, programs may be managed according to consumer health needs (e.g., diabetes, cancer), consumer age (e.g., elderly, neonates, women), services (e.g., addictions, rehabilitation), medical specialty (e.g., neurosciences, endocrinology), or geography (e.g., catchment areas). Although the corporate structure is shared,

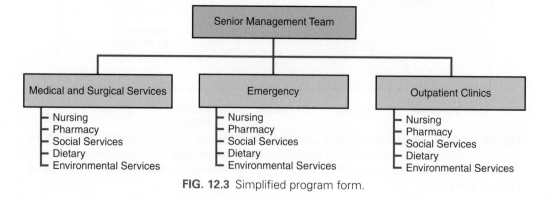

FIG. 12.3 Simplified program form.

each program tends to operate as a semiautonomous unit with its own management team composed of medical, administrative, and nursing representatives (Charnes & Tewksbury, 1993). Professionals who work in program organizations may not report to a discipline-specific supervisor.

Program designs can optimize service delivery because local experts with accountability for costs, outcomes, and staffing control resources and can make timely operational decisions (Leatt et al., 1994). Patients can access integrated services from an array of health professionals with specific clinical expertise. With the program form, there is a push toward a multidisciplinary team approach. However, clients who require access to more than one program may find it difficult to coordinate services among different programs. Integration by program occurs at the expense of decreased coordination among programs (Charnes & Tewksbury, 1993). Although organizational relationships with medical staff are enhanced when programs are grouped by medical specialty, health care professionals may be isolated from their colleagues in other programs, and this has been associated with job dissatisfaction and lack of professional development opportunities (Young et al., 2004). For nursing, the concern is that no organization-wide mechanisms would exist to systematically handle professional nursing issues in terms of standards, resources, or professional advocacy. Because each program operates independently, processes and procedures are likely to be duplicated, and programs may compete for resources or develop goals that diverge from the corporate mission (Leatt et al., 1994).

Parallel Form

To address the challenges of purely functional forms, mechanisms in the parallel form assist in coordinating across functional departments (Charnes & Tewksbury, 1993). These mechanisms can include teams, specialists, task forces, liaison roles, and standing committees. For example, rather than each functional department separately establishing procedures to hire staff, a specialized human resource department may be created to deal with recruitment and employment issues across the organization. Another example is a rapid response team in a hospital that is composed of intensive care physicians and nurses and respiratory therapists. This team assists staff throughout the hospital in detecting and managing imminent patient deterioration and in resuscitating

compromised patients. Likewise, in home care, nurses with particular expertise such as wound care or palliative care might be responsible for referrals across multiple areas. Task forces bring together members from various divisions in an organization to address a concern. For example, developing and implementing critical pathways, evidence-based practices, disease management initiatives, case management projects, or outcomes management efforts generally require an interdisciplinary team of specialists. These types of mechanisms foster collaboration and cross-fertilization of knowledge across divisions and can reinforce consistency in clinical and management practices by standardizing procedures.

Modified Program Form

To offset the fragmentation and isolation of functions in pure program structures, organizations maintain the program structure and develop integrative mechanisms to unify functions and occupations across programs (Charnes & Tewksbury, 1993). For example, a nurse executive could address professional nursing issues related to standards, educational resources, and research activities across the organization. Unlike his or her counterpart in a functional nursing department who has line authority, a nurse executive in a modified program would not directly control operations, finances, or personnel issues (known as *staff authority*). A nurse executive with staff authority must use personal influence and leadership skills to effect change.

Matrix Form

In a pure matrix form, people and work are organized along both functional and program dimensions (Charnes & Tewksbury, 1993). Essentially, the program form overlays the functional form (Fig. 12.4). Although some employees may have dual reporting relationships, staff members are evaluated by both supervisors. The budget and decision making are shared between functional and program divisions. A matrix configuration has the flexibility to adapt to change and to deliver services innovatively and efficiently by drawing on a varied talent pool (Hatch & Cunliffe, 2013). In contrast, innovation in program forms is costly because additional cross-coordination may be required across functional divisions, or specialists may need to be hired for each program. However, true matrix forms are rarely seen and are difficult to maintain because the additional management infrastructure is costly and dual reporting relationships may

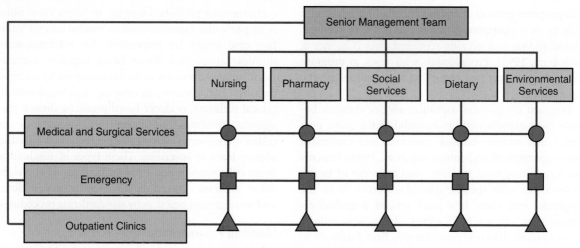

For example, team members for Outpatient Clinics (▲) are drawn from different functions.

FIG. 12.4 Simplified matrix form.

be ambiguous and lead to conflict (Charnes & Tewksbury, 1993). Success requires well-educated workers who can handle a multifaceted communication and authority web. Nurses in matrix organizations need strong interpersonal and teamwork skills to negotiate these complex environments.

ORGANIZATIONAL CHARTS

Hierarchy reflects the *formal* structure of the organization, which can be identified on an organizational chart. An organizational chart is a visual display of the organization's positions and the intentional relationships among positions. The organizational chart reflects the various positions and the formal relationships between and among the positions and, by extension, the people who are a part of the organization. The organizational chart generally presents the line positions, linked together by solid lines to show the flow of authority. Administrative roles are generally shown in vertical and horizontal dimensions. Staff positions or advisory bodies may be depicted on the chart with dotted lines to show consultative relationships. Organizational charts help with administrative control, policy making and planning, and the evaluation of the organization's strengths and weaknesses. They clearly depict who reports to whom. Charts are used to orient personnel because relationships and expected patterns of interaction within the formal organization are made clear. For

example, an organizational chart of a matrix structure may show dotted lines for the project or interdisciplinary team relationships. Dotted lines mean that a relationship to the position or the group would form for a project. In the process of applying for a job, obtaining the employer's organizational chart will help understand the relative positioning of individuals within the organization and how the organization is structured—or at least how decision makers believe it is structured.

In addition to a *formal* structure, organizations are characterized by an *informal* structure. The *informal* structure is simply the network or pattern of social relationships and friendship circles that are outside the formal structure. It is an interconnected web of relationships that operate in and around the formally designated lines of communication. The *informal* structure does not appear on the *formal* organizational chart.

ORGANIZATIONAL SHAPES

The shape of an organization structure can be described as relatively tall or flat. Several structural factors influence the shape of an organization. The formal reporting relationships among positions ensure the assignment of responsibility, authority, and accountability and result in hierarchical levels. The **span of control** of managers—the number of employees reporting directly to a management position—also influences organizational shape (Meyer, 2008). For instance, when managers on average have fewer direct-report staff, the organizational shape is relatively taller. Another structural factor involves decisions about the number of management layers in the hierarchy (i.e., the **scalar principle**). Increased layers of management help the organization cope with increasing work complexity and extended time lines (Jaques, 1990). A tall organization structure assumes a pyramidal shape with multiple management layers (Fig. 12.5). In contrast, a flat organization structure has minimal management layers (Fig. 12.6). Advantages and disadvantages associated with tall and flat organizational shapes are summarized in Table 12.2. However, a narrow focus on the hierarchical structure of an organization without attention to the people and processes within the organization or the outcomes achieved can be misleading. For instance, factors that can potentially offset the effects of tall organizations include the competence and leadership of members, the use of merit-based rewards, the effectiveness of reporting

relationships, and the sharing of information and authority (Jaques, 1990).

Span of management refers to the number and ordering of management positions and resources relative to other personnel and can be measured at organizational, departmental, managerial, work group, or employee levels (Meyer, 2008). There are many competing arguments about factors influencing the span of management, and decisions about the amount, type, and distribution of nursing management resources within health care organizations are influenced by a multitude of factors at the consumer, nurse, work group, manager, organizational, and regional levels (Meyer, 2008). A key controversy about the span of control of nurse managers relates to supervisory responsibilities. On the one hand, wider spans of control for managers are proposed because nurses and other health care professionals are experts committed to professional codes of ethics and regulated standards, therefore requiring less direct supervision (Meier & Bohte, 2003). On the other hand,

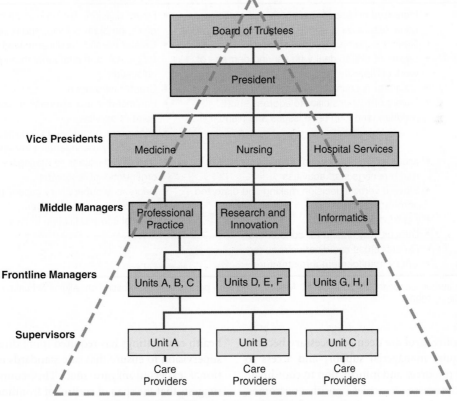

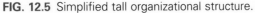

FIG. 12.5 Simplified tall organizational structure.

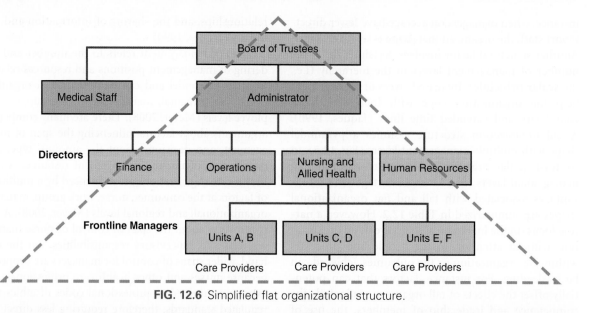

FIG. 12.6 Simplified flat organizational structure.

TABLE 12.2	Comparison of Flat and Tall Organization Structures	
	Tall Organization	**Flat Organization**
Advantages	• Increased access to managers and organizational resources • Greater supervisory capability • Layers of skill to deal with varying degrees of work complexity • Layers of accountability for work completion • Layers of responsibility to address short, medium, and long-term issues and planning	• Fewer divisions facilitate streamlining of goals, problem solving, and resource use • Greater hierarchical decentralization; potential for greater staff autonomy through increased delegation • Greater innovation • Enhanced responsiveness to consumers at point of service • Less cross-coordination required • Less costly management infrastructure
Disadvantages	• More hierarchical centralization; potential to micromanage staff activities • Slowed vertical decision making and distorted communication • Less innovation • Difficult way-finding for consumers • Greater cross coordination required • Costly management infrastructure	• Decreased access to managers and organizational resources • Decreased supervisory capability • Overextension of managers • Vertical communication delays

Compiled by the author. Copyright 2012 Raquel M. Meyer. Used with permission. Table based on: Alidina & Funke-Furber, 1988; Jaques, 1990; Pabst, 1993.

narrow spans of control are deemed necessary because (1) nurses require managerial support and access to organizational resources and information to coordinate complex work processes to achieve positive outcomes, and (2) the introduction of unlicensed workers into health care settings has required more direct, hands-on supervision to ensure that care standards and organizational expectations are met. This counterargument suggests that the span of control of frontline nurse managers should factor in the needs of staff nurses for their manager's support and supervision. In nursing, relationships between the span of control of frontline managers and manager, nurse, and clinical outcomes have been investigated (see Research Note).

STRUCTURAL POWER

Within the objective perspective, power has been conceptualized as a resource. Kanter's (1977) classic theory of the structural determinants of behavior in organizations has been investigated in nursing systems (Laschinger, 1996). For Kanter (1977, p. 166), power refers to "the ability to get things done, to mobilize resources." It is not the power to control or dominate others. When power is shared, rather than monopolized, employees are empowered and the organization is more likely to benefit. More activity can be accomplished by organizational members, and the capacity for effective action is increased. Kanter (1977) described three work empowerment structures: opportunity, power, and proportion. The structure of *opportunity* refers to expectations and future prospects (e.g., opportunities for growth, mobility, job enrichment). The structure of *power* stems from access to information, support, and resources. The structure of *proportion* denotes the social composition of the organization's workforce (e.g., gender, minorities). Empowered work environments are those in which all employees have access to opportunities to learn and grow and to information, support, and resources necessary for the job. Indeed, frontline nurses' job-related or structural empowerment has been linked to positive nurse outcomes, including greater nurse job satisfaction (Cicolini et al., 2014; Wong & Laschinger, 2013), increased organizational commitment (Smith et al., 2010: Yang et al., 2013), feelings of trust and respect in the workplace (Laschinger et al., 2014), lower job and career turnover intentions (Choi et al., 2014; Laschinger & Fida, 2014), and lower burnout and workplace incivility (Laschinger et al., 2013). Nurses who occupy positions at higher levels in the nursing hierarchy report increasingly greater degrees of empowerment (Laschinger et al., 2012), which may mean that nurses in management positions are likely to perceive greater access to opportunity and power structures than frontline nurses.

In Kanter's (1977) study, effective leaders were seen as both competent and powerful. Sensitivity with subordinates was secondary to having upward credibility within the organization; leaders to whom others listened, who accessed resources, and who produced results within the broader organization were perceived to be effective. Kanter (1977) proposed that effective leadership evolves from both *formal* and *informal* sources of power in the organization. *Formal* power is derived from work that is relevant to pressing organizational issues and that provides opportunities to perform extraordinary and highly visible activities; *informal* power comes from relationships and alliances with people in the organization.

Kanter (1977, p. 168) also theorized that "power begets power." Research indicates that nurses who are managed by empowered leaders are also empowered (Laschinger, 1996). For example, frontline nurses in organizations in which chief nurse executives had line authority reported significantly greater global empowerment with respect to resources than their counterparts in organizations in which chief nurse executives had staff authority (Matthews et al., 2006). The authors suggested that the *formal* power accessible to nurse executives with line authority enabled them to secure the staffing resources necessary for frontline nurses to provide high quality of care. Magnet hospitals typically consist of flat organizational structures with nursing councils that empower nurses through decentralized decision making. This structure engages staff nurses in decisions affecting their work, for example, when interprofessional staff work together to redesign workflow. Considered overall, the research suggests that empowerment structures have a positive impact on both nurses and managers and can inform the design of the organizational structures in which nurses work.

LEADERSHIP AND MANAGEMENT IMPLICATIONS

The global and local challenges for nursing within organizations and across systems are numerous. Leaders and managers can influence the structure in which goals are accomplished. In fact, determining the structure is a key responsibility of leaders and managers in planning an organization that is conducive to high-quality nursing care. As environments and technologies evolve, the leadership and management team may need to rethink and redesign the organization and work group structures to better match the changing conditions and achieve the desired outcomes. In nursing, determining the structure is a planning and organizing aspect of the management process that can be informed by evidence and theory from the management field.

Leaders and managers may be involved in revising or changing organizational structures. *Restructuring* means revising or modifying the structure to reshape it or switch to another structural form. Restructuring efforts have typically been geared toward fixing existing operational processes. Lean, decentralized, self-governing organizations that empower first-line caregivers are the preferred structures. To begin anew, processes are analyzed from the point of view of the consumer (patient and family) as well as the requirement to achieve greater cost containment, quality, service, and speed. User-friendly processes, efficiency, and economy are key ideas. Job redesign focuses on who does what tasks and on maximizing flexibility, cross-training, and productivity.

Changes to organization structure afford opportunities to empower nurses. Strategies include maximizing nurses' scope of practice, creating autonomous and visible nursing roles relevant to organizational priorities, and providing more leadership opportunities for nurses at all levels. Fiscal and material resources can also be deployed to empower nurses by facilitating access to knowledge-development opportunities (e.g., courses, conferences) and by providing adequate resources for job completion (e.g., staffing). A decentralized, participative structure can be promoted through coordination mechanisms that involve nurses in shared governance councils and task forces (e.g., related to clinical practice or nurse retention) and in information exchange (e.g., newsletters, open forums, web technologies).

A transparent and participative approach to the development of programming devices to standardize work processes (e.g., clinical protocols, electronic health records) can be used to build shared goals for interdisciplinary teams. Organizations can also deliberately foster informal coordination mechanisms to enhance the relational and functional networks in which work is accomplished (Hatch & Cunliffe, 2013). For example, physical colocation, communal space, communities of practice, rotational job assignments, electronic chat groups, and interdisciplinary training programs can foster spontaneous interactions and relationships across functional, professional, and geographical silos, resulting in knowledge sharing, problem solving, and innovation.

Hierarchical reporting relationships can be greatly enhanced by transformational leaders who establish trust with nurses by communicating role and behavior expectations, giving constructive performance feedback, and recognizing and rewarding successes (Wong & Laschinger, 2013). When workers fall outside organizational lines of authority (e.g., outsourced services, nursing agencies such as travelers), managers and leaders need skills in negotiating standards and performance outcomes, in resolving problems across organizational boundaries, and in building relationships and shared goals to overcome differing alliances (Porter-O'Grady & Malloch, 2014).

In more highly matrixed organizations, nurse managers and leaders must network with interdisciplinary stakeholders within and across programs and support services. Success for leaders with line authority requires strong relational skills, credibility, an ability to link resource use to outcomes using a business model, and an in-depth understanding of the needs of clients and staff (Lorenz, 2008). The trends toward increased outsourcing, decreased reliance on traditional inpatient services for revenues, and increased specialization of health services require an entrepreneurial skill set and innovative leadership roles to build business partnerships and alliances and to foster change at the point of service delivery (Porter-O'Grady, 2015). In the context of nurse and manager shortages, organizations need to recruit and deploy management resources in line with objectives by reevaluating the number of management layers and the span of control of individual positions, as well as by developing a nursing leadership succession plan. To be supportive of nursing staff, nurse managers need access to the support and information of senior management and peers, professional development and mentorship, an office that is easily accessible to staff, administrative support, and a strong and shared organizational culture.

Organizational Assessment

Nurse leaders can use organizational assessment to generate data needed for analysis that serves as the foundation for planning and change management as well as to identify the status of quality and safety efforts. Organizational assessments focus on assisting teams, departments, organizations, and systems to better understand the organization as it is and to continuously improve by indicating areas in need of further development. There are a variety of organizational assessments. Some are commercial and not in health care, like the Organizational Effectiveness Survey from Dale Carnegie Training

(2016). Some are both in business and industry as well as health care, such as the Malcolm Baldrige National Quality Award (ASQ, n.d.), which recognizes US companies that have implemented successful quality management systems. Some focus specifically on the unit, such as the Dartmouth Institute's (2010) Microsystems at a Glance and the Institute for Healthcare Improvement's (IHI) 2016 Clinical Microsystem Assessment Tool. In nursing, the Magnet Recognition Program® only focuses on the quality of nursing services and resources for nurses.

CURRENT ISSUES AND TRENDS

During the 1990s, health care systems in many developed countries were subjected to restructuring, decentralization, specialization, and performance management, resulting in the de-layering of management structures in an effort to contain costs and achieve outcomes (Mahon & Young, 2006). Those managers remaining in the system faced expanded roles. Instead of a traditional head nurse position responsible for patient care on a single unit, the role of the nurse manager typically grew to encompass the management of finances, operations, and human resources across multiple clinical areas and services in program management structures with regulated and unregulated multidisciplinary staff.

The twenty-first century has ushered in significant concerns related to the global community and public safety. These issues are intensified by calls for transparency, accountability, and public reporting in the management of health care services, which in turn have increased demands on the internal structures and external boundaries of organizations. In addition, at a societal level, preparedness for disasters, bioterrorism, and pandemics has required health care organizations, communities, and jurisdictions to pool resources and coordinate activities along the external boundaries of organizational structures. Furthermore, large companies in the business world have been working to eliminate *vertical* and *horizontal* boundaries within and to break down *external* barriers between the company and its customers and suppliers. This **boundaryless** organization seeks to eliminate the hierarchical chain of command, replace departments with empowered teams, and promote learning in order to keep pace with rapid change (Hatch & Cunliffe, 2013). Although achieving a boundaryless state may never be completely actualized, especially in health care organizations, there is evidence of moves to create better integration of care delivery processes across care sectors and organizations within health systems (Edgren & Barnard, 2012).

Attempts to remove vertical boundaries, flatten the hierarchy and implement cross-functional and cross-organizational teams (which include senior executives, middle managers, supervisors, employees, and care recipients), participative decision-making practices, and boundary-spanning leadership practices are being implemented in health care to break down vertical and horizontal boundaries (Shirey & White-Williams, 2015). With wide-ranging changes introduced with the Affordable Care Act (ACA) of 2010 and the Institute for Healthcare Improvement's (IHI's) Triple Aim framework for optimizing health system performance, a focus for organizations is on improving individual patient and family care experiences, increasing the health of populations, reforming primary care, and reducing overall costs. All of these priorities require high levels of system integration and even transformation (Shirey & White-Williams, 2015). One solution has been a rise in the number of health care organizations (hospitals, ambulatory facilities, continuing care homes, and home health) merging not only to achieve economies of scale but as also as a way of better organizing the clinical functions across different sites and locations (Kerfoot & Luquire, 2012; Shirey & White-Williams, 2015). With the emergence of these larger health systems, the role of the system chief nurse executive has increased (Bradley, 2014).

At a global level, increasing shortages of nurses and other health care professionals has engendered a call for developed countries to create self-sufficient and sustainable nursing workforces by increasing domestic supply (Gantz et al., 2012). At the organizational level, employers need to attract and retain nurses through changes to work conditions and structures such as creating full-time positions, re-dividing work to continue to remove non-nursing tasks, supplying adequate staffing and material resources to accomplish the work, and improving work climates that support exemplary professional nursing practice (Gantz et al., 2012). These strategies are necessary to stabilize the nursing workforce within organizations and to ensure that the knowledge, skills, and competence that nurses possess are retained and appropriately deployed in the organization.

Increased awareness and disclosure about medical errors and preventable adverse events have encouraged organizations to address consumer safety through risk reduction and the development of cultures of safety (DiCuccio, 2015). To address safety, new coordination mechanisms and explicit safety standards are based on the science of human factors engineering, which takes a systems approach to understanding and preventing critical incidents (Carayon et al., 2014). A systems approach considers how adverse events occur in relation to management, organization, and regulatory factors such as policies and procedures, information technology, staffing practices, and physical structures. Recall that policies, procedures, and information systems are coordination devices. For instance, safety risks may be reduced when nurses standardize care through the use of evidence-based clinical protocols. Organizations are also compelled to collaborate in the development and sharing of safety innovations. The Center for Quality Improvement and Safety in the United States and the Canadian Patient Safety Institute in Canada are examples of how safety innovations can be widely shared and standardized across organizations.

RESEARCH NOTE

Source
Wong, C.A., Elliot-Miller, P., Laschinger, H.K., Cuddihy, M., Meyer, R., Keatings, M., et al. (2015). Examining the relationships between span of control and manager and unit work outcomes in Ontario academic hospitals. *Journal of Nursing Management, 23*(2), 156–168.

Purpose
The aim of this study was to examine the effect of front-line manager (FLM) personal characteristics and span of control (SOC) on their job and unit performance outcomes.

Description
Health care downsizing and reform have contributed to larger spans for FLMs in Canadian hospitals and increased concerns about manager workload. Despite increased awareness of SOC issues among decision makers, there is limited research evidence related to the effects of SOC on outcomes. A non-experimental predictive survey design was used to examine FLM SOC in 14 Canadian academic hospitals. Managers (n = 121) completed an online survey of work characteristics and The Ottawa Hospital (TOH) SOC tool. Unit turnover data were collected from organizational databases.

Results
In this study, a multidimensional measure of SOC was used rather than the number of direct reports, which has been used in most studies documenting FLM SOC. The combination of SOC and manager core self-evaluation significantly predicted manager role overload, work control and job satisfaction, but only SOC predicted unit adverse outcomes, and neither significantly predicted unit turnover.

Application to Practice
Findings demonstrated the advantage of going beyond the number of direct reports in defining managers' SOC. TOH's span tool was a more robust indicator of span because it includes not only number of direct reports but also the skill, stability, and diversity of staff; the complexity of unit(s) managed; and the budget and diversity of the program for which the manager is responsible. The overall TOH score was a valid predictor of manager job outcomes. Chief nurse executives can use this tool to assess manager SOC within their organizations and generate conversations regarding the relevance and reasonableness of current spans and what resource supports might be necessary to ensure managers can manage their spans effectively.

The finding that the *TOH* score positively predicted higher frequency of adverse outcomes suggests a possible link between FLM SOC and patient and staff safety. In addition, increased resource supports predicted decreased adverse outcomes, which suggests the positive role of infrastructure supports in reducing the frequency of medication errors, nosocomial infections, staff work-related injuries, and other safety outcomes. The fact that managers in this study perceived only moderate work control suggests that organizations may need to examine manager role responsibilities as well as ensure that managers have adequate authority to carry out their work. The importance of adequate infrastructure such as administrative, clerical, charge, and clinical practice roles to alleviate the impact of large spans was underscored in these findings. Organizations need to put in place the necessary clinical, educational, clerical, and technological supports in line with manager SOC and also regularly monitor the effectiveness of those supports.

CASE STUDY

Bed Turnaround

Between 11 AM and 8 PM, as many as 17 patients will be discharged and new patients will be admitted on a 34-bed medical–surgical unit. The support associate (SA) is responsible for patient transport and housekeeping duties, including cleaning rooms. The SA is pulled away four or five times per room to transport patients for discharge or to and from ancillary testing. Meanwhile, new admissions are held in the emergency department or outpatient center while they await a clean bed. A centralized housekeeping team is often STAT-paged to clean the room.

Further analysis identifies that the lack of trust between departments in this facility often results in sending out a staff member to other units to "truly assess" bed status. Lack of teamwork exists between the SAs and housekeeping personnel. The average bed turnaround time from the point of patient discharge to the bed being ready for occupancy is 82 minutes.

As a result, a multidisciplinary team is formed to identify options for reducing bed turnaround time and to evaluate the SA role. Team members consist of an administration representative, the medical–surgical unit manager, three SAs, two housekeeping personnel, a unit clerk, the house-wide bed coordinator, and one registered nurse (RN).

Through this team, the reporting relationship of the unit-based housekeeper responsible for cleaning the common areas (e.g., nurses' station, waiting rooms, and hallways) is changed to a matrix reporting structure in which the housekeeper reports directly to the director of environmental services but also has a dotted-line relationship to the individual department director. In addition, a centralized support associate STAT team is initiated to work from 1 PM to 11:30 PM, Monday through Friday, and 7 AM to 3 PM on Saturdays. Dispatch of the STAT team is delegated to the charge RN via a beeper as opposed to going through the centralized environmental services department. On the off-shift, the STAT SA team reports to and is dispatched by the off-shift supervisor. Finally, one SA per unit is assigned to perform strictly discharge room cleaning, which eliminates transport interruptions. As a result of these structure and role changes, the time from discharge of a patient to the time a bed is ready is decreased 53% to 38 minutes.

CRITICAL THINKING EXERCISE

Nurse manager Jane McClelland has just received a new assignment from her immediate supervisor, the director of the surgical program at a community acute care hospital. She is being moved from her current unit to become the new manager for a new unit, which will mean planning and implementing the merging of two former 25-bed inpatient units into one large unit of 40 beds in a recently renovated area of the hospital. In order to achieve efficiencies and reduce the overall number of beds, the new unit will incorporate two surgical subspecialties, thoracic and vascular surgery. Jane's responsibilities include creating a plan for the integration of the two units, and determining the administrative structure including required unit support roles, the overall staffing requirements, and how the two care teams will be integrated on the new unit.

1. What elements of organizational design does Jane need to take into consideration in formulating her plan?
2. How does she approach the problem of integrating the two teams and what coordinating mechanisms might be important?
3. How can the manager's authority, responsibility, and accountability for this project be explained?
4. What principles of organizational structure could be helpful in this situation? Which could be barriers?
5. What challenges do you think the manager faces in bringing together these two teams?

Decentralization and Shared Governance

Cheryl Hoying

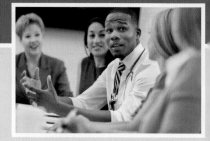

(e)http://evolve.elsevier.com/Huber/leadership

Efforts to reshape health care have been underway with renewed momentum since the Institute of Healthcare Improvement's (IHI, 2016) Triple Aim was established in 2008. The three aspects of the Aim are to improve the patient experience of care, improve the health of populations, and reduce the cost of care. Since then, innovations in health care abound, "including e-ICUs, telestroke programs, e-visits for primary and specialty care, telerounding, video-connected postsurgical transfers and follow-up, and urgent care" (Aston, 2015). Creative solutions to access to care for patients, such as telehealth, are often accomplished with a shared governance approach, which places decision authority over practice at the lowest operational level: direct care nurses.

DEFINITIONS

Centralization and Decentralization

Hospitals are organized and their work is structured around a guiding philosophy. The philosophy serves as the institutional framework that shapes the direction of knowledge and skill acquisition. It is the pivotal factor in the long-term development of the institution.

The **mission,** core values, and **vision** are the instruments that give voice to the organization's philosophy. "The mission is a simple and direct expression of a company's goals and objectives. . . . It defines what a company stands for" (Kurian, 2013, p. 186). The vision is the formulation of ideas, plans, or dreams that "help shape the

future and ability to persuade colleagues and associates to share those dreams" (Kurian, 2013, p. 287). Likewise, the **organizational chart** is a diagrammatic representation that displays "the flow of authority, chain of command, titles and functions." (Kurian, 2013, p. 202).

Centralization and **decentralization** are organizational philosophies about power distribution that pertain to the hierarchical level of decision-making authority in the institution and are manifested in the organizational structure as where the locus of decision power resides. Centralization ("Centralization," 2016) means that the power of planning and decision making are exclusively in the hands of top management. Decentralization ("Decentralization," 2016) means that planning and decision making are disseminated throughout the organization. Fig. 13.1 illustrates examples of each.

BACKGROUND

As seen in Chapter 12, organizations have an identifiable structure that affects decision-making authority and the power that nurses have to control and make improvements in their practice. The higher the degree of decentralization in an organization, the more decision making is done at the point of activity. Institutions organize and structure themselves by defining departmental function and authority to achieve a more coordinated effort. This drives plans and decisions about responsibilities and who reports to whom.

Centralization and decentralization are relative terms when applied to the operating philosophy of institutions. In institutions where the executive leader retains

---

Photo used with permission from asiseeit/Getty Images.

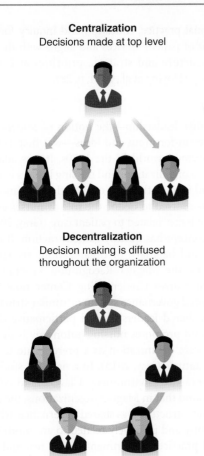

Centralization
Decisions made at top level

Decentralization
Decision making is diffused
throughout the organization

FIG. 13.1 Centralization and decentralization.

more decision-making authority, the operation takes on a more centralized philosophy. As institutions evolve into more complex global operations, the amount of information for which staff are accountable grows exponentially.

An institution with centralized decision making is demonstrated in this first scenario:

> Abigail Hutton is the nurse manager in the primary care clinic, a medical nursing unit in General Medical Center. Once a candidate is screened for a position by the human resources department, Nurse Hutton interviews applicants to fill open nursing positions in the clinic. At the conclusion of the interviews, she decides whom to hire and notifies human resources.

Although this is a somewhat simplistic example, of note is that the decision-making authority is vested solely in the nurse manager. That example is compared with the following second scenario:

> Jordan Jones is the nurse manager of 4 East, a medical nursing unit in City Hospital. With three staff nurse positions vacant, he posts the openings and asks the unit council—made up of nurses and other staff on the unit who have had human resources training on behavioral interviewing—to act as part of the selection committee. Based on the needs of the nursing unit and the availability of nursing applicants who match those criteria, human resource staff screen the files of the applicants. They pass on the applications of those nurses who meet the requirements for the positions to the selection committee, who then schedules interviews with the applicants. Once the selection committee has interviewed the candidates, they decide on the best candidate for each position. The committee's recommendations, along with the rationale for its choices, are relayed to the manager. The manager (1) meets with the candidates and takes into consideration the recommendations by the selection committee, (2) interviews them, and (3) makes the job offers.

In this second scenario, the staff nurses are involved in making a hiring decision that directly affects their work environment. This scenario clearly illustrates a more decentralized organizational philosophy. In such an organization, decision-making authority rests in levels closer to the point of service rather than in the executive levels. Decentralization encourages and facilitates greater innovation, more input, and faster response times because staff who are directly responsible for implementing changes and delivering care are a major part of decision making at the point of implementation.

It is important to note that although the two staffing scenarios depicted would appear distant from one another, many organizations exhibit varying degrees of centralization or decentralization. Here's an example of how decentralization works in a large, non–health care organization:

> At multinational giant W.L. Gore, an American manufacturing company with 10,000 employees, all decision making is accomplished through self-managing teams of 8 to 12 people. CEO Terri L. Kelly believes that "It's far better to rely upon a broad base of individuals and leaders who share a common set of values and feel personal ownership for the overall success of the

organization. These responsible and empowered individuals will serve as much better watchdogs than any single, dominant leader or bureaucratic structure" (Kastelle, 2013).

SHARED GOVERNANCE

Shared governance is an accountability-based system that empowers individuals within the decision-making system and increases staff's authority and control over their practice. In this model, staff are empowered through autonomy and accountability.

Shared governance is an ideal example of decentralization. It is described as "an organizational innovation that gives health care professionals control over their practice and extends their influence into administrative areas previously controlled only by managers and supervisors" (Swihart & Hess, 2014, p. 80). In a shared governance environment, staff take ownership of decision making. This is "a dynamic staff-leadership partnership that promotes collaboration, shared decision making and accountability for improving quality of care, safety, and enhancing work life" (Mathias, 2015).

For shared governance to be effective, decision making must be shared by empowered staff at the point where patients receive care. This requires a decentralized management structure. "All care team members—not just physicians, but also nurses, dietitians, pharmacists, occupational therapists, and others—can help make shared decision making a reality in all clinical settings. Furthermore, adopting an approach that involves all team members in the shared decision-making process can further efforts to improve care coordination and reduce fragmentation by helping break down the silos that divide various health professions" (Legare & Witterman, 2013, p. 281).

Empowered staff is a major outcome of true shared governance. A prime example is Cincinnati Children's Hospital. "Cincinnati Children's Hospital and Medical Center has a long history of embracing empowerment of all care team members through shared decision making . . . Shared governance is a vital facet to our operational effectiveness, from the unit to the divisional level," according to senior vice president Cheryl Hoying (Hoying et al., 2014, p. 28). The medical center's "Patient Care Governance Council, which has representatives from nursing, allied health, medicine, and the patient advisory council, ensures the accountabilities of interdisciplinary professional practice, education and inquiry for the department of patient services and aligns with the institutional structure and strategic priorities at Cincinnati Children's" (Hoying et al., 2014, p. 28).

History

Participative leadership—the notion of leaders turning to their team for input and ideas—was first introduced to the business world in the 1970s. It was adapted by health care organizations and nursing leaders in the early 1980s and formed the basis of shared governance, which today has evolved to define the role of nurses as well as to resolve issues related to patient care (Gray, 2013).

The concept has quickly gained traction. It is a centerpiece and hallmark of organizations recognized as Magnet by the Magnet Recognition Program®. "The American Nurses Credentialing Center now requires that a shared governance system or similar structure that supports shared leadership and participative decision-making and promotes nursing autonomy is in place at a health care organization as a prerequisite to seeking Magnet status" (Gray, 2013). In a national study of the nursing practice environment, Clavelle and colleagues (2013) found that in Magnet organizations, the primary governance structure was shared governance, which was significantly and positively related to an improved professional practice environment. To be real and make a difference for nurses, the shared governance needs to be manifested through point-of-care structures where direct care nurses make decisions about patient care and unit operations. Unit practice councils (UPCs) are an example.

Challenges

Effective shared governance is an ongoing process. Both staff and unit managers need to become comfortable with how governance is shared. Development is gradual and time consuming. To be successful, shared governance structures need leaders who are role models and mentors. Staff and management must be dedicated to coaching and continuous learning.

Implementing a shared governance structure can take years; it does not happen overnight. It takes commitment, ongoing education, transparency, time, and dedication. "Shared Governance is not easy to develop . . . It takes time to be effective. Neither staff nor leaders/managers should assume that the approach relieves leaders and managers of their responsibility to do their jobs"

(Finkelman & Kenner, 2016, p. 457). "The biggest barrier to shared governance is having dedicated time for meetings and for work on projects" (Mathias, 2015). Additionally, the financial commitment must be there to dedicate time and resources for staff to be involved in meeting time. Paying nurses for committee work time and arranging for coverage to attend meetings are organizational strategies to boost effectiveness and participation. Both affect perceptions of managerial support, which in turn affects staff nurse participation (Wilson et al., 2014). In some places there is a planned committee meeting day once a month so that managers can plan staffing coverage for important shared governance activities.

The degree to which nurses are engaged in decision making can affect the effectiveness of shared governance. The National Institutes of Health's Clinical Center had a robust shared governance model, yet nurses indicated they were only moderately satisfied with decision making and autonomy. In a survey, "the nurses responded that they had a high degree of satisfaction in other areas, such as nurse–physician collaboration, so decision making and autonomy became a focus of improvement efforts" (Jordan, 2016, p. 15). The decision was made to expand the current shared governance model to include UPCs. The purpose of the UPC is described as being "part of the shared governance structure to promote shared decision making at the unit/clinic/program of care level. To make and implement recommendations to improve practice, processes, and outcomes" (Jordan, 2016, p. 16). Extensive staff education and a thoughtful marketing campaign were planned. Although too soon to tell, "We're optimistic that the addition of UPCs to our Shared Governance structure will increase our nurses' satisfaction with decision making and autonomy" (Jordan, 2016, p. 18).

At Cincinnati Children's Hospital Medical Center, staff in the patient services division can submit a problem or an idea to the Nursing Professional Coordinating Council. "This is indicative of the highly collaborative nature of Cincinnati Children's Shared Governance structure," noted Hoying. "Accessed online via the Shared Governance webpage, the submission process gives everyone a voice" (Davidson et al., 2016, p. 184). Each submission's progress is charted in an online database; 70 to 80 submissions are received each year.

French-Bravo and Crow (2015, p. 8) found that without staff buy-in, shared governance may not bring about desired change: "Buy-in is the difference between an engaged nursing staff and employees who are disengaged or are just going through the motions . . . Nurse leaders can maximize their efforts to ensure buy-in by: a) promoting psychological meaningfulness, safety, and availability and b) spurring initial engagement and trust, helping employees understand the balance of options faced by the organization, creating positive personal connections built on mutual trust, and making time available for initiative success. Leaders have the obligation to ensure that employees have the necessary knowledge, skills, abilities, and time to meet the complex needs of the patients and families they serve."

Brull (2015) believed that a deliberate education strategy is necessary to successfully implement shared governance, particularly when the implementation timetable is brief. In such instances, "Unfortunately many hospitals 'give up' or stop providing the necessary resources and financial assistance needed to ensure Shared Governance is in place. This often leads to . . . 'We have tried this before and it didn't work'" (Brull, 2015, p. 314).

Wilson and colleagues (2014) wondered if direct care nurses and nurse managers had varying perceptions of factors affecting direct care nurses' participating in unit-based and general shared governance activities and nurse engagement. They found some significant differences, concluding that "nurse managers and unit council leaders/members should evaluate their nurses' perceptions of manager support, teamwork, lack of disruption to patient care, and pay for their participation in Shared Governance–related activities. These research findings can be used to facilitate evaluation of hospital practices for direct care nurse participation in unit-based Shared Governance activities" (Wilson et al., 2014, p. 22).

LEADERSHIP AND MANAGEMENT IMPLICATIONS

Although shared governance shifts decision making away from a health care organization's leader and into the hands of empowered staff, shared governance does not mean that leaders can ignore their responsibility in the decision-making process. Nor does it mean, of course, that all decisions are made by nurses. To be effective, leaders must be ready—and accepting of this shift. So too must leaders be prepared to empower staff. They have good reason:

Staff who experience empowerment feel that they are respected and trusted to be active participants.

Staff who feel empowered also demonstrate a positive image to other healthcare team members, patients and their families, and the public. Nurses who do not feel empowered will not be effective in conveying a positive image, because they will not be able to communicate that nurses are professionals with much to offer. Empowerment that is not clear to staff is just as problematic as no staff empowerment. Empowered teams feel a responsibility for the team's performance and activities, which in turn can improve care and reduce errors (Finkelman & Kenner, 2016, p. 457).

Organizations that are successful in implementing and maintaining a shared governance culture can see evidence of nurses who demonstrate empowerment, autonomy, and commitment to the organization through improved staff nurse retention. Nurse leaders and managers who rule autocratically present a hindrance to this culture.

In organizations that practice shared governance, staff as well as nurse managers and leaders are responsible for innovation. As noted in Chapter 2, innovation is considered crucial to safely and effectively solve complex care problems. The entire team is responsible for unit outcomes, not just the individual manager. The manager is primarily responsible for mentoring, facilitating, enabling, and supporting. Experts recommend an inter-professional approach to shared governance:

An interprofessional approach to Shared Governance must be embedded throughout the organization adopting it, from the clinical decisions at points of service to the strategic priorities placed on interprofessional issues by senior leadership. A cornerstone of this approach to practice may be the inclusion of patients and families as full partners on both care teams and planning groups. Respecting and valuing the knowledge and service of all team members contributes to a trusting, openly communicative, learning environment and positive patient care and practice outcomes (Swihart & Hess, 2014, p. 87).

An inter-professional approach "often engages patients and families as partners. Keys to successful implementation…include active participation of all team members contributing to mutually respectful, trusting, collaborative, openly communicative, safe, and effective learning environments of care and practice across disciplines and departments. Interprofessional Shared Governance provides a unique structure for shared decision-making reflective of the current and devolving demands of an increasingly diverse and integrated care delivery system" (Swihart & Hess, 2014, p. 4).

To sustain a culture of shared governance, it is important to recruit leaders who support the concept. Education and encouragement of active participation in making decisions must be ongoing. For example, Cincinnati Children's Hospital Medical Center created the role of facilitator to ensure standardization of development and implementation of shared governance across the medical center. Responsibilities of this position included (1) developing council leaders and members who can effectively use their voice to influence decision making, (2) keeping the work of councils moving forward, and (3) ensuring that council goals are integrated with strategic initiatives of the medical center (Hoying & Allen, 2011).

Once implemented, shared governance can become the motivation for development of a new practice model. This was the case at Cincinnati Children's. Before 2012, many of the medical center's professions were guided by their own practice models. Knowing that migration toward accountable care organizations was imminent, in 2012, Hoying and colleagues "urged the patient care governance council to develop a new practice model that aligns various professional practices with one common language and goal: patient-centered care" (Hoying et al., 2014, p. 29). The resulting practice model (Fig. 13.2) was developed and implemented to catalyze value-based care.

Nurses' involvement in governance is an important component of the American Nurses Credentialing Center's Magnet Recognition Program® (see Chapter 3). "Research is proving that Magnet hospitals score higher in nurse job satisfaction (attributed to increased autonomy, structural empowerment, and a positive work environment) and thus demonstrate lower RN turnover and vacancy rates" (Elsevier, 2014) (see Chapters 10 and 12 for more on structural empowerment). Additionally, patients treated in Magnet hospitals had 14% lower odds of mortality and 12% lower odds of failure-to-rescue (McHugh et al., 2013).

The recognition as Magnet, now given to more than 440 organizations representing six countries (including 7.6% of US hospitals), honors health care organizations for quality patient care, nursing excellence, and innovations in professional nursing practice (American Nurses

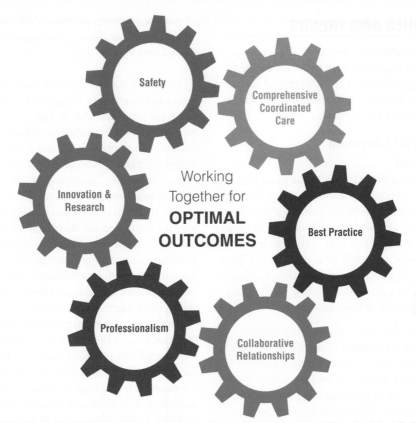

FIG. 13.2 Cincinnati Children's Hospital Medical Center Interprofessional Practice Model. (Courtesy Cincinnati Children's Hospital Medical Center, 2013.)

Credentialing Center, 2016). To earn the recognition, organizations must demonstrate evidence of formal structures of empowerment and nurses' involvement in governance regarding their practice. Organizational structures that foster empowerment are essential to achieve a professional practice model.

Shared governance has far-reaching implications for leaders in today's health care environment, in which the focus is to provide patient care safely, efficaciously, and efficiently. Organizational benefits include increased commitment of staff to the organization; accountability of the nurse; a new level of professional autonomy; a more efficient model for point-of-service decision making; more expert involvement at the point of service; a more assured, confident patient advocate; and improved financial outcomes. Patients benefit from a more efficient model of health care service, more committed health care professionals, quicker responses at the point of service, and a more assured, confident patient advocate.

Leaders stand to realize numerous organizational gains as professional nurses embrace the quest for empowerment and professional autonomy. However, the journey to shared governance can be both invigorating and tedious, as staff are groomed for opportunities of empowerment and accountability and are taught how to manage these responsibilities. Guiding counsel from the nursing profession's most nurturing leaders is needed to support both staff nurses and nurse managers as they cope with the change from a hierarchical system to one of shared leadership. Mentoring by clinically credible role models will be an important facet of the transformation toward shared governance. The goal is to transfer leadership wisdom not only to aspiring leaders but also to all employees. The role of today's leaders is to encourage transformation through their own commitment to the journey and to coordinate and facilitate the efforts of others (Porter-O'Grady & Malloch, 2015).

CURRENT ISSUES AND TRENDS

Health care is ever changing. Some of the issues and trends that are shaping health care now and in the future and have an impact on shared governance include inter-professional education and collaboration, whole-system integration, and engagement.

Inter-Professional Education and Collaboration

"As multiple clinicians provide care to the same patient or family, clinicians become a team—a group working with at least one common aim: the best possible care—whether or not they acknowledge this fact. Each clinician relies upon information and action from other members of the team" (Mitchell et al., 2012, p. 2). This inter-professional approach to patient care is ideally introduced to health care students while in the classroom. One example of how this can work is:

> In an unpublished study of the effectiveness of interprofessional teamwork at Cincinnati Children's, 26 nursing and medical students worked together in three pediatric simulation training exercises over an eight month period. Results indicated their learned scores were higher than control groups who did not train in an interprofessional setting. Nursing students demonstrated a higher score on teamwork and collaboration and positive professional identification compared to medical students in both groups. Plans to continue simulation training in an interprofessional environment are underway with a goal to boost teamwork among all hospital professions (Davidson et al., 2016, p. 186).

An article on the website of the American Nurses Association (2015) explained why inter-professional collaboration may be valuable in the future:

> One of the byproducts of the Affordable Care Act is that the way hospitals get paid for services is changing, with hospital reimbursements based more on how the patient flows through the episode, says Peggy Crabtree, MBA, RN, vice president of The Camden Group. As a result, nurses will have a bigger say in how care is provided to their patients. That change will offer more opportunities for nurses to collaborate with doctors to ensure the patient is getting the best care—and at the same time, make certain money and resources aren't being wasted. It's a natural extension for nurses, who know more than anyone where the waste is happening and what is and isn't working for patients, Crabtree says.

Education is a major part of inter-professional collaboration as nurses play a larger role in making sure that patients are ready and able to take care of themselves after they are released from the hospital or another health care facility. With the prevalence and costs of chronic diseases, nurses increasingly will be tasked with making sure patients stay healthy. "According to the Centers for Disease Control and Prevention, chronic diseases were responsible for 7 of 10 deaths in 2010, and treating people with chronic diseases accounted for 86 percent of the nation's health care costs" (American Nurses Association, 2015). Decentralization is an organizational structure suited to fostering nursing and health care delivery. For nurses, shared governance addresses the need for inter-professional teams to be able to work together both rapidly and effectively.

Clinical process management (CPM) is an allied concept that takes a holistic view of clinical processes, deals with complexity, promotes interdisciplinary shared governance, uses clinical workflow analysis, and leverages health information technology to evaluate when processes are working well or whether they can be improved. The extent to which health information technology can support the work and clinical processes is an important factor in CPM and is central to effective process management. For example, interdisciplinary teams can bring their clinical expertise and partner with health information technology personnel to achieve quality yet efficient work flows.

Whole-System Integration

Some see the benefits of decentralization and the shared governance model extending beyond nurses and all care providers to all employees. "As for the future of Shared Governance, Susan Allen PhD, RN, (assistant vice president, Cincinnati Children's Hospital) says it would be ideal to see whole-system integration involving all hospital staff. But will Shared Governance ever be the sole governing system or will there always be a traditional system to manage operations? Shared Governance would have to be highly integrated, says Allen" (Gray, 2013). Clearly, the next steps in this vision are to include patients and the community more deliberatively into the shared governance model. Allen says Cincinnati Children's Hospital has a family advisory council and a teen council that get involved in projects, including reviewing potential educational materials and designing a new learning center (Gray, 2013).

Engagement

An ongoing challenge among US employers, including health care systems, is to keep employees engaged. A Gallup poll (2014) indicated that only 31.5% of employees in the United States report they are "engaged at work," meaning they are committed to their job and making positive contributions. Fifty-one percent reported they are "not engaged at work," meaning they are not likely to put effort into organizational goals. Seventeen and a half percent are "actively disengaged," described as unhappy, unproductive and likely to spread negativity. Shared governance is the gold standard for engaging nurses in solving problems at the point of care.

Perhaps improved technology can also make a difference. According to the American Hospital Association (2016), "almost 30% of clinicians aren't satisfied with technology used by their organization." It will become more and more important for nurses to leverage the power of shared governance to improve practice and help deliver desired outcomes. Nurses need to both structure and participate in shared governance as a routine part of their work life.

RESEARCH NOTE

Source

Clavelle, J.T., Porter-O'Grady, T., & Drenkard, K. (2013). Structural empowerment and the nursing practice environment in Magnet organizations. *Journal of Nursing Administration, 43*(11), 566–573.

Purpose

One component of a Magnet organization is structural empowerment. This study was conducted to identify the characteristics of shared governance and its relationship with the nursing practice environment in Magnet organizations.

Discussion

The study's authors e-mailed surveys to chief nursing officers (CNO) and the leaders of nursing practice councils (NPC) in 344 Magnet organizations. The surveys used the Index of Professional Nursing Governance (IPNG) and the Nursing Work Index – Revised (NWI-R). The research questions asked were:

1. What are the characteristics of nursing shared governance in Magnet organizations?
2. What are the characteristics of the professional nursing practice environment (NPE) in Magnet organizations?
3. Is there a relationship between nursing shared governance, the professional practice environment, and organizational outcomes in Magnet organizations?

Measurement tools used were the IPNG, an 86-item instrument that measures perceptions of governance using six subscales, and the NWI-R, which measures characteristics of the nursing professional practice environment in four subscales.

Results

Responses were received from 107 chairs of nursing practice councils and 95 chief nursing officers for a 31.1% and 27.6% response rate, respectively. IPNG results indicated that the following were within the shared governance range: access to information, participation, resources supporting practice, control over practice, and goals and conflict resolution. Control over personnel, however, was within the traditional governance range, with management/administration as the dominant controlling group. A highly significant, moderate, and positive correlation was found between total IPNG score and total NWI-R score (r = 0.416, p <0.001). In addition, highly significant and small to moderate positive correlations were found to exist between the NWI-R subscales and the IPNG subscales. The strongest relationships were found in these areas:

- NWI-R subscale of organizational support and the IPNG subscale of control over personnel (r = 0.42, p <0.001),
- NWI-R subscale of autonomy and IPNG subscales of control over practice (r = 0.367, p <0.001) and resources supporting practice (r = 0.365, p <0.001),
- NWI-R subscale of organizational support and IPNG subscale of control over practice (r = 0.365, p <0.001).

All of the other NWI-R subscales and IPNG subscales revealed smaller but highly significant positive correlations with the exception of the NWI-R subscale nurse–physician relationships and with these exceptions of the IPNG subscales: control over personnel, access to information, resources supporting practice, participation, and goals and conflict resolution. The only small, significantly positive relationship found was between the NWI-R subscale of nurse–physician relationship and IPNG subscale of control over practice (r = 0.255, p = 0.014). A statistical relationship was not found among IPNG total and subscale scores, NWI-R total and subscale scores, and organizational, CNO, and NPC variables.

Continued

RESEARCH NOTE—cont'd

Application to Practice

It is important to note that survey results were received from less than one-third of all Magnet organizations, which limits generalized conclusions. However, this study does support the notion of a positive relationship between nursing shared governance and the nursing practice environment. It points out the important role of chief

nursing officers in transforming the nursing work environment: leading the design, implementation, and evaluation of shared governance structures and enabling others to act with impact. The authors of this study concluded that when nurses are engaged in shared governance, they actively participate in improving their own nursing professional practice environment.

CASE STUDY

The purpose of this case study is to consider one example of shared governance in action in a large academic pediatric medical center in Cincinnati, Ohio, that has had shared governance in place in nursing since 1989. The case study describes the decision to institute daily chlorhexidine bathing to applicable patients as related by Kneflin and colleagues (2016).

Several questions arose from direct care nurses about unwarranted variations in bathing practices across settings and whether bathing standardization could help address prevention of infections of patients with central lines. Shared governance council members identified daily chlorhexidine bathing as a potential intervention to standardize bathing across the hospital. At the time, chlorhexidine bathing had been widely adopted in adult hospitals but was less commonly practiced in pediatric institutions.

The inter-professional shared governance model used at the medical center is designed around three cornerstones of quality care: practice, education, and research. Various levels of shared governance councils include direct care providers, managers, and other professionals with roles that are essential to robust, informed discussion.

The Nursing Professional Practice Council (NPPC) leadership team consists of the chair (a direct care nurse), the chair-elect (a direct care nurse), a nursing leadership representative and a shared governance facilitator. Through a structured online referral process available to all clinical staff, the NPPC team received numerous referrals related to bathing practices. The NPPC members identified two themes: (1) unwarranted variations in bathing practices across settings and (2) the desire to decrease incidence of central line–associated bloodstream infections (CLABSIs). One referral proposed chlorhexidine gluconate (CHG) bathing as a possible practice change.

1. Based on the information presented thus far, is the nursing department centralized or decentralized? What factors do you look for when determining whether an institution has a centralized or decentralized organizational structure?

2. Describe the value of a structured online referral process for clinical staff.

Recognizing CHG bathing as a potential solution, the NPPC decided they needed an evidence synthesis about CHG bathing to make an informed evidence-based decision about the standardization of bathing practices. The NPPC sent the CHG bathing referral to the Nursing Professional Inquiry Council (NPIC) asking for an evidence-based recommendation about the use of CHG for daily bathing in children. An NPIC subgroup performed a thorough search of evidence. They found two studies of pediatric patients, both supporting the intervention of CHG to reduce the incidence of bloodstream infections. Because of the small number of studies conducted with pediatric patients, a review of adult literature followed. The subgroup found many studies that supported the intervention of daily CHG to reduce the incidence of bloodstream infections in adults. Ultimately, NPIC reached consensus and wrote this statement of recommendation to NPPC: It is strongly recommended that patients older than 2 months of age in a critical care setting receive a daily bath using CHG to decrease the risk of bloodstream infections. It is recommended that the Neonatal Intensive Care Unit Practice Council make its own decision regarding patients older than 2 months due to their unique environment.

The NPPC took the recommendation to stakeholders, including MDs, infection control leadership, and pediatric experts, for input and discussion. With significant expert input, the NPPC made the decision to standardize best practice to include daily CHG baths. Within months the Nursing Professional Education Council launched mandatory education about CHG bathing, and the practice changes were fully implemented across the medical center.

1. How might a shared governance committee including allied health personnel, physicians, and families differ from a committee composed solely of nurses?

2. What key factors in the case study help you determine whether this shared governance structure is successful?

3. The process described in this case study took 18 months to achieve. Do you think the outcomes would be compromised if the pace was faster? What would you suggest to speed up the process?

CRITICAL THINKING EXERCISE

Joshua Jackson and a number of other staff on the unit complain after seeing the online staffing schedule. Once again, they are scheduled to work on days that were requested off, and now Joshua has to reschedule his dentist appointment for the second time. Lately staff have been absent from work, and the Hospital Care Assurance Program scores are decreasing.

1. What are the areas of concern in this scenario?
2. With shared governance in mind, what should Joshua do? What would you do?
3. How would the nurses go about initiating and implementing a shared governance structure? Do they need a consultant?

14

Strategic Management

Mary G. Harper

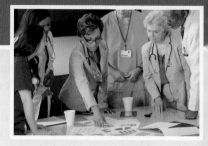

http://evolve.elsevier.com/Huber/leadership

Thinking and behaving strategically are prime methods for nurses to be proactive in a complex, fast-changing, rapid-cycle environment. Arising from the business field, strategic management has made its way into health care leadership, including nursing. The leadership role of nurses has become an area of increasing focus since the Institute of Medicine (IOM, now called the National Academies of Sciences, Engineering, and Medicine, Health and Medicine Division), in its 2011 *Future of Nursing* report, called for increased leadership development and participation in leadership among nurses. Evaluation of progress toward the *Future of Nursing* goals indicates that although leadership development opportunities have been created since the release of the IOM report, insufficient data exist to determine progress toward nurses serving on "executive management teams and other key leadership positions" (National Academies of Sciences, Engineering, and Medicine, [NAM], 2015). Leadership development and participation continues to be an area of focus for nursing as the profession strives to fulfill the IOM goals.

In order to be effective leaders, nurses must gain competence in a variety of areas. The American Organization of Nurse Executives (AONE) divided these competencies into five broad categories: communication and relationship management, knowledge of the health care environment, leadership, professionalism, and business skills and principles (AONE, 2015). One key area of business skills includes strategic management. Competencies that align with strategic management consist of several processes, including organizational assessment, planning, management of implementation, and evaluation.

In alignment with the competencies developed by AONE (2015), strategic management involves conducting an environmental scan, knowing the competition, establishing goals, setting targets, developing an action plan, implementing the plan, and evaluating success (Management Study Guide, n.d.; Pearce & Robinson, 2012). This approach has long been used in business to ensure a competitive advantage over similar enterprises. Issues in the health care industry, including the Hospital Consumer Assessment of Healthcare Providers and Systems (HCAHPS) and the Hospital Value-Based Purchasing Program, among others, require health care organizations to function as businesses to obtain and maintain a competitive advantage. The success of a health care enterprise depends on this competitive advantage of how well it does something compared with similar efforts and how well it is able to continuously achieve superior performance. Those enterprises that do not do so fail to remain viable for long.

Strategic management involves strategic planning and implementation. It provides a "blueprint" for operating a business, establishing a competitive position, ensuring customer satisfaction, and reaching strategic objectives or goals. Although most strategic planning occurs at the "macro" level (i.e., the executive levels of the health care institution), its implementation typically becomes the responsibility of the "micro" level, such as the nursing division, department, or unit. As a result, success depends on the engagement of the entire workforce (Jasper & Crossan, 2012). Fortunately, strategic management prepares nurses to adapt to the current health care environment and helps them achieve their goals, whether related to the workplace or to the profession.

Photo used with permission from asiseeit/Getty Images.

DEFINITIONS

A review of literature by Jasper and Crossan (2012) determined that strategic management is a multifaceted concept that is difficult to define. These authors embraced the definition of **strategic management** offered by Nag and colleagues (2007), which asserts that "strategic management deals with the major intended and emergent initiatives taken by general managers . . . involving utilization of resources, to enhance the performance of firms in their external environments" (p. 944). This definition encompasses the five characteristics of strategic management found by Jasper and Crossan (2012):

- Engagement of the entire workforce in organizational leadership
- Alignment with the external environment
- Future orientation
- Use of change management strategies to achieve performance goals
- Facilitation of decision-making with well-communicated decisions

The concept of strategic management includes strategic planning and strategy implementation (Management Study Guide, n.d.). Additional terms associated with an organization's use of strategy include *organizational mission and vision, core values, core purpose, strategy, tactics, strategic plan, objectives,* and *stakeholders.* The **organizational mission and vision** collectively is a guiding framework that describes the organization's purpose and future direction (Society for Human Resource Management [SHRM], 2012). **Core values** define the characteristics or beliefs that underlie the organization's activities. The **core purpose** is the reason the organization is in business. **Strategy** is a competitive move or business approach designed to produce a successful outcome. **Tactics** are operational choices for action that are made to implement a strategy. A **strategic plan** is a document that specifies a plan for actualizing the mission. A strategic plan may also involve a *business plan* or an *action plan* (either as part of the strategic plan or as an adjunct to it) that consists of the who, what, by when, where, and in general terms, the costs involved in implementing the activities identified as objectives in the strategic plan. **Objectives** are defined as the targets an organization wants to achieve. These can be financial or performance based with short-range or long-range targets. Finally, **stakeholders** are individuals, groups, or another institution with a financial interest in—or who are affected by—what happens with the organization ("Stakeholder," n.d.).

STRATEGIC PLANNING PROCESS

Strategic management generally begins with a strategic planning process, triggered by recognition of the need for an organization to establish its competitive position in the marketplace or to address some other perceived need (e.g., seeking Magnet Recognition from the American Nurses Credentialing Center's Magnet Recognition Program®, [2013], applying to become a Certified Comprehensive Stroke Center through The Joint Commission [2016], or simply establishing future directions). These are questions to be answered in the strategic planning process: Where are we currently? Where do we want to go? How will we get there?

The components of the nursing process—assessment, planning, implementation, and evaluation—are similar to those employed in strategic management. Although a variety of strategic planning frameworks exist, they include the following six components, as shown in Fig. 14.1:

- Creating strategic mission and vision
- Assessing the environment
- Setting objectives
- Developing strategies to achieve the objectives
- Planning for implementation
- Planning for evaluation

The strategic plan provides a framework for strategic management, considering both external and internal environmental factors. Although the strategic planning process may appear to be sequential, it may be iterative as each stage illuminates new ideas for consideration.

Creating Mission and Vision Statements

The first step of the strategic planning process is to formulate or review and update as needed the organization's mission and vision in alignment with the organization's core purpose and values. The mission delineates what the

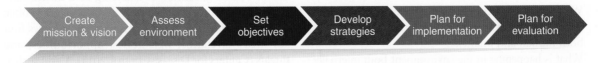

| Create mission & vision | Assess environment | Set objectives | Develop strategies | Plan for implementation | Plan for evaluation |

FIG. 14.1 Strategic planning process.

organization does, while the vision articulates the preferred future state of the organization (SHRM, 2012). This step requires a determination of what the organization is, what business it is in and for whom, and where the business seeks to be in the future. The documentation of the mission and vision serves to communicate both purpose and direction to all stakeholders.

The mission and vision are informed by the core values of the organization. The core values held by an organization are those values that are held regardless of whether circumstances—either internal or external—change. They provide a standard for decision-making processes (SHRM, 2012). These core values are so embodied in the culture of the organization that even if they were seen as a liability, they would not be abandoned. Core values do not change even if the industry in which the organization operates changes. Thus, in health care, the organization that has as its core values quality care, patient safety, integrity, and social responsibility would retain those core values despite internal changes (e.g., changes in chief executive officers [CEOs]) or external changes (e.g., reimbursement, the nursing shortage).

The organization's core purpose is the reason the organization exists. The mission defines what the organization does, and the core purpose delineates why (Jones, 2015). The core purpose, like the core values, is relatively unchanging. It provides direction to the organization and contributes to the articulation and implementation of its mission.

In the strategic planning process, the following questions can help develop or revise vision and mission statements:

- What business are we in now?
- What business do we want to be in?
- What do our customers expect of us now?
- What will the customers' expectations be in the future?
- Who are our customers now?
- Who will our customers be in the future?
- Who are our current stakeholders (other than customers)?
- How will those stakeholders change in the future? What about their expectations?
- Who are our primary competitors currently?
- Who will our competitors be in the future?
- What about partners, now and in the future?
- What will the effect of technology be?
- What are the available and the needed resources, both human and financial?
- What is happening in the environment both internally and externally, now and in the future, that may affect us?

In many cases, the core values and the core purpose of the organization may have been defined previously, but if not, planners engaged in the strategic planning process should develop them using questions such as the following:

- What are the values on which we base our work?
- How central or essential are these to the organization?
- Would these values be supported if circumstances changed, or if the industry in which we currently operate changes?

The core purpose can be defined and refined by asking, "Why are we in business?" As a result, the initial response, "We are in the business of health care," may be further refined to "We want to contribute to the community in which we exist." Thus asking "why" may result in the core purpose of providing needed health care services to the community in which the organization is located.

Responses to these questions by the principals involved in an organization (e.g., executive management, supervisory staff, department heads) shape an organization's mission, vision, strategic plan, and, as a result, its strategic management. However, involving individuals at all levels of the organization (e.g., staff nurses, clerical workers) in addition to those at the top of the hierarchy ensures a variety of perspectives and more buy-in to the final product. Such inclusion also engages all levels of staff in helping make the vision a reality. When everyone involved in an institution shares the same vision, individuals know where the organization is going and can be instrumental in helping it get there through their daily activities. As the old saying goes, "If you don't know where you're going, then any path will take you there." Conversely, if all of the individuals in the institution know the mission and vision, they are more likely to take the same path. Thus, although it is tempting to skip the mission, vision, and values review, sound strategic planning is premised on a firm linkage to them so that the plan then makes sense and flows out from this core.

Assessing the Environment

A key component of the strategic planning process is to assess the environment. This assessment, called environmental scanning, consists of analyzing both internal and external environmental factors. A SWOT analysis is often used in the environmental assessment and reviews four key areas: strengths, weaknesses, opportunities, and threats (Centers for Disease Control, 2015). A grid such as the one seen in Table 14.1 is often used for documenting

TABLE 14.1	**SWOT Analysis Template**	
Internal Factors	Strengths	Weaknesses
External Factors	Opportunities	Threats

the SWOT analysis. In this approach, strengths and weaknesses internal to the organization are identified. These strengths and weaknesses are generally related to resources, programs, and operations in key areas of the organization, examples of which are the following:

- *Operations:* efficiency, capacity, processes
- *Management:* systems, expertise, resources
- *Products:* quality, features, prices
- *Finances:* resources, performance

Once identified, these components are analyzed for the purpose of drafting a picture of the critical features of the organization, its achievements and failures, and its good points and bad points.

The external components are described as opportunities and threats, and they are identified in the same manner as the internal factors. Opportunities and threats may include changes in industry, marketplace, economy, political climate, technology, and competition.

Once identified, these strengths, weaknesses, opportunities, and threats must be analyzed for their impact on the organization. Next, priorities are established for the critical issues so that strategies are based on the priority issues. For example, a change in the market for the organization's services may be a threat but a low priority, so the organization determines it is not essential to target resources (e.g., human, financial) to deal with the threat when a higher priority is to take advantage of an opportunity involving technology. The SWOT analysis often leads to strategies in which the organization determines to build on strengths, resolve or minimize weaknesses, seize opportunities, and avoid threats.

The strategies identified through the SWOT analysis help shape the strategic plan on which strategic management is based. The more carefully the analysis is conducted, the more reliable the strategic plan. A plan based on faulty assumptions or careless analysis does not serve the organization well and indeed may lead eventually to its demise.

There are a variety of methods used to analyze and craft a strategic plan. Besides the SWOT analysis, the SOAR (**s**trengths, **o**pportunities, **a**spirations, and **re**sults) planning model has been used in nursing to encourage innovation (Wadsworth et al., 2016). SOAR is a more positive alternate to the more traditional SWOT,

places greater emphasis on the organization's future, and encourages employee involvement.

In addition to a SWOT or SOAR analysis of the current environment, individuals engaged in the strategic planning process must project the future. The assessment of future environmental impact takes the form of assumptions. These assumptions encompass the sociodemographic, political, economic, and technological aspects of the external environment. Of course, these assumptions are merely best guesses, because it is impossible to predict the future with certainty.

Setting Objectives

Once the organization's mission and vision have been established and the environmental assessment conducted, the next step in strategic planning is to develop the ways and means to achieve the vision. Strategic goals and objectives are crafted in this step. These objectives generally define the "who," "what," and "where" of the strategies to be implemented. Clearly defined objectives allow individuals to recognize where the organization wants to go and how much time it will take to get there. Absence of strategic objectives results in individuals trying to move in too many directions without a coordinated plan or not moving at all because of confusion about the organization's direction.

Strategic objectives provide a way of converting the rather abstract mission and vision of an organization into concrete terms. These are targets of performance that when taken together will achieve the mission and vision. Objectives also offer a way of measuring progress toward achieving the organization's mission and vision. These objectives generally are written to reflect not what *is* but what *should be*—activities that encourage the individuals implementing them to be creative, stretch beyond their current limits, and challenge themselves to improve their performance. These objectives must be achievable, however, lest individuals lose faith that they can accomplish them. If the strategic objectives are challenging but achievable, they prevent employees of an institution from becoming complacent or settling for the status quo.

Objectives may be written in terms of financial outcomes that relate to improvements in an organization's fiscal health and result in a stronger position for the institution in the industry. For example, a hospital may set a financial objective to decrease expenses by a specific percentage each year. This objective may be accomplished through tactics to decrease length of stay or prevent hospital-acquired conditions such as pressure ulcers (HAPU) or ventilator-associated pneumonia (VAP). In addition, the organization may have objectives to enhance their position as a health care provider or employer of choice. These objectives may relate to obtaining high scores on publicly reported data such as HCAHPS or achieving quality recognition such as Magnet designation.

Developing Implementation Strategies

Objectives are the targeted results and outcomes, and strategies are actions taken to achieve those outcomes. The strategies must be aligned with the organizational culture. In addition, they must be realistic, planned, and intentional, yet flexible enough to respond to unanticipated events.

In the strategic management process, tactics need to be developed with patient safety and quality care as the guiding force (Jasper & Crossan, 2012). Operational strategies need to be evidence based and engage employees at all levels of the organization. Because of this, individuals who develop implementation strategies need to be cognizant of the organizational culture and the impact of changes on those who are tasked with carrying out the plans. As Jasper and Crossan (2012, p. 843) stated, "if we accept that part of the organization's culture is a sense of agreement among staff as to what constitutes the best way forward in any given situation then acknowledgment of those values and beliefs when formulating strategy will be key to successful implementation."

Plans that engage employees are realistic. The need for realistic yet flexible plans is emphasized by the American Nurses Association's (ANA, 2013) Leadership Institute Competency Model. This model identifies the leadership competency of strategic planning as the ability to "translate vision into realistic business strategies" (ANA, 2013, p. 9). Behaviors that demonstrate this competency include:
- Adjusting plans as needed based on circumstances
- Developing plans with consideration for organization-wide needs
- Formulating realistic tactical plans that align with organizational strategies
- Creating contingency plans
- Balancing "long-term goals with immediate organizational needs" (ANA, 2013, p. 9).

This ability to rapidly adapt to changing environmental influences is referred to as *strategic agility* (Kotter, 2014; Shirey, 2015). Kotter maintains that organizations that are not able to shift their operational focus quickly are at risk in an environment of ever-increasing change. Strategic agility has become a key to organizational success. A flexible

implementation plan helps an organization remain strong enough to withstand competition, overcome obstacles, and achieve peak performance. The organization's strategy must be flexible to respond appropriately to the following:
- Evolving needs and preferences of customers and stakeholders
- Advances in technology
- Changes in political climate and regulatory requirements
- New opportunities
- Altered market conditions
- Disasters and crises

Planning for Implementation

Once the strategies have been delineated, the next step in the strategic planning process is planning for implementation. Implementation involves trying out the activities in a way that determines how best to close the gap between how things are done and what it takes to achieve the strategy. For example, given an objective related to improvement of the financial bottom line, the first step is to determine current cost and then compare it with desired cost to decide what needs to be changed to reach the desired lower cost.

If strategies are to be effective, they must be implemented proficiently, efficiently, and in a timely manner. For this to occur, the organization must attend to its capabilities, the reward structure, available support systems, and the organizational culture. For example, if employees are not rewarded in ways that are meaningful to them, they are unlikely to initiate or maintain efforts to implement the strategy. If the organizational culture does not support innovation or risk taking, or if the prevailing attitude is "if it's not broken, don't fix it," then efforts to improve performance or outcomes may be doomed. Support systems such as education, policies, and procedures must be developed to support the implementation plan.

Implementing strategy is closely linked to an organization's operations; it involves managing, budgeting, motivating, changing culture, supervising, and leading. Strategic planning and implementation are managerial processes that accomplish the following:
- Demonstrate leadership in implementation of the strategy
- Reward those who carry out the strategy successfully
- Allocate necessary resources to activities critical to the strategy
- Formulate policies and procedures that support the identified strategy
- Initiate continuous quality improvement activities

- Develop and reward best practices
- Maintain a culture that supports the strategy

Effective implementation is more likely when an action plan is developed with input from the individuals who are responsible for implementing the strategic plan. The action plan should include a priority order for achieving the strategic objectives or outcomes, the determination of who (individual or group) is responsible for achieving these objectives, an indication of available or necessary financial support, and a timetable outlining when achievement of the objectives can be expected. If the strategic objective is long term or complex, it may also be advisable to include interim activities and time frames so that progress can be evaluated.

Planning for Evaluation

The final step in the strategic planning process is developing the evaluation design. Planning for evaluation is imperative to ensure that systems and measurements are in place to determine whether the strategic plan has been achieved. During the strategic planning process, measures of success are delineated, responsible individuals are identified, and frequency of evaluation and reporting of these measures is determined. If these progress reports reveal that the measures of success are not being achieved, further evaluation—such as environmental scanning with additional SWOT analysis—may be indicated.

Strategic plan progress reports may appear in a variety of formats from a simple narrative to use of complex strategic management software. Whatever format is used, it should clearly indicate the organization's progress toward its strategic goals.

ELEMENTS OF A STRATEGIC PLAN

Strategic planning results in a written document called the strategic plan. This document may be written by the individuals involved in the strategic planning process or by the individual who facilitated the process (e.g., consultant). Strategic plan documents generally contain the following sections:

- *Executive summary:* A two- to three-page synopsis of the plan, written in language understandable by all potential readers
- *Background:* A description of the institution, its history, and current state, including its accomplishments, as well as the situation that prompted the strategic planning process

- *Mission, vision, and values:* A description of the philosophy of the organization
- *Goals and strategies:* A list of the target objectives and the strategies identified to ensure achievement of the objectives
- *Appendices:* All additional documentation related to the strategic planning process to provide the background information used by the strategic planners to arrive at the final plan

Appendix materials may include the annual reports of the institution, SWOT analysis results, financial information, environmental scan results, staffing information, and current and projected programs and services. Other materials may be included as desired. Caution should be exercised, however, to not include confidential data that should not be viewed by individuals outside of the organization.

The strategic plan should be disseminated widely throughout the institution. However, the document does not need to be reproduced in its entirety for everyone in the institution. A decision needs to be made about which parts of the strategic plan are appropriate for the individuals who will receive them. Some may need the entire plan, others may need only the executive summary, and still others may need only the goals and strategies.

In any case, the strategic plan should be communicated to stakeholders: board members, management, and staff. Copies should be included in orientation programs for new employees. The institution's vision and mission—including the core values—should be displayed in public areas (e.g., waiting rooms, cafeteria), as well as in areas reserved for employees. The core values can be listed on employee identification badges and printed in all marketing materials for the organization. The strategic plan tenets should be incorporated into all of the institution's policies and procedures.

Copies of the plan may also be provided to trade or professional organizations with which the institution is associated. The public relations or community outreach department in the institution can use the strategic plan as the basis for a media campaign to educate the community and other stakeholders and audiences about the institution's vision and mission. Patients may be provided with a condensed summary of the strategic plan on admission, particularly those sections related to their care. Patients should be informed of the institution's core values as well.

IMPLEMENTATION OF THE STRATEGIC PLAN

At this point, strategic management often fails. Strategic plans are developed and then allowed to languish as the necessary commitment to implementation is not realized. Often competing priorities impede implementation of the plan. Executives and staff in health care organizations have numerous responsibilities, and implementing strategic objectives adds another burden to an already overwhelming workload. To overcome this obstacle, the strategic plan must be integrated into the organization's daily activities. Everyone must be committed to implementing the strategic plan, from the leaders to the staff at all levels and in all departments. Focusing on the strategic plan and its meaning to the viability and future of the institution is imperative.

An action plan is key to maintaining focus on implementation of the strategic plan. The action plan breaks the strategic plan into manageable components, particularly for those individuals who were not directly involved in crafting the strategic plan. During implementation, the action plan must become a living document that is constantly referenced, consulted, and discussed. The action plan should be reviewed and updated at regular intervals. Actions that have been completed or those that do not move the organization toward achievement of its goals should be deleted, and new actions based on existing environmental conditions should be added. It may also be necessary to readjust the timeline for completion of some activities in response to external or internal factors that affect the ability to accomplish the desired activities.

Ensuring that the action plan remains at the forefront of daily activities—whether in an institution as a whole, a department, or a unit—often requires a "champion." This champion is an individual who is passionate and committed to the implementation process and who can inspire others. Often a champion appears as the strategic planning process unfolds; generally, this individual contributes freely, is engaged in the work groups, and expresses interest in the process. Champions can be selected as well, but those who volunteer are usually more enthusiastic about the work than those who are "drafted."

LEADERSHIP AND MANAGEMENT IMPLICATIONS

Strategic management is useful for nursing leaders and managers because it can be used to analyze the environment for opportunities and threats; to set measurable, achievable goals and strategies; and to help determine the future of the nursing department or unit. Nursing departments do their own strategic plan for nursing. This plan needs to link and relate to the organization's overall mission, vision, and values. Success in strategic planning and implementing the strategic plan will position nursing well in an institution. The process provides an opportunity for nursing to shine, because the similarities between the nursing process and the strategic planning process allow nurses to shortcut the learning curve and begin to move forward with the implementation phase while others may still be grappling with the planning process. Nursing skills and abilities make it relatively easy to plan strategically, and nurses, as 24-hour workers, can approach implementation as an ongoing, continuous, and seamless process. Nurses' involvement with continuous quality improvement and performance improvement systems provides a basis for participation in strategic planning that is systematic and thorough.

Implementation of the organization's strategic plan can be useful in unifying staff on a nursing unit or in a department. Collaboration and cooperation among staff generally are required to accomplish strategic objectives. Working together to accomplish a strategic objective keeps staff engaged. Involvement in decisions that ultimately will affect them is essential and often results in positive spin-offs; for example, staff members feel a sense of ownership in the process and pride in their accomplishments.

CURRENT ISSUES AND TRENDS

Many current issues and trends affect the strategic management process in health care organizations and nursing. These trends include a focus on the Institute for Health care Improvement's (IHI) Triple Aim, the effect of the Patient Protection and Affordable Care Act (ACA), and continued attention to the goals of the IOM's *Future of Nursing* report.

First proposed in 2008, the Triple Aim established by the IHI includes goals related to population health, improving the patient experience, and decreasing per capita cost (IHI, 2016; Whittington et al., 2015). The IHI posits that these goals can strengthen other health care reform measures such as accountable care organizations (ACOs), bundled payments, and avoidance of penalties for preventable events such as hospital readmissions or hospital-acquired infections. Strategic management in health care organizations requires attention to these goals in order to maintain optimal reimbursement and remain financially viable.

Tenets of the Triple Aim were incorporated in the ACA, another trend that affects strategic management in health care organizations. Provisions of the ACA, which was implemented in 2010, continue to evolve (Rand Health, n.d.). Overall, the ACA has resulted in fewer uninsured individuals but has also affected hospital and provider reimbursement. As the ACA's mandates continue to be phased into practice, health care organizations must strategically manage their impact on overall operations.

Finally, the continued focus on the IOM's (2011) *Future of Nursing* goals drives the strategic goals of health care organizations and nursing practice. Elimination of barriers to practicing at the full scope of practice, advancing educational preparation of nurses, creating diversity in the nursing workforce, leading change to promote health, and improving collection of nursing workforce data all require continued effort (NAM, 2015). However, the shifting health care environment requires more interprofessional collaboration and mandates that organizations and nursing professionals engage with a broad base of stakeholders to promote the Triple Aim targets of population health, patient satisfaction, and decreased costs of health care.

CONCLUSION

Strategic planning is not reserved for activities such as seeking recognition through the ANCC Magnet Recognition Program® or for ameliorating workforce issues in a particular institution. Any business venture benefits from having a strategic plan. The plan provides for assessment of the environment, including current and future opportunities, and identification of specific, measurable, realistic ways of taking advantage of those opportunities. Most importantly, perhaps, the strategic plan answers the question, "What business are we in?" Clearly defining a mission and vision helps a nursing unit or department focus its efforts on its core business.

Strategic planning and strategic management are necessary components of business in today's competitive and highly unstable health care environment. Strategic planning is a process similar to the nursing process, with defined and specific steps to be taken to ensure that a comprehensive and thorough process occurs. Strategic management involves implementation of the strategic plan to ensure that the organization is responsive to changes in its environment as well as to internal events.

Strategic planning and strategic management are not reserved exclusively for organizations. Individuals such as nurses can use these techniques to determine their own direction and establish objectives to ensure that they meet the goals they have set for themselves. Nurses in all areas of practice and in all employment settings can use the principles of strategic planning to explore programs, projects, and services and to advance their careers. Nurses who are involved in any aspect of an institution's strategic planning efforts should incorporate those activities into a personal portfolio (Oermann, 2002) and use those activities to reflect their competence and expertise as well as their own professional development.

◢ RESEARCH NOTE

Source

Titzer, J., Phillips, T., Tooley, S., Hall, N., Shirey, M. (2013). Nurse manager succession planning: Synthesis of the evidence. *Journal of Nursing Management, 21,* 971–979.

Purpose

The authors conducted a review of the literature to determine best practices for succession planning for nurse managers in order to identify strategies to increase the number of nurses prepared to assume unit-level leadership positions.

Discussion

Current challenges in the health care environment make strategic planning for nurse manager succession imperative. With high numbers of nurse managers facing retirement and many younger nurses lacking the desire to advance into nursing management due to the heavy demands placed on the unit leader, there are inadequate numbers of replacement nurse managers available. Despite the positive impact that effective nurse managers have on patient outcomes, research indicates that health care organizations do not routinely include nurse manager succession planning in their strategic plans.

Thirteen articles published between 2007 and 2012 were reviewed and synthesized. The articles included were all peer reviewed and included both formal research and anecdotal reports. Four common themes of succession planning were identified from the articles: current practices, elements, evaluation, and barriers.

The articles reviewed demonstrated that succession planning for nurse managers is not a common element in

Continued

RESEARCH NOTE—cont'd

strategic plans, and most nurse managers are selected based on clinical expertise or longevity. As a result, they are inadequately prepared and lack basic management competencies. The time new managers spend gaining competency in their roles is deleterious to patient outcomes, staff satisfaction, and productivity. The eight elements of succession planning identified included strategic planning, delineation of desired leadership competencies, projection of key positions for vacancy, identification of potential candidates, mentoring, professional development, allocation of necessary resources, and outcomes evaluation. In addition, evidence from this literature reviewed indicated that strategic succession planning included formal processes for evaluation. Evaluation methods consisted of use of management and leadership skills inventories, qualitative interviews and surveys, and organizational cost savings based on staff retention. Finally, identified barriers to succession planning included a failure to recognize the need, unwillingness of

current leadership to identify or develop potential leaders, lack of resources, challenges of the current health care environment, and the stresses on the nurse manager.

Application to Practice
The synthesis of evidence from the 13 reviewed articles resulted in the development of a nurse manager succession planning model consisting of the elements identified from the literature. One key element of the model is strategic planning and includes the role of current nurse leaders to act as "strategic thinkers" to ensure nursing input in the strategic decision-making process. These strategic decisions must include a formal process for succession planning for nurse managers that is supported by appropriate resource allocation and evaluation processes. This deliberate, proactive succession planning process will help organizations "manage environmental challenges effectively, while ensuring leadership continuity and strategic alignment" (p. 977).

CASE STUDY

Community General Hospital has had excessive unplanned 30-day readmissions of patients with congestive heart failure (CHF) over the past year and is facing a maximum 3% penalty from Medicare. One of the hospital's strategic goals is to maximize Medicare reimbursement. The chief nursing officer (CNO) has been assigned responsibility for implementation of this goal. The CNO challenges the nurse manager and staff of the medical cardiac unit to identify specific strategies to reduce the CHF readmission rate.

Recognizing that multiple disciplines care for patients with CHF, the nurse manager forms an inter-professional task force to address the high rate of readmissions. An initial 4-hour meeting for the team is scheduled to allow for team-building exercises and to give the team members an opportunity to consider the complexity of the issue. In preparation for this initial meeting, the nurse manager

asks each team member to document his/her role in caring for patients with CHF in order to discuss it with the other team members during the meeting.

During the initial meeting, after an interactive team building exercise, the nurse manager leads the team in sharing their roles and responsibilities in caring for CHF patients. This sharing leads to a discussion of the following questions:
• Where are we currently?
• Where do we want to go?

The team agrees that the current rate of readmissions is unacceptable in terms of quality patient care, which is a core value of the organization. In addition, the loss of revenue negatively affects the hospital's ability to fulfill its mission and vision. All members of the team agree to collaborate to identify strategies to reduce the readmission rate.

CRITICAL THINKING EXERCISE

Pursuant to the initial CHF readmission team meeting, the nurse manager of the cardiac medical unit arranges for additional weekly meetings for the team to conduct a SWOT analysis and develop strategies to address the high 30-day readmission rate for patients with CHF. Each team member researches the latest evidence-based practice guidelines for their discipline's contributions to the care of the patient with CHF.

1. What team members/disciplines should be included in this CHF readmission team? Why?
2. Once a plan is developed for reducing 30-day CHF readmissions, what elements of strategic management may be helpful to ensure implementation of the plan?
3. What should be included in the evaluation of the plan for reducing 30-day CHF readmissions?

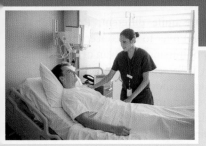

Professional Practice Models

Maura MacPhee, Farinaz Havaei

http://evolve.elsevier.com/Huber/leadership

The goals of safe and successful patient care delivery include high-quality and low-cost care with the achievement of patient and family outcomes and satisfaction levels. The ability to reach these objectives depends on the organization's approach to the matching of human and material resources with patient characteristics and health care needs via a model of professional practice for care delivery. Due to rising health care costs and global health provider shortages, many health care systems have had to transform themselves to find more efficient, effective ways to deliver safe, quality patient care with limited resources. Health care transformation has many names, such as redesign and restructuring. Responsible redesign is associated with quality improvement (QI). There are many QI tools and methods to assist organizational leaders with identification, implementation, and evaluation of care delivery innovations that yield positive, sustainable benefits to patients, providers, and organizations. One well-known conceptual framework by Donabedian (1988) is frequently used to "map" or determine what structures and processes promote positive outcomes.

The Donabedian (1988) three-concept framework is composed of **s**tructures, **p**rocesses, and **o**utcomes (S-P-O), and these three components are causally linked. Specific organizational structures are needed to support necessary care delivery processes to attain desired patient, provider, and organizational outcomes (White & Glazier, 2011). Structures include the way that care delivery is organized (e.g., team nursing, total patient care), the

types or classifications of staff providing care (i.e., skill mix), and the numbers of different types of staff (e.g., nurse–patient ratios, staffing levels). There are two broad categories of health care processes: clinical processes or services and interpersonal processes, such as collaborative teamwork, patient–provider communications, cultural sensitivity of care, and patient education. Outcome quality indicators are categorized by patients (e.g., falls, hospital-acquired infections, satisfaction with care), staff (e.g., job satisfaction, burnout), and the organization (e.g., hospital-wide performance measures).

Health care transformations often target the organization of nurses' work, particularly patient care delivery models. Responsible transformation, however, requires skilled leadership and application of QI tools, such as Donabedian's (1988) S-P-O framework. An example is culture change initiatives within nursing homes. A directive from the Patient Protection and Affordable Care Act of 2010 was to "transform both institutional and community-based long-term services and supports into a more person-centered system" (Grabowski et al., 2014, S65). There is considerable evidence to support the uptake of person-centered care delivery, including better resident and staff outcomes. Despite a federal directive, successful and sustainable culture change has been slow and difficult to sustain in the United States, and fewer than 2% of nursing homes succeeded in a culture shift over a 7-year period. In many instances, failures were due to lack of visionary leadership and lack of serious investment in the structures and processes necessary to reach desired outcomes (Grabowski et al., 2014).

Nursing care delivery model redesign is happening globally, and many of these initiatives have been tied to

Photo used with permission from JohnnyGreig/Getty Images.

safe staffing (MacPhee, 2014). At the unit level, the process of making safe staffing assignments depends on accurate assessments of patient care needs and shared decision-making processes between direct care nurses and management. International incidents related to safe staffing have raised professional and public awareness of the importance of safe staffing. For example, in the National Health Service of England, registered nurses (RNs) were replaced with unlicensed care aides across patient care sectors (e.g., long-term care, acute care). Unsafe RN staffing levels and introduction of RN-care–aide skill mix resulted in unnecessary patient injury and deaths. A government-commissioned public inquiry revealed erosion of safe staffing, leading to the implementation of national safe staffing policies (MacPhee, 2014). In the United States, the proposed Registered Nurse Safe Staffing Act (S.1132 — 114th Congress [2015–2016]) would mandate that each state ensure appropriate nurse staffing that meets patients' needs (American Nurses Association, 2015).

Care delivery model structures, processes, and expected outcomes have evolved over time to keep pace with the complexity of health care environments and patients, public and health policy mandates, and national and international health care trends. Some notable changes have been culture shifts toward patient-centered care/person-centered care philosophies (Epstein & Street, 2011; Grabowski et al., 2014) and interdisciplinary collaborative teamwork (Landman et al., 2014). Despite ongoing transformations of patient care delivery models, nurses need to ensure the presence of solid links between care delivery models and nursing professional practice models. Care delivery models represent the "nuts and bolts" of patient health care provision at unit or facility levels. Professional practice models act as an organizational umbrella for unit-level care delivery models, embodying the philosophy and essence of nursing's contributions to patient care. It is easy to get caught up in the functional or instrumental aspects of care delivery and overlook nursing's unique, carative role. Nurse leaders play a critical role in forging those solid links between a nursing vision and mission and the day-to-day, unit-by-unit delivery of care (Jost & Rich, 2010).

DEFINITIONS

There is confusion over the differences between the terms *professional practice models* and *care delivery models*. These concepts are often used interchangeably,

yet their meanings are quite different. **Professional practice models (PPMs)** refer to the conceptual framework and philosophy of nursing within an organization. One PPM definition is "a schematic description of a system, theory, or phenomenon that depicts how nurses practice, collaborate, communicate, and develop to provide the highest quality of care for those served by the organization" (Murphy et al., 2011, p. 67).

The core elements of a PPM include nursing values, leadership, the care delivery model, collaborative relationships and decision making, and professional development opportunities (Luzinksi, 2012). Many organizations have visual or pictorial representations of their PPMs. These may be found on websites or in organizational documents and reports such as nursing's annual report.

Care delivery models are the operational mechanisms by which care is actually provided to patients and families. Well-designed models maximize the quality and safety of nursing care. Functional care delivery models focus on management of nursing tasks or instrumental functions such as medication administration. Professional models acknowledge the complexity of nurses' work and provide opportunities for nurses to engage in "knowledge work" such as shared governance structures and processes (Dubois et al., 2013).

BACKGROUND

Executive leadership is responsible for making decisions about and designing strategies to create innovative work environments that support nurses' work. Work environments exert a strong influence over the safety and quality of patient care delivery (Aiken et al., 2013; Stimpfel et al., 2014). Professional practice models represent the importance and the valuing of nurses within an organization (Luzinski, 2012). Nursing care delivery models represent the organization of nurses' work at a unit level, and for management, they can be seen as the dynamic balance between routine resource management and the structure, process, and outcomes of practice. Given the complexity of nurses' work and the myriad factors that influence patient outcomes (not to mention staff and organizational outcomes), managers must actively collaborate with direct care nurses to determine what types of work organization will deliver the best outcomes (MacPhee, 2014). Due to financial constraints and workforce shortages, health care organizations are faced with strategic decisions that involve nurses, such as redesign of care delivery models with subsequent impacts on staffing, scheduling, and work flow. If these decisions are made only by management, quality improvement is less likely to occur.

Professional Practice Models

One important predictor of RN job satisfaction is the presence of a nurse professional practice model (PPM). Nurse job satisfaction is directly associated with nurse turnover, a significant human resource challenge for management (Hayes et al., 2012). Professional practice models consist of structures, processes, and values that support nurse control over practice and enhance job satisfaction and retention (Erickson & Ditomassi, 2011). The concept of "magnetism," arising from the Magnet Recognition Program®, addresses organizational attributes necessary for attracting and retaining nurses. There are five components of the Magnet model, and one of them is "exemplary professional practice." This component focuses on the PPM and its enactment within an organization (Luzinski, 2012).

Professional practice models are often associated with a theoretical framework, such as the Magnet model (Luzinski, 2012) or the American Association of Critical-Care Nurses' (AACN) Synergy Model (AACN, n.d.). Nurse-driven PPMs only flourish when nurse leadership/management at all levels of the organization support nursing professional practice. Evidence of professional practice support includes active shared governance councils and resources for nurse engagement in quality improvement. PPMs also flourish when there are strong links between the PPM and the organizational vision/mission statement and core values. Links between nursing values and organizational values better support an organization-wide culture of excellence (Luzinski, 2012). Mission, vision, values, and philosophy also are fundamental to strategic planning (see Chapter 14). Because they are foundational to PPMs, they are briefly reviewed here.

Mission Statements

Within an organization there is an established framework for management, typically represented by an organizational chart for each organization, and a characteristic collective of power and authority is vested in the managerial hierarchy. This legitimate authority, given by position, enables managers to meet the organization's goals. The purpose or goal of an organization is expressed by its *mission statement*. For health care organizations, the major purpose or mission is patient care delivery. Publicly posted mission statements inform key stakeholder groups, such as the public and employees, of the organization's key goals. Stakeholders are those individuals or groups who are affected by the organization and have a vested interest in its purpose and goals (MacPhee, 2007). Mission statements provide information and support an organization's public relations. For management at all levels of an organization, the mission statement acts as a blueprint or foundational guide for developing specific measurable objectives and actions.

Measurable *objectives and actions* associated with the mission statement explicitly represent what the organization is trying to do, and they help keep an organization on track by providing yardsticks and indicators for measuring present performance. Nurse managers need to ensure that their departmental/unit goals and performance measures are in alignment with the organization's mission. Lack of goal alignment across an organization can trigger conflict and slow progress toward goal completion (Porter, 2010). A common source of conflict related to goal achievement within complex health care environments is resource allocation, such as nurse staffing. An important leadership responsibility is to ensure that stakeholders agree with mission statement goals and support their enactment.

Vision Statements

Vision statements are often confused with mission statements. The vision statement is focused, however, on the future direction of the organization. Vision statements are crafted to describe the most desirable state at some future point in time, and they are meant to be an inspirational tool for organizational leadership to reenergize and motivate stakeholders, particularly if/when stakeholders are complacent, cynical, or start to disengage from the organization. Transformational nurse leaders often use imagery, stories, and participative strategies such as appreciative inquiry to sustain the vision and re-motivate disengaged staff (Brookes, 2011).

Values Statements

Core *values* are strongly held beliefs and priorities that guide organizational decision making. Core values are things that do not change. They are anchors or fundamentals that hold constant and relate to mission and purpose, whereas operations and business strategies change. Values drive how people truly act in organizations. Adams (2004, p. 2) stated, "Articulating values provides everyone with guiding lights, ways of choosing among competing priorities, and guidelines about how people will work together."

Philosophy

A statement of *philosophy* is defined as an explanation of the systems of beliefs that determine how the mission and vision will be achieved. The philosophy is abstract; it describes an ideal state and gives direction to achieving the purpose. It may begin with "We believe that . . ." For example, the system of beliefs, or philosophy, might be stated in any of the following ways:

- We believe that everyone has a right to the highest quality of client care.
- We believe that we have an obligation to render quality client care at a cost-effective price.
- We believe that any person who presents for care should receive care, regardless of his or her ability to pay.

The philosophy has implications for a nurse's practice role. If an organization's stated mission includes patient care, teaching, and research, then all employees will be expected to be involved in all three aspects of the mission. Part of the nurse's job will be to teach students and be involved in research. In one longitudinal study, more than 400 hospital-based nurses completed a questionnaire on ethical conflict, work-related stress, and organizational commitment. Nurses reported three types of ethical conflict with their places of employment: patient care values, value of nurses, and staffing policy values. A year later the researchers queried these same nurses about turnover intention and actual turnover. All three types of ethical conflict were significantly related to actual turnover (Gaudine & Thorne, 2012). Nurse leaders, therefore, need to identify values misalignment and address possible sources of ethical conflict before nurses take action and leave.

Policies and Procedures

Policies and procedures are two functional elements of an organization that are extensions of the mission statements. Both are written rules derived from the mission statement. Together they determine the nursing systems of the work unit and the department of nursing. The purpose of policies and procedures is to provide some order and stability so that the unit functions in a coordinated manner within the larger structure of nursing

and the institution. Organizations need to integrate the behaviors of employees to prevent random chaos and maintain some order, function, and structure. These plans are often referred to as *standard operating policies and procedures*. They guide personnel in decision making (Huber, 2013).

Policies

A **policy** is a guideline that has been formalized. It directs the action for thinking about and solving recurring problems related to the objectives of the organization.

There will be specific times when it is not clear who is supposed to do something, under what circumstances it should be done, or what should be done about unusual circumstances. For example, there are often controversies about the dress code because of disagreements about the definition of what is appropriate. This occurs, for example, when the dress code says, "Nurses will come to work dressed in appropriate attire." In response, organizations may, by policy, standardize the dress code. For example, all nurses wear gray scrubs and all housekeepers wear plum-colored scrubs.

Policies direct decision making and serve as guides to increase the likelihood of consistency in decisions and actions. Policies should be written, understandable, and general in nature to cover all employees. If written, they are *formal policies*. They should be readily available in the same form to all employees. Policies should be reviewed during employee orientation because they indicate the organization's intentions for goal achievement.

After institutional approval, policies need to be collected in a manual or computerized database with an online portal that is indexed, classified, and easily retrievable. Policies so organized can be easily replaced with revised ones, which often become necessary in light of new environmental circumstances such as changes in laws or regulations. Policy formulation in any organization is an ongoing core process. Hospitals will have a standing committee for the review of policies as a part of the organizational structure. Policies establish broad limits on and provide direction to decision making, yet they permit some initiative and individuality for unique circumstances.

Policies can be implied, or unwritten, if they are essentially established by patterns of decisions that have been made. In this situation, the *informal policies* represent an interpretation of observed behavior. For example, the organization may expect caring treatment for all clients.

BOX 15.1   Policies

- Serve as guides
- Help coordinate plans
- Control performance
- Increase consistency of action
- Should be written
- Usually are general in nature
- Refer to all employees

BOX 15.2   Procedures

- Provide step-by-step methods
- Are written in detail
- Provide guidelines for commonly occurring events
- Provide a ready reference
- Guide performance of an activity
- Should include the following:
  - A statement of purpose
  - Identification of who performs activity
  - Steps in the procedure
  - A list of supplies and equipment needed

This expectation may not be written as a policy of the organization. However, by the decisions and disciplinary actions that occur, an employee can infer that there is a policy that will be enforced even though it is not written. The vast majority of policies are and should be written, however. Informal and unwritten policies are less desirable because they can lead to systematic bias or unfairness in their application and enforcement (Box 15.1).

Some general areas in nursing require policy formulation. These are areas in which there is confusion about the locus of responsibility and in which lack of guidance might result in the neglect, malpractice, or "malperformance" of an act necessary to the patient's welfare. For example, clear policies need to be in place about medication error reporting and follow-up. A policy is necessary in those areas in which it is important that all persons adhere to the same pattern of decision making given a certain circumstance. Areas pertaining to the protection of patients' or families' rights should also have written policies. For example, the use of restraints to manage difficult patients came under scrutiny as the Omnibus Budget Reconciliation Act of 1987 (OBRA) pushed restraint-reduction strategies and created policy revisions. Other examples are policies related to "do not resuscitate" and end-of-life care. Areas involving matters of human resource management and personnel welfare, such as vacation leave, should have written policies. Many conflicts arise about the scheduling of vacations. How many people can be off at any one time? How long in advance must a vacation request be made? How is the priority for granting requests to be determined (e.g., by seniority or order of request)? The policy provides explicit criteria to inform management's decisions (Huber, 2013).

Procedures

Procedures are step-by-step directions and methods for actions to follow in common situations. **Procedures** are descriptions of how to carry out an activity and should be evidence based. They are usually written in sufficient detail to provide the information required by all persons engaging in the activity. This means that procedures should include a statement of purpose and identify who is to perform the activity. Procedures should include the steps necessary and the list of supplies and equipment needed. They help achieve regularity and serve as a ready reference for all personnel (Box 15.2).

The similarities between policies and procedures are that both are a means for accomplishing goals and objectives. Both are necessary for the smooth functioning of any work group or organization. The difference between a policy and a procedure is that a policy is a directive that must be followed, such as use of restraints, and a procedure provides direction, such as evidence-based steps for performing a urinary catheterization. There are legal implications to the application of policies and procedures. For example, the nurse may be held liable for failing to follow written policies and procedures. Thus it is important for nurses to be informed about the policies and procedures governing practice in an institution. In addition, both policies and procedures need regular, periodic reviews (Huber, 2013).

Clinical Protocols

The variety of types of clinical protocols have been called *structured care methodologies* (SCMs). SCMs are streamlined interdisciplinary tools used to "identify best practices, facilitate standardization of care, and provide a mechanism for variance tracking, quality enhancement, outcomes measurement, and outcomes research" (Cole & Houston, 1999, p. 53). Examples of SCMs are *critical pathways, evidenced-based algorithms, protocols, standards of care, order sets,* and *clinical practice guidelines.* All forms of clinical protocols need to be evidence based. The use of best evidence is considered the gold standard to reduce practice variation in an environment focused on patient outcomes. Critical paths outline time and the sequence of events for an episode-of-care delivery. Resources appropriate in amount and sequence to a specific case type and individual client are managed for length of stay, critical events and timing, and anticipated outcomes. A *critical path* is a written plan that identifies key, critical, or predictable incidents that must occur at set times to achieve client outcomes within an appropriate length of stay in a hospital setting. As a pathway, it is a tracking system for the timing of treatments and interventions, health outcomes, complications, activity, and teaching/learning (Huber, 2013). Pathways are also considered a method of quality improvement to assist health care providers with clinical process innovation (Vanhaecht et al., 2010). Pathway effectiveness has been questioned for complex care situations and concerns that they are driven by a cost-cutting managerial agenda (Watts, 2012). In an exploration of end-of-life care pathways to promote a "good death," Watts argued that a potential benefit of this type of pathway is raised awareness of meaningful care interventions that offer dignity and quality of care to dying individuals and their families. A concern, however, is that end-of-life pathways within a biomedical framework may encourage one conceptualization of "good death" and dying "management."

Healthy Work Environments

Positive work environments are also known as **healthy work environments** (see Chapters 3, 4, and 8) or quality practice environments, and they are often found in Magnet-designated organizations. Magnet hospitals are known for their excellent nursing care, leadership, and superior patient outcomes—such as lower mortality and morbidity rates—over non-Magnet hospitals (McHugh et al., 2013). Magnet hospitals' work environments have specific structures and processes that support nursing professional practice (Houston et al., 2012; Stimpfel et al., 2014). Kramer and colleagues (2010) did an analysis of the healthy work environment literature using the Donabedian's (1988) S-P-O framework. Box 15.3 summarizes organizational structures associated with Magnet-like healthy work environments.

Stimpfel and colleagues (2014) found that a significantly greater proportion of nurses in Magnet hospitals described their quality of care delivery as excellent compared with nurses in non-Magnet hospitals. Another key study finding was the important role of the work

---

> **BOX 15.3   Organizational Structures for Healthy Work Environments**
>
> - Effective leaders at all levels of the organization
> - Professional development opportunities
> - Staffing structures that consider nurse competencies, patient needs, and teamwork
> - Interdisciplinary collaboration
> - Empowered, shared decision making
> - Patient-centered culture/culture of safety
> - Quality improvement infrastructure, evidence-based practice
> - Visible acknowledgment of nursing's unique, valued contributions (e.g., professional practice model, vision/mission/philosophy statements)

---

environment. The presence of a supportive, professional practice environment was the key factor differentiating between nurses' reports of quality of care. Of note is that most Magnet-like characteristics are easy to adapt to different work contexts, such as involving nurses in patient care delivery decisions and offering regular nurse in-services and workshops on evidence-based practices. Aiken and colleagues (2011) conducted a study in more than 600 US hospitals to determine the impact of nurse staffing, nurse education, and types of work environments on patient mortality rates. A survey tool was used to determine nurse workloads, defined as nurse–patient ratios. The Nurse Work Index (NWI) assessed nurses' work environments on five Magnet-like characteristics, including nurse leadership, nurse participation in hospital affairs, and professional development opportunities. The researchers classified work environments as good or poor, depending on NWI scores. Across all hospitals, the presence of nurses with baccalaureate education significantly decreased the risk of patient death. The effect of decreased workloads only made a difference in positive work environments. The researchers concluded that the impact of improved nurse staffing is diluted by poor work environments. Efforts to address nurse workloads by adding more nurses, therefore, may fail to influence patient outcomes if other Magnet-like aspects of the work environment are not addressed beforehand.

TYPES OF CARE DELIVERY MODELS

There are a variety of patient care delivery models. Care delivery model redesign is influenced by fiscal responsibility, accountability to the consumer, available resources, and quality and safety considerations. Although all models have their advantages and disadvantages, there is no one right way to structure patient care. The appropriate care delivery model is the one that maximizes existing resources while meeting organizational goals and objectives (i.e., the mission). Quite often, aspects of older, previous models are incorporated into new delivery models. It is important, therefore, to understand the variety of models available, both old (traditional) and new (evolving and innovative). Pure nursing models (effective in less complex times) have yielded to collaborative practice and interdisciplinary approaches with the proliferation of health care provider roles, expedited care processes, and increased patient acuity and needs. Knowing history helps nurses understand what has been done before and better analyze options for current suitability.

Traditional Nursing Care Delivery Models

Historians mark the emergence of modern nursing from the time of Florence Nightingale's work in the Crimea. Nightingale believed that nursing care of patients included spiritual well-being as well as the environment. The evolution of nursing models of care has resulted from the impact of economic, social, and political agendas over the past century. There are five traditional nursing models of care: (1) private duty, (2) functional, (3) team, (4) primary, and (5) case management. Of these, functional, team, primary, and case management were and are currently associated with hospital nursing practice. Private duty and case management were associated with public health, home health care, and community health but have been adapted to the inpatient setting. Private duty, later called *case* or *case management,* was the original way nursing care was delivered; it later became the foundation for public health nursing and community service delivery (Huber, 2013).

Private Duty Nursing

Private duty nursing is sometimes called *case nursing,* because it is based on the case method where each patient is a case. Another term is *total patient care.* There are two ways of thinking about total patient care. One approach is holistic care of the total patient, including mind, body, and spirit. Another approach is functionally based, where a nurse assumes total care for one patient. Private duty nursing is the oldest care model in

the United States. Between 1890 and 1929 in the United States, graduate nurses acted as private duty nurses, caring for patients in their homes (Shirey, 2008). They did the cooking, cleaning, bathing of wounds, and organizing of the household functions, basically functioning as a home manager. A form of hospital case nursing evolved between 1900 and the 1930s. When the Great Depression hit, most families were too poor to afford private duty nurses and so nurses were without jobs. Hospitals then began to employ graduate nurses. As the graduate nurses who had been doing private duty moved into the hospital, they wanted to retain the type of care model to which they had become accustomed. Private duty was transplanted into hospital settings for as long as nurses were paid by clients. When nurses became employees of hospitals, the kind of client care that private duty allowed was not possible within the organizational structure of hospital staff nursing (Huber, 2013; Reverby, 1987).

The advantages of private duty nursing were one-to-one care, fostering close nurse–patient relationships. This model also allowed nurses a great degree of autonomy. The disadvantages were the high cost and low efficiency associated with this model. With the shift to hospital-based care, nurses' job security was also questionable (Reverby, 1987; Shirey, 2008).

Two main variations on the basic pattern of private duty nursing developed within hospitals.

Group nursing was a care model proposed in the 1930s by Janet Geister, then the executive director of the American Nurses Association (ANA). Defined as nursing group practice, the idea of group nursing in hospitals was similar to divisional private duty in which several clients shared a private nurse. The plan was to reorganize private duty from individual to group practice both inside and outside the hospital. The intention was to link a group practice registry of private duty nurses to a community's public health nursing service, but the plan died after political pressure. Hospitals also experimented with a group nursing care modality, described as being halfway between a private duty arrangement and graduate nurse hospital staff nursing. Under this plan, clients were grouped together in a special unit in which several clients shared a private nurse. Thus three nurses could do 8-hour shifts for two clients instead of four nurses being needed for 12-hour shifts. The hospital paid the nurses' wages but charged the clients directly as a surcharge on the hospital bill. The advantages included shorter hours for nurses, order and regularity in hospital staffing, steady employment for nurses, slightly cheaper rates for clients, and responsibility for the total care of several clients for the nurse. Nurses had the autonomy and care delivery method of private duty without its isolation and uncertainty. Nurses were members of the hospital's staff, yet their time was specifically allocated only to a set number of clients who paid for this service directly. However, economic and political pressures for more efficiency, productivity, and service cut off the adoption of this system in hospitals (Reverby, 1987). It is interesting to note the parallels between group nursing and what eventually came to be the way physicians organized themselves (Huber, 2013).

Total patient care initially occurred in intensive care, hospice care, and home health care. The term *total patient care* has come to mean the assignment of each client to a nurse who plans and delivers care during a work shift (Minnick et al., 2007). This model is also known as patient allocation (Tran et al., 2010).

Functional Nursing

Functional nursing emerged as a care model in the 1940s. In this model, the division of labor is assigned according to specific tasks and technical aspects of the job, such as medication administration and taking vital signs. Under functional nursing, the nurse identifies the tasks to be done for a shift. The work is divided and assigned to nursing and support personnel, such as care aides.

Functional nursing was the norm in US hospitals from the late 1800s through the end of World War II. In the early 1900s, business and industry concepts of "scientific management" emphasized efficiency. The efficiency was gained by breaking down a work process into its component task steps and then analyzing and timing the steps, establishing standards, and determining the best way to perform each task. Thus managerial control over the planning and execution of work could be established. Assembly lines in factories were one result. Functional nursing was developed as a result of this concern for task analysis and proper division of the nursing workload. Under this model, there might be a "temperature nurse," a "medication nurse," a nurse for the right side of the hall, and a nurse for the left side of the hall (Huber, 2013; Reverby, 1987). This model enabled hospitals to improve service efficiency and control labor costs by requiring fewer RNs. Another advantage of this model was clear division of labor. Over time, with the increased complexity of patient care needs, the functional model has become less favored due to the fragmentation of care and patient exposure to multiple care providers. The focus on tasks diminishes nurse critical thinking and the patient-centered approach of care delivery (Shirey, 2008).

Team Nursing

Team nursing is a care model that uses a group of people led by a knowledgeable nurse. It is a delivery approach that provides care to a group of patients by coordinating a team of RNs, licensed practical nurses, and care aides under the supervision of one nurse, called the *team leader*. Team nursing developed in the early 1950s in response to a shortage of RNs and in reaction to the dissatisfaction with functional nursing (Shirey, 2008).

Team nursing is designed to make use of each member's capabilities to meet the nursing needs of his or her group of clients. The nurse leader considers the scopes of practice and expertise for each team member when making team assignments. Each team member has his/her own patient assignments, and team members are expected to assist and support each other as needed. This model requires effective team leadership, collaboration, and frequent communication. A smoothly functioning team provides extra surveillance for patients and greater support for novice nurses (Fernandez et al., 2012). Blurring of scopes of practice along with educational preparation and training in professional and specialty silos are significant challenges for team nursing models (MacPhee, 2014). The research literature suggests that teams with a greater proportion of RNs or richer skill mix have better patient outcomes (Aiken et al., 2011). Kalisch and Lee (2011) found that nurse reports of more collaborative or "higher" teamwork were associated with better staffing levels and richer skill mix.

Primary Nursing

Primary nursing began in the 1970s as a way to overcome the discontent with functional and team nursing's emphasis on tasks and discrete functions that directed nurses' attention away from holistic care of the patient. This matched a societal trend toward accountability, as well as nursing's rising level of professionalism. In this model, the primary nurse has 24-hour-per-day accountability for the patient's plan of care from admission to discharge. Associate nurses oversee patient care delivery when the primary nurse is not on shift, although associate nurses are expected to follow the primary nurse's plan of care. This model enhances continuity of care; maximizes RN utilization of professional competencies, such as critical thinking, collaboration, and teaching; and philosophically complements holistic, patient-centered care. Although this model is favored by RNs and patients due to its relational nature, it takes time and energy investment to have 24-hour accountability. Implementation of this model is threatened when nurses are required to care for too many patients (Shirey, 2008). Primary nursing was initially associated with all-RN staffing due to the greater depth of RNs' formal educational preparation. Due to cost containment measures since the 1980s, this once-popular model is used less for care delivery (Shirey, 2008).

A systematic review of care delivery models' effect on nurse and patient outcomes was conducted by Fernandez and colleagues (2012). More than 3000 studies were published on care delivery models between 1985 and 2011. The final review focused on 16 studies with strong methodologies, and the majority of these were comparative studies in acute care settings. The most popular models (or variation of them) in the literature were team nursing and total patient care. Studies comparing team nursing with other models (e.g., total patient care, primary nursing) found little differences between them with respect to quality of communication among staff, nurse job satisfaction, absenteeism rates, and role clarity (Fernandez et al., 2012). Impact on patient outcomes was equivocal. Team nursing was associated with significantly decreased medication errors, less fewer adverse events involving intravenous management, and lower pain scores for patients, although there were no differences for patient fall rates. Overall, the researchers concluded that team nursing is often preferred when there are staff with less experience or skills levels on a particular unit. Nine studies in a systematic review on primary nursing models between 1990 and 2013 met inclusion criteria (Mattila et al., 2014). One study found that the primary nursing model was less costly than a team nursing model. In two studies within maternity care units, primary nursing was associated with mothers who reported less breast discomfort and engaged more effectively in breastfeeding. Another study found that nurses on primary nursing units reported higher quality care delivery than nurses on team nursing units. The researchers emphasized that primary nursing, especially in areas such as maternity, should be family centered. Studies in the review focused on individual patients and nursing staff.

Case Management

Case management as a nursing model of care evolved in the late 1980s. It has been defined as both a process (it is a provider intervention) and a care delivery model. Case management has developed as a method to manage care. The Case Management Society of America (CMSA) is the professional organization representing case managers in practice. It is a multidisciplinary organization. The CMSA definition of case management is "a collaborative process of assessment, planning, facilitation, care coordination, evaluation, and advocacy for options and services to meet an individual's and family's comprehensive health needs through communication and available resources to promote quality, cost-effective outcomes" (CMSA, 2016). **Managed care** is care coordination that is organized to achieve specific patient outcomes, given fiscal and other resource constraints (Huber, 2013).

Case management and care coordination have been the care delivery models used for years by public health and community health nurses, although case management can occur in any health sector (e.g. acute care, community), extend across the health care continuum, or be linked to a population focus, such as school nursing (Engelke et al., 2008). In the face of strong economic external forces, acute care hospitals turned to case management to help reduce provider practice variation and to ensure the appropriateness of care. The risk with case management models is that communication and coordination infrastructures may not be available or integrated for effectiveness (Huber, 2013).

Case management has components of health services delivery, coordination, and monitoring, through which multiple service needs of clients are met. Hospital-based acute care nursing case management focuses on an entire episode of illness, crossing all settings in which the client receives care. Care is directed by a case manager, who is not always a nurse, and can be unit or population focused (Huber, 2013). An example is a nurse-led case management program for patients requiring peritoneal dialysis (Chow & Wong, 2010). An intervention study compared successful transition from hospital to home for patients with end-stage renal failure: 42 patients in a control group received routine discharge services, and 43 patients participated in a comprehensive education program with case manager follow-up by phone at regular intervals. The Kidney Disease Quality of Life short form tool was used to assess patients' general health and specific concerns of dialysis patients. Study patients had reduced anxiety, increased confidence and coping with fluid and dietary restrictions, and were more engaged in daily activities. The researchers surmised that the nurse case management approach, a collaborative and holistic approach to care management, "humanize[d] medical technologies" and provided a "supportive and empowering environment" for patients (Chow & Wong, 2010, p. 1790). Other research has shown that care delivery models with an RN case manager who interacts with other team members and involves the patient and family in care planning are associated with improved patient outcomes (Hajewski & Shirey, 2014).

EVOLVING MODELS

Nursing shortages and health care reform will continue to have a strong impact on the creation of **current and evolving types** of patient care delivery models. Nurse staffing models were retooled in the late 1980s as a result of a severe nursing shortage and in an attempt to complement the work of the professional nurse with the use of nursing extenders (Fernandez et al., 2012; Shirey, 2008). Many of the resulting structures for patient care are skill mix models or mixed models where nurses are partnered with a variety of "extenders" or multi-skilled workers. Outcome studies have clearly demonstrated the negative impact of "substitution models" in which extenders have not been used to complement nurses but rather served as replacements (MacPhee, 2014). The seminal and replicated work of Aiken and Colleagues (Aiken et al., 2011, 2013, 2016) contributes a body of evidence that richer RN-specific skill mix reduces patient mortality. Care delivery model redesign needs to always be considered with respect to nursing's professional practice standards and code of ethics.

Patient- and Family-Centered Care

Patient-centered care (PCC) or family-centered care has been in the health care literature for more than 50 years. When the Institute of Medicine (IOM, now called the National Academies of Sciences, Engineering, and Medicine, Health and Medicine Division) (2001) included PCC as one of its major goals for twenty-first century health care improvement, many health care organizations based it on their strategic vision, mission, and core values. PCC is "care that is compassionate, empathetic, and responsive to the needs, values and expressed preferences of each individual patient; patients should be

> **BOX 15.4   The Eight Dimensions of Patient-Centered Care**
>
> 1. Respect for patient preferences, values, needs
> 2. Information, education, communication
> 3. Coordination, integration of services
> 4. Emotional support
> 5. Physical comfort
> 6. Family/close other involvement
> 7. Continuity, safe transitions between care settings (e.g., hospital to home)
> 8. Access to care and services

informed decision-makers in their care" (Rathert et al., 2013, p. 2). Family-centered care is often understood to be an integral component of PCC, where family members are considered critical supports and advocates for the patient. Family-centered care also highlights the importance of helping families cope and recognizes the diverse cultural and ethical beliefs of each patient and family (Gooding et al., 2011). The IOM (2001) used eight dimensions to operationalize PCC (see Box 15.4).

Underlying PCC is nurses' determination of patient preferences, their provision of realistic care options, and their assistance with making care decisions based on patient values versus provider values (Burman et al., 2013). A number of decision support tools have been created to assist nurses and other health care providers with guiding patients and their families through decision making (Légaré & Witteman, 2013), and decision aids are available for patients and families as well (Stiggelbout et al., 2012).

INNOVATIVE AND FUTURE MODELS

The complexity of health care delivery necessitates dynamic, flexible models. The IOM's 2001 report *Crossing the Quality Chasm: A New Health System for the 21st Century* describes the need for sweeping change and redesign of patient care delivery models to foster innovation and improve the delivery of care. Nurses have opportunities to lead innovative model redesigns. In the United States and other countries, many older citizens suffer from multiple chronic conditions that involve the interactions of physical, cognitive, and emotional health problems. These individuals have frequent care transitions (e.g., from home to hospital to assisted living) that involve many health care providers in many different settings. This population is particularly vulnerable to breakdowns in PCC. A number of new care models, known as "transitional care," have emerged to promote safe passage of senior patients between different providers and services (Naylor, 2012).

One well-studied model is the *transitional care model* (TCM), a nurse-led, team-based care delivery model for chronically ill older adults. The transitional care nurse leader (TCN) is typically master's prepared with population-specific clinical expertise. Three National Institute of Nursing Research–funded randomized controlled trials using TCM have demonstrated improved quality of care outcomes and cost savings. Some notable outcomes are reduced numbers of unnecessary hospital readmissions and enhanced patient satisfaction (Naylor, 2012).

A related care delivery model is the *patient-centered medical home* (PCMH). The PCMH was originally designed by the American Academy of Pediatrics to care for children with special needs. This model refocuses patient care from the hospital to the primary care setting. The current model has expanded to include PCC across the life span (Jackson et al., 2013). Approximately 25% of primary care patients have one or more psychiatric disorders, such as depression and anxiety. This population often has chronic conditions such as diabetes and heart disease, and psychological disorders often impair these patients' capacity to manage their own care or care of others. The PCMH is being trialed with this population to decrease unnecessary primary care/specialty care visits and hospitalizations and to improve self-care management with diet, exercise, and medication adherence. The PCMH for this population uses a nurse (i.e., care manager) to promote education and shared decision making with respect to treatment adjustments (e.g., medication management), and to track common psychiatric disorders such as depression. The nurse care manager connects weekly with a psychiatric consultant and updates the PCMH primary care provider as needed. Nurse care managers are tasked with monitoring patients to ensure no one "falls through the cracks." In one pilot (Katon et al., 2010) with specially trained medical nurse care managers, PCMH patients had decreased depression scores and improved physiological parameters (e.g., blood pressure, glycemic control) versus patients receiving usual care. In addition, this pilot was associated with significant cost savings over a 2-year period.

Health care reform efforts, such as the TCM and the PCMH, preceded the passage of the federal 2010 Patient Protection and Affordable Care Act (ACA). Federal interest was in new payment and delivery models with proven successes (e.g., positive patient outcomes, cost savings) (Katon & Unutzer, 2013). Continuity of care, with seamless communication and care coordination, became new imperatives under the ACA. The primary goal of this statute was to improve access to health care through insurance reforms. An outcome of the ACA, however, has been the generation of many new care delivery models that integrate health care services (Hardcastle et al., 2011). The ACA has prompted a shift toward primary health care, emphasizing disease prevention and health promotion. The focus for too long has been on health care services that treat disease symptomology. More than 50% of all deaths in the United States are due to preventable conditions that result from individual behaviors (e.g., smoking, diet, inactivity), the environment (e.g., contaminated water, food, pollution), and the social determinants of health (e.g., income, housing, education). Thus new care models focus on prevention. Preventive interventions that target root causes are responsible for 80% of successful reductions in morbidity and mortality; health care services that treat disease are responsible for less than 20% of morbidity/mortality reduction (Hardcastle et al., 2011). The ACA helped to forge integration of services at the care delivery model level, and it was the catalyst at higher levels for policies that integrate public health and health care.

Customer Satisfaction

A valuable outcome of PPMs is customer satisfaction. Patient satisfaction or customer satisfaction are measured in a variety of ways. For example, in health care, the Hospital Consumer Assessment of Healthcare Providers and Systems (HCAHPS) is a national, standardized survey of patients' perspectives about hospital care and is used by the Centers for Medicare & Medicaid Services (CMS) and endorsed by the National Quality Forum. Hospitals in the United States and Canada are publicly reporting patient satisfaction scores for accountability and accreditation purposes, such as the Hospital Report Series in Canada (Canadian Institute for Health Information, 2017).

PCC or family-centered care has been studied for its relationship to patient satisfaction. A systematic review of PCC studies between 1990 and 2012 yielded over 1200 studies. Forty of these studies were methodologically rigorous (Rathert et al., 2013). Regardless of methodology, there were positive relationships between PCC and patient satisfaction and patient reports of well-being. Some research suggests that patient satisfaction and well-being are associated with patient compliance and self-management behaviors (Rathert et al., 2013).

LEADERSHIP AND MANAGEMENT IMPLICATIONS

Fundamentally, a care delivery model is the way patients' needs are matched to health care resources to achieve positive clinical outcomes. Through many complex relationships, the care delivery model influences the quality of nursing care provided and its cost. A number of nursing care models have been developed, and there is evidence of evolutionary changes underway. Traditionally, care delivery was provided within a pure nursing framework. Over time, nursing care delivery methods were adapted to better fit external forces and the balance of the needs of patients and the needs of employing organizations. With these changes came variations in modes of delivery (e.g., team nursing, total patient care), skill mix, staffing levels, and nurse roles and accountabilities. Nursing care delivery has become more complex as integration with other provider disciplines—such as through interdisciplinary teams—is essential to meet the patients' needs through the entire continuum of care. Future trends point to greater integration and inter-professional team collaboration models as health care reform drives changes within the health care industry.

"The Affordable Care Act is altering the way healthcare is delivered" (Katz & Frank, 2010, p. 82). The IOM's vision for the future, with a key feature being new models of care, has been carried forward in the ACA. The themes of integration and coordination of care, addressing needs in a comprehensive manner with patients as key partners, and providing services efficiently continue to predominate and trigger a radical shift in the delivery of health care toward primary health care. Reimbursement structures and incentives to health care providers are incentivizing new models and offering leadership opportunities for nurses (Huber, 2013).

Nursing leaders and managers must have a broad vision to facilitate the design of care delivery models that meet the objectives of cost containment, patient satisfaction, quality, and safety outcomes over the course of the care cycle. Nursing leaders are in the perfect position to lead the changes essential in care delivery redesign. Nursing, as a major percentage of the health care labor force, must be able to demonstrate its effectiveness in producing financial as well as clinical outcomes. The challenge to prove "value" will continue.

Mentoring staff to participate in the creation of new care delivery methods is an aspect of effective leadership. Many factors, including the environmental context, influence successful implementation of new models, and nurses need to be engaged in these quality improvement initiatives. There is evidence to show that professional practice models, particularly their valuing of nursing and their shared governance structures and processes, are critical to nurse satisfaction and retention. Further, there is evidence that care delivery models, a component of professional practice models, are associated with nurse, patient, and organizational outcomes. Nurses and nurse leaders, therefore, need to be front and center when planning patient care delivery strategies at all levels of the organization. The leadership and management challenge is to balance risk taking and adoption of innovations with the pragmatic necessity to be systematic, evaluative, and realistic. The American Organization of Nurse Executives (AONE) (2012) has developed a *Guiding Principles for the Role of the Nurse in Future Care Delivery* toolkit to help organizations design and build the best location-specific care delivery model.

CURRENT ISSUES AND TRENDS

The challenges for patient care in the future are massive. The work environment of the nurse is dramatically different now. Cost containment and demands for quality and safety outcomes will continue to drive care delivery model redesign. The Donabedian S-P-O framework can be used to plan and test model structures and processes associated with quality, safe care delivery outcomes.

Clearly, forces and pressures outside of professional nursing influence care models. It is not known which is the best model for each patient care setting, and research evidence to support specific inpatient nursing care models is seriously limited (Fernandez et al., 2012). Nurses are urged to examine their patient populations, come to grips with the business aspects of health care, and remain vigilant in analyzing emerging economic and clinical trends in order to be active participants in the creation of patient care delivery models of the future.

A final trend worth noting is the shift toward interprofessional collaborative leadership. In complex health care environments, nurses and nurse leaders must learn to work constructively in intra-professional and inter-professional teams. "We" forms of leadership need to replace "I" forms of leadership (MacPhee et al., 2014). Nurses play a critical role in facilitating this transition by encouraging knowledge exchange, shared problem solving, and the creation and reinforcement of patient-centered/family-centered goals. Traditional hierarchies in health care will only be replaced when true collaboration exists within the organization. Nurses are exceptionally skilled at building informal and formal relationships across levels, permitting more rapid coordination and service integration and more effective communication. Nurse leaders, therefore, have the capacity to lead the way in care delivery model redesign and innovation.

RESEARCH NOTE

Source

Dubois, C-A., D'Amour, D., Tchouaket, E., Clarke, S., Rivard, M., & Blais, R. (2013). Associations of patient safety outcomes with models of nursing care organization at unit level in hospitals. *Journal of Quality in Health Care, 25*(2), 110–117.

Purpose

Dubois and colleagues used a care delivery model taxonomy with five dimensions to study the influence of different types of functional and professional care delivery models on patient outcomes. They applied their taxonomy to 22 medical units in 11 Canadian hospitals and identified four distinct types of care delivery models: two functional models and two professional models. The researchers classified the functional models as basic or adaptive. Adaptive models were characterized by an expanded scope of practice where practical nurses performed a broader array of patient care tasks. Among the professional models, there were basic and innovative models. The innovative models involved RNs in expanded roles, including oversight for quality improvement initiatives.

Patient outcomes were measured as six types of nurse-sensitive adverse events, or those events directly related to the quality of nursing care. The six adverse events were medication administration errors, falls, hospital acquired pneumonia, urinary tract infections, pressure ulcers, and unjustified restraint use. The five taxonomy dimensions were staffing intensity (care hours per patient day), skill mix (proportion of RN hours/total nursing hours), education level (proportion of university graduate hours/total nursing hours), scope of practice, and the practice environment (Dubois et al., 2013). Scope of practice was assessed with the Actual Scope of Nursing Practice Questionnaire that categorizes the degree to which nurses maximize their use of professional competencies (e.g., assessment, planning, teaching, and communications). Practice environments were assessed with the well-known Nursing Work Index.

Discussion

Table 15.1 summarizes the performance of the four care delivery models with respect to the five taxonomy dimensions. A key finding of this study was that patients' risk for experiencing adverse events was significantly lower in both professional models versus the two functional models. There are multiple factors that influence patient safety outcomes. The innovative professional model was associated with the least number of patient adverse events. This model also had a richer skill mix, higher staffing intensity, more university-educated nurses, and a positive practice environment with RNs in expanded roles, including leadership

TABLE 15.1 **Performance of Four Care Delivery Models**				
	FUNCTIONAL MODELS		**PROFESSIONAL MODELS**	
Care Delivery Model Dimensions	**Basic**	**Adaptive**	**Basic**	**Innovative**
Staffing Intensity	Low	High	Low	High
Skill Mix	Low	Low	High	High
Education Level	Low	Low	Low	High
Practice Environment (positive, less positive)	Less positive	Less positive	More Positive	More positive
Capacity for Innovation (High to Low)	Low	Low	Low	High
Scope of Practice	Low	Low	Moderate	Moderate

Continued

RESEARCH NOTE—cont'd

and quality improvement. The innovative professional model is most closely aligned with the Magnet model of professional practice environments. The findings in this paper are supported by other research where richer skill mix, better staffing levels, baccalaureate nurse preparation, and Magnet-like environments are known to produce better patient outcomes. This study put all these factors together, illustrating the validity and reliability of these findings, and challenging us with the complexity of today's health care delivery.

Application to Practice
Nurse leaders need to use research evidence to deliberately structure and advocate for work environments and nurses' work organization (i.e., care delivery models) that are associated with quality, safe patient care delivery.

CASE STUDY

Overview
Memorial Medical Center is a 400-bed teaching hospital. The care delivery model for all areas is total patient care, with RNs of different experience levels having shift responsibility for a group of seven to eight patients on medical and surgical floors. The third floor is a general medical unit with 72 beds. Patient diagnoses include cardiovascular (with telemetry monitoring), renal, pulmonary, oncology, and gastrointestinal diagnoses. An interim patient care manager has responsibility for the unit. Charge nurses are responsible for daily operations and frequently have patient assignments. Novice nurses account for 30% of the staff. Certified nursing assistants (CNAs) are occasionally assigned to a nurse but are more likely to be assigned tasks. Their responsibilities include basic custodial care, and they are frequently assigned as "sitters."

There have been many patient and physician complaints regarding the nursing care provided. Reporting of significant incidents and "near misses" have increased. The nursing director for the area recently conducted a comprehensive assessment of patient care to determine whether changes in the method of care delivery are needed.

Assessment and Findings
The director's assessment found that patient care delivery at Memorial Medical Center is fragmented, with functions being performed among multiple caregivers with little communication and coordination. Nursing assessments and reassessments are not timely or complete, and evidence of nursing care planning is limited in the clinical documentation. Nurses are frequently unaware of the patient's diagnosis and medical plan of care. Nursing tasks are the focus of care, and evidence of critical thinking for decision making is lacking, especially among novice nurses. Care coordination is performed by the case manager, but the manager rarely communicates with point-of-care nurses. Discharge planning is usually not considered at time of admission, frequently delaying discharges.

Communication of the plan of care from shift to shift and from caregiver to caregiver is inadequate because of a lack of continuity (with 12-hour shifts), problem identification, and prioritization. Inter-professional communication between providers (including physicians and nurses) is sporadic and incomplete; nurses rarely use tools such as SBAR and handoff reports to standardize and share critical information. Nurses are not comfortable with delegation of tasks to CNAs and frequently assume non-nursing functions. There is no mechanism for oversight or support for novice or temporary nursing staff. Professional development opportunities are lacking, and some staff feel that their assignments are beyond their scope.

Care Delivery Redesign
The nursing director and the nursing vice president agree that care delivery redesign is necessary to meet the objectives of quality patient care. The nursing director initiates a redesign process by forming a team of intraprofessional (i.e., members of the nursing care team, such as RNs and CNAs) and inter-professional care providers from the third floor. The team plans and introduces a quality improvement project that includes provider focus groups, discussions with a patient representative for the unit, an environmental scan of other hospitals' care delivery models, and a focused literature review. Staff meetings include time to brief everyone on planned changes and obtain feedback; openness and transparency are ground rules for this initiative.

A collaborative decision is made to use modular nursing, given the spatial layout of the third floor. Modular nursing is a form of team nursing that takes advantage of a unit's structural features or physical floor plan where clusters of similar patients are cared for within structural modules. The third floor unit is split into two separate units to maximize exposure to, and "knowing" of, specific patient populations. Patients are aggregated based on intensity of service, acuity,

CASE STUDY—cont'd

and diagnosis (cardiovascular/pulmonary and oncology/renal, with telemetry available on the cardiovascular unit). Staff members are assigned permanently on each unit based on preference but with an understanding that rotation to the sister unit is available after a pilot period of 6 months. Each module consists of 16 to 20 patients, and an experienced nurse is partnered with novice or agency nurses and one or two CNAs. Complete inter-shift report is taken by the module members, facilitating communication and continuity if one staff member is off the unit or not scheduled the next day. Daily inter-professional care planning rounds, facilitated by nursing, are established for each module. The practices of hourly nurse rounding and focused assessments are instituted to improve monitoring and surveillance of rapidly changing patient conditions.

A new level of CNA is established to increase simple skills performance, and competency assessments are done in the skills labs. A third floor shared governance council determines what CNA skills are most needed to reduce nurses' non-nursing tasks. Nurses and CNAs attended team-building workshops to facilitate understanding of delegation responsibilities and roles. The patient care manager remains responsible for both modules. However, a permanent charge nurse position without direct patient care responsibility is established on each module to facilitate communications and resource and staffing availability.

Evaluation

Process, quality, safety, and financial outcome indicators are established and clustered into a dashboard as an integral component of quality improvement. Because clinical outcomes must follow successful implementation of processes, a project team decision is made to measure process indicators for 6 months and then quality indicators at 6 months, 1 year, 18 months, and 2 years.

Fast Forward: The End of the First Year

Nursing satisfaction and perceptions of quality care delivery are improved, including facilitation of assessment, monitoring, achievement of care goals, organization of care, delegation, patient teaching, documentation, and continuity of care delivery. Agency usage is down, and attrition of new graduates is reduced by 20%. Patient satisfaction scores are beginning to demonstrate improvement with regard to pain management, discharge preparation, and meeting of care needs. Although the incidence of pressure ulcers remains constant, the number of patient falls is reduced.

Conclusions

Careful and deliberate planning with the participation of stakeholders can result in a successful project. In this instance a care delivery model redesign (and quality improvement initiative) was successfully carried out through collaborative planning, implementation, and evaluation.

CRITICAL THINKING EXERCISE

PCC philosophy puts patients and families first regarding their values, beliefs, and preferences. Your organization has recently gone through a strategic redesign, and PCC has been incorporated in the organizational vision/mission statement and core values. You are the manager for a critical care unit, and you use the S-P-O Donabedian framework to determine what structures and processes need to be in place within your work environment to support PCC outcomes. To determine your outcomes or goals, you do a patient/family survey to find out priority care preferences and needs. Major care preferences for patients and families are: regular, frequent communications with the health care team; more family involvement in hands-on care for patients; 24/7 close family

visitation; and patient/family collaboration in making decisions. In this unit, current policies limit family visitation and participation in care delivery.

1. What evidence-based structures are necessary to meet your PCC goals or outcomes?
2. What evidence-based processes are necessary to meet your PCC goals or outcomes?
3. PCC is sometimes used as the theoretical framework for Magnet hospitals' nursing professional practice models. What Magnet-like factors can you use to shift your work environment's culture (medical model) toward PCC? Hint: Consider using a matrix or table such as:

Structures   Processes   Desired Outcomes

16

Case and Population Health Management

Ellen Fink-Samnick, Teresa M. Treiger

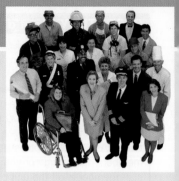

ⓔhttp://evolve.elsevier.com/Huber/leadership

Events of recent decades have thrown the health care system into a radical reformation. This revolution continues to unfold in ever-changing ways. Care delivery has shifted from acute institution-based interventional care to a patient-centered primary care model where quality-driven prevention and outpatient management are the preferred method of operating. Case and population health management are multidisciplinary by nature. Nurses provide these services and work in these care delivery models, as do many other disciplines (see Chapter 15).

The modern era of case, disease, and population health management began in the early 1990s. The effectiveness of what was called case management (CM) in producing quality and cost containment outcomes began to be noticed anecdotally by providers in the field. More importantly, it was noticed by health insurance companies that came to believe it worked. However, CM services were rarely paid for outside of rehabilitation and some social services areas, which severely limited the widespread implementation of CM and inhibited care integration. Despite funding restrictions, the belief in the effectiveness of CM spurred research and the development of the knowledge base and evidence for practice. Major professional, certification, and trade associations have also grown over the last 20 to 25 years.

The field split first into CM and disease management (DM) (Huber, 2005). With the criticism that not all health conditions, such as behavioral health, are "diseases," the term **disease management** was dropped in favor of **population health management (PHM)**. Rigorous research and

federal government–funded demonstration grants continued to solidify the evidence base for practice.

When necessary services other than acute care are actually added to/provided for in the mix of health care, it is difficult to demonstrate cost savings. However, CM, DM, and PHM strategies all have shown positive clinical outcomes. What is clear is that **care coordination** is the core element common to all provider interventions in CM, DM, and PHM.

DEFINITIONS

Case management (CM): "A collaborative process of assessment, planning, facilitation, care coordination, evaluation, and advocacy for options and services to meet an individual's and family's comprehensive health needs through communication and available resources to promote patient safety, quality cost-effective outcomes" (Case Management Society of America, 2016a).

Disease management (DM): "Disease management is a system of coordinated health care interventions and communications for populations with conditions in which patient self-care efforts are significant" ("Disease management," n.d.).

Population health management (PHM): "Population health management is an approach that aims to improve the health status of the entire population through coordination of care across the continuum of health in order to improve behavioral/lifestyle, clinical and financial outcomes" ("Population health management," n.d.). A more succinct definition is "the process of addressing population health needs and controlling problems at a population level" (Nash et al., 2016).

Photo used with permission from Photos.com.

BACKGROUND

Distinguishing Components of the Health Care Management Continuum

This chapter primarily discusses CM and DM. Before launching into these individual areas, it is essential to frame the health care management continuum and provide perspective on where CM and DM reside within and relate to the whole of PHM.

The health care management continuum (or spectrum as it is sometimes referred) is not synonymous with the continuum of health care practice settings or continuum of care. Although health care management is practiced across the continuum of care, the depth and scope of these services are often driven by the primary purpose of the organization or department (e.g., acute care hospital, emergency department, managed care organization) and the organizational resources available to take on the challenge of these services.

The health care management continuum is better known as PHM. PHM is the overarching umbrella under which CM and DM exist, along with a number of other health management initiatives.

Generally speaking, CM programs serve a smaller percentage of the overall population. Enrollees are complex from a medical–behavioral, health–social vulnerability perspective. Health plans often target the top 5% to 10% of their entire population for CM consideration. The case manager performs an initial screening followed by an in-depth individual assessment involving the client, family caregiver, and other care team members. From the information gleaned, a CM plan of care is developed. This plan includes highly individualized goals and desired outcomes. DM programs serve a larger percentage of patients whose main problem is one or more chronic condition(s). These individuals generally have similar primary needs regarding health condition education and accommodation strategies. Assessments focus on health condition–specific issues, and programs take a more standardized approach to education and resources (Chen et al., 2000). Table 16.1 contains definitions and additional distinguishing characteristics.

TABLE 16.1 Case Management, Disease Management, and Population Health Management Side by Side

Case Management	Disease Management	Population Health Management
". . . a collaborative process of assessment, planning, facilitation, care coordination, evaluation, and advocacy for options and services to meet an individual's and family's comprehensive health needs through communication and available resources to promote patient safety, quality cost-effective outcomes."*	"Disease management is a system of coordinated health care interventions and communications for populations with conditions in which patient self-care efforts are significant" ("Disease management," n.d.).	"Population health management is an approach that aims to improve the health status of the entire population through coordination of care across the continuum of health in order to improve behavioral/lifestyle, clinical and financial outcomes" ("Population health management," n.d.).
• CMSA definition is used by URAC and NCQA although multiple CM definitions exist • Relies on client-centered assessment, planning, facilitation, care coordination, evaluation, and advocacy • Standards of practice • Individual certifications • Program accreditation and certification available	• Multiple DM definitions • DM program usually focuses on single condition • Relies on a structured system of interventions that focus on a specific condition • No standards of practice • Program content and interventions are evidence and guideline based • Individual certification • Program accreditation and certification available	• Multiple PHM definitions • PHM is a term that overarches the spectrum of health care management • Practice standards exist for components within PHM • Certification and accreditation programs exist for components within PHM

DM, Disease management; *NCQA,* National Committee for Quality Assurance; *PHM,* population health management; *URAC,* Utilization Review Accreditation Commission.
*Data from Case Management Society of America (CMSA). (2016a). *CMSA standards of practice for case management.* Little Rock, AR: Author; Disease management. (n.d.). In Population Health Alliance *PHM glossary.* Retrieved from http://www.populationhealthalliance.org/research/phm-glossary/d.html; Population health management. (n.d.). In Population Health Alliance *PHM glossary.* Retrieved from http://www.populationhealthalliance.org/research/phm-glossary/p.html

CASE MANAGEMENT

CM evolved from a chain of social developments and historical events that made apparent the health, social, and human service needs of disadvantaged, ill, and injured populations through the identification and provision of social services and coordination of care (Treiger & Fink-Samnick, 2013, 2016). Although initially not formally labeled as CM, this history provides a rich context for understanding how CM evolved into what it is today, intertwined with social and legislative events, trends, and changes.

Before government-sponsored interventions, government programs were not addressing the most basic human needs in an organized manner. The federal government had not yet expanded into areas of social support or health care realms, and so efforts to provide social assistance and supportive services for individuals in need were humanitarian and grassroots in nature.

Charitable and community-based organizations with wealthy benefactors began to address and fill the local population's needs. The history of caring for the disadvantaged arose from the context of social–political–industrial changes, which piqued more liberal attitudes of social consciousness.

Landmark Legislation

A major influence on CM practice was the continuous stream of socially motivated legislation beginning with the 1935 Social Security Act. These laws put both federal and state governments—as well as newly created regulatory agencies—in a position of responsibility for support and care of the general population. Accompanying these major pieces of legislation was the demand for accountability, service quality, and consumer protection. The role of the case manager (also identified as a service coordinator), was first seen in the school setting (Education for All Handicapped Children Act, 1975). Passage of federal and state law mandated CM services for elders (Older Americans Act, 1965), the mentally ill (the Community Mental Health Centers Act, 1963), and the developmentally disabled (the Developmentally Disabled Assistance and Bill of Rights Act, 1975) (Weil & Karls, 1985).

Case management is not merely the outcome of a single event, piece of legislation, company's risk reduction strategy, or a particular professional affiliation. CM is an organically developed practice specialty; it is an insightful response to the interplay of biology, psychology, sociology, health care system factors, and the influences exerted on individuals with complex illnesses and injuries.

Case Management Models

As has long been noted, a single and universally accepted CM model does not exist (Huber, 2002). Huber noted that the diversity of practice models stems from there being multiple definitions of CM. Having infiltrated virtually every practice setting and area of specialization across the health care continuum, it seemed to be an unrealistic expectation that a single model could garner global agreement. However, this assumption hinged on the definition and characteristics of the practice models themselves. Among other influencers is the lack of title protection for case managers, resulting in the widespread misapplication of the case manager job title.

Contemporary approaches, defined on a foundation of practice competencies, have been introduced. One model sparked the notion that a universal practice paradigm is not only possible but is essential to the continued growth of professional CM practice. This section addresses the background and characteristics of CM models and highlights the current trend of practice models being general to practice settings and competency-based practice models.

Practice Models Background

There are a very large number of identifiable CM practice models. Some are nursing models, others are non-nursing models, and still others are team oriented. The core elements of CM models center on a case manager who coordinates and monitors care rendered to clients by multiple health care providers and services in an attempt to decrease service fragmentation and improve the quality of care (Rheaume et al., 1994).

By definition, CM is identified as a cycle. The CM process steps align with components of the nursing process. The CM process identifies needs, risks, and resources, and coordinates care and services while educating the client–caregiver to be better self-advocates for health care. CM is designed to support and foster an individual through the health care system using patient-focused care coordination strategies. "Case management should be considered a bridge, not a crutch" (Treiger, 2012). The CM process may be identified differently because of proprietary branding, and it is affected by legislation, regulation, organizational policy, and care setting. However, at its foundation is an approach that defines the various parts of the CM process. Voluntary practice standards provide a frame for qualifications and expectations in all health care practice settings.

Weil and Karls (1985) identified eight main service components common to all CM models:

1. Client identification and outreach
2. Individual assessment and diagnosis
3. Service planning and resource identification
4. Linking clients to needed services
5. Service implementation and coordination
6. Monitoring service delivery
7. Advocacy
8. Evaluation

These components remain a part of the basic CM process framework to the present day.

CM exists in many contexts, settings, and programs. This includes but is not limited to inpatient care, payer-based, accountable care organizations (ACOs), employer-based, workers' compensation, social services, independent practice, for-profit companies, non-profit organizations, patient-centered medical homes (PCMHs), nursing practice, public health nursing, home health care agencies, maternal–child care, and behavioral health settings.

CM programs incorporate a variety of key activities, some of which vary according to practice setting. These activities include (but are not limited to):

- Identification and screening of participants
- Assessment
- Needs identification
- Planning
- Service and product acquisition and implementation
- Coordination of care
- Ongoing monitoring

These and other activities focus on the achievement of client and organizational outcomes that should be accomplished within effective and appropriate time frames and through efficient utilization of available resources. The time span for CM engagement may be for an episode of care in a single care setting (e.g., acute hospital, rehabilitation) lasting a few days/weeks or may span across care settings (e.g., ACOs) over a number of years or for life. In the setting of patient-centered primary care, a client may engage with a case manager for multiple distinct episodes of care or for years of management due to the client's complexity of needs profile.

A model of CM may be designed for a large, rather generic target group or population (e.g., hospitalized, long-term care, chronic care, rehabilitation) or for a specified segment on the health care continuum (e.g., an episode in one setting, in one organization, or for the whole continuum). Historically, these CM models specify organizational policies and processes for care delivery, resource use, and job responsibilities based on general position descriptions. Depending on the organization's care process, the case manager may or may not be a direct care provider.

Many types of CM models and labels are found in literature. There are discipline-specific models as well as generally accepted overarching models. Two factors are common across all CM models: The core component is coordination of care, and the core principle is advocacy. There are fairly common process elements in CM models in addition to coordination of care, advocacy, brokering of services, and resource management. Models may be tailored to fit unique target groups (e.g., vulnerable populations, care setting) or discipline-specific factors.

Nursing and health care models tend to focus on the management of health/illness or disease or the rehabilitation needs of an individual or population. These models are sometimes called medical models, medical–social models, acute care nursing CM models, or disease management models. There has been some confusion in the nursing literature about whether CM is a care delivery model or an intervention that entails a process. In both nursing and social work, there is a differentiation between CM designed to deliver services and CM designed to coordinate the provision of services (Ridgely & Willenbring, 1992).

Several frameworks and other methods of classifying activities have been considered when discussing CM models. Because of the variability in how CM programs are designed and administered, classification into models helps describe—as well as compare and contrast—each type. Using distinctive classifications, CM models may be understood relative to perspective (e.g., organization, setting based), scope (e.g., services delivered within an organization, cross-continuum), and time (e.g., single or multiple episode of care). A methodology for consistent classification of CM practice models has neither been proposed nor accepted. The likelihood of universal acceptance is dim within the current health care context due to the issues associated with the variety of professions practicing CM, competing professional organizations, and the multitude of available individual certifications, among a number of other important influences. Unfortunately, there is no common understanding about what is meant by "doing case management."

Seminal Nursing Case Management Models

There are two nursing CM programs often cited in nursing literature as forerunners of modern-day nursing CM. These programs are the *New England Medical Center (NEMC) model* and the *Carondelet St. Mary's model*. The NEMC model is considered to be acute care nursing CM, whereas the Carondelet model is a community-based model.

The NEMC model is an extension of primary nursing methodology referred to as nursing CM. It focuses on the acute care episode (Zander, 2002). In the mid-1980s, this model was introduced at the NEMC, located in Boston, Massachusetts. This model exemplifies an organization-specific model; it is hospital-based CM. It is best known for how it structures the episode of care. It leverages principles of planning and management from engineering and other fields to extend primary nursing into outcomes management. The goals seek to balance cost, process, and outcomes.

The NEMC model is a client-centered approach instituted during episodes of acute illness. It focuses on resource utilization, nursing accountability, and outcomes. Written, standardized documents such as CM plans, timelines, and critical paths were developed and evolved into CareMap tools, forming the basis for a comprehensive hospital-wide CM system at the NEMC. The complete CareMap system includes variance analysis, use of an outcome–time focus in all multidisciplinary communication, case consultation and health care team meetings for clients at more-than-acceptable variance, and continuous quality improvement.

Carondelet St. Mary's Community Nursing Network, or the Arizona Model (Forbes, 1999), used professional nurse case managers (baccalaureate and master's level) organized as a nursing health maintenance organization (HMO) at the hub of a network to broker services. This model type is known as a beyond-the-walls, medical–social, across-the-continuum of care model. It is best known for its innovative work in moving beyond the inpatient episode of care and into across-the-continuum of care. This hospital-to-community model used case managers to follow the movement of high-risk clients from acute care to community to long-term care settings. Case managers are responsible for clients with chronic health problems and the relationship is long term in nature (Clark, 1996).

Social Work Models

CM has been integral to social work since the founding of the profession (Herman, 2013). From roots in charitable efforts there has been considerable evolution in CM models in use across the social work profession. Originally known as "social casework," the intervention was used to track the growing needs, progress, and changes for each person. Casework typically focused on enhancing an individual's self-reliance and independence as well as coordinating and integrating care (Ridgely & Willenbring, 1992). The emphasis has traditionally been on society's most vulnerable populations. These persons are at risk of poor physical, psychological, or social health, based on the World Health Organization's definition of health as a state of complete physical, mental, and social well-being (Young, 2009). Examples include individuals with chronic physical and/or mental illness, intellectual and/or physical disability, and housing insufficiency.

Social casework was especially helpful in marshalling scarce resources to the best advantage and minimizing the duplication of effort by those involved. By the 1960s, the role expanded in response to large numbers of persons with chronic and severe mental illnesses being transitioned from hospitals to the community (deinstitutionalization) and the mandate for skilled personnel trained to coordinate the unique scope of care, which included linkage to needed resources, ensuring referrals to existing service agencies, providing advocacy, and teaching (Summers, 2016).

By the 1980s, use of the term caseworker was on the wane as use of the term case manager was on the rise. These individuals were afforded expanded responsibility to manage society's continued generations of those in need (Summers, 2016). A new population of patients living with chronic and terminal illness (e.g., HIV/AIDs) appeared across the country, particularly in urban centers. The latitude offered through CM met the needs of community agencies tasked with monitoring the holistic needs of focused populations. Case managers were able to address a wider scope of issues beyond the single presenting problem identified by the patient (Summers, 2016).

The function of CM remains part of most social work jobs, and constitutes a core function of—and specialty within—social work practice. In 2013, standards of practice were developed by the National Association of Social Workers (NASW) to further elaborate on the distinctions for CM from the lens of social work. The six guiding principles are (1) person-centered services, (2) primacy of the client–social worker relationship, (3) person-in-environment framework, (4) strengths perspective, (5) collaborative teamwork, and (6) intervention at the micro, mezzo, and macro levels of practice (NASW, 2013, p. 17).

More than a dozen different models of contemporary social work CM have been identified in the literature (including medical, social advocacy, managed care, outreach, ecological, intensive, and clinical) (Berger, 2009; Fleisher & Henrickson, 2002; Herman, 2013; Summers, 2016). Those most commonly mentioned include: brokerage, primary therapist, interdisciplinary team, comprehensive, and strengths.

The **brokerage model** emphasizes the case manager's traditional linkage function. Clients are linked to a network of providers and service coverage using assessment and referral and ensuring the availability of service activities (Raiff & Shore, 1993). The case manager plans a comprehensive service package and negotiates through barriers that prevent clients from accessing needed services. Cost savings may or may not be an explicit goal, but such savings may be expected because the case manager facilitates better access to cost-effective alternatives, achieves better coordination and less duplication of services across agencies, reduces use of more expensive and less effective sites of care or services, and diverts clients from admissions (Ridgely & Willenbring, 1992).

In the **primary therapist model**, the case manager's relationship to the client is primarily therapeutic, and CM functions are undertaken as a part or an extension of therapeutic intervention. The client has one person to relate to about treatment, service access, and case coordination. However, the therapist may feel that CM is a secondary activity to therapeutic work (Weil & Karls, 1985).

The **interdisciplinary team model** uses a specialized team of various professional disciplines in which each member has a specific responsibility for service activities in his or her area of expertise. Team approaches are increasingly being used to maximize opportunities instead of competition over turf (Berger, 2009). Team structures vary considerably. In some, all case managers on the team are interchangeable and serve the total group of clients. Other programs consist of multidisciplinary teams of up to six different professions, often driven by client-specific issues and needs. One team member is identified as the lead, with the other members combining their knowledge to share information about the client. The best approach to the delivery of care is ultimately defined by group consensus (Berger, 2009).

The **comprehensive service center model** is used in agencies that provide comprehensive services and community-based programming that can include psychosocial support, vocational training, rehabilitation, and care coordination. Examples of settings include community health centers, community-focused programs, continuing care communities (e.g., nursing homes, assisted living facilities), and public housing programs. Case managers in these practice settings may engage in high levels of advocacy, often interacting with members of the client's health care team from other agencies and/or programs (Young, 2009). A personal **strengths model** may be used to further help clients in recovery to focus on and achieve goals (Huber, 2005).

Interdisciplinary Models

A growing number of interdisciplinary models for CM collaboration exist across practice settings. These models blend the unique competencies and knowledge that underlie nursing and social work education, a full listing of which are shown in Box 16.1. The strength of the social work profession is in its ability to assess the social environment of patients and families from a multidimensional perspective, which includes the biological, psychological, sociological, and spiritual domains (Ashford & LeCroy, 2013). Social workers are thus skilled in the evaluation of the premorbid condition of a client's unique situation and possess an understanding of what services are available in the community and how to access them (Robbins & Birmingham, 2005). Nursing education addresses understanding of the pathophysiology of illness with the core of practice to deliver holistic patient-focused care incorporating assessment, diagnosis, outcomes/planning, implementation, and evaluation (American Nurses Association [ANA], 2016).

The CM **dyad team model**—composed of a nurse case manager and social worker—has been widely adopted in hospitals. The dyad structure presents an opportunity for nurses and social workers to integrate their strengths and expertise in a collaborative patient-centered effort (Carr, 2009). These two helping professions align the power of their respective clinical knowledge: social work's proficiency in psychopathology, psychosocial issues, and resource linkage with nursing's emphasis on pathophysiology and the disease process. Both disciplines share the innate value of expertise in empathic listening, advocacy, and critical thinking. This skill set is a forceful combination when used to collaborate with team members in their efforts to evaluate, manage, plan, treat, and coordinate important aspects of the patient's care (Carr, 2009). There is some variation in roles and functions assigned to each discipline, with the distinct scope of job responsibilities defined by each organization.

Through its unique structure, the nurse and social work dyad provides the implementation of collaborative interventions that focus on (1) minimization of inpatient transitions, (2) reduction of cost by decreasing the length of stay, (3) promotion of patient and family satisfaction through efforts of advocacy, and (4) enhanced discharge planning (Carr, 2009).

Hospitals are also increasingly motivated to address readmissions and safe care transitions. Both of these issues are greatly affected by *social determinants*. Social determinants of health are defined by the World Health Organization (2016) as "the conditions in which people are born, grow, live, work and age. These circumstances are shaped by the distribution of money, power, and resources at global, national and local levels." Current literature has identified that inclusion of these factors can lead to a pronounced effect on calculated hospital readmission rates for patients across disease states (Gillespie, 2016; Hu et al., 2014; Nagasako et al., 2014; Rice, 2016). When barriers to access to care (e.g., poverty, housing insufficiency, health literacy, medication adherence) are clearly identified by the nurse and social worker, specific goals can be established, system processes can be developed or changed, and initiatives can be set into motion to provide patients with safe transitions (Ellsworth, 2015).

Another model presented for nurse–social worker collaboration is used in managed care (Hawkins et al., 1998). Called the **Biopsychosocial Individual and Systems Intervention Model,** it is derived from a combination of interdisciplinary collaboration models at the organizational and administrative levels and a CM intervention approach for individuals and small systems levels. Nurses and social workers are assumed to collaborate as equal partners in interdisciplinary team CM using a transdisciplinary model.

The one general, overarching interdisciplinary model that is becoming widely accepted as the generic CM model is Wagner's **Chronic Care Model** (Improving Chronic Illness Care, 2006–2016). The Chronic Care Model addresses concerns about how to manage chronic illnesses. The six elements of the health care system that encourage quality chronic illness care are the community, the health system, self-management support, delivery system design, decision support, and clinical information systems. The specific concepts related to the six elements are patient safety, cultural competency, care coordination, community policies, and CM. Chronic disease/illness care is important because almost one-half of all Americans (133 million people in 2005; estimated to be 171 million by 2030) live with a chronic condition. Almost half of those with a chronic illness have multiple conditions (Improving Chronic Illness Care, 2006–2016). This order of magnitude has generated great interest in strategies to be proactive and focused on keeping people as healthy as possible. CM is an attractive strategy because it is aimed at care coordination and decreased system-related fragmentation.

A close relative of the Chronic Care Model is the **Collaborative Care Model.** The latter is actively being implemented in primary care practices to address the increased costs for and numbers of patients with cooccurring physical and mental health needs. Patients who have a cooccurring behavioral health condition receive intervention from the health care system significantly more frequently, with bills that are anywhere from 50% to 175% higher than similarly ill patients without a behavioral health condition (Gupta, 2015; Milliman, 2014). The general features of Collaborative Care models are (Butler et al., 2008, Zimmerman & Dabelko, 2007):

- Integration of mental health professionals in primary care medical settings
- Close collaboration between mental health and medical/nursing providers
- Shared responsibility in the planning, delivery, and evaluation of health services
- Focus on treating the whole person and whole family

In the Collaborative Care Model, dedicated team members address the needs of patients though a comprehensive and strategic care delivery process. Included in the team are a primary care provider, a case manager who is trained in behavioral health, and psychiatric consultants and/or behavioral health specialists (Unützer et al., 2013). This comprehensive approach to care serves as a proactive means to screen and track mental health conditions within the primary care setting.

Outcomes identify the Collaborative Care Model as clinically sound and cost effective in treating patients with comorbid conditions, including depression and/or anxiety, along with a chronic medical condition (e.g., diabetes, congestive heart failure) (Eghaneyan et al., 2014; Fortney et al., 2015; Robert Wood Johnson Foundation, 2011; Unützer et al., 2013). Hospital readmissions have been reduced by nearly 40%, with a significant decrease in associated costs of care (Epstein Becker Green, 2015).

The new generation of inter-professional teams. The concept of the **inter-professional team** is rapidly emerging in the literature. The Health and Medicine Division of the National Academies of Sciences, Engineering, and Medicine (formally the Institute of Medicine) discussed the obligation of academic health centers to conduct interdisciplinary education and patient care (Interprofessional Education Collaborative [IPEC], 2011).

Concerns have been raised about how the terminology of multidisciplinary, interdisciplinary, and related team approaches were used interchangeably, but there is no resolution (Canadian Interprofessional Health Collaborative [CIHC], 2010; IPEC, 2011; Treiger & Fink-Samnick, 2016).

In 2007, representatives from health organizations, health educators, researchers, professionals, and students from the health care sector convened in Canada. The CIHC developed a seminal report, *Interprofessional Education (IPE) and Core Competencies: A Literature Review.* A main theme of the study was how shared accountability to achieve competency mastery belongs to all professional stakeholders: educators, learners, and practitioners (CIHC, 2010). The IPE imperative was subsequently adopted by the World Health Organization (WHO) (2010), which saw the promise of the process for the next generation of health care students. The group established the goal to prepare health professions students for deliberately working together, with the common aim of building a safer and better patient-centered and population-oriented United States health care system (IPEC, 2011).

Inter-professional teams refer to care delivered by intentionally created, usually relatively small work groups in health care. The teams are recognized by others, as well as by themselves, as having a collective identity and shared responsibility for a patient or group of patients. Examples include distinct teams for rapid response, palliative care, and primary care (IPEC, 2011). These teams are different from many teams found in interdisciplinary models, where members of only two different disciplines (such as nurses and doctors) might partner with or communicate with each other about the care of select patients. The four competencies identified for inter-professional teams are: values/ethics for inter-professional practice, roles/responsibilities, inter-professional communication, and teams and teamwork.

Outcomes demonstrating the success of inter-professional teams are in the early stages, with the verdict still out on long-term acceptance across the industry. The implications for CM are vast, particularly with close alignment of its standards of practice with the IPEC principles. Sustainability will ultimately be driven by how the health care sector and its unique stakeholders interpret and operationalize the new term *inter-professional* as a construct (Treiger & Fink-Samnick, 2016). A number of demonstration projects are in process. Reports and funding opportunities are available on the IPEC website *(https://ipecollaborative.org).*

Competency-based Models

In order for CM practice to progress in step with or ahead of general health care evolution, thought leaders must continuously generate theoretical frameworks and practical solutions to address the challenges of health care delivery, including definition of best practice, terminology (e.g., common language), dedication of resources (e.g., dosage), expected outcomes, and qualifications for professional practice (e.g., education, experience, credentials). In order to provide high quality care continuity, case managers need to speak the same language across the care continuum (Treiger & Fink-Samnick, 2016).

Rather than focus on care setting or organizational priorities as the driver of CM scope and practice, competency-based models approach practice through a lens of qualities and characteristics that contribute to practice excellence. As noted by the Case Management Society of America (CMSA, 2017), case managers require specific knowledge of the CM process as well as a variety of skills in order to apply their expertise effectively. The two recognizable CM-specific competency frameworks are COLLABORATE and e4.

The COLLABORATE model. This model builds and supports competent professional practice through the identification and application of essential skills, behaviors, and characteristics. Because it is a model based on characteristics and key elements, the paradigm integrates into existing CM processes and programs across the entire care continuum (Treiger & Fink-Samnick, 2016). COLLABORATE is an acronym identifying the competencies that are important to master for professional CM practice. The acronym stands for **C**ritical thinking, **O**utcomes-driven, **L**ifelong learning, **L**eadership, **A**dvocacy, **B**ig picture orientation, **O**rganized, **R**esource awareness, **A**nticipatory, **T**ransdisciplinary, and **E**thical–Legal.

Independent of health care's ongoing challenges, case managers must be sufficiently agile to frame (and reframe) professional practice in order to facilitate a client's best outcomes. This is why defining a competency-based CM model, which fits into any setting of care and applies to all populations, is essential. Ultimately, this competency-based model elevates the quality of practice and contributes to optimal CM and health care outcomes (Treiger & Fink-Samnick, 2013). Each competency and the associated key elements of the COLLABORATE model are displayed in Table 16.2.

e4 framework. This framework introduced by CMSA assists "individuals to identify and develop the knowledge and skills needed to be an effective case management practitioner and deliver sustainable business performance. Of equal importance, these cross-sector frameworks sets out competencies, employers should expect from professionals in case/care management" (CMSA, 2016b).

CMSA categorizes practice essentials under main headings: CM Concepts, Knowledge and Understanding, Communication, Outcomes Improvement, and Leadership. CM Concepts addresses CM process, competency validation, and critical and analytical thinking. Knowledge and Understanding is inclusive of the domains of legal/ethics, regulatory, professional education, and business management. Communication includes effective engagement and empowerment as well as relationship management. Outcomes Improvement incorporates research and quality as well as implementing value-added solutions. Finally, Leadership addresses change management and workforce development (CMSA, 2016a). Each of these categories describes the expectation of individual competence and spans six levels of practice experience/position.

Other Case Management Models

CM is practiced in ACOs, PCMHs, primary care, long-term care, rehabilitation, occupational health, workers' compensation, and pharmacy. A different setting of care does not necessarily mean another CM model has been created. That said, there are many care settings in which CM is practiced. In some models, the functions of CM, utilization review (UR), and disease management (DM) overlap. The overlap and distinctions between these areas result in organizational challenges. Policies, procedures, and processes are designed to clarify desired work flow in order to eliminate the risk of redundancy.

Insurance models may be divided into brokerage, gatekeeper, catastrophic, managed care, and government models. The **brokerage model** includes an emphasis on linkage to resources but with no provision of direct services. It is similar to the broker in other social work models except for a strong emphasis on conserving benefits utilization.

A **gatekeeper** model is defined as an informal, though widely used, primary care CM model health plan. In this model, all care from providers other than the primary care provider (except for true emergencies) must be authorized by the primary care provider before care is rendered (Kongstvedt, 2013). Gatekeeper models manage access to services and promote the use of cost-effective alternatives to expensive services (Ridgely & Willenbring, 1992). Cost savings are realized by managing care, including advocating for less costly but more appropriate services by not authorizing the requested higher-cost services. Rather

TABLE 16.2 COLLABORATE Competencies and Key Elements

Acronym	Competency	Key Elements
C	Critical thinking	Out of the box creativity Analytical Methodical approach
O	Outcome driven	Patient outcomes Strategic goal setting Evidence-based practice
L	Lifelong learning	Valuing: • Academia and advanced degrees • Professional development • Evolution of knowledge requirements for new and emerging trends (e.g., technology, innovation, reimbursement) • Practicing at top of licensure and/or certification • Acknowledging no one case manager can and does know all
L	Leadership	Professional identity Self-awareness Professional communication: verbal/non-verbal Team coordinator: a unifier rather than a divider
A	Advocacy	Patient Family Professional
B	Big picture orientation	Bio-psycho-social-spiritual assessment Macro (policy) impact on micro (individual) intervention
O	Organized	Efficient Effective
R	Resource awareness	Utilization management Condition/population specific Management of expectations per setting
A	Anticipatory	Forward thinking Proactive versus reactive practice Self-directed
T	Transdisciplinary	Transcending • Professional disciplines • Across teams • Across the continuum
E	Ethical–legal	Licensure Certification Administrative standards Organizational policies and procedures Ethical codes of conduct

Data from Treiger, T.M., & Fink-Samnick, E. (2016). *COLLABORATE for professional case management: A universal competency-based paradigm.* Philadelphia, PA: Wolters Kluwer.

than facilitating access, gatekeepers restrict access as a means to control utilization, which ostensibly controls costs but may just control short-term expenditures. The ability of managed care case managers to create savings depends on the availability of appropriate cost-effective alternatives, the case manager's authority within the care system, and the case manager's ability to control financing for the care deemed appropriate (Ridgely & Willenbring, 1992). Although there are variations in department configuration, many managed care plans have a medical management department under which a complex—also referred to as catastrophic—CM team exists.

Catastrophic CM is focused on complex and **catastrophic** illness or injury (e.g., spinal cord injury, traumatic brain injury, chronic degenerative neurological disease, medical–behavioral health dual diagnoses) and applies primarily to managed care, workers' compensation, and life-care planning. It is designed to manage and maximize insurance and health care benefits, which may be capped at a lifetime maximum. Screening, data mining, referrals, and other red flag strategies are leveraged to detect the potential for high-cost cases and to interact with clients and service providers proactively to optimize and economize the health services used (CMSA, 2016a; Cline, 1990).

In **managed care** models, prospective or capitated reimbursement systems often place providers in the position of carrying financial risk. This creates pressure on providers to control total costs, provide and promote prevention-oriented services, and substitute lower-cost services, preferably without sacrificing quality. An example of this is integrated health care, defined as a network of organizations that provides or arranges to provide a coordinated continuum of services to a defined population and is held accountable for the population's health status (Shortell et al., 1993). The type of managed care organization dictates the degree to which case managers directly interface with clients and providers. For example, in a staff model HMO, the case manager and provider are employees of the same organization. The working relationship is collegial in nature. There is regular face-to-face contact between the case manager, provider, and client. However, in an independent provider organization (IPO), the IPO contracts with an HMO to provide health care services to its members. The providers are primarily affiliated with their medical group practice, whereas the case manager is employed by the health plan. The working relationship between provider and case manager tends to be more adversarial, because the allegiance of provider and case manager are to different organizations. In this model, the case manager's primary mode of contact with the client is via telephone. However, this varies because in some instances the case manager works within the four walls of the medical group or at an acute care setting.

In the **government model,** federal, state, and local agencies manage and reimburse health care via programs such as Medicare, Medicaid, and workers' compensation. Often management of these programs is handled by established health plans that create separate lines of business for government plans.

Case Management Practice Standards and Code of Conduct
Practice Standards

CM practice has expanded at an accelerated rate in order to meet the evolving needs of health care and social services and proliferated across various health care and payer settings and practice models. It is essential to recognize that although these programs were frequently referred to as CM, the actual functions and activities of staff were often not reflective of the full scope of CM practice. Department and job titles were often grouped together within overarching care management strategies due, in part, to name recognition. It appears that little attention was given to ensuring CM departments and jobs were aligned with CM practice standards (Treiger & Fink-Samnick, 2013).

CM **standards of practice** are offered by two different CM-related organizations: CMSA and the American Case Management Association (ACMA). Other CM practice standards are offered by the US Department of Veterans Affairs (VA), which apply to CM practice within the VA system, and the NASW, which apply only to social workers. The American Nurses Association (ANA) offers overarching standards and scope of practice for nurses but does not offer CM-specific practice standards. In addition, there is no CM-specific professional society affiliated with the ANA.

CMSA's *Standards of Practice for Case Management*, originally released in 1995, is in its fourth revision. Each revision was undertaken to address ongoing growth and expansion of CM across the continuum of care and into virtually every care setting. In addition to the standards, the document addresses definition, philosophy and guiding principles, practice settings, roles and responsibilities, and components of the CM process (CMSA, 2016a).

Standards of Practice & Scope of Services for Health Care Delivery System Case Management and Transitions of Care (TOC) Professionals comes from the ACMA (2013). This version includes education, care coordination, compliance, transition management, utilization management, and standards of practice (including accountability, professionalism, collaboration, care coordination, resource management, and certification). ACMA focuses on CM practiced within the health care delivery system, inclusive of transition management. As a result, the standards are applicable to a limited array of care settings. The ACMA certification standard focuses on its own Accredited Case Manager (ACM) designation.

Code of Professional Conduct

Although adherence to practice standards is often considered to be voluntary, one exception is the Commission for Case Manager Certification's *Code of Professional Conduct* (CCMC, 2015). Adherence to this code is mandated for individuals possessing the certified case manager (CCM) credential. It is important to recognize that in a situation where legal action against a case manager occurs, attorneys and the court look at practice standards (in addition to other documents and guidelines) as a means of determining whether the actions of a case manager were aligned with accepted practice. In the case of a nurse case manager, these additional documents include one's own state practice act or remote practice act (when practice involves the Nurse Licensure Compact), applicable nursing standards of practice, CM standards of practice, and organizational policy and procedure.

The most recognizable code of conduct for case managers is the *Code of Professional Conduct for Case Managers with Standards, Rules, Procedures, and Penalties*, produced by the Commission for Case Manager Certification (CCMC, 2015). The objective of the code is to protect the public interest. The code is divided into sections, including principles, rules of conduct, scope of practice, definitions, standards for board-certified case manager conduct, and procedures for processing complaints (CCMC, 2015).

The Case Management Process

The **CM process** focuses on the identification of individuals who would benefit from CM services and the activities of assessment, problem identification, care planning, care delivery, advocacy, monitoring, and evaluation of the care provided, specifically for its relevance to the needs of the patient and caregiver as well as for the health care team's ability to meet the desired outcomes and established goals (CMSA, 2016a; Tahan, 2017).

Although the process is presented as having a different number of phases, both CMSA and CCMC have supported following an organized iterative process. A consideration relating to the CM process is that of care setting. Care setting often dictates the type of interaction between case manager and client. For example, the acute care setting generally ensures face-to-face interaction, whereas the managed care setting varies and may be a combination of telephonic, face-to-face and/or Internet chat. The manner in which each case manager

interacts with a client not only affects the ability to objectively assess that person but also influences how the relationship will evolve.

Commission for Case Manager Certification

CCMC defines the CM process as it applies to case managers who have achieved the CCM credential as being collaborative in nature. The phases of this process meld seamlessly and aim to support the patient, caregiver, support system, and care team members in addressing health and related issues (CCMC, 2016).

According to CCMC (2016), the process is divided into nine phases: screening, assessing, stratifying risk, planning, implementing (care coordination), following up, transitioning (transitional care), communicating post transition, and evaluating. The CCM navigates CM process being cognizant of the client and caregivers' cultural beliefs, interests, wishes, needs, and values. Because the CM process is an iterative cycle, each phase is revisited as necessary until desired outcomes are achieved and the client's interests are met (CCMC, 2016).

Case Management Society of America

CMSA also stipulates that the CM process is cyclical and recurrent, rather than linear or unidirectional. The CM process incorporates critical thinking and evidence-based knowledge and is carried out within the ethical and legal constructs of a case manager's scope of practice. The steps of the CM process as defined in the CMSA's *Standards of Practice for Case Management* (2016a) are client identification and selection, assessment and opportunity identification, development of the CM plan, implementation and coordination of CM plan interventions, monitoring and evaluation of the CM plan, and closing of the CM engagement.

Table 16.3 elaborates the CM process phases and notes the similarities between CMSA, CCMC CM, and nursing processes.

Case Management Program Development and Implementation
Case Management Program Development

CM programs are structured around roles and functions of case managers. The case manager's role balances the aspects of provider, care coordinator, and financial manager. Frequently identified case manager roles are advocate, facilitator, provider, liaison, coordinator, collaborator, broker, educator, negotiator, evaluator, communicator, risk

TABLE 16.3 Nursing and Case Management Processes

Nursing	CCMC	CMSA	Comments
	Screening	Client identification and selection	Screening and/or selection is specific to case management (CM) where access to a case manager is limited according to the capacity, policy, or practice scope of an organization or department.
Assessment	Assessing	Assessment and opportunity identification	
Diagnosis			The CM process does not include a diagnosis phase, but there are some similarities that align in the opportunity identification and planning phases.
	Stratifying Risk		• CCMC defines stratifying risk as the classification of a client into one of three risk categories (low, moderate, and high) in order to determine the appropriate level of intervention based on the client's situation and interests.*
			• In some CM settings, each client's stratification risk is set by the use of predictive modeling software. Subsequent risk score may be edited by the case manager based on client's current status (e.g., health, psychological health, social needs, complexity of care).
Outcomes/ Planning	Planning	Development of the CM plan	• Despite minute differences, a planning phase is intended to assimilate assessment findings into a workable plan of care for both nurse and case manager.
			• A CM plan includes overall goals and desired outcomes for identified needs.
Implementation	Implementing (care coordination)	Implementation and coordination of CM plan interventions	The implementation phase puts the plan into action.

CCMC, Commission for Case Manager Certification; *CMSA,* Case Management Society of America.
*Commission for Case Manager Certification (CCMC). (2016). *Case management body of knowledge (CMBOK).* Mount Laurel, NJ: Author.

manager, mentor, consultant, and researcher. CM functions are often identified as care coordination, facilitation and linkage, education, advocacy, discharge planning, resource management, and outcomes management.

For provider-based case managers, a CM program may be built based on CMSA's *Standards of Practice for Case Management* (2016a). The practice components identified in these standards are authoritative statements that are reflective of the unique roles and responsibilities for which case managers are held accountable. As a result, they can be used as an outline to establish step-by-step processes. In addition, the standards reflect how exclusive values and priorities of practitioners are operationalized and understood by mutual stakeholders (Treiger & Fink-Samnick, 2016).

CM programs are developed using a number of situation-specific elements. Two initial assessments are helpful: assessment of the organization and assessment of client populations. The *organizational assessment* focuses on identification of resources, whereas the client population assessment focuses on how care is experienced by clients and the characteristics of client populations served by the organizations. Box 16.2 lists related assessment questions. If CM is used for specific client populations, priority would go to clients who have a high rate of recidivism or frequent emergency department encounters; have unpredictable needs for care; have significant complications, comorbidities, or variances in usual care patterns; fall into high-risk profiles; and/or are high cost.

BOX 16.2 Case Management Assessment Questions

Organizational Assessment
- What clinical and support services are needed?
- When in the client experience are services most appropriately provided?
- How should services be provided?
- Where are services best delivered?
- Who are the most appropriate providers?
- Where and by whom are services best managed?

Client Assessment
- What are the major client populations served by the organizations—by volume, diagnosis, cost, payer mix, and high-intensity/resource use outliers?
- What is the service path followed by client populations—by entry point, internal flow, discharge, and recidivism?
- What groups of clients fall into high-risk categories—by volume?
- What clients are at risk for less-than-desired outcomes—by morbidity, mortality, infection rates, falls, and clinical outcomes?

The general process for the development of a CM program is to:

1. Assess the organization and the client population served. This assessment provides a baseline for implementation.
2. Identify high-volume or high-risk case types. This assessment will indicate priority areas for care coordination.
3. Determine the usual client care problems, issues, or difficulties related to the high-volume or high-risk case types, with desired goals.
4. Form an interdisciplinary care team of the interrelated care providers who will be involved with the case types.
5. Develop and design an interdisciplinary critical pathway for each selected case type. The path should outline and specify measurable clinical outcomes, key professional care processes, and exact corresponding timelines as based on practice patterns, professional standards of care, and length-of-stay parameters. The input and involvement of the client and each provider group need to be clearly specified in relation to actions for achieving client outcomes. The pathway would mark the occurrence of routine treatments, tests, consults, client activities, medications, diet, educational

interventions, and discharge planning. Variance from the path triggers analysis and intervention.
6. Develop a pilot program or trial site.
7. Evaluate the pilot program and consider system-wide implementation. Review the pilot program's articulation with the existing mode of nursing care delivery.

CM program development processes emphasize the potential of inter-professional team approaches by involving engaged disciplines in establishing treatment plans and completion of outcomes. They also highlight the importance of preparing patients, professionals, and the organization to facilitate success.

CM has become a popular and effective means to manage patients across populations and practice settings. In hospitals, it has decreased length of stay and secured important outcomes (Daniels, 2015; Watson, 2016). In the newest generation of CM settings, including primary care practices, ACOs, and PCMHs, quality and outcomes are being emphasized more than ever (Watson, 2016). Persuasive arguments exist for implementing CM programming. For example, close follow-up, continuous reinforcement, and systematic treatment adjustments facilitated by case managers contributed to improvement for adult clients with diabetes, heart failure, and comorbid physical and mental health conditions (Advancing Integrated Mental Health Solutions [AIMS] Center, 2016; Stellefson et al., 2013; Takeda et al., 2012; Unützer et al., 2013).

CM has equally been identified as a major strategy for cost containment, which also incorporates quality control. Given the vast financial impact for all practice settings, the case manager shoulders significant responsibilities for tracking both quality and outcomes in addition to targeting improvements. These actions are completed as a means to verify the case manager's own performance, the performance of the team, and to some extent the entire organization (Watson, 2016). Research has emerged over the past decade to substantiate savings from CM interventions, including studies on effectiveness from across the industry (Kolbasovsky et al., 2012; Momany et al., 2006; Stellefson et al., 2013).

Case Management Outcomes

Two basic outcomes categories to be captured are clinical outcomes and financial outcomes. For clinical outcomes, Braden (2002) identified these six direct outcomes of CM: (1) patient knowledge, (2) patient involvement, (3) patient participation in care, (4) patient empowerment, (5) patient adherence, and (6) coordination of care.

Improvement in a key indicator (e.g., patient knowledge) can be a direct measure of the clinical effectiveness of a CM intervention. The effectiveness of CM is further strengthened when the outcome of improved patient knowledge is linked to research evidence pertaining to improved patient knowledge reducing chronic relapse or use of health care resources.

Proving financial gain has been somewhat more problematic for CM, although the tide is turning. There has been acknowledged value and acceptance of CM in some areas, such as diabetes, congestive heart failure, and other chronic diseases (Kolbasovsky et al., 2012; Momany et al., 2006; Stellefson et al., 2013). In mental health and substance use, the outcomes are becoming more visible (Fortney et al., 2015; Unützer et al., 2013). A robust amount of literature has emerged courtesy of demonstration projects associated with the Collaborative Care Model out of the University of Washington's Advancing Integrated Mental Health Solutions (AIMS) Center (2016). A full listing of these programs is available on the AIMS Center website *(http://aims.uw. edu/projects).*

DISEASE MANAGEMENT

DM has been acknowledged as a payer strategy to prevent or manage one or more chronic conditions, improve care quality, and reduce costs (Ahmed, 2016; Treadwell & Bean, 2009; Walters et al., 2012) Since DM's entrance into the health care market, the term has experienced a fair level of transition. DM advanced from identification of persons at risk for one chronic condition to reflect a more comprehensive view of the customer base and is one indicative of a global focus on care for entire populations (Ahmed, 2016; Goodman et al., 2014; Rushton, 2015; Walters et al., 2012).

The terms DM and PHM appear throughout this section. However, on the health care management continuum, the overall umbrella concept is better known as PHM. Both CM and DM are segments of the PHM spectrum.

History and Background

DM programs were developed and implemented largely as managed care health plan initiatives. The rise of DM occurred in the late 1980s and into the 1990s in the US health care delivery system. Nested within the general evolution of CM practice, managed care organizations and health plans began to look closely at DM after

initial CM programs had been active for decades. Further refinements in program quality and cost savings were desired by employer group purchasers of health coverage., The unique challenges of chronic conditions occurring on a large scale needed to be addressed. Prior experiences with CM became the platform. In pharmaceutical companies, DM emerged as a way to encourage medication adherence.

Growth of Managed Care Systems and a Focus on Quality Care

Two major forces triggered the rise of a DM perspective: (1) the abundance of managed care systems as a prevailing form of organized health care delivery (the influence of health plans), and (2) the national attention generated by *Crossing the Quality Chasm,* a health care quality initiative of the Institute of Medicine (IOM, now called the National Academies of Sciences, Engineering, and Medicine, Health and Medicine Division). Health plans led the charge to address the care coordination and service integration needs of clusters of members who had identifiable health conditions that are generally chronic in nature. In 1996 the Health and Medicine Division of the National Academies of Sciences, Engineering, and Medicine launched an ongoing effort focused on the assessment and improvement of the quality of health care in the United States. Their 2001 report *Crossing the Quality Chasm: A New Health System for the 21st Century* (IOM, 2001) highlighted the need for profound changes in the environment of care, including revamping practices that fragment the care system. The coordination of care across patient conditions, services, and settings was viewed over time as a major organizational challenge, yet a key dimension of patient-centered care.

DM evolved into proven and effective strategies to make groups of individuals healthier while saving scarce health care coverage dollars (Lipold, 2002). In the early 2000s, the federal government's Centers for Medicare & Medicaid Services (CMS, 2003) took notice of DM programs, sponsored DM demonstration projects, and encouraged contracting with DM vendors for outsourced medical management programs because DM was found to be effective in select populations.

Disease Management Transitions to Population Health Management

Moving into the 21st century, DM's identity shifted because of societal transitions. The community had become a more viable focus for health care services, prompting the need to expand DM's perspective. Social and economic pressures demanded that health care organizations focus on ways to provide cost-effective, population-based care. Roughly 40% of deaths were found to be caused by behaviors that could be modified by preventive, population-based intervention. Although these cases only accounted for a small percentage of health spending, the death and disability prevention aspect was important (Berwick et al., 2008; Shaljian & Nielsen, 2013).

The next generation of health care began to explore the care process across the entire continuum. **Continuum of care** is a concept involving a system that guides and tracks patients over time through a comprehensive array of health services to span all levels and intensity of care (Young et al., 2014). The services incorporated in each patient's unique continuum vary based on the individualized health and/or behavioral health needs of each person.

Prevention and early detection programs (e.g., parenting, wellness), family and community services, pharmacies, behavioral health, and end-of-life care have also been incorporated as components of the continuum of care. Persons who are homeless and those on domestic and/or international travels are also factored into the equation, as are the services incurred during their experience (Young et al., 2014).

Building an effective continuum of care involves understanding the true health needs of an individual community. Emphasis on the health of a community is anchored in a rich history of innovations in community and public health methods and programs directed at reducing risk factor prevalence, decreasing acute and chronic disease burden and injury occurrence, and promoting health (Goodman et al., 2014).

Community health involves meeting the collective needs of a group or individual community by identifying problems and managing interactions both within the community and between the community and the larger society. Risk factors, health status indicators, functional ability levels, health promotion, health outcomes, and prevention of identified chronic diseases are the focus of data gathering, program planning, and implementation processes and activities. The term *community health* has experienced some evolution in recent years to account for the expansion into public health practice settings and the importance of community engagement as a core element (Goodman et al., 2014).

The evolution is further understood by the need for health care professionals to focus more intentionally on both cultural diversity and the social determinants of health, which are key factors for successful patient engagement and activation (Ashford & LeCroy, 2013; Gillespie, 2016; Goodman et al., 2014; Hu et al., 2014).

As the scope of DM grew, a grander scale of attention beckoned for health care professionals interested in addressing societal trends and implications of chronic illness. In the emerging context of wellness and prevention for society, the term population provided a wider lens and presented as a more logical way to refer to the next wave of health management.

A **population** refers to a group of individuals—in contrast to the individuals themselves—organized in many different units of analysis, depending on the research or policy purpose (Kindig, 2007). The **population health** perspective explores beyond a biomedical model of individual health and allows providers to consider what makes some groups of people healthier than other groups of people (Young, 2004). The emphasis by the industry on the impact of socioeconomic factors on hospital readmissions speaks to a population health focus (Hu et al., 2014). Applying population health across the continuum entails the goals of (Nash et al., 2016, p. xvii):

1. Keeping the well, well
2. Reducing health risks
3. Providing quick access to care for acute illness so that health does not deteriorate
4. Managing chronic illness to prevent complications
5. Getting those with complex or catastrophic illness to centers of excellence or compassionate care settings

Accomplishing these goals involves both community participation and partnership, which are key concepts to PHM. Active participation in decision-making processes through a concerted and combined effort induces a vested interest in the success of any effort to improve the health of a community. For nurses, the concept of community as client directs the focus to the collective or common good instead of individual health. Population-based care draws on partnership and community-as-client concepts.

Chronic Health Conditions Align With Population Health Management

Chronic health conditions have long posed a formidable challenge to the health care delivery system. They affect almost half of the adult US population, with 25% having more than one chronic illness (Ward et al., 2013). The management of chronic conditions has been a particular burden for health care payers and employers. Chronic disease creates two particular difficulties for businesses. First, these conditions in the workforce lead to diminished productivity. Second, these conditions result in a greater portion of the business's revenue being diverted to health care expenditures. Further effects have an impact on the health care delivery system, society, and individuals' functioning and activities.

Population and health trends are tracked by governmental agencies such as the US Census Bureau, Centers for Disease Control and Prevention (CDC), Bureau of Labor Statistics (BLS), and Health Resources and Services Administration (HRSA), as well as private foundations and organizations. Clearly, health and health care delivery systems data are continually in flux. However, the available statistics are impressive. Costs are a considerable pressure, because on average individuals with chronic conditions cost 3.5 times as much to serve as others and they account for a large proportion of services (80% of all bed days and 69% of hospital admissions) (Nobel & Norman, 2003). According to the CDC (2012, p. 1):

> Chronic diseases—such as heart disease, cancer, and diabetes—are the leading causes of death and disability in the United States. Chronic diseases account for 70% of all deaths in the U.S., which is 1.7 million each year. These diseases also cause major limitations in daily living for almost 1 out of 10 Americans or about 25 million people. Although chronic diseases are among the most common and costly health problems, they are also among the most preventable. Adopting healthy behaviors such as eating nutritious foods, being physically active, and avoiding tobacco use can prevent or control the devastating effects of these diseases.

The chronic conditions that pose a particular economic burden but can be helped by PHM are characterized by high prevalence, high expense, relatively standardized treatment guidelines, and a significant role played by the individual's behavior on the progression of the condition.

It is widely recognized that health care delivery can and must be improved. The pressures to provide access to care, maintain a high level of quality, and control expenditures are converging on a traditionally fragmented and acute care–focused system. Projections are that sociodemographic and economic tidal waves are set to converge in a "perfect storm" of crisis over health care in the near future. These tidal waves include the aging of the US population, the effect of the maturing of the baby boom generation, high pharmaceutical costs, advancing medical technology, dramatic increases in chronic health conditions, and US government budget deficits.

The solutions are not easy or obvious. However, PHM is now being viewed as a major health care strategy to improve health outcomes across multiple populations while lowering costs and improving patient satisfaction. It is one of the Institute for Healthcare Improvement's (2017) Triple Aims and is an important aspect of ACOs. PHM has demonstrated effectiveness across disease states, including integrated behavioral health, chronic illness (e.g., diabetes, congestive heart failure), and assorted payers (e.g., Medicare, Medicaid, third party populations) (Fortney et al., 2015; Lyles, 2016; Rushton, 2015; Sidorov & Romney, 2016). Attractive features include effective population management, coordination of care for chronic conditions, consistency of care for at-risk populations, customization of care support, encouragement of adherence to treatment, and proactive interventions.

Population Health Management Practice Approaches

Early DM programs offered by health plans were developed in house or purchased either from a vendor or another organization such as a hospital. The newest generation of PHM programs involves proactive outreach. Nursing outreach programs are the core element. Personal communications (usually via telephone) between an expert nurse and the health plan participant build a personal relationship, help identify knowledge deficits and counseling needs, facilitate close monitoring and progress toward goals, enhance treatment adherence, and promote clinical and cost stabilization.

Functioning as a personal health advisor, the health coach, case manager, or care coordinator establishes a single point of contact and coordination of care and service for patients having health problems and promotes a trusting relationship. Whether employed by a health plan or a contracted outside vendor, the PHM provided by nurses functioning as personal health advisors and advocates is central to effective outcomes.

The core of the DM concept was to comprehensively integrate care and reimbursement based on a disease or health condition's natural course. Both clinical and nonclinical interventions are timed to occur where and when they are most likely to have the greatest impact. This sequencing and targeting ideally prevents occurrences or exacerbations, decreases the use of expensive resources, and creates positive health outcomes through the use of prevention and proactive CM strategies. Chronic conditions are the focus, and the methods use systematic ways of delivering health care interventions to patients with similar characteristics. PHM models focus on the identification, standardization, and coordination of services across the continuum of care and for populations with the same or similar health care needs. Several program examples are discussed in the following sections.

The Population Care Coordination Process

Rushton's (2015) *Population Care Coordination Process* provides a scalable framework for providers and/or organizations (e.g., single offices or larger ACOs) to provide multilevel care based on population- and patient-centered principles. It involves care coordination, CM, and PHM to maximize health outcomes and resource utilization for populations and the individuals within them. The process involves six phases to focus on coordinating care for the entire population with individualization of that care: data analysis, selection, assessment, multidisciplinary planning, implementation/intervention, and monitoring/evaluation (Rushton, 2015).

Care of Mental, Physical and Substance Use Syndromes

Identified as one of the largest Collaborative Care population health implementation initiatives, the Care of Mental, Physical and Substance Use Syndromes (COMPASS) initiative included over 4000 Medicare and Medicaid patients across 187 clinics in seven states: California, Colorado, Massachusetts, Michigan, Minnesota, Pennsylvania, and Washington (Fortney et al., 2015). A core systematic case review (SCR) team intervened with chronically ill patients who were diagnosed with uncontrolled depression and uncontrolled diabetes and/or heart disease. The following program components were included:

- An initial evaluation to measure condition severity and assess the patient's readiness for self-management
- A computerized registry to track and monitor the patient's progress
- A care manager to provide patient education and self-management support, coordinate care with the primary care physician and consultants, and provide active follow-up.
- A consulting psychiatrist and consulting medical physician to review cases with the care manager and

recommend changes in treatment to the primary care physician
- Treatment intensification when there is a lack of improvement
- Relapse and exacerbation prevention

Overall aggregated results from all 18 participating regional groups demonstrated that goals were exceeded for depression, heart disease, and diabetes improvement (Advancing Integrated Mental Health Solutions, 2016; Fortney et al., 2015).

Evolving Practice Standards and Guidelines

Unlike the clear and prevalent industry practice standards for CM, PHM is just achieving its stride with respect to established professional guidelines. The *Population Health Alliance Outcomes Guidelines, Vol. 6,* was released in 2015 and serves as a basis for many PHM programs throughout the industry (Population Health Alliance [PHA], 2015). For professional certification, the Chronic Care Professional (CCP) Certification has been offered since 2004 to eligible professionals working in health care or a health-related field. Non-clinical team members (e.g., community health educators, program leaders, or consultants who support health and chronic care improvement) may also apply (Health Sciences Institute, 2016).

Since 2002, The Joint Commission (TJC, 2016) has offered Disease-Specific Care (DSC) Certification. The program "is designed to evaluate clinical programs across the continuum of care." TJC-accredited health care organizations may seek a 2-year certification for care and services provided for virtually any chronic disease or condition. In addition, an advanced level of certification is available to programs that meet the requirements for DSC certification plus additional clinically specific requirements and expectations. The available advanced certification programs include: acute stroke ready hospital, chronic kidney disease, chronic obstructive pulmonary disease, comprehensive stroke center, heart failure, inpatient diabetes, lung volume reduction surgery, palliative care, perinatal care, primary stroke center, and ventricular assist device (TJC, 2015, 2016).

The American Organization of Nurse Executives (AONE, 2015) developed *Nurse Executive Competencies: Population Health.* Leadership from the nurse executive is viewed as vital to the development, execution, and refinement of PHM programming. As an advocate for community health needs and patient populations, the nurse executive—and his or her role as an agent of change—is viewed as paramount (AONE, 2015).

The National Association of Chronic Disease Directors (NACDD, 2016) is a non-profit public health organization committed to serving chronic disease program directors of each state and US jurisdiction. NACDD works to provide educational and training, develop legislative materials, educate policymakers, provide technical assistance, develop partnerships and collaborations, and advocate for the use of epidemiological approaches in chronic disease services planning and chronic disease data. Moving forward, it is expected that the industry will see the further development and evolution of more standards, organizations, and certifications specific to PHM.

Disease Management Process, Program Development and Implementation

The goal of DM is to maintain or improve the current state of chronic disease(s) through the systematic use of evidence-based interventions. DM uses risk assessment, education, and risk factor reduction strategies to influence behaviors toward the goals of improving outcomes and reducing cost (Ahmed, 2016). DM has been a pivotal health care strategy for decades. However, unlike CM there does not appear to be a single endorsed DM process that is consistently referenced in texts or journals. The general components associated with a DM program include population risk analysis, identification, stratification, enrollment and engagement, program delivery, outcomes and effectiveness evaluation, and reporting. Each of these components is displayed in Fig. 16.1 and is amplified further in this section.

Before identification of a specific population eligible for a DM program, health plans and DM companies analyze claims data to identify the conditions that are prevalent in a given population. This is completed using coding conventions such as the International Classification of Diagnosis (ICD) and Current Procedural Terminology (CPT). This, combined with claims expenditure data, reveals disease classifications that most affect a covered population. From this perspective an organization is able to determine its strategic and tactical priorities for program development.

Disease Management Program Components
Population Risk Assessment

The aggregate health care costs of chronic conditions increase yearly as individuals grow older. Older individuals tend to have chronic conditions that require complex care. It is estimated that one-third to one-half of all health care spending is consumed by the elderly. With the shift in demographic trends toward increasing numbers of elderly, there is a shift in the need for preventive care and chronic illness management services (Coleman, 1999). To meet this challenge, managed care organizations have created infrastructures of population-based risk assessment, demand management (self-management and decision support systems such as call centers), DM, and CM.

To be effective at individual and population-based care management, both CM and DM programs need to identify, assess, and define the populations to be served early in the program planning effort. This component represents the effort to assess the health of a specific population (e.g., patient panel, enrollment). This assessment typically "triangulates" by drawing on available types of information (e.g., self-reported health questionnaires, health insurance claims, laboratory and pharmacy data, and clinician documentation). Once the population is defined, individuals within the population must be selected and assessed as to which program and level of intervention will optimally meet the most pressing needs. Factors that are included in an individual profile include age, number of chronic illnesses, and number of medications (CCA, 2012a).

Identification

The participant identification process is driven by algorithms or other logic frameworks that are applied to claims data and look for specific diagnosis codes. In addition, predictive modeling tools (e.g., artificial intelligence, neural net logic) are leveraged to harvest information beyond simple diagnosis. *Predictive modeling* is "a commonly used statistical technique to predict future behavior. Predictive modeling solutions are a form of data-mining technology that works by analyzing historical and current data and generating a model to help predict future outcomes" (Gartner, 2016). Predictive models have been used in other industries and businesses, such as credit card companies and retailers, for years. In health care, these methodologies look for experience and other red flags that indicate an individual is at risk and to what extent. The case-finding techniques help to identify individuals who appear to be in most need of additional support in order to stem worsening health conditions and resource expenditures. The identified individuals are then screened by intake specialists to determine the best match between program intensity and client need (Ahmed, 2016).

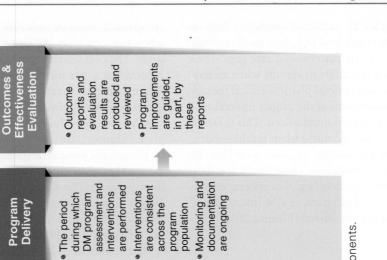

FIG. 16.1 Depiction of disease management program components.

Population Risk Analysis
- Process to identify, assess, and define the population
- Individuals assessed for the need of CM or DM intervention
- Sometimes considered part of **Identification**

Identification
- Process of claims data used to identify conditions or therapies (or gaps in therapies) in a targeted population
- Consumers are evaluated through stratification to determine risk and level of DM support
- Sometimes considered part of **Risk Analysis**

Stratification
- Process of sorting a population of eligible consumers into groups based on relative need versus the total population
- May integrate a variety of available data (e.g., claims, pharmacy, laboratory, health risks, consumer-reported) and individual assessment to assign level

Enrollment & Engagement
- Process of assignment and/or outreach to qualified candidates
- Includes passive and active engagement
- May be opt-in or opt-out strategy
- Individual consent to participate is usually voluntary and may be rescinded

Program Delivery
- The period during which DM program assessment and interventions are performed
- Interventions are consistent across the program population
- Monitoring and documentation are ongoing

Outcomes & Effectiveness Evaluation
- Outcome reports and evaluation results are produced and reviewed
- Program improvements are guided, in part, by these reports

Additional cycles of predictive modeling help to stratify each person's risk level (e.g., low, medium, high) as well as to look at care patterns and care gaps. These programs also have the ability to identify when an individual is not receiving optimal pharmaceutical therapy, is not having provider visits at the proper interval, or is not receiving the proper immunizations. This information is available to the DM nurse when reaching out to clients, providers, pharmacies, or other providers involved with the individual's care. These results also drive the intensity of intervention (e.g., reminders, risk reduction measures, DM program, or CM interventions) that an individual may be offered (Plocher, 2013).

Stratification

The next step in the population health process is to stratify patients into meaningful categories for patient-centered intervention targeting that uses information collected in health assessments (CCA, 2012a). In population health management, **stratification** has two meanings (PHA, 2015): a method of randomization and a process for sorting a population of eligible members into groups relating to their relative need for total population management interventions. Stratification may be based on the integration of a variety of data, if available, including claims, pharmacy, laboratory, health risks, or consumer-reported data such as health assessments. The stratification process harvests information that can be used to divide the patient population into different levels to ensure a return on investment (ROI) based on resources allowed.

Enrollment and Engagement

Once individuals are identified and stratified, those who appear to qualify for DM intervention receive an outreach notification (e.g., telephone call). The opportunity to enroll in a condition-specific program is offered during this initial contact. The program is explained, and consent to participate is requested. Although the enrollment process sounds straightforward, there are a number of barriers to overcome in getting individuals on-boarded into a program, such as inaccurate data, incorrect contact information, and outright refusal (Plocher, 2013).

One factor that is at the root of some nonenrollment is consumer mistrust of the insurance company's motives for contact. This concept contributes to unwillingness to participate in programs offered by the insurance company. Consumer mistrust is especially important when one considers the cost of delivering a DM program. The cost relating to a DM program is frequently reported at a per-member-per-month (PMPM) level. The expense of creating and maintaining such programs is borne by the insurance company regardless of whether the individual actively participates in the program (Ahmed, 2016).

Historically, program engagement has been a challenge, as typically only about 20% of those eligible participate in these programs (Brown et al., 2012; Schore et al., 1999). Despite these programs being established for decades, research on why people opt out or do not participate is limited (Hawkins et al., 2014).

The results of a 2014 study that examined factors driving engagement suggest that individuals most motivated to engage are those who are well informed of the program benefits and have a perceived need that would benefit from said program (e.g., living alone, needing a supportive person to discuss ideas) (Hawkins et al., 2014). Recruitment and engagement strategies continue to evolve, but the challenges facing this component of DM programming include privacy, meaningful engagement, and physician integration (Plocher, 2013).

Program Delivery

Whenever possible, the components of DM should be delivered by leveraging a variety of communications and interventions. This mixed mode approach optimizes the resources and outreach and accommodates the preferences and technological abilities of recipients with the ultimate goal of increased engagement and self-management (CCA, 2012b). This also takes into account that communication preferences vary based on generational differences. Although demographic splitting by age groups may not lead to absolute accuracy, it is generally accepted that communicating with a baby boomer versus a millennial requires consideration of a variety of channels (e.g., social media, hard copy print, telephone calls).

Interaction and management. Communication is a means of interaction and management for program delivery. It mostly involves the program participants, primary care providers, and program staff. There are a number of communication channels used to enhance interaction between the plan and both member and provider. The choice of modes used depends on the organization's ability to maintain compliance with the

Health Insurance Portability and Accountability Act of 1996 (HIPAA) across each channel, financial resources to establish and maintain each channel, understanding of a given population's communication preferences, and other factors. Examples of communication options include (Plocher, 2013):

- Mailings
  - Information to enrollee: welcome packet, interval updates and results, reminders
  - Information to provider: orientation packet, periodic progress updates, periodic guideline recommendations
- Outbound telephone calls and interactive voice response (IVR) (e.g., initial welcome, assessments, progress checks, coaching)
- Inbound calls from participants to address condition and DM care plan questions
- Internet-based text and video chats for progress updates, reminders, condition and DM care plan questions
- Home telemonitoring devices for home device connection to monitor real time results. Frequently transmitted biometrics are weight, vital signs, and pulse oximetry.
- Medication adherence tools with pill box monitoring support for complex medication regimens
- Technology platforms (e.g., web portals) for secure messaging
- Face-to-face conversation for assessment, progress updates, and coaching

As technology continues to develop, so too will communication options. Technology is a core expectation of DM programs. Organizations have invested millions in developing technology to support DM programs from front (e.g., population assessment to identify prevalence, risk stratification) to back (e.g., reporting, effectiveness, outcomes analysis).

Outcomes and Effectiveness Evaluation

Program outcomes and effectiveness reports are an evolving source of information. Before-and-after program enrollment comparison is a common method of demonstrating program impact, but these often require at least a year of continuous participant enrollment to be deemed significant. In addition, the Healthcare Effectiveness Data Information Set (HEDIS®) requires this time span for data collection. These metrics look at testing frequency or certain drugs being prescribed, instead of test result improvement, such as hemoglobin A_1C, low density lipoprotein (LDL) cholesterol, appropriately prescribed angiotensin converting enzyme inhibitor, and appropriately prescribed beta blockers.

In today's lightning-fast, results-driven environment, waiting a full year to see results of an investment is difficult to sell. Metrics of interest include PMPM cost, episode-of-care cost, and utilization (e.g., hospital admissions, inpatient days) (Plocher, 2013). This imperative has spurred on the use of "big data" analytics. For example, at Geisinger Clinic in Pennsylvania, the big data approach was eyed to better manage patients with chronic conditions. Big data is defined as the large volume of structured and unstructured data that swamps businesses on a day-to-day basis (SAS, 2016). Much of the data collected about patients lies dormant and is not used in routine analytic methods. Geisinger undertook a process redesign with its coronary artery disease (CAD) program that eliminated waste, automated processes where possible, and delegated tasks to appropriate staff. Geisinger accelerated the delivery of care through continuous use of data and informatics and addressed nine patient-oriented goals focused on improving the health of nearly 17,000 patients with CAD. The goals were measured in an "all or none" bundle to encourage team-based workflows rather than measures that focused on a particular team member's performance (e.g., prescribing rate). The measures addressed care issues faced by all patients with CAD. The bundled approach to care measures realized a 300% improvement. The use of big data analytics was anticipated to harvest even more significant improvements in patient care (Graf et al., 2014). The use of big data is poised to flourish in all areas of health care, translating massive amounts of unusable data into useable information.

Reporting

In their 2015 joint report, the Health Enhancement Research Organization (HERO) and Population Health Alliance (PHA) published a core guide to metrics, the *Program Measurement & Evaluation Guide: Core Metrics for Employee Health Management*. The categories included financial, health outcomes, participation, satisfaction, organizational support, productivity and performance, and value on investment framework. The report was framed by the following statement, "HERO and PHA are responding to employers who seek a greater level of clarity regarding the value of their wellness efforts. Thus we recommend an initial set of measures to assess the impact of the health management programs offered to employees. The results are better informed business decisions and boardroom discussions" (HERO-PHA, 2015). Although aimed at employer groups, these metrics are solid indicators of PHM program impacts. These metric categories may be applied in whole or in part to measure program impacts and as a means for classifying areas requiring further performance improvement.

When designing and implementing a DM program, use of a detailed project plan is essential to develop and maintain. This is done to track progress toward completion and hold stakeholders accountable for completing assigned tasks. Once implemented, in addition to program metrics, the project plan gives way to more simplified tools such as checklists. Table 16.4 depicts one such checklist. It is strongly recommended that tools such as this be customized to each unique program.

LEADERSHIP AND MANAGEMENT IMPLICATIONS

Nurses who manage client care are clinical managers. The shift to managed care in integrated health systems and ever-expanding care settings (e.g., ACO, PCMH) highlights CM as a key strategy for nursing practice management and empowerment of nurses. It also has made care team collaboration an imperative. Leadership roles for nurses are essential because of the need for care continuity.

Future CM effectiveness is thought to be based on decisions about what types of organizational structures and nursing care delivery systems best enable nurse-managed client care and best support nurses in practice. One related question is, "How much management structure does a nurse require to be effective?" One assessment is the extent

TABLE 16.4 Checklist to Evaluate Disease Management Programs		
Component	Present (Yes); Absent (No)	Specific Method or Metric Used
Population identification and selection		
Risk assessment		
Risk stratification		
Use of evidence-based practice guidelines		
Type of practice model		
Collaborative mechanism		
Single-discipline predominates (identify)		
Patient self-management		
Education		
Primary prevention		
Behavior modification		
Lifestyle change motivation		
Telephone contact		
Health advocates		
Compliance/adherence		
Surveillance		
Process, outcomes management		
Process identification and measurement		
Process evaluation		
Outcomes identification and measurement		
Outcomes evaluation		
Process and outcomes management		
Feedback loop		
Communication to:		
Patient		
Physician		
Health plan		
Ancillary providers		
Practice profiling		

From Coggeshall Press. (2017). *Care for the total population.* Coralville, IA: Author.

to which a nurse provides client care or manages the care of clients. CM is one specific approach to redesigning care delivery for client care improvement. This may mean that some traditional management practices need to be changed or discarded. CM has come to be a part of care delivery management that emphasizes the expertise of nurses (see Chapter 15).

CM is practiced beyond the walls of the acute care setting. There is no single way to go about identifying how much management structure is necessary because of the variety of care settings and associated bureaucracy. CM leader-managers need to examine the state of health care management in their organizations and develop strategies to implement coordination of care models to best meet client, organizational, societal, and professional priorities, often referred to as patient-and-family-centered models. Given the interdisciplinary nature of CM, model development and success may require a buy-in by other health care disciplines and other organizational stakeholders. Physicians and hospital administrators are crucial stakeholders for the success of CM programs. The CM leader-manager needs to master communication, collaboration, and advocacy skills in order to effect changes within his/her own department as well as across the organization.

Partnering With Human Resources

Another CM leader-manager challenge is the human resources department itself. Now more than ever the question "Who is qualified to be hired as a case manager?" is one that needs careful consideration. In today's outcomes-driven health care environment, it is important to have the right people in the right positions to maximize their experience, knowledge, and skills. In short, competence should be the driver of personnel changes.

The CM leader-manager works closely with a human resource specialist (HRS) to clarify department structure, mission, and vision. Job descriptions should clearly distinguish position types and grade levels. New position descriptions should provide the required experience, knowledge, and skills that a qualified candidate should possess. CM position descriptions must reflect education level and credential requirements, being mindful to distinguish requirements from preferences so as to simplify the candidate screening process.

Individual Suitability for Case Management

CM leader-managers need to evaluate employees in existing positions who are considered as case managers. In many situations, job titles and/or responsibilities change over the years regardless of whether the employees are well suited for their new scope of work. In other instances, department reorganizations have allowed people to retain the coveted case manager job title despite the position's purpose having changed significantly. There must be an objective process in place in order to fairly evaluate existing employees. Reassignments may be necessary after such an evaluation process. The evaluation process is stressful on staff and management. The CM leader-manager needs to have a clear vision, strategy, and a proactive communication plan in order to move the department through the change management process.

It is important to clarify the requisite experience and credentialing required to fill the CM job. Certification is typically an official credential awarded to an individual by a nationally recognized professional organization based on eligibility and passing a standardized examination. The credential affirms a baseline degree of education, experience, and knowledge. Individual certification is a mark of professional achievement, and although it is difficult to attain, certification is a floor—not a ceiling—of achievement.

CURRENT ISSUES AND TRENDS

There are constant pressures that affect CM practice, including the lack of title protection, which allows misuse of the case manager designation; the inflow of unlicensed and inexperienced individuals performing CM tasks; and challenges with licensure portability affecting individuals' ability to work seamlessly to provide care coordination services across state lines. This section is devoted to select challenges currently challenging the CM workforce.

Branding and Lack of Universal Definition

Health care reform has amplified the number of career options for the CM workforce, especially with the expansion of ACOs, PCMHs, and integrated behavioral health programs. These opportunities span business models, practice settings, professional disciplines, and across the transitions of care. Yet a double-edged sword exists with regard to the vast number of CM-associated titles, roles, functions, and job descriptions that have followed suit. Experts challenge that this expansion has contributed to a paradoxical effect on CM's identity (Treiger & Fink-Samnick, 2013; 2016).

Patients and family caregivers, employers, and other stakeholders with a vested interest are consistently challenged to comprehend the similarities and differences among the many job titles for CM (e.g., case manager, care manager, geriatric care manager, care coordinator, case worker, care advocate, advanced life care planner, patient advocate, patient navigator, health care coach). This role multiplicity is one more obstacle to CM's maturity from advanced practice to established profession (Treiger & Fink-Samnick, 2013; 2016). It also serves to splinter rather than forge a strong foundation for professional CM practice.

Influx of Unqualified, Non-Clinical Workers

Maintaining a workforce consisting primarily of licensed and/or certified clinical professionals is an expensive proposition. In spite of geographical variation, RNs and SWs are justifiably compensated for their clinical and health care system knowledge. Historically, organizations employed RNs and SWs in CM positions. Later, when organizations became more focused on cost-savings and efficiency, they began to use non-clinical staff to perform CM activities or applied the case manager job title indiscriminately in order to attract candidates with a desirable position. The impact of this staffing methodology on care quality or value for service delivered has not been clearly or consistently demonstrated (Treiger, 2011).

The economics of maintaining a workforce largely made up of clinical professionals continues to force review of hiring practices and raises questions pertaining to required qualifications of individuals working in CM. To reduce program costs, some organizations opt to hire individuals for care coordination positions who lack a professional degree and/or have limited if any clinical experience necessary to handle the complexity of CM functions. In one Midwestern health system, this hiring strategy was brought to an abrupt halt when leaders realized that the staff hired to coordinate care were not qualified to perform an independent assessment, unable to clearly identify patient care challenges and needs as an outcome of the independent assessment, and unqualified to develop a CM care plan to address individual challenges and needs. The failure was corrected by hiring appropriate staff (e.g., RN, SW) for CM positions. However, this was not without some pain and lost time in having to rework an otherwise well-considered corporate revitalization. CM leader-managers need to continue to advocate for a strong workforce made up

largely of professional case managers who are qualified to maintain CM practice integrity.

Legislative and Regulatory Disruptors
Licensure Portability and the Nurse Licensure Compact

Current regulations continue to be grossly out of sync with practice realities for health care professionals, particularly nurses engaged in CM. Many case managers experience huge challenges and potential violations for practicing without a license in a state where the patient is. The case manager may not be licensed to practice in that particular state, and/or their scope of practice fails to allow for telehealth practice (Fink-Samnick & Muller, 2015). This has been a chronic issue, particularly for those nurses employed by national managed care and/or workers' compensation organizations, multihospital systems, or other health and behavioral health providers. For example, tele-management assessment is not permitted consistently across all professional disciplines or states. As a result, nurses are encouraged to check the websites for their respective individual professional state licensure boards and/or certifications on a regular basis to accurately define their individual scope of practice (Fink-Samnick & Muller, 2015).

The **Nurse Licensure Compact** (NLC) gives multistate rights to RNs and licensed practical/vocational nurses (LPN/VN) residing in a member state. Advance practice nurses (APN) maintain a separate compact. The NLC allows nurses to have one multistate license with the ability to practice in both their home state and other compact states (National Council of State Boards of Nursing, 2016). The advancement of the NLC across states has been a vital factor to promote the legal practice of CM across state lines. A current map of NLC member states is available (*https://www.ncsbn.org/nurse-licensure-compact.htm*).

Measuring and Sharing Case Management Outcomes

In 2010, the Agency for Healthcare Research and Quality (AHRQ) issued the comparative effectiveness report *Outpatient Case Management for Adults With Medical Illness and Complex Care Needs* (Hickam et al., 2013). The report focused on this single segment of practice and specific questions pertaining to case management as an intervention strategy for chronic illness outpatient management. The findings clearly note that there was a wide diversity in the included study populations, interventions, and outcomes. That notwithstanding, the overall conclusion was that case management demonstrated limited impact on patient-centered outcomes, quality of care, and resource utilization among patients with chronic medical illness (Hickam et al., 2013). It is important to sort out the conflicting literature on CM outcomes because direct cause-and-effect may not capture the actual importance of CM to clients and because cost reduction or ROI is hard to demonstrate when a labor-intensive service like CM is added.

These findings need to be leveraged to identify and implement program modifications as well as determine measures that accurately capture CM as value-added irrespective of monetary ROI. Sharing of program metrics across the health care continuum is one way in which research-generated evidence will influence practice moving forward. CM leader-managers undertaking quality and process improvements within a CM department must remain mindful of the importance of the evidence generated from these efforts because it is valuable to the entire CM community.

Treatment Adherence

Treatment adherence continues to be a driver of disease cost and a needed focus of intervention with patients. Medication adherence alone is estimated to have an annual cost of $100 billion in the United States (Lee, 2016). *Adherence* refers to the extent to which the patient continues a negotiated treatment. The topics of treatment adherence and patient engagement are major drivers in ensuring successful outcomes and establishing a PHM program's ROI.

Health risk behaviors (e.g., smoking, inactivity, poor diets, or nonadherence to prescribed therapies) significantly contribute to a population's overall morbidity, disability, mortality, reduced productivity, and escalating health care costs (Lee, 2016; Prochaska & Prochaska, 2016). Intense employer focus on wellness and prevention has escalated the importance of and growth of PHM programs. Studies show as many as 73% of companies are offering workplace or employee wellness to incentivize engagement in healthy lifestyles (Lee, 2016). Identified reasons for low ROI for early DM programs have included late identification of patients, turnover rate, lack of benefit coordination (especially when using an outside DM vendor), and the presence of comorbidities (Ahmed, 2016).

More engaged patients incur lower costs, whereas less engaged patients can generate up to 21% higher health care costs (Calhoun et al., 2016). Successful interventions with nonadherent patient populations include using the transtheoretical model of behavior change, which integrates advising, guiding, and supporting patients through the six stages of health behavior change: precontemplation, contemplation, preparation, action, maintenance, and termination. Key strategies and processes have been identified that work best at each stage to reduce resistance, facilitate progress, and minimize relapse (Prochaska & Prochaska, 2016) (see Chapter 2).

There are planned updates to popular health risk assessments over the next few years toward a more conclusive assessment that takes into account determinants of health and performance (e.g., advances in technology, use of smartphones, and new research) (Edington et al., 2016). All health care professionals, especially nurses, can develop the skills to engage patients in the care process through leveraging meaningful use goals (e.g., health IT) and delivering adherence interventions (Calhoun et al., 2016; Prochaska & Prochaska, 2016).

Conclusion

Health care's strong fiscal imperatives have the industry well aligned with the business sector. Organizations strive to align overall goals, financial drivers of care, and department staffing in way that demonstrates ROI as a marker for financial viability. As a result, leaders need to ensure solid processes are in place to guide the development of department programming, provide clear job descriptions for those to be hired, and render a comprehensive means to identify and promote performance quality.

Despite the widespread dissemination of CM and DM as an intervention and system-wide strategy, a number of challenges remain specific to program development and implementation. Organizations struggle with a number of issues including whether and how to internally combine or separate functions. With an emphasis on financial viability or profit margin, CM and DM programs have been analyzed, challenged, redesigned, and reinvented under different labels in order to justify the allocation of scarce resources to them. Where CM is concerned, continued confusion over definitions, evolution and expansion of titles, and ongoing licensure and reimbursement challenges further contribute to constant changes within CM departments and programs.

RESEARCH NOTE

Source
Katon, W.J., Lin, E.H., Von Korff, M., Ciechanowski, P., Ludman, E.J., Young, B., et al. (2010). Collaborative care for patients with depression and chronic illnesses. *New England Journal of Medicine, 363*(27), 2611–2620.

Purpose
Patients with depression and poorly controlled diabetes, coronary heart disease, or both have an increased risk of adverse outcomes and high health care costs. Care for patients who have multiple chronic illnesses (43% of Medicare beneficiaries) accounts for more than 80% of Medicare health care costs. Major depression is especially prevalent among patients who have diabetes and coronary heart disease. Major depression is also a risk factor for poor self-care, complications, and death.

A study was conducted to determine whether coordinated care management of multiple conditions improves disease control in these patients. A single-blind, randomized, controlled trial was implemented across 14 primary care clinics in an integrated health care system in Washington state. It involved 214 participants who had poorly controlled diabetes, coronary heart disease, or both, along with coexisting depression. Patients were randomly assigned to either the usual care group or to the intervention group, in which a medically supervised nurse worked with each patient's primary care physician. Patients in the intervention group also received guideline-based, collaborative care management, with the goal of controlling risk factors associated with multiple diseases.

The primary outcome was based on simultaneous modeling of glycated hemoglobin, low-density lipoprotein (LDL) cholesterol, and systolic blood pressure levels and Symptom Checklist-20 (SCL-20) depression outcomes at 12 months; this modeling allowed estimation of a single overall treatment effect.

Discussion
At the end of the 12 months, changes were noticed with respect to both behavioral and medical adherence. An intervention involving nurses who provided guideline-based, patient-centered management of depression and chronic disease significantly improved control of medical disease and depression compared with those assigned to the usual care group.

Patients in the intervention group (37%) were also more likely than patients who received usual care (22%) to meet guideline criteria or achieve clinically significant improvement from baseline values for control of glycated hemoglobin, LDL cholesterol, and systolic blood pressure and to have a decrease in systolic blood pressure of 10 mm Hg or more and a 1% or greater decrease in the glycated hemoglobin level.

Nurses enhanced patient self-care with education encompassing self-monitoring, behavioral activation (e.g., increase in enjoyable activities), goal setting, and problem solving to improve medication adherence. Weekly supervision and case reviews by attending physicians and nurses provided timely support for the primary care physician in adjusting medications to achieve specific clinical goals.

Application to Practice
DM and PHM involved strategic interventions targeted to a defined population. An intervention involving proactive follow-up by nurse care managers working closely with physicians, integrating the management of medical and psychological illnesses, and using individualized treatment regimens guided by treat-to-target principles improved both medical outcomes and depression in depressed patients with diabetes, coronary heart disease, or both.

CASE STUDY

Having formed an ACO, the Helping Hands Health System has taken on accountability for behavioral health for its population. There are too few psych/mental health providers, fewer beds available, and the hospital's emergency department (ED) has been forced to board psych patients for up to 7 days in the ED due to physicians deeming them not safe for discharge. This is exacerbated by the state-run chronic mental health institution's location nearby, because patients from the institution come to the ED when they have comorbid physical health issues.

Nurse Mike Catney has been called back from retirement to address the issues because of his years of psych/mental health experience and certification as an ARNP. His challenge is to set up a comprehensive PHM program that meets quality and cost goals. He searches the literature, reviews the history of CM models, and chooses the Collaborative Care Model as the basis for design of the new program, which will coordinate the provision of services using social casework and PHM principles. He first needs to implement the model using professional nurse and social worker case managers. Policies and procedures need to be in place. Meanwhile, he needs to use a robust IT platform and begin to use data analytics for decision making. He decides to use the seven steps of the general process for development of a CM program and begins with assessing the organization and the client population and looking for high-volume and high-risk case types.

CRITICAL THINKING EXERCISE

Nurse Chun Li works in maternal–child health and has a special focus on high-risk pregnant teens. She also is currently in a master's program and taking a leadership class. She has a class assignment to design a new program for her population of interest. The problem she has identified is that the pregnant teens exhibit apathy and lack of engagement in the educational and social support activities already set up to teach them parenting skills, yet these activities are designed to prevent poor outcomes after the baby is born. Nurse Li knows that something different needs to be done, and she wants to be creative. She thinks perhaps a different model is needed but is confused among the various types of CM, DM, and PHM programs.

1. What is the problem?
2. Why is it a problem?
3. What information does Nurse Li need to proceed?
4. What should Nurse Li do first?
5. What CM and PHM strategies might be useful?

Evidence-Based Practice: Strategies for Nursing Leaders

Laura Cullen, Kirsten Hanrahan, Nathan Neis,
Michele Farrington, Trudy A. Laffoon, Cindy J. Dawson

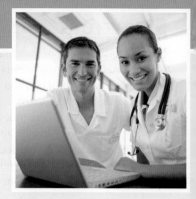

http://evolve.elsevier.com/Huber/leadership

Nursing has a long history of using research to improve practice beginning with Florence Nightingale's work, re-emphasized with research utilization efforts from the 1980s, and progressing to the current trend in using best evidence to engage patients in guiding patient care. There is now a rising expectation by consumers as well as in regulatory standards that evidence-based knowledge be used in health care. Despite national and international policy and research agendas, provision of evidence-based care does not meet expectations, and a continued gap exists between the conduct and application of research findings (Atamna et al., 2016; Ball et al., 2016; Ivanovska et al., 2016; Von Korff et al., 2015; Wieczorkiewicz & Zatarski, 2015). Using the evidence-based practice (EBP) process to answer clinical and operational questions can be challenging.

Nurses in leadership positions have responsibility for building and expanding use of EBPs in care delivery to improve patient and organizational outcomes (Baggett et al., 2014; Dogherty et al., 2012; Everett & Sitterding, 2011; Forberg et al., 2014; Gifford et al., 2013; Hauck et al., 2013; Matthew-Maich et al., 2013; Melnyk et al., 2016; Parkosewich, 2013; Stetler et al., 2014; Taylor et al., 2015; Tonges et al., 2015). A number of models are available to provide direction for use of the EBP process for individual projects. Implementing EBP initiatives as an organizational program requires additional strategies for success. Information is not as readily available to guide nurse executives in building EBP programs within health care organizations. Given this challenge, a systematic approach is outlined to provide guidance.

Although the demand for EBP has grown, implementation science on which EBP work is based is still developing. The application of EBP is the responsibility of every nursing leader, especially those in the nurse manager role. This chapter outlines successful strategies used to expand an EBP culture and program for a clinical setting and an organization.

The best process to use when addressing clinical or operational issues depends on the question at hand and the extent of research or other evidence available on the topic. Several processes may be used to improve care, from quality/performance improvement to EBP or conduct of research. For questions that can be addressed through quality improvement (e.g., efficient throughput), improvements may be quickly brought to the patient level. Clinical questions with little or no research that include patient risk may be appropriate questions to answer by conducting research. EBP offers the benefit of using existing evidence for effective interventions, implementation, and in guiding how to avoid unintended consequences.

DEFINITIONS

An understanding of evidence-based practice and related concepts requires knowledge of a variety of terms. **Evidence-based practice** is a process of shared decision making in a partnership between patients and clinicians that involves the integration of research and other best evidence with clinical expertise and patient values and preferences in making health care decisions (Sackett et al., 2000; Sigma Theta Tau International Research and Scholarship

Photo used with permission from Photos.com.

Advisory Committee, 2008). This emphasizes inclusion of the best available evidence (e.g., research informed by lower level evidence). EBP is a scientific process for improving health care quality and safety by building on what is learned from—as well as influencing—quality improvement and conduct of research.

Additional terms are also important to understand. **Best practice** is a popular term, but the definition remains elusive. Use of the term may describe innovative practices that are recognized by peer organizations and that contribute to quality or fiscal goals. Although "best practice" and "evidence-based practice" are sometimes used interchangeably, the extent that "best practices" are evidence based is often unclear. To promote understanding, it is recommended that when using scientific evidence for guidance, the term evidence-based practice provides better clarity.

A **clinical practice guideline** is a statement designed to assist providers and clients in making decisions about appropriate health care for specific clinical circumstances (Institute of Medicine, 2011a). Guidelines are systematically developed, link evidence with health outcomes (benefits and harms), and continue to require subjective judgments when applied to patient care. Guidelines are developed with the intent to influence clinician behavior by making clear practice recommendations. A rigorous scientific process used to combine findings from research (usually randomized controlled trials) into a powerful and clinically useful report to guide practice is known as a **systematic review.** Standard components of a systematic review are processes for (1) initiating, (2) finding and assessing individual studies, (3) synthesizing the body of evidence, and (4) reporting using a standard format (Institute of Medicine, 2011b). Rigor varies considerably in development of systematic reviews and other reports that synthesize evidence.

Translational research includes testing the effect of interventions that promote the rate and extent of adoption of EBPs by nurses, physicians, and other health care providers and describing organizational, unit, and individual variables that affect the use of evidence in clinical and operational decision making (Baggett et al., 2014; Clay-Williams et al., 2014; Taylor et al., 2015; Titler, 2004; Titler, 2014; Titler & Everett, 2001). Translational research provides guidance about effective strategies for implementing EBP. *Translational research* is often used interchangeably with *implementation science* and *knowledge translation* in different regions across the globe.

Implementation science offers great opportunity to learn effective strategies to promote EBP as the standard for health care delivery.

"Implementation science is the study of methods to promote the integration of research findings and evidence into health care policy and practice. It seeks to understand the behavior of health care professionals and other stakeholders as a key variable in the sustainable uptake, adoption, and implementation of evidence-based interventions. As a newly emerging field, the definition of implementation science and the type of research it encompasses may vary according to setting and sponsor. However, the intent of implementation science and related research is to investigate and address major bottlenecks (e.g., social, behavioral, economic, management) that impede effective implementation, test new approaches to improve health programming, as well as determine a causal relationship between the intervention and its impact" (NIH Fogarty International Center, 2016).

Knowledge translation refers to the process of putting scientific knowledge into practice (Harrison et al., 2013; Straus et al., 2011). After initial pilot implementation and evaluation, the process used to promote integration of EBP is called **reinfusion.**

Sustaining EBP changes is the goal of implementation. **Sustainability** refers to long-term use of the practice recommendation following implementation of the innovation and indicates the new practice has been hardwired as the new standard of care (Ament et al., 2015; Maher & Gustafson, 2010). This reversal of current practice requires **de-implementation** or de-adoption, which is a new area of research (Montini & Graham, 2015; Niven et al., 2015). In addition to integration and sustaining EBP, additional roll-out or **scaling up** refers to the systematic process used to expand the reach of effective clinical interventions in new settings or with new target populations (Milat et al., 2015; Milat et al., 2014).

Organizational context refers to the health system environment in which the proposed EBP is to be implemented. The core elements that help describe the organizational context include the prevailing culture of the system (e.g., patient centered); the nature of human relationships in the system, including the leadership styles that are operational (e.g., team work, clear role delineation); and the organization's approach to routine monitoring of systems and services within the organization (Clay-Williams et al., 2014; Harvey & Kitson, 2016; Stetler et al., 2014).

Informal leaders who influence peers by evaluating innovations for use in certain settings and promoting clinicians' use of evidence in clinical decision making are referred to as **opinion leaders.** Opinion leaders are likeable, trustworthy, informative, and influential (Flodgren et al., 2011). **Academic detailing** or **educational outreach** is a marketing strategy provided by a trained person meeting one on one with practitioners in their setting to provide information about the EBP. This may include feedback on the provider's performance. The detailer may be from inside or outside the provider's organization, and the information may be tailored to address site-specific barriers (Avorn & Soumerai, 1983; Van Hoof et al., 2015; Yeh et al., 2016). The terms *academic detailing* and *educational outreach* are used interchangeably. Opinion leaders using additional strategies, such as academic detailing, can be effective for implementing EBP.

MODELS

A variety of models now exist for translation of knowledge into practice (Davison et al., 2015). Many work well to guide research but lack step-by-step guidance for the EBP process. Several EBP process models can guide implementation and sustained organizational change (Table 17.1). These models have been used successfully to improve adoption of EBP recommendations and improve patient and health care outcomes (Block et al., 2012; Farrington et al., 2015). The Iowa Model (The Iowa Model Collaborative, In review; Titler et al., 2001) is one example. Recently updated to reflect the current environment in health care and emergence of implementation science, the Iowa Model-Revised (The Iowa Model Collaborative, In review) is used to guide clinician decision making in a variety of health care settings. Additional details and comparisons of select models are summarized elsewhere (Dang et al., 2011; Rycroft-Malone & Bucknall, 2010; Schaffer et al., 2013).

The challenge for clinicians is to identify a model that guides the EBP process and promotes successful translation and implementation of EBP changes (Block et al., 2012; Dang et al., 2011; Farrington et al., 2015). Adoption of one EBP model across the organization (Hanrahan et al., 2015) for inter-professional initiatives (Farrington et al., 2015; Rockafellow et al., 2014) is one strategy for promoting continuous learning and coordination of efforts across a system. EBP models tend to follow a basic problem-solving process and can be used

parallel to other quality improvement processes (e.g., Six Sigma). Senior leadership support for EBP can be leveraged by outlining the similarities between EBP and quality improvement processes, structures, and resources for comprehensive improvement in clinical and organizational outcomes.

STEPS FOR PERFORMING EVIDENCE-BASED PRACTICE

Students and novice nurses can learn and practice the basic steps for EBP. It begins with a question that arises out of nursing practice. Formulating a clinical question is aided by the PICOT format: P (patient/disease), I (intervention), C (comparison), O (outcome desired), and T (time for intervention to achieve outcomes). These five elements are answered in specific detail. Then, appropriate resources for searching for evidence are determined and a search strategy is developed. There are many databases to use, such as PubMed, MEDLINE, CINAHL, OVID, and the Cochrane Database of Systematic Reviews, to name a few. Use of keywords or Medical Subject Heading (MeSH) headings helps to focus the literature search. A librarian can be very helpful at this stage. There are websites that offer training in the use of these databases.

There is a hierarchy of evidence that indicates the level and quality of the evidence. The seven levels (from highest to lowest) are (1) systematic review or meta-analysis, (2) randomized, controlled trial, (3) controlled trial without randomization, (4) case-control or cohort study, (5) systematic review of qualitative or descriptive studies, (6) qualitative or descriptive study, and (7) opinion or consensus (Stillwell et al., 2010). This is important because nurses need to have confidence that what they have is the best evidence for making decisions for clinical practice. Which research methodology gives the best evidence depends on the type of clinical question. For example, a systematic review—especially of randomized, controlled trials—or a meta-analysis are the most desirable study designs when looking at what intervention is the best one for a given situation. Once the search is conducted, there is a need to evaluate the results and do further refinements, such as restriction to date ranges or more specific keywords. Depending on the clinical question and the situation, a search for best practice guidelines, clinical practice protocols, or documents from relevant professional organizations may be important.

TABLE 17.1	Select Evidence-Based Practice Models	
Model	**Citation**	**Sample Report**
Iowa Model-Revised	The Iowa Model Collaborative. (In review). The Iowa Model-Revised: Development and Validation. Available at: *https://www.uihealthcare.org/otherservices.aspx?id=1617* Titler, M.G., Kleiber, C., Steelman, V.J., Rakel, B.A., Budreau, G., Everett, L.Q., et al. (2001). The Iowa Model of Evidence-Based Practice to Promote Quality Care. *Critical Care Nursing Clinics of North America, 13*(4), 497–509.	Farrington, M., Hanson, A., Laffoon, T., & Cullen, L. (2015). Low-dose ketamine infusions for postoperative pain in opioid-tolerant orthopedic spine patients. *Journal of PeriAnesthesia Nursing, 30*(4), 338–345.
Johns Hopkins Nursing Evidence-Based Practice (JHNEBP) Model	Newhouse R.P., & Johnson, K. (2009). A case study in evaluating infrastructure for EBP and selecting a model. *Journal of Nursing Administration, 39*(10), 409–411.	Mori, C. (2015). Implementing evidence-based practice to reduce infections following arthroplasty. *Orthopedic Nursing, 34*(4), 188–194. doi:10.1097/NOR.0000000000000157.
Stetler Model	Stetler, C.B. (2001). Updating the Stetler Model of research utilization to facilitate evidence-based practice. *Nursing Outlook, 49*(6), 272–279. PMID: 1753294	Velez, R.P., Becker, K.L., Davidson, P., & Sloand, E. (2015). A quality improvement intervention to address provider behaviour as it relates to utilisation of CA-MRSA guidelines. *Journal of Clinical Nursing, 24*(3–4), 556–562. doi:10.1111/jocn.12684.
Advancing Research and Clinical Practice Through Close Collaboration (ARCC) Model	Melnyk, B.M. (2012). Achieving a high-reliability organization through implementation of the ARCC model for systemwide sustainability of evidence-based practice. *Nursing Administration Quarterly, 36*(2), 127–135. doi:10.1097/NAQ.0b013e318249fb6a.	Melnyk, B.M., & Fineout-Overholt, E. (2011). *Implementing evidence-based practice: Real life success stories.* Indianapolis, IN: Sigma Theta Tau International.
ACE Star Model of Knowledge Transformation	Stevens, K. (2013). The impact of evidence-based practice in nursing and the next big ideas. *OJIN: The Online Journal of Issues in Nursing, 18*(2), 4.	Farra, S.L., Miller, E.T., & Hodgson, E. (2015). Virtual reality disaster training: Translation to practice. *Education in Practice, 15*(1), 53–57. doi:10.1016/j.nepr.2013.08.017.
Promoting Action on Research Implementation in Health Services (PARIHS) Framework	Harvey, G., & Kitson A. (2016). PARIHS revisited: From heuristic to integrated framework for the successful implementation of knowledge into practice. *Implementation Science, 11*(1), 33. doi:10.1186/s13012–016–0398–2.	Powrie, S.L., Danly, D., Corbett, C.F., Purath, J., & Dupler, A. (2014). Using implementation science to facilitate evidence-based practice changes to promote optimal outcomes for orthopedic patients. *Nursing, 33*(2), 109–114. doi:10.1097/NOR.0000000000000036

IMPLEMENTING AND SUSTAINING EVIDENCE-BASED PRACTICE CHANGES

Implementation of EBP changes can be challenging in complex health care settings. Despite research supporting use of effective strategies for implementing EBP changes, use of ineffective implementation strategies persists. As an example, education is a common and essential first step to develop an understanding of why evidence supports a practice change, but education alone does little to change practice (Clay-Williams et al., 2014; Rangachari et al., 2013). A large variety of implementation strategies support adoption of EBP. Strategies need to target both clinicians and the health care system (Cullen & Adams, 2012; Rogers, 2003; Titler, 2014).

The Diffusion of Innovations Model (Rogers, 2003) provides a well-recognized theoretical framework with strong research support guiding the hard work of implementation (Chun et al., 2016; Greenhalgh et al., 2005). Planning for implementation requires use of effective implementation strategies across adoption phases. Although strong evidence supports use of some strategies that promote integration of EBP in health care, other strategies need further testing. The Evidence-Based Practice Implementation Guide (Fig. 17.1) was developed to assist nurse leaders with planning and use of effective implementation strategies through a process of active diffusion: creating awareness and interest, building knowledge and commitment, promoting action and adoption, and pursuing integration and sustained use (Cullen & Adams, 2012). The Evidence-Based Practice Implementation Guide can be used as a planning tool with EBP process models.

Multiple interactive and reinforcing strategies, as outlined, promote adoption of EBP recommendations (Chun et al., 2016; Cullen & Adams, 2012). Strategies to capture a busy clinician's attention are important to include early in implementation planning. Nurse leaders can identify additional strategies when working across phases. Strategies are added to create a cumulative and comprehensive implementation plan to garner momentum before, during, and after implementation.

A number of strategies have good evidence and are particularly effective. Academic detailing, or educational outreach, is an implementation strategy that is effective in promoting adoption of EBP recommendations (O'Brien et al., 2007; Yeh et al., 2016) by increasing knowledge and commitment to the change. Academic detailing involves a strategic approach to communication and discussions with clinicians. Clinicians tend to buy into the need for the practice change when there is a strong evidence base, the topic addresses an identified need, data demonstrate an opportunity for practice improvement within the clinical area, and the practice change offers a relative advantage. Localizing or adapting practice recommendations to fit the local setting and culture is an essential step in the process and the role of the opinion leader and team of local experts (Cahill et al., 2014). When done by an opinion leader, academic detailing with a performance

gap assessment is a highly effective example of using multifaceted interactive strategies in promoting adoption of EBP (Dogherty et al., 2012; Mwaniki et al., 2014; Paparone, 2015). This approach can be used in practice to increase knowledge and garner consensus from an interprofessional team by leading discussions using these strategies. Some strategies are essential to carry out across phases (e.g., highlight advantages, academic detailing) to achieve sustainability.

Once the practice has been adapted and is ready for piloting, additional planning is needed for implementation and evaluation. Development of a fluid action plan can keep the team on task and collectively moving forward (Cahill et al., 2014; Cullen & Adams, 2012; Johnson et al., 2014). Common strategies used for sustaining EBP include adapting the practice recommendation, trending evaluative data, ongoing training, champions and leaders across all levels, aligning project work with organizational priorities, having sufficient resources allocated, and communicating and partnering with stakeholders (Doyle et al., 2013; Hakko et al., 2015; Hulscher et al., 2013; Luke et al., 2014; Maher & Gustafson, 2010; Ogden et al., 2012; Pronovost et al., 2013; Schell et al., 2013; Wiltsey Stirman et al., 2012).

The sustainability step in implementation is one of the most difficult in the EBP process. Audit and feedback of key indicators remains a necessary component of an integration plan (Ivers et al., 2012). Key indicators to monitor are drawn from the pilot data and include process (i.e., knowledge, attitudes, and practices) and outcomes (Bick & Graham, 2010; Parry et al., 2013), including balancing measures (Institute for Healthcare Improvement, 2015a). Integration also requires linkages across the governance structure (Berenholtz et al., 2011; Davies et al., 2010; Spyridonidis & Calnan, 2011; Stenberg & Wann-Hansson, 2011; Stetler et al., 2014; VanDeusen Lukas et al., 2010). An important strategy is to link within the quality improvement methods and infrastructure (Hulscher et al., 2013). This promotes essential influence needed from senior leadership (Doyle et al., 2013; Ogden et al., 2012; Spyridonidis & Calnan, 2011). Change can only be complete and sustained using a combination of implementation strategies (Cullen et al., 2012; Davies et al., 2010; Hanrahan et al., 2015; Maher & Gustafson, 2010). These principles are highlighted in the following EBP exemplar.

Implementation Strategies for Evidence-Based Practice

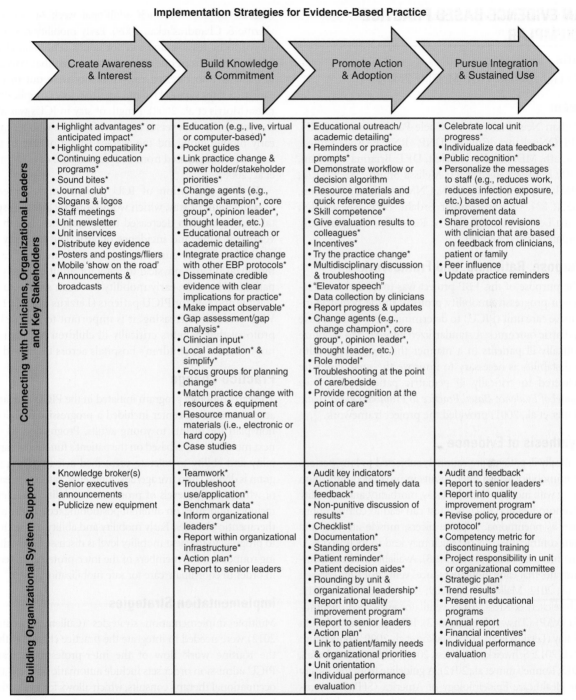

	Create Awareness & Interest	Build Knowledge & Commitment	Promote Action & Adoption	Pursue Integration & Sustained Use
Connecting with Clinicians, Organizational Leaders and Key Stakeholders	• Highlight advantages* or anticipated impact* • Highlight compatibility* • Continuing education programs* • Sound bites* • Journal club* • Slogans & logos • Staff meetings • Unit newsletter • Unit inservices • Distribute key evidence • Posters and postings/fliers • Mobile 'show on the road' • Announcements & broadcasts	• Education (e.g., live, virtual or computer-based)* • Pocket guides • Link practice change & power holder/stakeholder priorities* • Change agents (e.g., change champion*, core group*, opinion leader*, thought leader, etc.) • Educational outreach or academic detailing* • Integrate practice change with other EBP protocols* • Disseminate credible evidence with clear implications for practice* • Make impact observable* • Gap assessment/gap analysis* • Clinician input* • Local adaptation* & simplify* • Focus groups for planning change* • Match practice change with resources & equipment • Resource manual or materials (i.e., electronic or hard copy) • Case studies	• Educational outreach/ academic detailing* • Reminders or practice prompts* • Demonstrate workflow or decision algorithm • Resource materials and quick reference guides • Skill competence* • Give evaluation results to colleagues* • Incentives* • Try the practice change* • Multidisciplinary discussion & troubleshooting • "Elevator speech" • Data collection by clinicians • Report progress & updates • Change agents (e.g., change champion*, core group*, opinion leader*, thought leader, etc.) • Role model* • Troubleshooting at the point of care/bedside • Provide recognition at the point of care*	• Celebrate local unit progress* • Individualize data feedback* • Public recognition* • Personalize the messages to staff (e.g., reduces work, reduces infection exposure, etc.) based on actual improvement data • Share protocol revisions with clinician that are based on feedback from clinicians, patient or family • Peer influence • Update practice reminders
Building Organizational System Support	• Knowledge broker(s) • Senior executives announcements • Publicize new equipment	• Teamwork* • Troubleshoot use/application* • Benchmark data* • Inform organizational leaders* • Report within organizational infrastructure* • Action plan* • Report to senior leaders	• Audit key indicators* • Actionable and timely data feedback* • Non-punitive discussion of results* • Checklist* • Documentation* • Standing orders* • Patient reminder* • Patient decision aides* • Rounding by unit & organizational leadership* • Report into quality improvement program* • Report to senior leaders • Action plan* • Link to patient/family needs & organizational priorities • Unit orientation • Individual performance evaluation	• Audit and feedback* • Report to senior leaders* • Report into quality improvement program* • Revise policy, procedure or protocol* • Competency metric for discontinuing training • Project responsibility in unit or organizational committee • Strategic plan* • Trend results* • Present in educational programs • Annual report • Financial incentives* • Individual performance evaluation

*=Implementation strategy is supported by at least some empirical evidence in health care.

FIG. 17.1 Evidence-based practice implementation guide. (Reproduced with permission from Laura Cullen, DNP, RN, FAAN, and the University of Iowa Hospitals and Clinics. From Cullen, L., & Adams, S. [2012]. Planning for implementation of evidence-based practice. *Journal of Nursing Administration, 42*[4], 222–230.)

AN EVIDENCE-BASED PRACTICE EXEMPLAR

Title

No Lion Around: PICU Mobility Protocol

Team

Nathan Neis, BAN, RN; Michele Farrington, BSN, RN, CPHON; Laura Cullen, DNP, RN, FAAN; Sameer Kamath, MD, MS; Kayla Priest, DPT; Brianna Clarahan, DPT; Matthew Reed, RRT; Melissa Smith, MS, OTR/L, CIMI; Angela Otto, BSN, RN, CNML; Amanda Houston, MSN, RN, CCRN; Jennifer Erdahl, BSN, RN, CCRN; Paula Levett, MS, RN, CCRN; Renee Kramer; Kimberly Jordan; Kristen Rempel

Purpose, Rationale, and Framework

The purpose of this EBP project was to initiate a nurse-driven progressive mobility protocol in the pediatric intensive care unit (PICU) to determine safety and improve pediatric outcomes. A standardized approach to mobilize critically ill patients in a manner that promotes health and stability is necessary to improve the quality of care delivered to critically ill pediatric patients. The *Iowa Model of Evidence-Based Practice to Promote Quality Care* (Titler et al., 2001) provided the project framework.

Synthesis of Evidence

Critically ill patients are routinely subjected to long periods of immobility, which often results in prolonged intubation along with increased length of stay, morbidity, and mortality (Zomorodi et al., 2012). Bed rest can lead to complications such as pneumonia, pressure ulcers, muscle atrophy, and joint contractures, any of which may lead to increased ICU length of stay (Rauen et al., 2008). Available evidence demonstrates that early mobility reduces ventilator time (Bassett et al., 2012; Malkoc et al., 2009; Ronnebaum et al., 2012; Schweickert & Kress, 2011), ventilator-associated pneumonia (VAP) (Titsworth et al., 2012), ICU and hospital length of stay (Letzkus et al., 2013; Malkoc et al., 2009; Ronnebaum et al., 2012; Schweickert & Kress, 2011), and cost (Lord et al., 2013; Ronnebaum et al., 2012). A guideline from the Society for Healthcare Epidemiology of America (SHEA) recommends early mobility to prevent VAP (Klompas et al., 2014).

Mobilization of critically ill patients is often perceived as a complex task, partly due to catheters, tubes, and life support equipment; therefore these patients are often on bed rest. Statistics show that after 1 week of bed rest, muscle strength decreases as much as 20% and continues to decrease by 20% for each additional week of bed rest (Perme & Chandrashekar, 2009). Early mobility has been shown to be feasible and safe for adults (Pohlman et al., 2010). Results from one study demonstrated that critically ill patients who received early mobility were out of bed earlier (5 days versus 11 days) and had low complication rates (Morris et al., 2008). Length of stay in ICUs was also shortened (5.5 days versus 6.9 days) for those who received early mobilization, and the average length of stay in the hospital was decreased from 14.5 days to 11.2 days (Morris et al., 2008).

Early mobilization of ICU patients may decrease overall length of stay, which would directly affect hospital costs related to decreased use of supplies, length of ventilator time, and incidence of VAP. The majority of available evidence currently focuses on benefits of early mobilization and physical therapy for adult critically ill patients. However, early mobility has been shown to be feasible and safe for PICU patients (Letzkus et al., 2013). With evidence increasing, it is important to establish a protocol that benefits critically ill children that can be implemented in children's hospitals across the world.

Practice Change

The early mobility program initiated in the PICU at a large academic medical center included a progressive mobilization plan for infants to young adults. Progression to the next mobility level is based on the patient's functional capability and ability to tolerate prescribed activity. The program is divided into five age/developmental categories, each of which has five levels of progressive mobility. Each level includes guidelines on different positioning techniques and therapeutic exercises. Early mobility and ability of the child to progress to the next mobility level is discussed daily during rounds among members of the inter-professional team in order to coordinate care for safe mobilization.

Implementation Strategies

Multiple implementation strategies (Cullen & Adams, 2012) were needed to integrate the practice change within the routine work flow of the inter-professional team. PICU admission order sets include automatic physical and occupational therapy consults, which allows for evaluation by the therapists the next day. The project team was led by a staff nurse and included leaders from all disciplines. Initial training was provided across all shifts during a set week. A group of staff nurses and the physical therapist served as champions. Champions did just-in-time training and troubleshooting to build confidence with using the practice change. A physician leader served as a critical champion, and training was provided at standing morbidity and mortality meetings. Monthly updates and daily follow-up, along with revisions to the admission order set, were provided to promote adoption as licensed independent practitioners rotated on service. The project slogan and logo stimulated important conversations among clinicians, and more importantly, engaged patients and families in planning mobility. A comprehensive list of implementation strategies used for this project is shown in Fig. 17.2.

Evaluation

Standard EBP evaluation components were collected, including process and outcome indicators. Process evaluation included clinician knowledge, attitudes, and behaviors (Bick & Graham, 2010; Parry et al., 2013). Outcomes were evaluated to demonstrate an impact on VAP rates and to determine whether revisions of the practice change or implementation plan were needed. Outcome measures also included relevant balancing measures (Institute for Healthcare Improvement, 2015a). Balancing measures were collected to reflect avoidance of undesirable consequences from early mobility (e.g., falls, unplanned extubation, inadvertent line removals).

Feedback from clinicians (staff nurses, respiratory therapists, physicians [attendings and fellows], nurse practitioners) was captured in a questionnaire distributed pre- and postimplementation of the practice change (n = 58 pre; n = 95 post). Results demonstrated that clinicians were very knowledgeable about immobility and the need for early mobilization both pre- and postpilot. Clinician perceptions improved regarding feeling supported in efforts to provide early mobilization for PICU patients (2.45 pre; 2.78 post; 1–4 Likert scale), having adequate resources for early

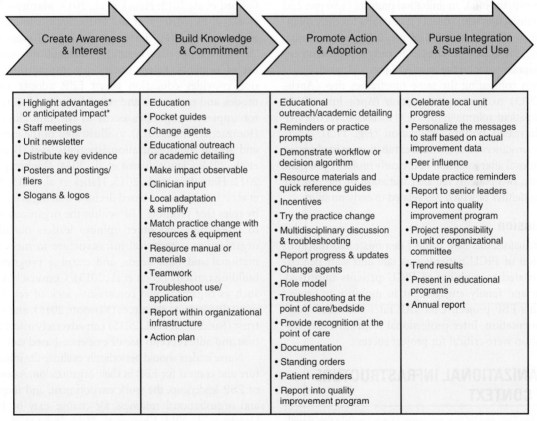

Create Awareness & Interest	Build Knowledge & Commitment	Promote Action & Adoption	Pursue Integration & Sustained Use
• Highlight advantages* or anticipated impact* • Staff meetings • Unit newsletter • Distribute key evidence • Posters and postings/fliers • Slogans & logos	• Education • Pocket guides • Change agents • Educational outreach or academic detailing • Make impact observable • Clinician input • Local adaptation & simplify • Match practice change with resources & equipment • Resource manual or materials • Teamwork • Troubleshoot use/application • Report within organizational infrastructure • Action plan	• Educational outreach/academic detailing • Reminders or practice prompts • Demonstrate workflow or decision algorithm • Resource materials and quick reference guides • Incentives • Try the practice change • Multidisciplinary discussion & troubleshooting • Report progress & updates • Change agents • Role model • Troubleshooting at the point of care/bedside • Provide recognition at the point of care • Documentation • Standing orders • Patient reminders • Report into quality improvement program	• Celebrate local unit progress • Personalize the messages to staff based on actual improvement data • Peer influence • Update practice reminders • Report to senior leaders • Report into quality improvement program • Project responsibility in unit or organizational committee • Trend results • Present in educational programs • Annual report

*=Implementation strategy is supported by at least some empirical evidence in health care.

FIG. 17.2 Implementation strategiespediatric intensive care unit mobility protocol. (Adapted and used permission from Laura Cullen, DNP, RN, FAAN and the University of Iowa Hospitals and Clinics. From Cullen, L., & Adams, S. [2012]. Planning for implementation of evidence-based practice. *Journal of Nursing Administration, 42*[4], 222–230].)

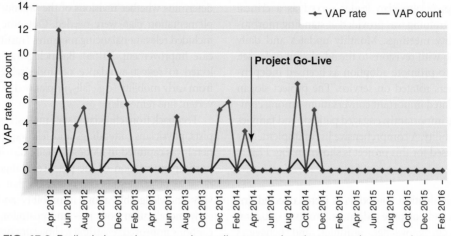

FIG. 17.3 Pediatric intensive care unit ventilator-associated pneumonia rate and count.

mobilization of PICU patients (1.98 pre; 2.45 post), satisfaction with the PICU mobilization protocol (1.96 pre; 2.52 post), satisfaction with collaborative efforts for early mobilization of PICU patients (2.08 pre; 2.44 post), and that engaging PICU patients/families in early mobilization enhances quality care on the unit (3.17 pre; 3.31 post).

When comparing the same timeframes pre- (April–June 2013) to postimplementation (April–June 2014), overall patient volume in the PICU increased, yet the VAP rate decreased postimplementation (Fig. 17.3). There were no instances of unplanned extubation or inadvertent line removal after initiation of the early mobility protocol. However, two patients fell after initiation of the practice change, neither of which was related to early mobility.

Conclusion

In conclusion, this EBP project demonstrated that mobilization of PICU patients was safe and staff perceptions related to mobility of PICU patients improved. Patient and family engagement in mobility improved with this EBP project. Unit VAP rates decreased postimplementation. Inter-professional teamwork and collaboration were critical for project success.

ORGANIZATIONAL INFRASTRUCTURE AND CONTEXT

Nurse leaders are in key positions responsible for developing and sustaining an organizational infrastructure and creating an environment that affects adoption of EBPs and improves patient outcomes (Dogherty et al.,

2012; Everett & Sitterding, 2011; Forberg et al., 2014; Gifford et al., 2013; Hauck et al., 2013; Matthew-Maich et al., 2013; Melnyk et al., 2016; Parkosewich, 2013; Stetler et al., 2014; Taylor et al., 2015; Tonges et al., 2015). A supportive organizational culture promotes use of evidence, values nurses questioning their practice, provides education about EBP, adopts an EBP model, and recognizes and rewards the work. Strategies for implementing EBPs occur at the unit/clinic level (Rangachari et al., 2013), as illustrated in the exemplar, and also at the organizational/systems level (Breimaier et al., 2013; Clay-Williams et al., 2014; Dogherty et al., 2012; Hanrahan et al., 2015; Hauck et al., 2013; Stetler et al., 2014). Evidence-based decision making is facilitated by roles that promote EBP within the organization, ties to researchers and other opinion leaders outside the organization, a technical infrastructure to meet informational and data needs, and training programs for building capacity (Ellen et al., 2013). Conversely, factors such as organizational constraints, lack of reimbursement, inadequate resources (Kissoon, 2015), and lack of trust (Sandstrom et al., 2015) can adversely affect adoption and adherence to use of evidence-based care.

Nurse leaders should periodically evaluate the infrastructure and context for EBP in their organization. Assessment of EBP leadership, the work environment, and individual and organizational readiness for change may be helpful (Jacobs et al., 2014; Khan et al., 2014; Pryse et al., 2014). Standards for a professional practice environment, such as those outlined through the Magnet Recognition Program®, provide guidance when evaluating an EBP program.

A strategic, systematic approach is needed for building EBP capacity (Hauck et al., 2013; Stetler et al., 2014; Titler, 2010). Leaders should integrate EBP at the organization or health system level, building infrastructure and creating a culture for change.

Mission, Vision, and Strategic Plan

Development of a mission, vision, and strategic plan inclusive of EBP language provides a sturdy foundation for this work at all levels of the organization and begins the process of building a culture in which evidence-based health care is the expected norm (Stetler et al., 2014). A **mission** statement defines the purpose and reflects the values of the organization. When a mission statement is developed, it should be clear that EBP and patient care outcomes are fundamental to the purpose and why the organization exists (Oster, 2011). The mission statement begins to create a culture of inquiry and set the expectation that clinicians will make decisions and practice based on evidence. The **vision** statement can further stretch the current boundaries of EBP and promote work that leads staff to reach for a higher standard. An example of a vision statement might be to develop a center of excellence for EBP in the organization and be seen as a leader in evidence-based care delivery. The **strategic plan** is a continuous and systematic planning process used to make the mission actionable and outcomes achievable. The strategic plan includes clearly articulated and measurable goals, objectives for meeting outcomes, metrics for measuring progress, a list of resources needed, and a timeline for completion. Attainment of strategic goals should be aimed at positioning the organization for success in a competitive, complex, rapidly changing health care environment (Oster, 2011). Goals and objectives should be consistent with the vision and values of the organization. Specific goals for EBP in the strategic plan provide structure for nurse leaders (Hauck et al., 2013). Action steps for creating a culture that values inquiry and innovation and provides leaders with a foundation of support for EBP are needed.

Shared Governance

To support the mission, vision, and strategic plan, an infrastructure that integrates the work of EBP in the organizational governance is needed. A shared governance system is based on the belief that nurses own their practice and are best informed for making decisions about and advancing it (Parkosewich, 2013). The right committee or council structure will vary in each organization but should include point-of-care clinicians and reflect the expertise, functions, and responsibility needed to promote EBPs (Cullen et al., 2012; Stetler et al., 2014). Practice change is best facilitated when documentation, policies and procedures, and education include the essential components of clinical practice guidelines. Clinical experts can provide an excellent critique of a new policy or procedure and make recommendations so policies link practices with evidence and support adaptation of guidelines for the organization. A clear path for communicating EBP work and necessary approvals between committees should be outlined within the governance structure. Discussion during committee meetings can stimulate interest in—and use of—EBP. One strategy is to include an EBP item on each agenda. Another key strategy is having a nurse leader on the Institutional Review Board and a clear process for determining research on human subjects, differentiated from EBP, with a clear process for organizational approvals (Foote et al., 2015; Ogrinc et al., 2013).

Performance Expectations and Appraisal

The value of EBP must be evident through the expected behaviors of nurses at every level in the organization. Critical skills for shared governance committee members who supplement point-of-care clinical experts include appraisal and synthesis of the evidence, development of an implementation and evaluation plan, statistical analysis for quality improvement, and reporting of results (Cullen et al., 2012; Cullen et al., 2010). Additional expertise can be developed through consultation and collaborations within a practice network, partnerships with academic institutions, or hiring nurse scientists (Debourgh, 2012; Duffy et al., 2016; Granger et al., 2012; Levin, 2014; Missal et al., 2010; Weeks et al., 2011). Performance appraisals based on job descriptions with EBP components are important for setting behavioral expectations. Inclusion of EBP components in performance appraisals across all job classifications—from top executives to all levels throughout the system—promotes positive reinforcement and priority setting in the busy work environment. Providing personal or group performance feedback helps clinicians be accountable for improving outcomes (Hoke & Guarracino, 2016; Kouzes & Posner, 2012; Ofek et al., 2015). EBP must be alive in daily practice, not just "pulled off the shelf" when organizational leaders appear in clinical areas.

Resources

EBP resources and time must be allocated by nurse executives and be accessible to clinicians (Aarons et al., 2014; Clay-Williams et al., 2014; Dogherty et al., 2012; Hauck et al., 2013; Melnyk et al., 2016; Ubbink et al., 2013). The organization can build an EBP culture during orientation for new hires, competency review for current employees, and ongoing training for senior leaders as well as clinicians. Recruiting and hiring nurses with interest in EBP will help build the desired culture and capacity. Orientation can contain basic EBP concepts and protocols, with new staff learning from colleagues who share experiences from EBP teamwork on their unit. This provides recognition for completed work, sets the expectation that EBP is important in clinical care, and demonstrates that nurses have authority over their practice. New graduates have developed skills that support EBP (QSEN Institute, 2012). Nurses in new graduate residency programs can stimulate new—or support existing—EBP work using their creativity, technical skills and supported time (Jackson, 2016). EBP mentors can be developed from successful projects and used to nurture the next generation of clinical leaders (Abdullah et al., 2014; Gagliardi et al., 2014; Hosking et al., In press).

Organizational information systems must be designed to incorporate EBPs into clinical work flow if adoption is to occur and best outcomes achieved (Piscotty et al., 2015). Electronic documentation systems, designed to support clinical practice, must capture essential elements of guidelines that clinicians are expected to perform. The documentation system can serve as a "trigger" to assess important risk factors (e.g., risk for falling, risk for pressure ulcer development), patient conditions (e.g., pain), and outcomes of care (e.g., unintended consequences or development of pressure ulcers or oral mucositis) (van Klei et al., 2012; Weiss et al., 2011). One strategy to promote integration of an EBP into daily work flow is to use clinical decision support, such as order sets and documentation prompts (Piscotty & Kalisch, 2014).

Reporting

Internal and external dissemination of project results is essential to promote adoption, share learning, garner continued support, and recognize success from the institution's EBP program (Dembe et al., 2014; The Iowa Model Collaborative, In review). Internal sharing of anticipated outcomes found in research reports can be helpful early in the process. Outcomes that target patients and families, staff, and finances are valued by the team and organization and need to be considered in evaluation planning (Dembe et al., 2014; Institute for Healthcare Improvement, 2015a; Parry et al., 2013; Stevens, 2013). Cost savings or cost avoidance may not be achieved with every project but should be calculated whenever possible (Sadler et al., 2009; Tucker, 2014). Large volumes of cost data are available in the literature and can be used to estimate cost savings (Agency for Healthcare Research and Quality [USPSTF], 2014) and generate interest in EBP changes.

Nursing leaders have a responsibility to clearly articulate EBP work in a way that will be heard by decision makers. Sharing results with senior leaders helps them recognize great work while reporting the business case for evidence-based care to governing boards (Aarons et al., 2014). Communication with boards about EBP goals and initiatives is an important strategy (Bisognano & Schummers, 2015; Institute for Healthcare Improvement, 2016; Mason et al., 2013). Three to five brief talking points or take-away messages should be shared, including reporting linkages between EBP and the organization's mission, vision, values, and strategic plan.

Linking quality improvement and EBP is another strategy for building a strong organizational context. Quality improvement programs have standardized forms, a reporting system, and an established process to use results for continuous improvement until the practice reaches an established goal and becomes integrated (Hulscher et al., 2013; Pronovost et al., 2013). Using the quality improvement system for reporting EBP changes provides efficient communication within the existing organizational infrastructure. The quality improvement process also supports ongoing planning, monitoring, and reinfusion of expected care delivery, supporting successful adoption and integration of EBPs.

Rewards

Successes need to be rewarded along the way. Celebrations help build a culture that supports and expects use of evidence in practice. Rewards should include formal recognition from high-level organizational leaders, visibility for inter-professional teams and project champions, accessibility to practitioners within the organization, and a clear articulation of the benefits of EBP. Celebrations provide an opportunity to put practitioners in the spotlight for doing great work. Recognition can clearly articulate the benefits to, and commitment of, the organization. Celebrating successes promotes buy-in and commitment by the organization to the EBP process and strengthens the foundation for future efforts.

LEADERSHIP ROLES IN PROMOTING EVIDENCE-BASED PRACTICE

Innovative organizations with responsive leadership that support staff will promote use of evidence-based care (Aarons et al., 2015; Aarons et al., 2014; Cullen, 2015). Leadership, both formal and informal, is essential across all organizational levels and nursing roles when implementing evidence-based changes (Aarons et al., 2015; RNAO, 2013; Stetler et al., 2014). Everyone (e.g., chief nurse executives, nurse managers, advanced practice nurses, point-of-care nurses) has an important role in EBP work that builds on individual as well as collective knowledge and skills (Balakas et al., 2013; Gifford et al., 2013; RNAO, 2013). Nurse executives have organizational responsibility for establishing the foundation for EBP by (1) developing and sustaining a vision and infrastructure inclusive of EBP, (2) creating a culture in which clinicians expect EBP, and (3) creating the capacity to accomplish EBP (Forberg et al., 2014; Hauck et al., 2013; RNAO, 2013; Stetler et al., 2014; Ubbink et al., 2013).

Strategies discussed in building an organizational infrastructure for EBP are effective in developing the culture, building the capacity, and sustaining the vision at both the organizational and unit level (Forberg et al., 2014; Matthew-Maich et al., 2013). Nurse managers are responsible, parallel to the nurse executive, for developing the unit culture supporting innovation and evidence-based care (Aarons et al., 2015; Cullen, 2015; Huis et al., 2013; Ubbink et al., 2013). Developing a positive unit culture for promoting EBP affects unit outcomes (Aarons et al., 2015; Ubbink et al., 2013). Managers' use of transformational leadership that is responsive and supportive will promote evidence-based care by point-of-care nurses (Aarons et al., 2014; Dogherty et al., 2012; Forberg et al., 2014; Gifford et al., 2013; Paparone, 2015; Stetler et al., 2014; Torrey et al., 2012). Nurse managers can facilitate and support EBP work in the following ways: set unit expectations, discuss importance of EBP with unit nurses and inter-professional team members, encourage and respond to new ideas, promote staff questioning practice, support the team with project work time, promote the project's importance, track progress, facilitate movement of the project through the institutional shared governance approval process, and allocate resources (Paparone, 2015; RNAO, 2013). When nurse managers encourage nurses to attend and disseminate project work at conferences, stimulate inquiry, and participate in research, point-of-care nurses will increase use of EBP (Dee & Reynolds, 2013). The nurse manager's commitment to improving quality and safety and performance feedback is critical to project success and can significantly affect project outcomes (McMullan et al., 2013; Paparone, 2015; Stetler et al., 2014).

Advanced practice nurses (e.g., clinical nurse specialists, unit practice leaders, advanced registered nurse practitioners) may partner with project team leaders and play an important role in project development, functioning as opinion leaders and facilitators throughout the process (Cullen et al., 2012; Dogherty et al., 2012; Gawlinski & Becker, 2012; McMullan et al., 2013). Capitalizing on their existing knowledge and skills will facilitate use of research findings in practice (Gerrish et al., 2012; Morgan, 2012). These nurses may act as mentors for the inter-professional team and/or project director (Dogherty et al., 2012; Gawlinski & Becker, 2012; Gerrish et al., 2012). Nurses in this role have the ability to take on the most challenging steps in the EBP process, such as leading a team, identifying potential roadblocks, facilitating problem solving during implementation and evaluation, reporting results, and providing expertise throughout the process. Critique and synthesis of evidence, development of an evaluation plan, and analysis of results are steps in the EBP process that use this expertise.

Point-of-care nurses are ideally positioned to identify important and clinically relevant topics that can be fully developed as EBP projects (Balakas et al., 2013; Crabtree et al., 2016; RNAO, 2013). These nurses are expert clinicians with the skills to collaborate and problem solve, often identifying creative solutions while providing quality care through implementation of EBP changes. Point-of-care nurses can function as change champions and core group members within their current role (Cullen et al., 2012; Mark et al., 2014). With appropriate coaching and support, these nurses can also function as opinion leaders and/or project directors (Balakas et al., 2013; Dogherty et al., 2012; Grimshaw et al., 2012). Use of a bottoms-up approach for topic selection and implementation by point-of-care nurses can facilitate adoption of the practice change (Aarons et al., 2014; Clay-Williams et al., 2014). Clinicians will "pull" the practice change into their care processes instead of having the change "pushed" in from above (Matthew-Maich et al., 2013). Programs with formal support are needed to help point-of-care nurses integrate EBP changes in care delivery (Clay-Williams et al., 2014; Matthew-Maich et al., 2013; Paparone, 2015; RNAO, 2013; Stetler et al., 2014). When point-of-care nurses receive sufficient support, they are effective at integrating EBP changes in care and are empowered by the experience (Abdullah et al., 2014; Block et al., 2012; Cullen et al., 2014; Farrington et al., 2015; Morgan, 2012; Rockafellow et al., 2014; Walter et al., 2014).

One important role that keeps projects moving forward is that of the project director. The project director is responsible for establishing meeting schedules and timelines with the inter-professional team, running meetings, updating the action plan, delegating work assignments, and overseeing the process and progress. As a key strategy for success, project directors need to focus on moving the project forward despite challenges. The project director may orchestrate discussions for identifying potential challenges, addressing those that cannot be avoided, but continuing to move forward despite distractions. Point-of-care nurses can function as project directors if given sufficient support and mentorship (Block et al., 2012; Cullen et al., 2014; Farrington et al., 2015; Rockafellow et al., 2014). Point-of-care nurses and nursing leaders must work together with complementary skills and expertise to address challenges and issues inherent in all EBP initiatives (Jackson, 2016).

LEADERSHIP AND MANAGEMENT IMPLICATIONS

Change is always difficult, which makes use of a multi-faceted approach by nurse leaders across roles imperative to integrating and sustaining EBP at the unit or organizational level (Clay-Williams et al., 2014; Cullen & Adams, 2012; Dogherty et al., 2012; Gifford et al., 2013; Matthew-Maich et al., 2013; McMullan et al., 2013; Paparone, 2015; Stetler et al., 2014). Identifying leaders within each discipline (e.g., nursing, medicine, pharmacy, physical therapy) who are innovative and influential among their peers to function as opinion leaders and change agents is important (Clay-Williams et al., 2014; Cullen & Adams, 2012; Cullen et al., 2012; Dogherty et al., 2012). Reporting internal data demonstrating a performance gap can motivate participation by team members (Cullen & Adams, 2012; Cullen et al., 2012; Dogherty et al., 2012; Paparone, 2015). Simple solutions should be sought first, and creativity should

be used to anticipate and address barriers. Point-of-care nurses can often bring fresh approaches to address challenges. Adding new graduates to the team creates a culture for EBP that builds on the knowledge and skills gained through academic programs (Mick, 2014) and resources obtained from new graduate nurse residency programs (American Association of Colleges of Nursing, 2015; Hosking et al., In press; Kramer et al., 2012; Mick, 2014). Strategic planning is essential for provision of evidence-based health care and for EBP to be strategically woven throughout the organization. Meeting these expectations is an essential component of a Magnet organization (American Nurses Credentialing Center, 2016; Balakas et al., 2013; Lewis, 2014).

Leaders influence an organization's capacity for EBP. Leadership that demonstrates and expects EBP will promote its use in clinical and operational decision making at the unit/clinic and organizational level. Prioritizing and facilitating leaders' and clinicians' ownership of EBP work is essential. Helping clinicians be accountable for EBP requires leaders to clear a path and remove obstacles (Kouzes & Posner, 2012).

CURRENT ISSUES AND TRENDS

There is a growing demand for patient-centered care, increased provision of EBP, and increasing public accountability and transparency for quality and safety (Centers for Medicare & Medicaid Services, 2015a; Centers for Medicare & Medicaid Services, 2015b; The Joint Commission, 2016). Pay for performance through the Centers for Medicare & Medicaid Services' value-based purchasing and accountable care organization alignment has grabbed the attention of health care leaders (Centers for Medicare & Medicaid Services, 2015b). New reimbursement structures reflect the importance of system redesign to improve coordination, efficiency, and provision of evidence-based care for improved population health. National patient safety goals established by The Joint Commission include a growing number of evidence-based standards. For example, recent standards for catheter-associated urinary tract infections reflect a growing intolerance for hospital acquired infections (http://www.jointcommission.org/topics/hai_cauti.aspx). Likewise, use of national benchmarks (https://data.medicare.gov/) promotes transparency and will likely add additional accreditation standards and quality indicators. The financial pressure for provision of EBP will continue to grow with demand from payers and patients.

Improving patients' experiences with health care is an area of growing investment (Centers for Medicare & Medicaid Services, 2011; Institute of Medicine, 2012). Patient engagement and provision of patient-centered care is now central to the national and international health care agenda (Balik et al., 2011; Centers for Medicare & Medicaid Services, 2011; RWJ Aligning Forces for Quality, 2013). Making progress is complicated when patients do not have a good understanding of EBP (Liira et al., 2015) and their preferences for health care are not understood by clinicians (Crowe et al., 2015; Milic et al., 2015), so it is essential to find new ways to engage patients and improve their participation in health care decisions (Advisory Board, 2015; Institute of Medicine, 2012; Ryan et al., 2014; Stacey et al., 2014). More research is needed to understand how best to facilitate patient decision making (Prochaska & Sanders-Jackson, 2016).

A long-standing challenging step in the EBP process continues to be appraisal and synthesis of the body of evidence when designing a practice change (The Iowa Model Collaborative, In review). Trends in evaluating evidence and making recommendations continue to evolve. In the past, meta-analyses and randomized controlled trials were considered essential for making practices changes. Inclusion of additional research designs and other supportive evidence for making practice changes is essential when designing practice changes that fit within the local setting and work flow. Accordingly, evidence grading systems have also changed. Whereas individual research studies were previously graded by research design and quality, the current trend is toward grading the body of evidence when making practice recommendations (Agency for Healthcare Research and Quality [USPSTF], 2012; GRADE, 2012).

After evidence is appraised and synthesized, a clinical practice guideline or a practice recommendation is made. There has been a proliferation of guidelines from federal agencies and specialty organizations. Instead of independently exploring evidence, nurse leaders can use clinical practice guidelines and tailor them to their organization, population, or setting. The National Guideline Clearinghouse *(http://www.guideline.gov/),* sponsored by the Agency for Healthcare Research and Quality, provides a large repository for international guidelines, offering free access to guideline summaries and links to full reports. The National Guideline Clearinghouse set new standards for accepting clinical practice guidelines only from professional organizations that follow IOM standards (Institute of Medicine,

2011a). This will make it easier to evaluate clinical practice guidelines for rigor, bias, and generalizability before adopting them. Tools for evaluating guidelines are now available, such as the AGREE II *(www.agreetrust.org).* Watch for emerging approaches to facilitate interpretation and application of practice recommendations (DECIDE, 2015).

Resources and standards available to promote evidence-based care are evolving. Additional resources are available through the Registered Nurses' Association of Ontario *(http://rnao.ca/)* and the Joanna Briggs Institute *(http://joannabriggs.org).* Also of note is the Guidelines International Network *(http://www.g-i-n.net/)* and other centers of excellence *(http://www.hopkinsmedicine.org/evidence-based-practice/jhn_ebp.html)* (Cullen et al., 2012). Likewise, the Institute for Healthcare Improvement *(http://www.ihi.org/)* has easily accessible resources that promote collaborative learning while continually raising the bar for health care delivery. Nursing leaders have a responsibility to stay abreast of the changing health care agenda and available resources.

The Future of Nursing report (Institute of Medicine, 2015b) is best known for the call to action for doctoral education in nursing. Trends now show growing enrollment in doctoral programs by nurses, particular the doctor of nursing practice (DNP) *(http://www.aacn.nche.edu/faculty/news/2015/enrollment)* (O'Connor, 2012). The report also highlighted the need for nursing leadership to improve quality care. DNP leadership is one solution to improve practice and promote inter-professional teamwork *(http://www.doctorsofnursingpractice.org/resources/dnp-scholarly-projects/).* However, varying expectations for student scholarship when leading implementation of evidence-based improvements (American Association of Colleges of Nursing, 2015) remain a national issue. Integration and approval for EBP and student project work is evolving (Foote et al., 2015; Office for Human Research Protections [OHRP], 2016; Ogrinc et al., 2013; Platt et al., 2013). Students need to be aware of policies and seek organizational approval. Integrating student work within the organizational system creates student learning about how organizations work and may facilitate sustainment of their practice changes. The result creates a win–win for students and organizations, which ultimately create a win for patients and families.

Student project work and organizational practice updates highlight the need to address developments at the federal level that affect delivery of evidence-based care. The Health Information Technology for Economic and Clinical Health (HITECH) Act was enacted as part of the American Recovery and Reinvestment Act (Department of Health and Human Services, 2009). The HITECH Act provides incentives for adoption and implementation of electronic health records (EHR) while enhancing privacy and security for patients and providing incentives to engage in meaningful use—now referred to as the EHR incentives program (Centers for Medicare & Medicaid Services, 2015c). The third stage of meaningful use continues to focus on improving patient outcomes and information exchange for coordination, efficiency, and effectiveness.

The EHR is expected to contribute to safety through access to stored health data, evidence-based clinical decision support, improved communication about patient's health and health care needs, and reduced risk of medical errors (Garcia et al., 2015). Opportunity for enhanced data mining of large health care databases will be a boon for researchers and nursing leaders to get real-time data to adopt, track, and trend provision of evidence-based health care. Nurses will play key roles in using these data to improve quality and manage cost (Bates et al., 2014; Borenstein et al., 2016; Roski et al., 2014; Schall et al., In review). Continued emphasis on data security and patient privacy remains a priority. EBP team leaders are responsible for obtaining and securing evaluative data to drive practice improvements, demonstrate an impact, and promote transparency, all while providing big data access to clinicians, researchers, and students.

The growth in doctorally prepared nurse leaders may improve application of resources through their expanded skill set. Sharing that learning with the larger nursing community is imperative. Disseminating EBP work promotes shared learning to move health care forward. Publication is still challenging when reviewers use research perspectives or research review criteria. Authors may facilitate sharing their learning with the larger nursing community by working with journal editors for better review criteria and examples (Adams et al., 2012; Standards for Quality Improvement Reporting Excellence [SQUIRE], 2015).

A continuing priority for implementation science is to better understand how nurse leaders can promote adoption of evidence-based health care to improve quality and reduce costs (Cullen & Adams, 2012; Forberg et al., 2014; Harrison et al., 2013; Stetler et al., 2014; Tucker, 2014). Understanding how to scale up and sustain EBP improvements is a critical priority with a young field of research calling for more evidence (Kruk et al., 2016; Proctor et al., 2015).

Nurses want to work in an organization that promotes innovation and EBP. Leadership continues to be an important contextual factor affecting an organization's ability to consistently use evidence in practice (Aarons, 2006; Aarons et al., 2015; Clay-Williams et al., 2014; Davies et al., 2006; Fleuren et al., 2004; Hauck et al., 2013; Vaughn et al., 2002; World Health Organization, 2007). An exhaustive body of research on barriers consistently finds that leadership support is essential. Yet research continues to be needed to identify the most effective leadership strategies, organizational context, and infrastructures (Forberg et al., 2014; Harrison et al., 2013; Stetler et al., 2014). The organizational context within which clinicians work is a complex and dynamic culture unique to each practice setting. Leaders are responsible for providing resources, structures, and processes that move teams beyond barriers to facilitate EBP. Research is still needed to better understand infrastructure design and effective strategies to affect organizational context, encouraging adoption and delivery of evidence-based care (Forberg et al., 2014; Institute of Medicine, 2015a; Jacobs et al., 2014; Sandstrom et al., 2015).

CONCLUSION

Nursing has a long history of valuing the provision of high-quality care and using the best evidence to improve care. Despite many years of work, there continue to be many challenges to using evidence-based care in the current health care environment. Nurses in leadership positions have responsibility for supporting evidence-based clinical care as well as evidence-based operational decision making. Models outline the process for updating applicable practices when addressing clinical and operational issues. Implementation is one of the most challenging steps in the EBP process. Multiple reinforcing and interactive strategies are needed in a phased approach for implementation and sustained improvement. Effective, evidence-based implementation strategies can be combined to create a highly influential implementation plan.

Step by step, nursing leaders can systematically build a strong program supporting evidence-based care delivery. Building on the organization's mission, vision, capacity, and value for reliable high-quality care provides a foundation for success. Nurse leaders need to connect their evidence-based initiatives to the organization's vision, mission, values, and infrastructure to garner support and resources for provision of EBP care delivery. Implementing EBPs is best accomplished by understanding the interplay between organizational and unit factors supported through the organizational infrastructure. The infrastructure supporting EBP is essential for creating the desired organizational and unit culture and capacity. Communicating the business case for EBP will help nurses articulate their impact in a way that will be heard by senior leaders. Leadership is a vital ingredient to success. Complementary skills are needed within all nursing roles to create effective EBP teams. Every nurse has a responsibility to support evidence-based care delivery to improve outcomes for patients and their families, staff, and the organization.

RESEARCH NOTE

Source

Herzer, K., Niessen, L., Constenla, D., Ward, W., & Pronovost, P. (2014). Cost-effectiveness of a quality improvement programme to reduce central line-associated bloodstream infections in intensive care units in the USA. *BMJ Open, 4*(9):e006065. doi:10.1136/bmjopen-2014-006065

Purpose

The purpose of this study was to describe a cost-effectiveness analysis outlining costs associated with implementation of an evidence-based central line insertion checklist and related cost savings from reduced hospital-acquired infections and avoidable deaths. The intervention includes implementation of a five-item checklist for central line insertion, which was compared with control units providing usual care.

Discussion

Program start-up costs and recurring costs were calculated to determine costs per patient for participating intensive care units (ICUs). Cost categories included capital items, supplies, personnel, education, and training of the team. Capital budget items included an insertion cart for convenient access to standardized supplies. Supplies included chlorhexidine, central line dressing kits, and oral care kits. Personnel costs for implementation represented the largest portion of investment costs and included nurses', physicians', respiratory therapists', infection preventionists', and pharmacists' time. Education and training costs were captured as start-up costs. Average cost per patient was $540.

Existing data were used to create a cost estimate of $18,793 for each central line bloodstream infection. The insertion checklist was estimated to reduce central line infections by 81%. For an ICU caring for 1000 patients per year with central lines, use of the insertion checklist had an estimated annual cost savings of $249,000.

Application to Practice

Leadership skills that support adoption of clinical practice guidelines in clinical settings should include a systematic evaluation. Nurse leaders have a significant opportunity to demonstrate the business case of providing evidence-based care (Tucker, 2014). Evaluation of EBP changes should include cost savings when appropriate, using a framework to calculate the return on investment from EBP initiatives (Sadler et al., 2009). Adoption of EBPs for central line insertion using checklists was associated with an estimated cost savings for hospitals through reduced rates of infection and death.

CASE STUDY

A member of the pain service approaches you with an idea to elevate nursing practice. This nurse wants to improve postoperative pain management for opioid-tolerant orthopedic spine surgery patients through expanded use of low-dose ketamine infusions. As a nurse manager, you recognize this as an opportunity to infuse EBP into the pain service. The following benefits are anticipated:

- Improving care
- Improving patient satisfaction
- Empowering staff nurses through innovative nursing practice

- Developing a culture for the pain service that uses evidence in daily practice

What Are Your Next Steps?
You recognize the need to form an inter-professional team, review evidence, revise the current policy and procedure, and create comprehensive implementation and evaluation plans. Partnering with experts in the organization will best match the skills and expertise needed. As a member of the pain service, the point-of-care nurse raising the question is already an opinion leader and ideally suited to lead

Continued

CASE STUDY—cont'd

the team; you are committed to assisting her. The team develops an action plan and divides responsibility for project work. Team members tackle each of the following:

• Reviewing the literature
• Developing a clinician questionnaire related to knowledge and attitudes regarding pain and ketamine infusions
• Developing a patient questionnaire related to pain and use of ketamine infusions
• Developing an educational presentation and poster based on the literature review
• Developing an implementation plan for strategies to promote adoption of the practice change

The practice change involved identifying potential orthopedic spine surgery patients during their preoperative appointment. A consistent referral process will be created that includes development of a practice alert in the EHR for patients taking an opioid medication and with an order for them to have surgery. An automatic consult is sent to the pain service pharmacist or attending physician to schedule a preoperative appointment or telephone consultation with the patient to collaboratively develop a surgical pain treatment plan.

This practice change is innovative and will require multiple strategies for implementation. A small number of patients will be involved in the pilot phase of the project, but the side effects of ketamine warrant special attention. The team decides to use the following strategies for implementation: highlight compatibility of the practice change, discuss at staff meetings, distribute key evidence, provide educational outreach or academic detailing, troubleshoot use/application, create resource materials and quick reference guides, change documentation and standing orders in the EHR, and revise the current policy and procedure.

Process and outcome indicators are included in the evaluation (Bick & Graham, 2010; Institute for Healthcare Improvement, 2015b; Parry et al., 2013). Knowledge and attitudes of the nurses and medical team related to pain and use of ketamine were measured. Data suggests overall clinician knowledge improved (72% preimplementation; 77% postimplementation) and attitudes are rated slightly higher on a 1 to 4 Likert scale, but both could be better. The inter-professional team determined that additional education and ongoing training and support should occur related to use of ketamine infusions with opioid-tolerant patients. Patient feedback obtained pre- and postimplementation of the practice change indicates that care during hospitalization likely improved, but the team now needs to prioritize time and attention on the follow-up care plan for pain after discharge.

This project successfully led to proactive identification of opioid-tolerant orthopedic spine surgery patients who may benefit from ketamine infusions and development of individualized pain treatment plans. Yet, like so many EBP changes, additional work is needed. The pain service nurses will now reinfuse and integrate the practice change across all adult inpatient units caring for patients with ketamine infusions. An innovative nursing practice has been introduced, and patient care improvements continue through the EBP process. The nurse manager facilitates project work and integration of the practice change by serving as a coach and team member throughout the EBP process. The manager serves a key role in establishing the priority for project work, finding resources, and guiding the team to maneuver through the system for adoption and dissemination of the practice change.

CRITICAL THINKING EXERCISE

You are the nurse manager in the surgical intensive care unit (SICU). At a staff meeting, a nurse named Karen, asks "Why do we have limited visiting hours for families? Where I used to work, families were not restricted to when they could visit." She further states, "AACN issued a call to expand open visitation in the ICU years ago" (AACN Practice Alert, 2011). Joe, a long tenured and informal historian on the unit states, "Well, that's just not how we have done it here, because we are a SICU, our patients are different, besides, we tried extending our visiting hours once, but it didn't work." Others agree with Joe that changing unit visitation practices would not be good. You ask your team about the evidence on visitation

in the SICU. Susan, who is in graduate school, says "evidence is strong for unrestricted visitation for families in general care areas, but I don't know the SICU literature." The team is uncertain but are now interested in learning more. You recognize current unit visitation practices are a sacred cow, an old practice habit that is considered routine and beyond dispute despite evidence for change (Hanrahan et al., 2015; Makic & Rauen, 2016). You realize this is potentially an EBP project that might even improve patient satisfaction or decrease falls on the unit.

How will you engage the team in this EBP project?
1. What are the issues for pursuing an evidenced-based, standardized practice for visitation?

2. Whom would you consider to be the project director to manage the project and why?
3. How can you help the team determine whether this is a priority for the organization?
4. Who are the stakeholders and potential team members?
5. How will you, as nurse manager, be involved in the project?
6. Why is a review of current literature specific to this population important?
7. Why is it important to adapt the practice to your unit?
8. How might staff learn more about patients and family preferences?

9. Knowing this is a sacred cow practice, what does this mean for implementing and sustaining the practice change?
10. After developing an evidence-based change in visitation:
   a. Who needs education?
   b. How can the change agent role benefit implementation?
   c. What are key process and outcome indicators to measure?
   d. How should the key indicators be measured?
   e. Who can assist with monitoring ongoing compliance with the practice change?

18

Quality and Safety

Luc R. Pelletier

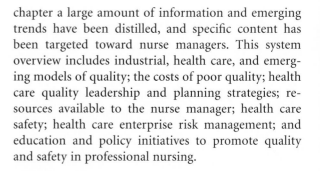

http://evolve.elsevier.com/Huber/leadership

In this era of continuing health care reform, quality and safety are sharing center stage. Quality and safety principles and practices form the foundation of an accessible, reliable health care enterprise. Health care quality is an art and science that continues to evolve. Its relevance was heightened with ongoing reports from the National Academies of Sciences, Engineering, and Medicine's Health and Medicine Division (HMD) (previously the Institute of Medicine [IOM]) and other national organizations related to health care and health care quality. Well before these reports were published, however, professional nurses assumed key roles in the business of measuring, monitoring, and improving health care quality and safety. Nurses have typically taken a leadership role in performance and quality improvement and continue to do so in their roles as board members, chief executives, chief quality officers, health care quality professionals, enterprise risk managers, and safety officers. It is important to note that identifying opportunities for improvement and continuously improving services is every health care professional's job. Patients and their families also have rights and responsibilities related to quality and safety. Where once there were dedicated quality departments in health care organizations, now best-in-class health care organizations train everyone in performance improvement models and techniques (e.g., Plan-Do-Study-Act [PDSA], Lean, Six Sigma). It would be difficult to describe the entire field of health care quality and patient safety in one chapter. In this

chapter a large amount of information and emerging trends have been distilled, and specific content has been targeted toward nurse managers. This system overview includes industrial, health care, and emerging models of quality; the costs of poor quality; health care quality leadership and planning strategies; resources available to the nurse manager; health care safety; health care enterprise risk management; and education and policy initiatives to promote quality and safety in professional nursing.

DEFINITIONS

There are many concepts and terms related to health care quality and safety. Definitions are:

In ambulatory care (and other settings), **benchmarking** "is the process of comparing a practice's performance with an external standard. Benchmarking is an important tool that facilitators can use to motivate a practice to engage in improvement work and to help members of a practice understand where their performance falls in comparison to others" (Agency for Healthcare Research and Quality [AHRQ], 2013a, ¶11).

Continuous quality improvement (CQI) is defined by the American Society for Quality (ASQ) as "a philosophy and attitude for analyzing capabilities and processes and improving them repeatedly to achieve customer satisfaction" (ASQ, n.d.a). **Evidence-based practice** was originally defined by Sackett and colleagues (1996) as "the conscientious, explicit, and judicious use of current best evidence in making decisions about the care of individual patients" (p. 71). A **fair and just culture** "is an approach to medical event reporting that emphasizes learning and accountability over blame and punishment" (California Patient Satisfaction Coalition [CAPSAC], 2016, ¶1).

Lean enterprise originated in manufacturing before being applied to health care. It is "a manufacturing company organized to eliminate all unproductive effort and unnecessary investment, both on the shop floor and in office functions" (ASQ, n.d.b).

Patient activation describes the degree of patient engagement, including "1) believing the patient role is important, 2) having the confidence and knowledge necessary to take action, 3) actually taking action to maintain and improve one's health, and 4) staying the course even under stress" (Hibbard et al., 2004, p. 1005). **Patient engagement** is defined as "actions an individual must make to obtain the greatest benefit from the health care services available to them" (Center for Advancing Health, 2010, p. 2). A more recent definition describes "a set of behaviors by patients, family members, and health professionals and a set of organizational policies and procedures that foster both the inclusion of patients and family members as active members of the health care team and collaborative partnerships with providers and provider organizations" (Maurer et al., 2014, p. 10).

Patient safety practices are "discrete and clearly recognizable processes or manners of providing care that have an evidence base demonstrating that they reduce the likelihood of harm due to the systems, processes, or environments of care" (National Quality Forum [NQF], 2009, p. 3).

A **performance measure** is "a quantitative tool (for example, rate, ratio, index, percentage) that provides an indication of an organization's performance in relation to a specified process or outcome" (The Joint Commission [TJC], 2016a). A **performance measurement system** is "an entity that has a set of process and/or outcome measures of performance; processes for collecting, analyzing and disseminating these measures from multiple organizations as well as disseminating the results of analysis to its client base; an automated database that can be used to facilitate performance improvement; and the ability to generate both internal comparisons of each participating organization's performance over time, and external comparisons of performance among participating organizations" (TJC, 2016b, ¶1).

A **performance/quality improvement program** is an overarching organizational strategy to ensure accountability of all employees, incorporating evidence-based health care quality indicators to continuously improve care delivered to various populations. It is the organization's blueprint for achieving and maintaining performance excellence. **PDSA** is an acronym for an improvement model for testing change, which includes "developing a plan to test the change (Plan), carrying out the test (Do), observing and learning from the consequences (Study), and determining what modifications should be made to the test (Act)" (Institute for Healthcare Improvement [IHI], 2016a, ¶1).

Quality refers to characteristics of and the pursuit of excellence. **Health care quality** is defined as "the degree to which health services for individuals and populations increase the likelihood of desired health outcomes and are consistent with current professional knowledge" (Lohr, 1990, pp. 128–129). Inpatient **quality indicators** are "a set of measures that provide a perspective on hospital quality of care using hospital administrative data. These indicators reflect quality of care inside hospitals and include inpatient mortality for certain procedures and medical conditions; utilization of procedures for which there are questions of overuse, underuse, and misuse; and volume of procedures for which there is some evidence that a higher volume of procedures is associated with lower mortality" (AHRQ, 2015, ¶1). The Agency for Healthcare Research and Quality (AHRQ) also has quality indicators for prevention, patient safety, and pediatric care.

Risk adjustment is a process in which differences among clients or variables such as age or disease severity are weighted or adjusted for in outcomes analyses or benchmarking efforts. **Enterprise risk management (ERM)** "in healthcare promotes a comprehensive framework for making risk management decisions which maximize value protection and creation by managing risk and uncertainty and their connection to total value" (Carroll, 2014, p. 5). An **ERM program** includes components of culture, strategy, objectives, appetite/tolerance, ERM structure and plans, communication and reporting plans, and oversight (Carroll, 2014, pp. 6–8).

A **sentinel event** "is a patient safety event (not primarily related to the natural course of the patient's illness or underlying condition) that reaches a patient and results in death, permanent harm, or severe temporary harm (critical, potentially life threatening harm lasting for a limited time with no permanent residual, but requires transfer to a higher level of care/monitoring for a prolonged period of time, transfer to a higher level of care for a life-threatening condition, or additional major surgery, procedure, or treatment to resolve the condition)" (TJC, 2016c, p. SE1).

Standards are defined as written value statements. These statements form the rules that apply to key processes and the results that can be expected when the processes are performed according to specifications. The three basic types of standards for health care quality are (1) structure, (2) process, and (3) outcome standards, following Donabeidan's (1980) quality framework. **Structure standards and measures** focus on the internal characteristics of the organization and its personnel. **Process standards and measures** focus on whether the activities within an organization are being conducted appropriately, effectively, and efficiently. **Outcome standards and measures** refer to a change in the patient's current or future health status that is attributed to antecedent health care and client attributes of health care.

Total quality management (TQM) is a term coined by the Naval Air Systems Command to describe its Japanese style management approach to quality improvement. "Since then, TQM has taken on many meanings. Simply put, it is a management approach to long-term success through customer satisfaction. TQM is based on all members of an organization participating in improving processes, products, services and the culture in which they work" (ASQ, n.d.c).

HEALTH CARE QUALITY IN THE TWENTY-FIRST CENTURY

Professional nurses have an obligation to reasonably ensure that the care they provide is evidence based (Sackett et al., 1996) and that work processes are consumer and family centric. Their interventions should be intentional, that is "purposeful, focused and determined" (Waddill-Goad & Langster, 2016, p. 169). Providing "quality" health care is "the degree to which health services for individuals and populations increase the likelihood of desired health outcomes and are consistent with current professional knowledge" (Lohr, 1990, pp. 128–129). As clinical leaders and managers, nurses have served as health care quality professionals and have promoted standardization, measurement, and continuous quality improvement in a variety of care delivery settings. Professional nurses have consistently held the practice of quality management in high regard and have the effective care of clients and families as their primary focus. Nurses are bound by their professional

association's *Code of Ethics* (American Nurses Association [ANA], 2015) and scope of professional standards to participate in the continuous improvement of the services they provide. Specifically, in Provision 3, the "nurse promotes, advocates for, and protects the rights, health, and *safety* of the patient" (Hegge, 2015, Set 2: slide 45). Recent health reform legislation serves as a call to action for professional nurses—from frontline clinicians to executives—to be actively involved in health care transformation. This includes ensuring that patients and families receive safe and effective health care (Institute of Medicine [IOM], 2011, p. 22).

Although the manufacturing industry has dutifully explored ways to enhance its business practices, health care has lagged behind, and only within the past 30 years or so has it embraced improvement concepts. Health care has borrowed and applied models of continuous quality improvement and total quality management with principles and practices originally developed for the manufacturing industry. *Continuous quality improvement (CQI)* is defined by the American Society for Quality (ASQ) as "a philosophy and attitude for analyzing capabilities and processes and improving them repeatedly to achieve customer satisfaction" (ASQ, n.d.a). *Total quality management (TQM)* is a Japanese-style management approach to quality improvement. It is a management approach to long-term success through customer satisfaction whereby all members of an organization participate in improving processes, products, services, and the culture in which they work. The methods for TQM are found in the teachings of such quality leaders as Philip B. Crosby, W. Edwards Deming, Armand V. Feigenbaum, Kaoru Ishikawa, and Joseph M. Juran (ASQ, n.d.b). As industry has had its quality gurus, so too has the health care quality movement been fostered by health care professionals who have focused on continuous improvement.

Donald M. Berwick, MD, co-author of the book *Curing Health Care: New Strategies for Quality Improvement* (Berwick et al., 1990), was an early pioneer in identifying how the concepts of TQM programs could apply to health care. In 1991 the National Demonstration Project on Quality Improvement in Health Care was conducted as a collaboration between members of the John A. Hartford Foundation, the Harvard Community Health Plan, the Juran Institute, the Hospital Corporation of America, and other health care organizations (IHI, 2004). The goal was to apply the methods and tools of industrial quality improvement in a variety of organizations to determine whether they could apply to a service industry. Berwick was a principal investigator for this project. As a result of this endeavor, the IHI was founded and became an early advocate for the concepts of process improvement and team problem solving in health care organizations. In 2010 Berwick was appointed by President Obama as administrator of the Centers for Medicare & Medicaid Services (CMS). He served for 18 months and was responsible for introducing the "Triple Aim": improving the patient care experience, improving population health, and reducing health costs (Berwick et al., 2008). His administration was also responsible for initiating major transformative changes under health reform legislation (Affordable Care Act).

In the mid-1990s The Joint Commission (TJC), a health care accreditation organization, began incorporating the principles of CQI in its revised standards. Starting in 1996 the IOM, through its Committee on Quality of Health Care in America (CQHCA), convened the nation's quality leaders and other public and private stakeholders to assess and improve health care for all. These leaders have promoted CQI in health care through education, research, and evaluation. Tenets promoted by these health care leaders and organizations—and embraced by health care professionals—include:

- Processes and systems are the problems, not people.
- Standardization of processes is key to managing work and people.
- Quality can be enhanced only in safe, non-punitive work cultures.
- Quality measurement and monitoring is everyone's job.
- The impetus for quality monitoring is not primarily for accreditation or regulatory compliance, but as a planned part of an organization's culture to continuously enhance and improve its services based on continuous feedback from employees and customers.
- Consumers and stakeholders must be included in all phases of quality improvement planning.
- Consensus among all stakeholders must be gained to have an impact on quality and safety.
- Health policy should include a focus on continuous enhancement of quality and safety.

A framework for understanding health care improvement was proposed by the IOM Committee on Quality of Health Care in America (2001) (Box 18.1). These six aims for health care quality improvement

---

BOX 18.1 Institute of Medicine's Specific Aims for Health Care Quality Improvement

- *Safe:* "Patients should not be harmed by the care that is intended to help them, nor should harm come to those who work in health care" (IOM, Committee on the National Quality Report on Health Care Delivery, 2001, p. 47).
- *Effective:* "Refers to care that is based on the use of systematically acquired evidence to determine whether an intervention, such as a preventive service, diagnostic test, or therapy, produces better outcomes than do alternatives—including the alternative to do nothing" (IOM, Committee on the National Quality Report on Health Care Delivery, 2001, p. 49). Evidence-based practice requires that those who give care consistently avoid both underuse of effective care and overuse of ineffective care that is more likely to harm than help the patient (Chassin, 1997).
- *Patient-centered:* "Refers to health care that establishes a partnership among practitioners, patients, and their families (when appropriate) to ensure that decisions respect patients' wants, needs, and preferences; and that patients have the education and support they need to make decisions and participate in their own care" (IOM, Committee on the National Quality Report on Health Care Delivery, 2001, p. 50).
- *Timeliness:* "Refers to obtaining needed care and minimizing unnecessary delays in getting that care" (IOM, Committee on the National Quality Report on Health Care Delivery, 2001, p. 53).
- *Efficient:* "Refers to a health care system where resources are used to get the best value for the money spent" (Palmer & Torgerson, 1999, p. 1136). "The opposite of efficiency is waste; the use of resources without benefit to the patients a system is intended to help. There are at least two ways to improve efficiency: (a) reduce quality waste and (b) reduce administrative or production costs" (IOM, CQHCA, 2001, p. 54).
- *Equitable:* "Providing care that does not vary in quality because of personal characteristics such as gender, ethnicity, geographical location, and socioeconomic status" (IOM, CQHCA, 2001, p. 6).

From Pelletier, L.R., & Hoffman, J.A. (2002). A framework for selecting performance measures for opioid treatment programs. *Journal for Healthcare Quality, 24*(3), 25. Reprinted with permission from the National Association for Healthcare Quality.

propose that health care systems ensure that care is safe, effective, patient centered, timely, efficient, and equitable.

COLLABORATION AND HEALTH CARE QUALITY AS PROFESSIONAL NURSING IMPERATIVES

Collaboration should be a goal of any interaction, regardless of the workplace or situation. Collaboration is an imperative set by the American Nurses Association (ANA). The ANA, in its current *Guide to the Code of Ethics for Nurses with Interpretive Statements,* proposed that "The nurse collaborates with other health professionals and the public to protect human rights, promote health diplomacy, and reduce health disparities" (Hegge, 2015, Set 3: slide 12). Collaborative partnerships are part of this imperative and shape the way professional nurses act clinically and how they participate in performance and quality improvement efforts. As the complexity of care increases, multidisciplinary and inter-professional teamwork is used to solve complex problems in practice. For example, nursing, medicine, pharmacy, and information technology (IT) personnel may form a team or committee to develop a risk screen and smart alert for patients at risk for delirium.

Collaboration is about relationships. Conflict is typically the result of an undeveloped or poor interpersonal relationship with a colleague. To overcome conflicts, it is necessary to strengthen, not shy away from, the relationship of the two opposing parties. As early as the late 1990s, the Pew Health Professions Commission (PHPC) talked about practicing relationship-centered care as one of 21 health profession competencies for the twenty-first century (O'Neil & PHPC, 1998). Relationship-centered care in this context surely involves nurse and client/family interactions, but it also stresses the importance of collaborative inter-professional relationships. These 21 competencies are necessary ingredients for effective professional relationships and can become guideposts for successful professional working relationships within a continuous improvement framework.

The 21 competencies also include a professional nurse's responsibility and accountability for health care quality. The specific statements related to health care quality include "take responsibility for quality of care and health outcomes at all levels" and "contribute to continuous improvement of the health care system" (O'Neill & PHPC, 1998, pp. 29–43) (Box 18.2).

BOX 18.2   Twenty-One Competencies for the Twenty-First Century

1. Embrace a personal ethic of social responsibility and service.
2. Exhibit ethical behavior in all professional activities.
3. Provide evidence-based, clinically competent care.
4. Incorporate the multiple determinants of health in clinical care.
5. Apply knowledge of the new sciences.
6. Demonstrate critical thinking, reflection, and problem-solving skills.
7. Understand the role of primary care.
8. Rigorously practice preventive health care.
9. Integrate population-based care and services into practice.
10. Improve access to health care for those with unmet health needs.
11. Practice relationship-centered care with individuals and families.
12. Provide culturally sensitive care to a diverse society.
13. Partner with communities in health care decisions.
14. Use communication and information technology effectively and appropriately.
15. Work in interdisciplinary teams.
16. Ensure care that balances individual, professional, system, and societal needs.
17. Practice leadership.
18. Take responsibility for quality of care and health outcomes at all levels.
19. Contribute to continuous improvement of the health care system.
20. Advocate for public policy that promotes and protects the health of the public.
21. Continue to learn and help others learn.

From O'Neil, E.H., & the Pew Health Professions Commission (PHPC). (1998). *Recreating health professional practice for a new century: The fourth report of the Pew Health Professions Commission.* San Francisco, CA: PHPC.

INDUSTRIAL MODELS OF QUALITY

Industrial models have heavily influenced the way quality is currently understood and measured in health care settings across the continuum. Industry leaders who have influenced nursing's understanding of health care quality include Walter Shewhart, Joseph Juran, Philip Crosby, and W. Edwards Deming. These leaders provided blueprints from which nursing performance and quality improvement programs have been derived. Understanding quality in health care is enhanced by understanding the development of models of quality.

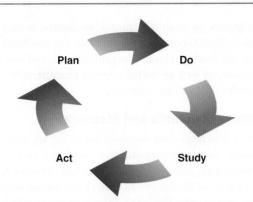

FIG. 18.1 PDSA (Plan, Do, Study, Act) cycle.

Shewhart explored causes of variation in core work processes. He quantified these variations, categorizing variables as common or special cause. His *Plan, Do, Check, Act (PDCA)* model was updated to the PDSA cycle and is probably the most frequently used improvement tool in health care quality settings today, as follows (Fig. 18.1): developing a plan to test the change (**P**lan), carrying out the test (**D**o), observing and learning from the consequences (**S**tudy), and determining what modifications should be made to the test (**A**ct) (IHI, 2016a, ¶1). Shewhart also provided the industrial community with statistical process control techniques that are used widely today. Deming (2000a, b) adopted his work and refined it.

Juran (1989) defined quality as "fitness for use." Quality, in his work, was defined as freedom from defects plus value and continuously meeting customer expectations. His approach to quality centered on the use of interdisciplinary teams that used diagnostic tools to understand why industrial processes produce a product not fit for use. His framework included a three-pronged approach: quality planning, quality control, and quality improvement. Quality planning:

establishes the design of a product, service, or process that will meet customer, business, and operational needs to produce the product before it is produced. Quality planning follows a universal sequence of steps, as follows:

- *Identify customers and target markets*
- *Discover hidden and unmet customer needs*
- *Translate these needs into product or service requirements: a means to meet their needs (new standards, specifications, etc.)*
- *Develop a service or product that exceeds customers' needs*
- *Develop the processes that will provide the service, or create the product, in the most efficient way*
- *Transfer these designs to the organization and the operating forces to be carried out (Juran Institute, 2009, ¶1–2).*

Crosby viewed quality in production terms of zero defects and measured quality in relation to conformance to requirements. He believed that the results or products of a company are made by people. He focused on systems and the consequences of poor quality. He emphasized doing the right thing the first time to prevent waste. Waste and rework were seen as costly, and good managers were those who prevented costly mistakes.

In addition to PDSA, Deming focused on statistical process control techniques and on continuous quality improvement through a culture of quality. He is credited as being influential in the success of Japanese industries post–World War II. He proposed 14 points to help management staff understand and commit to quality. These points are listed in Box 18.3 (Deming, 2000a, b) and have heavily influenced health care's adoption of quality principles.

STANDARDS OF QUALITY

Donabedian (1980) developed the initial theoretical model of health care quality standards: structure, process, and outcomes, which identified that quality can be measured using these three aspects. Donabedian's framework is the most widely referenced model of quality; professional nurses have used this model to develop performance and quality improvement programs and conduct evidence-based improvement studies and research. Standards essentially define quality, against which performance and outcomes are measured. Standards and measures are typically developed from *benchmarking* activities and reviews of best practices in best-in-class organizations. Therefore the selection of standards and measures is a critical activity in the performance and quality improvement process. Actually, standards establish the baseline against which measurement and evaluation are conducted. Therefore it is critical to decide who determines the standards and which standards are selected to define quality. Over the past 30 years, national groups have been formed to gain consensus on health care performance standards and measures. One such entity is the National Quality Forum (NQF), a not-for-profit, public–private membership organization created to

---

BOX 18.3   Deming's 14 Points for Quality

1. Create constancy of purpose toward improving products and services.
2. Adopt the new philosophy.
3. Cease dependence on inspection to achieve quality.
4. End the practice of awarding business on the basis of cost alone.
5. Improve constantly and forever every process for planning, production, and service.
6. Institute training on the job.
7. Adopt and institute leadership aimed at helping people do their jobs better.
8. Drive out fear by promoting two-way communication.
9. Break down barriers between departments.
10. Eliminate exhortations for the workforce in such forms as posters and slogans; these methods tend to create adversarial relationships.
11. Eliminate numerical quotas for productivity; instead have leaders promote continuous quality improvement (CQI).
12. Permit pride of workmanship by removing the barriers that prevent this.
13. Encourage education and self-improvement for all workers.
14. Define management's commitment to CQI and their obligation to implement these points.

From Deming, W.E. (2000a). *The new economics for industry, government, education.* Cambridge, MA: MIT Center for Advanced Engineering Studies; and Deming, W.E. (2000b). *Out of the crisis.* Cambridge, MA: MIT Center for Advanced Engineering Studies.

---

develop and implement a national strategy for health care quality measurement and reporting.

Structure Standards and Measures

Structure standards and measures focus on the internal characteristics of the organization and its personnel. They answer the following questions. Is an infrastructure in place and tools accessible to allow quality to exist? Is the structure of the organization set up to allow for the effective, efficient delivery of services? For example, a structural standard for a long-term care facility might be to have an adequate mix of registered nurses (RNs) and nursing assistants on site to ensure that comprehensive care is delivered. For specialized areas, structure standards may address whether there are enough specialists, "hospitalists," or "intensivists" to ensure quality care. Certain committees, policy statements, rules and regulations, or manuals, forms, or contracts may be needed. Structure standards regulate the environment to ensure quality. Human, organizational, and physical resources, as well as environmental characteristics, are examples of structure elements.

Process Standards and Measures

Process standards and measures focus on whether the activities within an organization are being conducted appropriately, effectively, and efficiently. Process measures focus on the behaviors of the professional nurse as a provider of care. The interventions recommended in a clinical practice guideline or best practice are examples of process standards. They relate to what the nurse will be doing and the process the nurse should follow to ensure effective, *evidence-based care.* Process standards look at activities, interventions, and the sequence of caregiving events, sometimes referred to as work flow. Typically, processes are assessed by audits, observational studies, or work flow analyses. Examples of process standards include the following: A nursing assessment is completed within 24 hours of admission, client calls are returned within 1 hour of the initial call, or a face-to-face assessment is completed within 1 hour for seclusion and restraints in a behavioral health setting.

Outcome Standards and Measures

Outcome standards and measures refer to whether the services provided by the organization make any difference: Were they effective? They answer important questions about the services that nurses provide. Did those services make a difference to the clients or to the health status of the population? Outcome standards address physical health status, mental health status, social and physical function, health attitudes/knowledge/behavior, utilization of services, and the client's perception and satisfaction with the care received. *Outcome process and measures* refer to a change in the current or future health status attributed to antecedent health care and client attributes of health care. Outcome standards present the possibility of measuring the effectiveness, quality, and time and resources allocated for care. Outcomes are reported as a rate per unit of measurement. Examples of outcome measures include the following: percentage of patients whose activities of daily living have improved by 80%, percentage of clients who have stopped smoking after 12 weeks of intensive psychoeducational therapy, and falls with injury per 1000 patient days.

BOX 18.4 Common Performance Measurement Selection Criteria*

- *Relevance:* The measure should address features of the health care system applicable to health professionals, policy makers, and consumers.
- *Meaningfulness and interpretability:* The measure should be understandable to at least one of the audiences. It should help inform them about the important issues or concerns.
- *Scientific or clinical evidence:* The measure should be based on evidence documenting the links between the interventions, clinical processes, and/or outcomes it addresses.
- *Reliability or reproducibility:* The measure should produce the same results when repeated in the same population and setting.

- *Feasibility:* The measure should be specified precisely. Collection of data for the measure should be inexpensive and logistically feasible.
- *Validity:* The measure should make sense (face validity), correlate well with other measures of the same aspects of care (construct validity), and capture meaningful aspects of care (content validity).
- *Health importance:* The measure should include the prevalence of the health condition to which it applies and the seriousness of the health outcomes affected.

*Criteria are listed in order of their frequency, with the one mentioned most often listed first. The same label for a criterion can have different meanings depending on the framework, because the criteria are not standardized. The definitions, rather than the labels, were used to construct the figure. Feasibility was used as a category covering several criteria in some of the frameworks and as a single criterion in others. Parts of this figure were adapted from NCQA's list of desirable attributes for HEDIS measures (IOM, Committee on the National Quality Report on Health Care Delivery, 2001, p. 81).
From Pelletier, L.R., & Hoffman, J.A. (2002). A framework for selecting performance measures for opioid treatment programs. *Journal for Healthcare Quality, 24*(3), 26. Reprinted with permission from the National Association for Healthcare Quality.

In measuring quality, both structure and process parameters are important, but they are not sufficient in determining whether the care led to an effective outcome or whether the client learned, recovered, or improved his or her health status. Over the years, the emphasis on structure, process, and outcome aspects of health care has varied. Ultimately, various stakeholders are interested in knowing whether care resulted in a positive, expected clinical outcome, based on objective, measurable criteria.

When developing a performance and quality improvement program, nurse managers are cautioned to not start by creating new standards and measures. Rather, a literature review will undoubtedly yield measures from which to choose (see Chapter 17). These measures have typically been tested for reliability and validity and have been piloted in the field. National repositories of performance measures can be found at:
- National Database for Nursing Quality Indicators (NDNQI) (Press Ganey, 2015)
- Agency for Healthcare Research and Quality's National Quality Measures Clearinghouse
- National Quality Forum
- Leapfrog Group
- National Guideline Clearinghouse
- The Cochrane Library
- Specialty professional associations and societies

Selection criteria can then be adopted and measures chosen for a specific intervention or program. A number of selection criteria guideline statements have been developed, including the performance measurement evaluation criteria from the NQF (2011). The performance measurement attributes common to these entities' guideline statements have been reported in the set of criteria proposed to be used for a national health care quality report (Institute of Medicine [IOM], Committee on the National Quality Report on Health Care Delivery, 2001). Common performance measurement selection criteria are listed in Box 18.4 (Pelletier & Hoffman, 2002). The adoption of these performance measurement selection criteria is the first step in developing a comprehensive performance measurement system.

EMERGING MODELS OF HEALTH CARE PERFORMANCE AND QUALITY MANAGEMENT

A number of industry-based models for quality management and measurement have been adopted by the health care industry over the past two decades. These include Six Sigma, Lean Enterprise, the Baldrige National Quality Award, high-reliability organizations, American Nurses Credentialing Center's Magnet Recognition Program®, and Planetree. These models are briefly described in the following sections.

Six Sigma

A strategy developed by Motorola and implemented successfully at General Electric (GE) and AlliedSignal Companies provided an innovative approach to reduce variation and error rates. Not surprisingly, the Six Sigma approach that these companies use is similar to tried-and-true approaches historically deployed by health care quality professionals. In the Six Sigma breakthrough strategy, errors are measured in defects per million opportunities (dpmo). Six Sigma is achieved when the organization reaches an error or defect rate of 3.4 or less per one million. Application of Six Sigma in health care can reduce patient waiting time in emergency departments, lost charges for billing in patient financial services, delinquent medical records, diagnostic result turnaround times, accounts receivable days, patients' length of stay, or medication errors (Ahmed et al., 2013). The Six Sigma strategy of **d**efine, **m**easure, **a**nalyze, **i**mprove, and **c**ontrol (DMAIC) (Harry &

Schroeder, 2000) is remarkably similar to Juran's problem-solving strategy (Plsek & Omnias, 1989) that has been applied to health care. Table 18.1 illustrates these similarities (Pelletier, 2000).

Lean Enterprise

Lean Enterprise is a model of quality measurement that was originally associated with Deming but was reintroduced to the United States by Womack in the mid-1990s (Jones & Womack, 2003). The premise of this model is that operational waste in an organization needs to be eliminated. A *lean enterprise* originated in manufacturing before being applied to health care. It is "a manufacturing company organized to eliminate all unproductive effort and unnecessary investment, both on the shop floor and in office functions" (ASQ, n.d.b). With a focus on core processes, "a perfect process creates precisely the right value for the customer. In a perfect process, every step is valuable (creates value for the customer), capable (produces a good result every time), available (produces the desired output, not just the desired quality, every time), adequate (does not cause delay), flexible, and linked by continuous flow" (IHI, 2005, p. 6). When any of these components are missing, the result is waste, which must be eliminated. Lean has wide applicability in health care where there are many opportunities to

TABLE 18.1   Comparison of Six Sigma Breakthrough Strategy and Juran's Problem-Solving Strategy

SIX SIGMA BREAKTHROUGH STRATEGY		JURAN'S PROBLEM-SOLVING STRATEGY	
Stage	**Step (Objective)**	**Phase**	**Step**
Identification	1. Recognize 2. Define (Identify key business issues)	Project definition and organization	1. List and prioritize problems 2. Define project and team
Characterization	1. Measure 2. Analyze (Understand current performance levels)	Diagnostic journey	1. Analyze symptom 2. Formulate theory of causes 3. Test theories 4. Identify root causes
Optimization	1. Improve 2. Control (Achieve breakthrough improvement)	Remedial journey	1. Consider alternative solutions 2. Design solutions and controls 3. Address resistance to change 4. Implement solutions and controls
Institutionalization	1. Standardize 2. Integrate (Transform how day-to-day business is conducted)	Holding the gains	1. Check performance 2. Monitor control system

From Pelletier, L.R. (2000). On error-free health care: Mission possible! (Editorial). *Journal for Healthcare Quality, 22*(3), 9. Reprinted with permission from the National Association for Healthcare Quality.

improve processes such as supply chain management or medication administration. By challenging and analyzing any work process, obvious wasteful rework is flushed out and then the process is redone to be both more efficient and effective. Nurses find it rewarding to reduce or eliminate unnecessary effort.

Malcolm Baldrige National Quality Award Program

The Baldrige National Quality Award (BNQA) establishes a set of performance standards that define a total quality organization. Named after the Secretary of Commerce, the BNQA "was established by Congress in 1987 to enhance the competitiveness and performance of U.S. businesses" (National Institute of Standards and Technology, 2007, p. 1). The standards in seven areas of excellence are (1) leadership, (2) strategic planning, (3) customer and market focus (focus on patients, other customers, and markets), (4) information and analysis, (5) human resource focus, (6) process management, and (7) business results (organizational performance results). Organizations committed to quality improvement choose to adopt the BNQA approach as another means of defining and improving their organizational processes to achieve quality outcomes. Manufacturing, service, and small business were the original award categories, but education and health care were added in 1999. With the trend in health care of adopting industry applications and measure sets for quality improvement, it was fitting that the health care industry was recognized as one that could benefit from participating in this program. It is appropriate for health care entities to strive to achieve internationally recognized standards for performance excellence that enable them to benchmark their "best practices" with others in the field. The first health care organization to apply and be awarded the BNQA in health care was the SSM system in St. Louis in 2002. The Alliance for Performance Excellence is a network of national, state, and local Baldrige-based organizations helping institutions achieve performance excellence using the Baldrige criteria (http://www.baldrigepe.org/alliance/). Various states have also developed quality awards based on the BNQA criteria. Hospital units can achieve the Baldrige Award.

High-Reliability Organizations

In their book *Managing the Unexpected* (2007), Weick and Sutcliffe described high reliability as involving anticipation and containment. They believed that an organization's "collective mindfulness" (Chassin & Loeb, 2013) ensured that potential problems are anticipated and that strategies are in place should an unexpected event occur. Anticipation has three elements: (1) preoccupation with failure—ever mindful of how complex their operations are and the fact that errors do occur, (2) reluctance to simplify—requiring staff to dig deep in understanding the cause of error versus overly simplified explanations (e.g., staff education), and (3) sensitivity to operations—always aware of structure and processes that are in place to effect desired patient outcomes. Containment has two elements: (1) commitment to resilience—having systems in place to return to normal operations quickly, and (2) deference to expertise—relying on and listening to frontline staff for their intimate knowledge about daily operations (Chassin & Loeb, 2013; Weick & Sutcliffe, 2007).

American Nurses Credentialing Center Magnet Designation

The American Nurses Credentialing Center's (ANCC) Magnet Recognition Program® recognizes health care organizations for "superior nursing processes and quality patient care, which lead to the highest levels of safety, quality, and patient satisfaction" (ANCC, 2016, ¶1). Magnet-designated hospitals "attract" staff and retain them due to their characteristics or "forces of magnetism," such as the quality of nursing leadership, professional models of care and quality of care, research and evidence-based practice (ANCC, 2016). The Magnet model includes the following components: transformational leadership, structural empowerment, exemplary professional practice, new knowledge, innovations and improvements, and empirical quality outcomes. Hospitals that embark on the Magnet journey first must assess where they are related to preestablished Magnet standards. Typically, nursing leadership staff complete a gap analysis to identify opportunities for improvement before submitting their application for designation. Organizations have used the journey to effect the rigor of research and inquiry (Erickson et al., 2015), shorten length of stay and lower costs (Yakusheva et al., 2014), lower mortality and failure to rescue in surgical patients (McHugh et al., 2013), and lower mortality in low-birth-weight infants (Lake et al., 2012).

Planetree

Since 1978, Planetree has designated health care organizations for patient-centered excellence. "Guided by a foundation of 10 components of patient-centered care, Planetree informs policy at a national level, aligns strategies at a system level, guides implementation of care delivery practices at an organizational level, and facilitates compassionate human interactions at a deeply personal level" (Planetree, 2014, ¶1). Its standards help organizations increase patient activation and staff engagement and foster staff and leadership development.

COSTS ASSOCIATED WITH POOR HEALTH CARE QUALITY

The cost associated with medical errors "in lost income, disability, and health care costs is as much as $29 billion annually" (Quality Interagency Coordination [QuIC] Task Force, 2000, p. 1) and plagues every sector in the health care industry. Policy experts have estimated that 30% of the $2.8 trillion spent on health care is attributable to waste (Roeder, 2014). Berwick and Hackbarth (2012) listed categories of waste as: failures of care delivery, failures of care coordination, overtreatment, administrative complexity, pricing failures, and fraud and abuse.

The number of medical errors was described as unacceptable in *To Err Is Human: Building a Safer Health Care System* (Kohn et al., 2000), an IOM report that has been referenced widely in the professional and consumer press since its release. The IOM report reached the highest levels in the federal government, but response to its findings and recommendations was lackluster at first. Health care organizations were slow to adopt its recommendations fully even 16 years later. Several reports on health care quality and safety have followed this landmark report.

The IOM reports defined specific strategies that could inform the development and refinement of health care safety systems nationwide. An important component of these reports is the mention of the error-reduction techniques of other industries. The federal reports provided another opportunity to advocate for patients, families, and populations. They gave health care quality professionals the evidence and research with which to defend a quality management budget, enhance information systems and technologies

to monitor and track errors, and further develop quality activities and studies using proven tools and techniques. The reports are also models in defining and describing cost/benefit analyses and return-on-investment scenarios for quality and performance improvement programs. In essence, they provided a business case for quality and safety.

The IOM report *Crossing the Quality Chasm: A New Health System for the 21st Century* (IOM, Committee on Quality of Health Care in America [CQHCA], 2001, p. 11) recommended that Congress establish a Health Care Quality Innovation Fund "to support projects targeted at (1) achieving the six aims of safety, effectiveness, patient-centeredness, timeliness, efficiency, and equity; and/or (2) producing substantial improvements in quality for the [15] priority conditions." The overall goal of the funding would be to produce a "public-domain portfolio of programs, tools, and technologies of widespread applicability" (p. 11). The report recommended an initial investment of $1 billion over 3 to 5 years to support this goal. Health care organizations could take the lead either by enhancing the current resources dedicated to quality and performance improvement in their organizations or by using the funds to finance regional collaborative health care quality projects. These successes could then be described in the literature for wider application.

Leadership by Example: Coordinating Government Roles in Improving Health Care Quality, the third in a series of IOM quality chasm reports, was released in 2002 (Corrigan et al., 2002). The original charge of the IOM Committee on Enhancing Federal Healthcare Quality Programs (CEFHQP) was to acknowledge that "The current federal quality oversight programs represent a patchwork of requirements and processes that have evolved over the last 30 to 35 years" (IOM, CEFHQP, 2002, p. 1). The committee was convened "to re-examine the various federal quality improvement and oversight programs to assess whether changes are needed to (1) provide adequate protection to beneficiaries, (2) provide strong incentives to providers to improve quality, and (3) improve the efficiency of the oversight processes by reducing redundancy" (IOM, CEFHQP, 2002, p. 1). In doing their work, the committee held workshops to obtain perspectives and information from various stakeholders with expertise in the fields of quality measurement, improvement, oversight, and research on ways to improve current federal programs (Medicare, Medicaid, Children's Health Insurance Program, Tricare, and Veterans Affairs). From his introductory remarks at the press briefing, the committee chair outlined the major findings of the study (Omenn, 2002, p. 2):

- There is a lack of consistency in performance measurement requirements both across and within these government programs.
- The programs are not using standardized measures.
- There is no well-thought-out conceptual framework to guide the selection of performance measures.
- Medicare, Medicaid, and the State Children's Health Insurance Program lack computer-based clinical data, which is seen as a major impediment.
- There is also a lack of commitment to transparency and openly sharing information on safety and quality.

These findings were not a surprise to many nurses and health care quality professionals who have been burdened with duplicative reporting for years. The positive message was that strong recommendations from this committee were sent to the federal government's leadership, asking them to attack these problems with a good deal of muscle to shape performance measurement for the whole health care sector. Standardization of protocols and measures is not a new idea (Pelletier, 1998). Reducing administrative burden and duplicative reporting could easily put time back in the hands of clinicians to do what they do best: provide direct health care services to individuals, families, and communities. Clinical standardization has become the focus of efforts to reduce variability in practice and health care costs, but the use of clinical practice guidelines is slow: from 35% in 2006 to 50% in 2011 (Lin, 2013).

LEADERSHIP AND MANAGEMENT IMPLICATIONS

Planning for Health Care Quality

An organization that adopts and nurtures a continuous performance and quality improvement culture (and rewards those who identify opportunities for improvement and their solutions) recognizes that change is an everyday event. One of the ways that change can be managed is to acknowledge it and make it a part of the organization's strategic planning process. Just as an organization defines its mission, vision, and core values, so too must change agents and teams define the purpose of the change (expected outcomes), the mission and vision of the change process, and the core values of the group that will be responsible for managing the change (see Chapters 2, 14, and 15).

An organization's mission is a concise statement that answers the question: What business are we in today? For example, Sharp HealthCare, a San Diego–based not-for-profit integrated regional health care delivery system that was the recipient of the Baldrige Award in 2007, stated that its mission is "to improve the health of those we serve with a commitment to excellence in all that we do. Our goal is to offer quality care and programs that set community standards, exceed patients' expectations and are provided in a caring, convenient, cost-effective and accessible manner" (Sharp HealthCare, 2016, ¶1). The Visiting Nursing Service of New York's (VNSNY) mission is "to promote the health and well-being of patients and families by providing high-quality, cost-effective health care in the home and community; to be a leader in the development of innovative services that enable people to function as independently as possible in their community; to help shape health care policies that support beneficial home- and community-based services; to continue our tradition of charitable and compassionate care, within the resources available" (VNSNY, 2016, ¶6).

An organization's vision should accurately depict what the company is striving to become. For example, Sharp HealthCare's vision is "to be the best health system in the universe" (Sharp HealthCare, 2016, ¶2). VNSNY's vision is "To become the most significant, best-in-class, nonprofit, community-based integrated delivery system providing superior care coordination and health care services to vulnerable populations across a broad regional footprint" (VNSNY, 2016, ¶1).

It is critical for mission and vision statements to be communicated effectively and widely to internal stakeholders (employees and management personnel) and to external stakeholders (investors, clients, patients, vendors, and accreditation agencies). In this way, the statements keep employees on a path to an attainable goal such as quality outcomes. Mission, vision, and values form the foundation for quality and safety and their management and improvement. Departmental mission and vision statements must be aligned with the organization's statements.

Core value statements frame the organization's culture in the same way mission and vision statements do. "Values are operational qualities used by organizations to maintain or enhance performance" (Harmon, 1997, p. 246). Values consciously and unconsciously guide a professional nurse's personal and professional behavior. His Holiness the Dalai Lama and Cutler (1998) said the following about values: "Higher stages of growth and development depend on an underlying set of values that can guide us. A value system that can provide continuity and coherence to our lives, by which we can measure our experiences. A value system that can help us decide which goals are truly worthwhile and which pursuits are meaningless. Values help us with the challenges of everyday life" (pp. 192–193).

Nurses' personal and professional values come from the experiences they have shared with others in interpersonal exchanges at work and at home. To identify a group's core values, investigate these questions: Which three people have had the greatest influence in your personal and professional life? What are the three most important values these influential people taught you? The answers to these questions can help inform the development of mission, vision, and core value statements. An example is a set of core values or "core principles" from the Mayo Clinic, as outlined in Table 18.2.

A Nurse's Health Care Quality Toolbox

Along with the paradigm shift from quality assurance to organizational performance improvement came the expectation that accredited organizations become skilled at the art and science of continuous performance and quality improvement. This included the concepts of leadership involvement, a commitment to customers' needs (i.e., patients and families), an understanding of the principle of process versus people, a devotion to data collection and analysis as the foundation for problem solving, and the view that inter-professional teams working within the processes that were under study were the experts and therefore best equipped to drive change and improvement.

Nurse managers in accredited organizations are expected to learn these principles and tools for quality improvement, educate staff—including nurses—in these tools and techniques, identify improvement opportunities on their units, and be able to speak to process changes that occurred as a result of data analysis. Nurses are tapped to participate in organization-wide improvement teams designed to address overarching problem resolution or process redesign projects. Many of the early quality leaders received training in facilitation and group meeting techniques in addition to the performance and quality improvement (PQI) tools. This enabled them to promote the team-based model of

TABLE 18.2   Mayo Clinic Value Statements

These values, which guide Mayo Clinic's mission to this day, are an expression of the vision and intent of our founders, the original Mayo physicians and the Sisters of Saint Francis.

Respect	Treat everyone in our diverse community, including patients, their families and colleagues, with dignity.
Compassion	Provide the best care, treating patients and family members with sensitivity and empathy.
Integrity	Adhere to the highest standards of professionalism, ethics and personal responsibility, worthy of the trust our patients place in us.
Healing	Inspire hope and nurture the well-being of the whole person, respecting physical, emotional and spiritual needs.
Teamwork	Value the contributions of all, blending the skills of individual staff members in unsurpassed collaboration.
Excellence	Deliver the best outcomes and highest quality service through the dedicated effort of every team member.
Innovation	Infuse and energize the organization, enhancing the lives of those we serve, through the creative ideas and unique talents of each employee.
Stewardship	Sustain and reinvest in our mission and extended communities by wisely managing our human, natural and material resources.

From Mayo Foundation for Medical Research and Education. (2016). *About Mayo Clinic: Mayo Clinic mission and values.* Rochester, MN: Author. Retrieved from http://www.mayoclinic.org/about-mayo-clinic/mission-values

cross-functional and inter-professional problem solving that became the standard for most organizations. Nurses in the new millennium continue to need skills and expertise in the concepts of team building, conflict resolution, statistical process control, customer service, and process improvement.

Nurses at all levels are affected by organizational quality efforts. Knowledge through continuous learning forms the backdrop for quality and safety. New nurses in nurse residency programs may undertake a small-scale, unit-based quality initiative or change project. Often the impetus arises from seeing a problem

in practice and then pursuing an evidence-based approach (see Chapter 17) and using PQI tools to analyze, plan, and take action through inter-professional teams and shared governance structures.

Health care quality professionals and nurses involved in performance and quality improvement activities have an enormous set of resources available to them as they plan for an enterprise-wide quality program. Tools and techniques that nurses can readily use are illustrated in Table 18.3. Figs. 18.2 through 18.7 illustrate examples of templates and forms to be included in a nurse's quality "toolbox."

TABLE 18.3 A Nurse Manager's Health Care Quality Toolbox

Tool	Description of the Tool	Example
Data-collection tools	Check sheets and checklists facilitate the gathering of data for eventual analysis and reporting. Good data collection tools can help to count and categorize data.	Sample data collection sheet for a nurse manager's quality toolbox (see Fig. 18.2).
Control chart	This tool includes data points and their placement on a graph to depict variation. Its purpose is to illustrate whether the process variation is expected ("common cause") or an unexpected or unusual variation ("special cause"). Included are three lines—the mean, an upper control limit (UCL), and a lower control limit (LCL). Generally, a process is considered "out of control" when the data points stray outside of the control limits or a series of data points follow a defined pattern that illustrates a lack of control in the process.	Sample control chart for a nurse manager's quality toolbox (see Fig. 18.3).
Cause-and-effect (or fishbone) diagram	This tool resembles diagramming sentences. The "effect" is illustrated in a box at the end of a midline (or "head" of the fish). The "causes" are generally four or five categories of elements that might contribute to the effect (e.g., machines, methods, people, materials, measurements) and the specific activities. Under each of these category headings, individual items that might lead to the effect are listed. By diagramming all of the possible contributors, the predominant or root causes may be found more readily.	Sample cause-and-effect diagram for a nurse manager's quality toolbox (see Fig. 18.4).
Detailed flowchart	Using various shapes, this tool is used to depict a work process, from start to finish, illustrating all of the processes' action steps, decision points, handoffs, or waiting stages. Flowcharts form the cornerstone of process improvement planning and analysis. The entire process must first be accurately defined to identify problems or process improvement opportunities.	Sample detailed flowchart for a nurse manager's quality toolbox (see Fig. 18.5).
Pareto chart	This bar graph can help depict the "80/20" rule. In the nineteenth century, it was used to show that 80% of the wealth was held by 20% of the people. In health care, typically 20% of the issues cause 80% of the problems. The use of this tool allows a performance improvement team to focus on the "vital few" causes of the problems in a process under study.	Example of a Pareto chart for a nurse manager's quality toolbox (see Fig. 18.6).

Continued

TABLE 18.3	**A Nurse Manager's Health Care Quality Toolbox—cont'd**	
Tool	**Description of the Tool**	**Example**
Scatter diagram	This graph describes the relationship between two variables that are continuous. It is used when the potential causes of effects under study cannot be easily categorized, such as in a Pareto chart or cause-and-effect diagram. Data points are plotted along the vertical and horizontal axes of the graph, and a correlation between the two variables can either be weak or strong, based on the pattern of the data points.	Example of a scatter diagram for a nurse manager's quality toolbox. (see Fig. 18.7).

Data Collection Sheet

Organization/Unit: _____   Date: _____

Process:_____

MEASURE	DATE	TIME	WHERE	WHEN

FIG. 18.2 Sample data collection sheet for a nurse manager's quality toolbox.

Control Chart

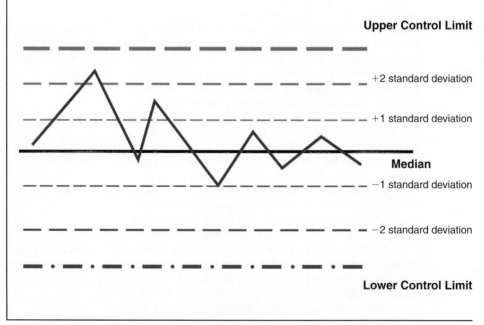

Upper Control Limit

+2 standard deviation

+1 standard deviation

Median

−1 standard deviation

−2 standard deviation

Lower Control Limit

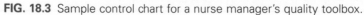

FIG. 18.3 Sample control chart for a nurse manager's quality toolbox.

Cause-and-Effect Diagram

Organization/Unit: _____ Date: _____

Process: _____

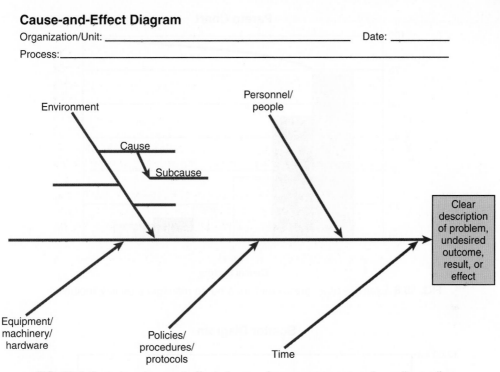

FIG. 18.4 Sample cause-and-effect diagram for a nurse manager's quality toolbox.

Detailed Flowchart

Organization/Unit: _____ Date: _____ Process owner: _____

Process: _____

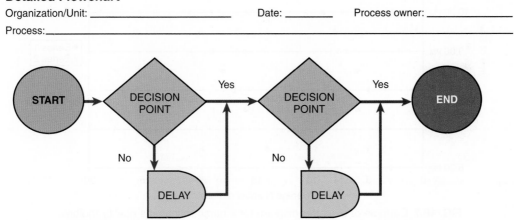

FIG. 18.5 Sample detailed flowchart for a nurse manager's quality toolbox.

One excellent resource for hospital-based quality programs is the National Database of Nursing Quality Indicators (NDNQI), which was developed by the American Nurses Association and now is owned by Press Ganey (Press Ganey, 2015). This database is composed of nurse-sensitive indicators collected at the nursing unit level and provides the ability for participants to benchmark performance with national averages. The NQF, in collaboration with the Robert Wood Johnson Foundation, has developed nurse-sensitive performance measures under its Core Measures for Nursing Care Performance Project (NQF, 2004, 2012).

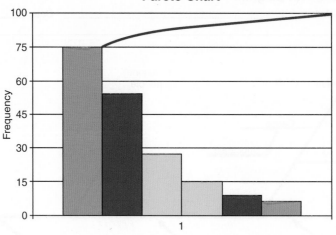

FIG. 18.6 Example of a Pareto chart for a nurse manager's quality toolbox.

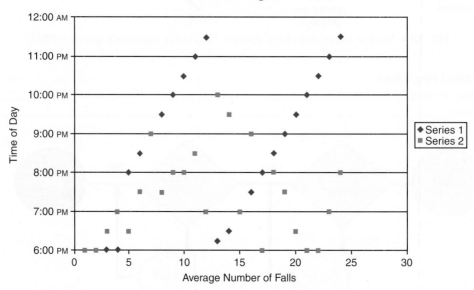

FIG. 18.7 Example of a scatter diagram for a nurse manager's quality toolbox.

Some of these measures have been endorsed by the NQF. They include falls and falls with injury, hospital-acquired pressure ulcers, health care–associated infections, nursing care hours per patient day, nursing care hours, nursing turnover, physical restraints, RN survey, and skill mix (Press Ganey, 2015). These "nurse-sensitive" indicators refer to the structure, process, and outcomes of professional nursing care. Because nursing care influences these outcomes (positively or negatively), they are called nurse sensitive.

In addition, the Internet can provide professional nurses with administrative and clinical tools to support a quality and performance improvement program regardless of the delivery setting. A health care quality glossary can also assist professional nurse managers in navigating the health care quality field. A glossary of frequently used terms is discussed in the Definitions section.

CURRENT ISSUES AND TRENDS

Health Care Safety and Health Care Enterprise Risk Management

Accreditation and Regulatory Influences on Quality

Quality and safety are crucial aspects of health care delivery. Yet how do consumers know if an organization is safe and of high quality? Health care organizations have always been required to meet standards for federal and state reimbursement regulations (Medicare and Medicaid) and state licensure rules and regulations in order to operate. These regulations have traditionally defined requirements for quality. However, the private accreditation process has probably had the most significant impact on the development of quality improvement systems in health care. It has been through organizations such as The Joint Commission (TJC, previously the Joint Commission on Accreditation of Healthcare Organizations), The American Osteopathic Association's Healthcare Facilities Accreditation Program (HFAP), CARF International, and the National Committee for Quality Assurance (NCQA) that performance standards have been promulgated and universally adopted. In each of these accreditation processes, the concept of system-wide quality improvement provides the framework for the standards. Although accreditation is not mandatory, eligibility to participate in and receive reimbursement from managed care organizations or federal and state program funding sources such as Medicare is often tied to the achievement of accreditation by one or more of the voluntary accreditation organizations.

Of all of these voluntary accreditation programs, TJC has had the greatest degree of impact on the health care industry. Founded in 1951, it led the way in establishing a set of performance standards for hospitals to follow to become accredited. Over the years, its accreditation standards and programs have evolved to reflect the many types of providers that now constitute the health care system, thus expanding its role beyond hospital accreditation. Currently, TJC sponsors accreditation programs for organizations that provide services in the areas of ambulatory care, assisted living, behavioral health, critical access hospitals, health care networks, hospitals, home care, laboratory, long-term care, and office-based surgery.

TJC has continually adjusted its performance standards for quality throughout its evolution. During the 1980s and the early 1990s, TJC promoted a "10-Step Process for Quality Assurance" that provided the framework for quality in hospitals. In 1994 TJC identified the need to enhance overall quality of care via an improvement in its own accreditation processes, and it completely revised the accreditation standards for all programs. Instead of chapters organized by department, the new approach revised and reorganized the requirements into cross-functional processes of care and services (e.g., Patients Rights, Patient Assessment, Patient Family Education) to more appropriately reflect the manner in which care is delivered. A new chapter titled "Improving Organizational Performance" was introduced that created specific standards focused on quality that were based on the principle of continuous improvement rather than on preestablished thresholds for performance of individual health care quality indicators. This change reflected the influence of the industrial quality movement on health care in the early 1990s.

With this major restructuring of TJC standards, the new era of thinking in terms of *process improvement* rather than quality assurance began not only for TJC-accredited organizations but also for other accrediting bodies. The description for this organization-wide programmatic approach, or *performance improvement* (PI), established the expectation that quality initiatives in the organization were no longer the responsibility of a single quality assurance nurse or department but instead the responsibility of the enterprise's leaders. Standards in the newly developed "Leadership" chapter established the expectation that the outcomes of performance improvement measures be elevated to review by the administrative and clinical leaders of the organization. This review of performance measurement at senior levels of the organization supplies the information that leaders require to provide oversight to the quality of care being delivered to all patients and families (customers).

The Joint Commission's PI standards delineate specific requirements for data collection in high-risk areas such as medication management, restraints, and blood transfusions. Beyond these mandatory quality indicators, the leaders of each organization are expected to set their own priorities for measurement that reflect the types of services provided to the various populations served by the organization. The PI and Leadership standards also expect that the outcomes of data analysis and the actions taken to address improvement opportunities should be communicated to staff. It is in this arena that a nurse manager can make the PI process come alive for nursing staff. Staff can relate to and understand data outcomes that are based on measurement of the everyday processes in which they work. The nurse manager needs to involve staff in identifying relevant and significant data collection measures for their unit/department that will have a direct impact on changing and continuously improving care processes. A sample data collection sheet is displayed in Fig. 18.2.

Nurse managers need to stay abreast of changes in the standards of their organization's primary accrediting and state and federal regulatory agencies to ensure that quality outcome measures for their units/departments remain current and viable. In addition to keeping up with these requirements, as previously described, many hospitals are pursuing or have plans to pursue Magnet designation of their hospital's nursing practice as awarded by the American Nurses Credentialing Center through its Magnet Recognition Program® (ANCC, 2016). To be positioned to score well on an application for the Magnet Recognition Program®, nurse leaders must take an active role in the development of robust and effective quality measures. A step further might be to participate in local, regional, and national committees that set performance standards. This can be done through professional associations such as the American Nurses Association, the National Association for Healthcare Quality, and the American Society for Professionals in Patient Safety. Certification programs are available through these professional associations.

Policies and procedures at the unit/department level must be updated and/or revised as new standards are introduced, either through participation in voluntary accreditation programs or because of regulatory requirements. Staff need to be educated about the impact and meaning of the standards that are applicable to the care they provide. Documentation requirements may change, and this may affect the outcome of clinical data measures and/or reimbursement. Nurse managers need to provide leadership in adopting and adapting to ongoing changes in these arenas. Many organizations do not have the luxury of devoting one individual or

department solely to managing accreditation or regulatory compliance processes. At best, in those organizations that have dedicated individuals or departments for this purpose, they serve as facilitators for the accreditation and licensing processes. Since 2006, TJC surveys have been conducted on an unannounced basis. This requires that managers throughout the organization be in a continual state of readiness (i.e., to have their departments and staff in compliance with all applicable standards at all times). Thus the onus of responsibility and accountability for continuous readiness has moved from a single regulatory or quality department to all leaders and managers in the organization.

Data Collection and Public Reporting of Quality Outcomes

By 1998, TJC developed a requirement for accredited organizations to participate in ORYX®, an antecedent to a core measure initiative. This program required accredited health care organizations to select six outcome measures that reflected the operations of their organizations and to choose a performance measurement vendor to aggregate and analyze the data and submit them on a quarterly basis to TJC. Similarly, since 1991, the Healthcare Effectiveness Data and Information Set (HEDIS) outcomes have been an integral part of the NCQA accreditation process for managed care plans. Of note, CARF International has required both program evaluation and quality outcomes measurement as components of its accreditation process since the 1980s, about a decade before the other accreditors.

One drawback to TJC's initial ORYX® process—and that of the quality reporting required by other accreditors—was an inability to compare performance outcomes across and among health care organizations. This was due primarily to the variability allowed in selection of measures and reporting systems. Also, as most organizations that analyzed their ORYX® data discovered, there was a limitation in identifying improvement opportunities with data that were purely outcomes based. In further refinement of its ORYX® process, TJC devised its Core Measures program. The initial measures were acute myocardial infarction (AMI), community-acquired pneumonia (PN), and heart failure (HF) and comprised 10 process measures, often referred to as the "starter set." In July 2002, accredited hospitals were required to begin collecting data on the Core Measures (with some exceptions, such as pediatric and psychiatric hospitals) and submit the data to TJC. Although participation in the ORYX® program was mandatory for each organization to be accredited, the results of Core Measures were not initially made public. The current Core Measure sets include: perinatal care, stroke, venous thromboembolism, substance use, tobacco treatment, hospital outpatient department, pneumonia measures, heart failure, acute myocardial infarction, surgical care improvement project, hospital-based inpatient psychiatric services, emergency department, children's asthma care, and immunization (TJC, 2016d). See Box 18.5 for sample Core Measures from the Hospital Compare database (CMS, 2016).

Since the 1980s, CMS has mandated that the cost and quality of services provided to its Medicare recipients be evaluated through its peer review organizations (PROs). These PROs evolved into state and regional quality improvement organizations (QIOs) that have continued their statutory mandate through the "Statement of Work" projects. The *Specification Manual for National Hospital Inpatient Quality Measures* is a guide that combines both the CMS measures and the TJC Core Measure sets "to achieve identity among common national hospital performance measures and to share a single set of common documentation" (TJC, 2016d).

CMS has historically mandated data submission programs for nonhospital health care organizations to qualify for participation in their Medicare programs. For long-term care facilities, CMS has required the submission of data through its Minimum Data Set (MDS)

program. For home health care, CMS required submission of data to the Outcome and Assessment Information Set (OASIS) that includes clinical quality, cost, and administrative measures. In both these initiatives, the results for individual health care organizations also were not originally made public. In fall 2001, the US Secretary of Health and Human Services announced the George W. Bush administration's commitment to quality health care through the publication of consumer information, along with quality improvement data, through CMS's QIOs. Their Quality Initiative program began in 2002 with the Nursing Home Quality Initiative (NHQI) and continued in 2003 with the Home Health Quality Initiative (HHQI). Its purpose was to allow consumers to make informed choices about their health care providers and encourage providers to improve their care. In 2004 the Quality Initiative was broadened to include renal dialysis or end-stage kidney disease (ESRD) and has now expanded to a Physician's Quality Reporting Initiative (PQRI).

In 2011, CMS developed the Hospital Value-Based Purchasing Program, which applied to payments beginning in fiscal year 2013 for discharges occurring on or after October 1, 2012. Under the program, CMS makes value-based incentive payments to 3500 acute care hospitals based either on how well the hospitals perform on certain quality measures or how much the hospitals' performance improves on certain quality measures from their performance during a baseline period. Reimbursement is based on quality of care, not quantity. The

---

BOX 18.5 Selected Hospital Measures Reported on the Hospital Compare Website

Survey of Patients' Experiences
- Patients who reported that their nurses "always" communicated well
- Patients who reported that they "always" received help as soon as they wanted
- Patients who reported that their pain was "always" well controlled

Timely and Effective Care
Heart Attack Care
- Average number of minutes before outpatients with chest pain or possible heart attack got an electrocardiogram (ECG)

- Heart attack patients given a procedure to open blocked blood vessels within 90 minutes of arrival

Complications
Health Care–Associated Infections
- Catheter-associated urinary tract infections (CAUTI) in intensive care units only
- Surgical site infections from colon surgery

Readmissions and Deaths
- 3-day unplanned readmissions and death by medical condition
- Heart attack
- Rate of unplanned readmission for heart attack patients

From Centers for Medicare & Medicaid Services. (2016). *Hospital Compare: Compare hospitals.* Retrieved from https://www.medicare.gov/hospitalcompare/search.html

higher a hospital's performance or improvement during the performance period for a fiscal year, the higher the hospital's value-based incentive payment for the fiscal year would be (CMS, 2015).

Initially health care providers were resistant and concerned about issues such as data integrity and the lack of risk adjustments that would ensure that the results were comparable. They were convinced that without safeguards built into state reporting systems, their organizations might look bad to the public. Data analysis systems have evolved and improved over the years to address these concerns. A majority of states have now enacted legislation requiring public reporting. With federal reporting requirements increasingly linked to reimbursement, providers must participate in data submission for public reporting or risk losing accreditation, income, and community status. As an example, organizations must be diligent in documentation of initial patient assessments, because care for patients with poor outcomes (e.g., skin breakdown) that are not recorded as being present on admission (POA), will no longer be reimbursed. Terms like "never events" represent a category of adverse outcomes that, in the view of insurers, should never happen and for which they are no longer willing to pay.

Nurses need to be cognizant of the variety of measures being collected for state, federal, and accreditation purposes that apply to their units and patients. Nurse managers and their staffs often have to participate in the data collection effort and discuss outcomes at quality improvement committees. Managers are held accountable to implement corrective action plans focused on their unit/department to address issues of noncompliance with quality indicators such as Core Measures (e.g., not documenting education about smoking cessation or offering tobacco replacement therapy for AMI patients). In the future, patients and families may inquire about the organization's publicly reported outcomes, so it is imperative that all nurses are engaged in quality initiatives and that managers are conversant with this topic.

Health Care Safety and Quality Improvement

A landmark report from the IOM launched a major national focus on the safety of health care systems and processes. In fact, the conclusion that 98,000 deaths in health care organizations were preventable was considered a call to action not only by health care providers

but also by business and government. Not surprisingly, health care safety became the focus as a key component of the accreditation process. Soon after the start of this millennium, new standards were established by TJC and other accrediting, regulatory, private, and public organizations to address the issue of safety within health care organizations.

In July 2001, new standards were introduced that required all hospitals accredited by TJC to establish and implement a formal patient safety program. Additional standards have been added over time to integrate health care safety programs in organization-wide processes. The components of a health care safety program are listed in Box 18.6. Those individuals and organizations

---

BOX 18.6   Components of a Health Care Safety Program

- Leadership commitment as evidenced through the allocation of resources for health care safety
- Assignment of individual(s) to manage the program
- Interdisciplinary (cross-organizational) participation, coordination, and communication about safety activities
- Education and involvement of patients and families in health care safety issues
- Disclosure of unanticipated outcomes of care to patients and families
- Education of staff on safety-related topics and training in team communication techniques
- Data collection and analysis in safety-related areas, including the following:
  - Incident/variance reporting
  - Medication errors, near misses
  - Infection surveillance and prevention
  - Facility/environmental surveillance
  - Staff willingness to report errors
  - Staff perceptions of and suggestions for improving safety
  - Patient and family perceptions and/or suggestions for improvement regarding safety
- Definition of terms related to safety, including sentinel events, "near misses" and what is reportable, and the development of policies and procedures to address each category of event
- Management of sentinel events
- Adherence to The Joint Commission National Patient Safety Goals
- Establishment of a risk reduction process to include Healthcare Failure Modes Effects Analysis (HFMEA)

committed to health care safety initiatives believe that a rigorous, ongoing, and proactive approach to the identification of risks will result in the prevention of errors as well as provide the framework to respond most effectively when errors do occur.

Just as a paradigm shift was required to move from a quality assurance mindset to one of performance improvement, the new paradigm for health care safety requires that organizations create a non-punitive culture for error reporting. This is application of the "process or system, not people" philosophy in its truest form. Systems that single out, blame, and punish caregivers who commit errors must be revamped. More importantly, nurse managers need to learn the principles of the non-punitive approach (i.e., they applaud and commend staff for reporting errors or "near misses"). In fact, in some industrial models, those managers or staff who detect and report errors or system failures in their areas are rewarded.

Personnel management regarding safety practices has generated the concept of a *fair and just culture* (Wise, 2014). A fair and just culture "is an approach to medical event reporting that emphasizes learning and accountability over blame and punishment" (CAPSAC, 2016, ¶1). Everyone throughout the organization is aware that medical errors are inevitable, but all errors and unintended events are reported—even when the events may not cause patient injury. This culture can make the system safer as it recognizes that competent professionals make mistakes and acknowledges that even competent professionals develop unhealthy norms (shortcuts or routine rule violations), but it has zero tolerance for reckless behavior. Health care organizations that have adopted a just culture typically have these characteristics (Wise, 2014):

- Mission and value statements are clear.
- Employees protect the organization's values by the choices they make and how they accomplish their duties.
- The organization has designed a system that catches errors before they become critical and designed recoveries to stop or reduce bad outcomes.
- The organization continuously refines its core processes from employee feedback and is always learning; employees feel safe in reporting errors or potential errors.

Health care organizations that embrace a fair and just culture identify and correct the systems or processes of care that contributed to the medical error or near miss. Managers believe that more health care professionals will report more errors and near misses when they are protected by a non-punitive culture of medical error reporting, and this will further improve patient safety through opportunities for improvement and lessons learned (CAPSAC, 2016). The American Nurses Association has endorsed just culture as a means of ensuring safe care (ANA, 2010).

The Veterans Affairs (VA) National Center for Patient Safety (NCPS) is an example of a large organization that has created health care safety programs and initiatives since the IOM reports were released. The NCPS is committed to the reduction of error and improvement of quality through proactive approaches to risk reduction (US Department of Veterans Affairs, 2015a). This is accomplished through focusing on prevention, creating non-punitive environments, and conducting safety research through such concepts as human factors analysis and studying high-reliability organizations (HROs) in other industries such as aviation and nuclear energy. The VA has created numerous educational programs through the NCPS and freely shares them with all health care providers who want to learn about health care safety tools and techniques. They have taken the lead in adopting the methodology and tools of Healthcare Failure Modes and Effects Analysis (HFMEA).

The National Quality Forum (NQF, 2004) is a consortium of public–private organizations that work collaboratively to address health care quality and safety. In 2003 the NQF published a list of 30 consensus standards to address safe practices that, if implemented, would yield improvements in the safety of health care. Examples of this initial list included establishment of a culture for safety, adoption of protocols to prevent wrong-side surgery, and implementation of effective admission assessments to identify and treat underlying conditions early in the care process. The NQF Safety Practices were updated in 2006, and a total of 34 practices were included in 2009 Safe Practices. New Safe Practices in the 2009 set were added in areas such as pediatric imaging, glycemic control, organ donation, catheter-associated urinary tract infection, and multidrug-resistant organisms. A number of previously endorsed practices were updated based on new evidence, including the pharmacist's role in medication management, pressure ulcers, and an entire chapter on health care–associated infections

(NQF, 2012). Current safety topics that the NQF has endorsed and recommend include implementation of effective handoff communication, initiation of rapid response teams, and management of methicillin-resistant *Staphylococcus aureus* (MRSA) infection.

Nurses and nurse managers can personally create an environment that is devoted to health care safety by doing the following:

- Learning the concepts and tools related to risk identification, analysis, and error reduction
- Adopting and embracing the concept of non-punitive error reporting
- Advocating for the establishment of a non-punitive culture if it is not currently a strong ideal within the organization
- Encouraging staff to be constantly vigilant in identifying potential risks in the care environment
- Creating a sense of partnership with patients and families to promote communication about safety concerns and soliciting their suggestions to correct and prevent potential risks
- Becoming a role model for staff and peers in practicing health care safety concepts

Sentinel Events

Organizational response to sentinel events is one element included in The Joint Commission standards in both the Leadership and Performance Improvement chapters. A *sentinel event* is defined by The Joint Commission as "a patient safety event (not primarily related to the natural course of the patient's illness or underlying condition) that reaches a patient and results in death, permanent harm, or severe temporary harm (critical, potentially life threatening harm lasting for a limited time with no permanent residual, but requires transfer to a higher level of care/monitoring for a prolonged period of time, transfer to a higher level of care for a life-threatening condition, or additional major surgery, procedure, or treatment to resolve the condition)" (TJC, 2016c, p. SE1).

Since 1999, TJC has required health care organizations to respond to sentinel events in a systematic and formal way (i.e., expecting that a root cause analysis [RCA] be conducted by administrative and clinical staff knowledgeable about the event). The detailed requirements for reporting and submitting RCAs are contained in the Sentinel Event policy and can be found on the TJC website (*http://www.jointcommission.org/sentinel_event_policy_and_procedures/*). Specific sentinel event outcomes are considered "reviewable" by TJC. Reviewable sentinel events are events that have resulted in an unanticipated death, permanent harm, or severe temporary harm and include:

- Suicide of any patient receiving care, treatment, and services in a staffed-around-the-clock care setting or within 72 hours of discharge, including from the hospital's emergency department (ED)
- Unanticipated death of a full-term infant
- Discharge of an infant to the wrong family
- Abduction of any patient receiving care, treatment, and services
- Any elopement (that is, unauthorized departure) of a patient from a staffed-around-the-clock care setting (including the ED), leading to death, permanent harm, or severe temporary harm to the patient
- Hemolytic transfusion reaction involving administration of blood or blood products having major blood group incompatibilities (ABO, Rh, other blood groups)
- Rape, assault (leading to death, permanent harm, or severe temporary harm), or homicide of any patient receiving care, treatment, and services while on site at the hospital
- Rape, assault (leading to death, permanent harm, or severe temporary harm), or homicide of a staff member, licensed independent practitioner, visitor, or vendor while on site at the hospital
- Invasive procedure, including surgery, on the wrong patient, at the wrong site, or that is the wrong (unintended) procedure
- Unintended retention of a foreign object in a patient after an invasive procedure, including surgery
- Severe neonatal hyperbilirubinemia (bilirubin >30 milligrams/deciliter)
- Prolonged fluoroscopy with cumulative dose >1500 rads to a single field or any delivery of radiotherapy to the wrong body region or >25% above the planned radiotherapy dose
- Fire, flame, or unanticipated smoke, heat, or flashes occurring during an episode of patient care
- Any intrapartum (related to the birth process) maternal death
- Severe maternal morbidity (not primarily related to the natural course of the patient's illness or underlying condition) when it reaches a patient and results in any of the following: permanent harm or severe temporary harm (TJC, 2016c, pp. SE2-SE3).

Time frames for concluding this analysis and guidelines for conducting a *thorough* and *credible* process are outlined in the current accreditation standards. The purpose of the RCA is to "drill down" to the most common cause(s), using flowcharting and cause-and-effect diagramming, for the event and determine what process improvements can be made to prevent the sentinel event from occurring in the future.

The action plan that results from the RCA must be robust and must be strong enough to sustain the prevention of such events from occurring in the future. The NCPS has developed an action hierarchy that outlines strong, intermediate, and weak actions (Box 18.7; US Department of Veterans Affairs, 2015b, p. 28).

The National Patient Safety Foundation has also developed a definitive guide on conducting RCAs (NPSF, 2016), which has been endorsed by TJC and other public and private patient safety organizations. The document provides teams with effective techniques to conduct comprehensive systematic reviews (RCAs) and develop sustainable actions to prevent

---

BOX 18.7 VA National Center for Patient Safety Action Hierarchy

Stronger Actions
- Architectural/physical plant changes
- New devices with usability testing before purchasing
- Engineering control, interlock, forcing functions
- Simplify the process and remove unnecessary steps
- Standardize on equipment or process or care maps
- Tangible involvement and action by leadership in support of patient safety

Intermediate Actions
- Redundancy/back-up systems
- Increase in staffing/decrease in workload
- Software enhancements/modifications
- Eliminate/reduce distractions
- Checklist/cognitive aid
- Eliminate look- and sound-alikes
- Enhanced documentation/communication

Weaker Actions
- Double checks
- Warnings and labels
- New procedure/memorandum/policy

From US Department of Veterans Affairs, VA National Center for Patient Safety, 2015b. Retrieved from http://www.patientsafety .va.gov/docs/joe/rca_tools_2_15.pdf

---

their future occurrence. See Fig. 18.8 for the *NPSF Root Cause Analysis and Action (RCA[2])* Process.

Organizations that have initiated comprehensive and robust health care safety programs are committed to the process of ongoing risk identification and prevention. These organizations encourage the staff to identify potential errors and report any "near misses" or "close calls" that occur. Even if an adverse event is not considered reviewable, such organizations conduct RCAs on these identified risks to prevent similar errors from occurring in the future.

The Joint Commission accreditation standards also require that organizations go a step beyond the RCA process in their health care risk reduction and management programs. A set of standards in the Patient Safety Systems chapter of the accreditation manual (TJC, 2016e) encourages leaders to maintain a safety system by promoting learning and motivating staff to uphold a fair and just safety culture, providing a transparent environment in which quality measures and patient harms are freely shared with staff, modeling professional behavior, removing intimidating behavior that might prevent safe behaviors, and providing the resources and training necessary to take on improvement initiatives (TJC, 2016f, p. PS-5).

One of the methods for proactive risk assessment that accredited hospitals are expected to implement is the process of Health Failure Modes and Effects Analysis (HFMEA). The expectation is that an HFMEA will be performed on at least one identified high-risk process annually. The HFMEA is conducted by an interdisciplinary team of professionals who own the process being studied and is facilitated by someone with knowledge and skills in quality improvement tools. The HFMEA begins with flowcharting the steps of the process being studied. The team assesses risk points within the process steps, and these key risk points are ranked in terms of their impact on the potential failure of the system. Scores for severity and probability are calculated to give a "hazard" score to the identified breakdown, and detectability of the failure mode is factored into the analysis of its impact on the overall process. The team then "designs out" the most critical of the potential failures and recommends process improvements for prevention of the failures. Once these prevention strategies are identified, action plans for implementing them are reported to the enterprise leaders and

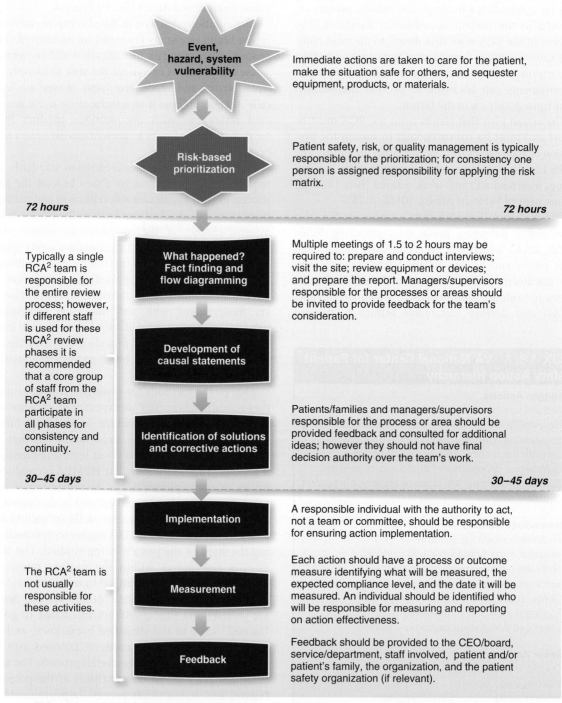

Event, hazard, system vulnerability

Immediate actions are taken to care for the patient, make the situation safe for others, and sequester equipment, products, or materials.

Risk-based prioritization

Patient safety, risk, or quality management is typically responsible for the prioritization; for consistency one person is assigned responsibility for applying the risk matrix.

72 hours   *72 hours*

Typically a single RCA² team is responsible for the entire review process; however, if different staff is used for these RCA² review phases it is recommended that a core group of staff from the RCA² team participate in all phases for consistency and continuity.

What happened? Fact finding and flow diagramming

Multiple meetings of 1.5 to 2 hours may be required to: prepare and conduct interviews; visit the site; review equipment or devices; and prepare the report. Managers/supervisors responsible for the processes or areas should be invited to provide feedback for the team's consideration.

Development of causal statements

Identification of solutions and corrective actions

Patients/families and managers/supervisors responsible for the process or area should be provided feedback and consulted for additional ideas; however they should not have final decision authority over the team's work.

30–45 days   *30–45 days*

Implementation

A responsible individual with the authority to act, not a team or committee, should be responsible for ensuring action implementation.

The RCA² team is not usually responsible for these activities.

Measurement

Each action should have a process or outcome measure identifying what will be measured, the expected compliance level, and the date it will be measured. An individual should be identified who will be responsible for measuring and reporting on action effectiveness.

Feedback

Feedback should be provided to the CEO/board, service/department, staff involved, patient and/or patient's family, the organization, and the patient safety organization (if relevant).

FIG. 18.8 NPSF Root Cause Analysis and Action (RCA²) Process. (Copyright 2015 National Patient Safety Foundation. Reprinted with permission of NPSF. All rights reserved.)

endorsed for implementation (US Department of Veterans Affairs, 2015c).

National Patient Safety Goals

Since the late 1990s, TJC has been collecting data on sentinel events and the outcomes of their RCAs for the purpose of sharing those data with health care organizations to prevent similar sentinel events from occurring. The results of the aggregation of these data are published by TJC in a series of newsletters titled *Sentinel Event Alerts*. These *Sentinel Event Alerts* address events such as preventing unintended retained foreign objects, preventing infection from the misuse of vials, safe use of health information technology, preventing falls and fall-related injuries in health care facilities, and detecting and treating suicide ideation in all settings (TJC, 2016g). The original intent of these alerts was for health care organizations to review the "lessons learned" from facilities that had experienced these sentinel events. With the emphasis on health care patient safety (including the adoption of their own set of patient safety standards), the impact of the IOM reports, and the industry-wide emphasis on error prevention as a backdrop, TJC formalized the information contained in their sentinel event database into a new accreditation requirement called the *National Patient Safety Goals* (TJC, 2016h).

In 2002, TJC's Board of Commissioners approved an initial list of six National Patient Safety Goals (NPSGs) that represented the most commonly occurring and/or serious events from its sentinel event database, combined with the recommendations of an interdisciplinary task force. Each goal had evidence-based or expert-based recommendations to define how to implement the goal successfully. The Joint Commission board re-evaluates the goals annually. New goals are added to the list if necessary, and/or existing goals may be replaced with new goals that reflect processes in which there are safety concerns (e.g., hand hygiene, goals for medication reconciliation and handoff communications, and a goal for anticoagulation therapy). Annually, the updated lists are published in the summer, with an implementation date of January 1 of the following year, providing a 6-month period in which accredited organizations must design and implement the processes necessary to become compliant with the new standards. Each organization must demonstrate compliance with all applicable NPSG recommendations during the time of their accreditation survey. These goals have become the underpinning of the survey process. Those organizations that effectively implement the NPSGs find that they are more apt to have a successful survey outcome in this era of unannounced surveys.

Nurse managers can serve as role models by fully embracing the NPSGs on their units/departments and communicating their belief that implementation of these standards leads to safer patient care. They are key to successful design and implementation of processes to address NPSGs.

The Accountability Imperative and Patient Engagement

Health care reform brings a heightened focus on accountability for health care professionals. A critical component of reform includes an emphasis on patient-centered care and patient engagement. The American Academy of Nursing has declared patient engagement and activation a health reform imperative for nursing (Pelletier & Stichler, 2013). *Patient engagement* is defined as "actions an individual must make to obtain the greatest benefit from the health care services available to them" (Center for Advancing Health, 2010, p. 2). A more recent definition describes "a set of behaviors by patients, family members, and health professionals and a set of organizational policies and procedures that foster both the inclusion of patients and family members as active members of the health care team and collaborative partnerships with providers and provider organizations" (Maurer et al., 2014, p. 10). Emphasis is on the actions of patients and families and their self-care behaviors. Engaging patients in their own care can affect inpatient safety in psychiatric inpatient settings (Pelletier, 2015; Polacek et al., 2015). Patient engagement in this context involves an active process of synthesizing health information, recommendations of health care professionals, and personal beliefs and preferences to manage one's illness.

Nurse leaders will continue to play an important role in designing care delivery systems that promote patient and family engagement (Pelletier & Stichler, 2014a). Various toolkits have been developed to assist staff nurses and managers who desire to engage patients and their families in hospitals (AHRQ, 2013c; Pelletier & Stichler, 2014b) and ambulatory and primary care (Caplan et al., 2014; Robert Wood Johnson Foundation, 2014). *Patient activation* describes the degree of engagement, including "1) believing the patient role is important, 2) having the confidence and knowledge necessary to take action, 3) actually taking action to maintain and improve one's health, and 4) staying the course even under stress" (Hibbard et al., 2004, p. 1005). Patient/consumer satisfaction is one common outcome measure of patient engagement, along with desired clinical outcomes.

Health Care Enterprise Risk Management

Enterprise risk management (ERM) "in healthcare promotes a comprehensive framework for making risk management decisions which maximize value protection and creation by managing risk and uncertainty and their connection to total value" (Carroll, 2014, p. 5). Risk management is an integral component of an organization's quality improvement and health care safety programs. An *ERM program* includes components of culture, strategy, objectives, appetite/tolerance, ERM structure and plans, communication and reporting plans, and oversight.

- **Culture:** A culture supporting ERM, including programs such as High Reliability Organizations (HROs), Crew Resource Management (CRM), TeamSTEPPS, Just Culture, and Mindfulness.
- **Strategy:** Management's game plan for strengthening enterprise performance, with an organizational strategy that is linked to vision, mission, goals, and objectives.
- **Objectives:** Ensuring that ERM objectives are SMART—specific, measureable, achievable, realistic, and timely.
- **Appetite/Tolerance:** Determining the desired level of risk the organization will take vis-à-vis its mission and threshold or qualitative range of risks taken in pursuit of the organization's strategy (tolerance).
- **ERM Structure & Plans:** Organization-wide communication and education plans that describe key roles and committee structures, employee engagement strategies, techniques to update employees on the progress of ERM initiatives, key performance and key risk indicators, and scenarios that highlight the value of ERM to the organization.
- **Oversight:** Acknowledging that the governing body is responsible for ERM oversight, leadership ensures that the governing body is regularly apprised of progress on risk strategies, status of key performance indicators (KPIs) and key risk indicators (KRIs),

emerging risks, and recommendations for new projects (Carroll, 2014, pp. 6–8).

ERM is a process whereby risks to the institution are evaluated and controlled to reduce or prevent future loss. Before the advent of comprehensive performance improvement and health care safety programs, one of the primary purposes of risk management was to prevent financial loss resulting from malpractice claims. The Joint Commission has traditionally required a risk management program for the entire organization as a part of its quality improvement efforts. Because a risk management program is structured to identify, analyze, and evaluate risks, these programs have now been incorporated as key components in organization-wide health care safety and PI programs. A risk manager is one of the "first responders" in a serious or sentinel event situation. Risk managers should facilitate the process by which the organization's definition of risk categories is established (i.e., what constitutes a "near miss," what is reportable on an incident report, what is included in the organizational definition of sentinel event). A new concept called "enterprise risk management" addresses the evaluation of all risks confronting an organization in order to maximize safety and risk reduction. The idea is to prevent undesirable events from happening and to minimize the impact of unpreventable risks. The concept of enterprise risk management dovetails with the overall requirements of a comprehensive organization-wide approach to health care safety.

Incident Reports

As tools for ongoing risk identification and reporting, *incident or occurrence reports* form the core of organizational reporting from a risk management perspective. The purpose of an incident/occurrence report is to provide a factual accounting of an incident or adverse event to ensure that all facts surrounding the incident are recorded. Key attributes of an effective incident reporting system include the following: (1) an institution must have a supportive environment for event reporting that protects the privacy of staff who report occurrences, (2) reports should be received from a broad range of personnel, (3) summaries of reported events must be disseminated in a timely fashion, and (4) a structured mechanism must be in place for reviewing reports and developing action plans (AHRQ, 2014, ¶2). A successful incident reporting process is one in which the majority of all appropriate incidents/adverse outcomes are reported by various health care professionals. However, fear of disciplinary action continues to be a reason for not reporting (AbuAlRub et al., 2015). Frequent reporting is more apt to be achieved in those organizations that have adopted a non-punitive culture for reporting errors.

The data contained in an incident/occurrence report also alert the risk manager about facts and circumstances that may contribute to a potential malpractice or lawsuit claim. Similar to quality improvement activities, the analysis of incident reports is the responsibility of the nurse managers in many organizations. The incident/occurrence reporting system provides the nurse manager with the opportunity to investigate all serious situations immediately. Data from incident reports are collated, analyzed, and used by unit nurse managers and risk managers to identify risk areas that have ongoing trends or to point to areas that have emerging risk potential. These data can inform the choices that the organization's leaders make in the selection of processes to target for HFMEA projects or to "drill down" further via an RCA to study an adverse outcome or "near miss" more fully. Aggregated data from the organization's health care ERM program are reported through the performance improvement and health care safety reporting systems to coordinate information about overall organizational risks. New performance measures defined in the action plan resulting from an RCA or HFMEA can be incorporated in a unit's/department's set of quality measures. Nurse managers can set the expectation for reporting of all risk events and "near misses" or "close calls" on their units/departments. Through diligent follow-up and the adoption of a non-punitive culture, managers can set the tone for a truly proactive and responsive ERM program.

In addition to internal reporting, many states (most via their health care licensure agencies, such as a department of health) have implemented mandatory adverse event reporting requirements, resulting in a new role for many health care risk managers. In organizations in these states, the risk manager is often accountable for the reporting of incidents that are on the mandated list. Most of these mandatory reporting programs also require the submission of formal RCAs as a follow-up to the initial report, including actions taken and assessment of the effectiveness of those actions. If the regulatory agency determines that the organization has not appropriately responded to the identified risks, it may result in further requirements for reporting and follow-up. This expanded role of the health care risk manager in external reporting creates a need for collaboration with the quality professionals in the organization. Working together as a team, the risk manager and quality manager will often share responsibilities for facilitation of RCA and HFMEA teams to meet all of the internal and external accreditation and regulatory reporting requirements.

The most frequently cited factor in medical errors is poor or inadequate communication. TeamSTEPPS, an evidence-based teamwork system, was designed for health care professionals by the US Department of Defense and the Agency for Healthcare Research and Quality to improve communication and teamwork skills among health care professionals (AHRQ, n.d.). The program provides a comprehensive suite of ready-to-use materials and a training curriculum to successfully integrate teamwork principles in all areas of a health care system (see Chapters 7 and 9).

Educating Nurses about Quality and Safety

Academia has confronted the challenge of educating nurses about quality and safety by developing formal curricula. Quality and Safety Education for Nurses (QSEN), funded by the Robert Wood Johnson Foundation, is a comprehensive resource for faculty to help new health care professionals learn the knowledge and skills necessary to lead and support quality and safety initiatives in health care organizations (QSEN Institute, 2014). QSEN has identified six core knowledge, skills, and attitude competencies related to quality and safety: "1) Patient-centered care: Recognize the patient or designee as the source of control and full partner in providing compassionate and coordinated care based on respect for patient's preferences, values and needs; 2) Teamwork and collaboration: function effectively within nursing and inter-professional teams, fostering open communication, mutual respect, and shared decision-making to achieve quality patient care; 3) Evidence-based practice: Integrate best current evidence with clinical expertise and patient/family preferences and values for delivery of optimal health care; 4) Quality improvement: Use data to monitor the outcomes of care processes and use improvement methods to design and test changes to continuously improve the quality and safety of health care systems; 5) Safety: Minimizes risk of harm to patients and providers through both system effectiveness and individual performance; and 6) Informatics: Use information and technology to communicate, manage knowledge, mitigate error, and support decision making" (QSEN Institute, 2014, ¶5).

These resources are free. Regional education sessions have provided the opportunity for the content to spread throughout nursing academia. Acknowledging the critical role that nurses play in improving the safety and quality of patient care, the AHRQ published *Patient Safety and Quality: An Evidence-Based Handbook for Nurses,* a comprehensive compendium of health care quality resources. Readers are provided with proven techniques and interventions they can use to enhance patient care outcomes (Hughes, 2008).

The Institute for Healthcare Improvement provides an "open school" for health professionals to learn about quality and safety. The IHI Open School for Health Professions is an inter-professional educational community that gives students the skills to become change agents in health care improvement (IHI, 2016b).

Advancing Quality and Safety Policy

The Nursing Alliance for Quality Care (NAQC) was established in 2010 at the George Washington University School of Nursing as a "bold partnership among the nation's leading nursing organizations, consumers, and other key stakeholders to advance the highest quality, safety and value of consumer-centered health care for all individuals, their families and their communities" (NAQC, 2016, ¶4). NAQC members include nursing professional associations and consumer groups such as ANA, AARP, American Association of Colleges of Nursing, American Academy of Nurse Practitioners, American Academy of Nursing, and Mothers Against Medical Error. The group proposes to set policy related to nursing's pivotal role in health care transformation. Since 2013, NAQC has been managed by the ANA.

Clearly, nurses have been accountable for health care quality and safety since the profession's inception. Over the years, nurses have assumed roles in various health care settings for oversight of quality and performance improvement, as well as health care risk management. The IOM reports, the CMS requirements for public data reporting, and recent health care reform legislation initiatives have raised public awareness about quality and safety outcomes in health care organizations. These quality and safety issues have challenged health care quality professionals and nurse managers for decades. A heightened public awareness, combined with increasingly stringent standards for reporting quality and safety outcomes, is driving the need for health care organizations to address these issues. Professional nurses in direct care, managerial, and executive roles need to continue to be at the forefront, leading the charge in adoption of quality and safety initiatives that continuously enhance the quality of care and services provided to patients/clients, families, and communities.

RESEARCH NOTE

Source

Zou, X.-J., & Zhang, Y.-P. (2016). Rates of nursing errors and handoffs-related errors in a medical unit following implementation of a standardized nursing handoff form. *Journal of Nursing Care Quality, 31*(1), 61–67.

Purpose

These nurse researchers conducted a prospective intervention study where rates of nursing errors were measured to determine the effectiveness of a standardized nursing handoff form (NHF).

Discussion

The authors designed a standardized NHF and trained nurses on an 80-bed medical unit in a tertiary hospital in China. Pre- and postintervention data on nursing errors were collected, and the incidence of nursing errors per 100 admissions was measured before and after implementation of the new, standardized NHF. There was a reduction in overall nursing error rates from 9.2 (95% confidence interval [CI], 8.0–10.3) to 5.7 (95% CI, 5.1–6.9) per 100 admissions ($P < .001$). Handoff-related error rates decreased in the areas of delayed (or omission of) medications/tests, pressure ulcers, inappropriate care of lines, and falls. The decrease in overall nursing and handoff-related errors indicated that the standardized NHF improved patient safety.

Application to Practice

Standardized communication tools such as the NHR are useful in providing a framework for nurses during handoff shift reports. Nurse leaders in various settings have an opportunity to develop standardized forms that highlight common high-risk handoff-related errors (medication omissions, pressure ulcers, and falls). A "Nurse Bedside Shift Report Implementation Handbook" has been developed by AHRQ (2013b).

CASE STUDY

Nurse Kathleen has been asked by senior leadership to spearhead a group to evaluate patient falls to decrease their frequency and ideally prevent them from occurring. Based on the ERM data available from incident/variance reports, she selects nurses and nurses' aides for her team from the patient care units in which patient falls are most prevalent. She adds a pharmacist and physician to the team to represent the inter-professional aspects of the fall issue. She also recruits a family member of one of the patients on an older adult unit to provide their perspective. Nurse Kathleen then applies the Plan, Do, Study, Act (PDSA) process to her project on patient falls.

In the "Plan" phase, she and the team use flowcharting to visually illustrate the steps that occur when a patient falls. Next the team brainstorms a list of all of the problems that are associated with a patient fall. From this list, Nurse Kathleen directs the team to categorize these factors in five or six groups using an affinity diagram. Once the categories are defined, the team uses a cause-and-effect (fishbone) diagram to identify all of the potential causes that lead to the eventual effect of a patient fall. From this fishbone diagram, specific factors are considered as potential root causes (e.g., no fall assessment, bed too high, patient confusion, slippery floors, poor lighting, medications that can cause dizziness, no assistance with ambulation, staffing and staffing mix, patient's lack of safety awareness, call bells not answered promptly).

Nurse Kathleen suggests collecting more data on each of these potential root causes. She further suggests that the data be stratified by patient age and gender, time of day, patient diagnoses, patient location, and staffing. She and the team design a data collection tool that will allow all of the data to be collected on one form.

After the data are collected, the team uses a Pareto chart to visually illustrate the most frequently occurring problems in descending order. By using this technique, they find that inadequate patient assessment and reassessment, call bells not answered promptly, and beds too high are the most common factors in patient falls. They also use Pareto charts to further define the stratification categories. When using this tool, they find that women older than 75 years with postoperative hip surgery seem most likely to fall on the evening shift. Most of the occurrences are on 4 South (the postsurgical unit).

During the "Do" phase, Nurse Kathleen and the team design an assessment tool for the older adult unit staff to collect data on all of the key factors identified earlier. For the trial, however, only the rooms of those female post–hip surgery patients older than 65 years are designated with a special symbol (a falling leaf) created by the team to represent a fall risk. Stickers with this symbol are also put on the call bell system lights for these rooms. Fall status is also included in the inter-shift report. Staff members are educated about the issue regarding quick call bell response and are requested to be especially vigilant in responding to the rooms with the special stickers. The data are collected for a 4-week trial period.

In the "Study" phase, the team reconvenes to evaluate the data collected in the trial. The data demonstrate a 37% reduction in patient falls from the same month in the previous year—just from addressing call bell response and none of the other factors.

Because the data on a sole factor demonstrated such a clear improvement, the team proceeds with development of a fall protocol, incorporating action plans to implement interventions for the other key factors identified earlier. The trial is expanded to another unit. When the data are analyzed for these two units and compared with the two other units with high fall occurrences, it is clear to the team that the protocol is having a positive impact on patient fall reduction. Throughout the process, nursing staff on the two trial units are solicited for feedback on the project, and their recommendations are incorporated in the protocol.

In the "Act" phase, the new fall prevention protocol is adopted. Before its official launch in the organization, physicians, pharmacists, and nursing personnel are educated on the protocol. Data are collected not only on the outcomes but also on compliance with the interventions included in the protocol. After 3 months, the data demonstrate that those units with the lowest frequency of falls were those that had adopted the new protocol with enthusiasm and commitment. Nurse Kathleen shares the data with the nursing leadership group using control charts to demonstrate the outcomes. Based on the results, and in consultation with the patient safety officer and the performance and quality improvement council, the group expands the definition of fall risk to include those patients who experienced a "near miss" (i.e., a fall in which the patient was assisted when falling and did not reach the floor). Data will now be collected on these patient occurrences and on their contributing factors. In so doing, leaders believe that overall patient safety can be further enhanced. Nurse Kathleen and her team receive an award at the hospital's annual Health Care Quality Innovations Day for contributing to significant improvements in patient safety and quality of care by reducing the number of falls in the organization.

CRITICAL THINKING EXERCISE

Nurse Manager Todd has just completed online courses on quality improvement and patient safety in health care from the Institute for Healthcare Improvement Open School. He has also served as the nursing department's quality improvement champion for 6 months, and he has been given accountability for program development. He thinks that some of the health care quality indicators that nursing is using are out of date and may not be evidence based. Furthermore, he does not see that the indicators address critical issues that the ANA (National Database of Nursing Quality Indicators), the VA, the NQF, and TJC have been emphasizing, especially in the areas of falls resulting in injury and fall prevention. He wants to ensure that the program is current, evidence based, and responsive to accreditation and other regulatory standards.

1. What should Nurse Todd do first to address this issue?
2. Describe the written materials he must prepare.
3. What sources can Nurse Todd investigate to find national standardized performance measures related to nursing?
4. How should Nurse Todd address resistance to change in this situation?
5. Describe the quality tools he could use to frame his project.
6. Describe the reports he will write about the project.

Measuring and Managing Outcomes

Sean P. Clarke, Lianne Jeffs, Abdullah S. Suhemat

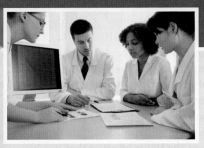

http://evolve.elsevier.com/Huber/leadership

Rising costs and demands for accountability in the health care system have led to an increased focus on measuring quality (National Quality Forum [NQF], 2015). Porter (2010) framed outcomes as a key part of *value* in health care. He defined value as the patient outcomes obtained in a health care setting divided by the costs incurred in providing the services, which places outcomes measurement and management at the heart of health care leadership. Outcomes research examines variations in the delivery and results of health care services that have particular relevance for clinicians and leaders alike. Health care leaders and researchers continue to be interested in quantifying the contribution of nurses and nursing interventions to various quality and safety outcomes and in building databases to enable benchmarked nursing-related outcomes across units, institutions, systems, regions and even countries (Jeffs et al., 2015a; Loan et al., 2011; Zrelak et al., 2012). Recent developments in the ever-evolving field of research include the emergence of Big Data, movement toward common data elements (CDEs) collected for large groups of patients, new emphasis on patient-reported outcome and experience measures (PROMs and PREMs), and the development of what is becoming known as symptom science. This chapter provides an overview of key concepts in outcomes and outcomes management, what outcomes research is and the challenges it involves, leadership and management implications, outcomes measurement and management, and current issues and trends.

Photo used with permission from Chagin/Getty Images.

DEFINITIONS

Key terms related to outcomes and their measurement and management include outcomes, indicators, CDEs, outcomes management, outcomes research, nursing outcomes research, and risk adjustment. Simply put, an **outcome** is the result or results obtained from the efforts to accomplish a goal. In proposing a three-part model of health care quality, Donabedian (1985) described outcomes as changes in the actual or potential health status of individuals, groups, or communities and contrasted outcomes with processes (what occurs in the delivery of health care) and structures (the organizational context and "raw materials" of health care delivery). Donabedian's classic framework is useful for understanding the relationship between outcomes and the structures and processes that have produced them. This suggests that nurses and nurse managers need to attend to structure and process factors as precursors to patient outcomes (Donabedian, 2005). A patient-focused definition of outcomes considers them "the results people care about most when seeking treatment, including functional improvement and the ability to live normal, productive lives" that are "inherently condition-specific and multidimensional" (International Consortium for Health Outcomes Measurement [ICHOM], 2016; Porter, 2010). In this chapter a purposefully broad definition of outcomes will be used that certainly does not exclude patient-reported experiences and endpoints that are especially meaningful to patients but might include measures that fit more closely with health care providers' and administrators' views of quality (for instance, financial outcomes/indicators).

Indicators are valid and reliable measures related to performance. They are specific markers used that make quality and quality differences visible to stakeholders in health care. Indicators can be used to measure all three of Donabedian's (1985) domains of quality: structure, process, and outcomes. Although patient outcomes are the focus of this chapter, other indicators such as structural indicators (staffing levels) or process indicators (the specific elements of care patients actually receive or do not receive) may be key to understanding and managing variations in outcomes indicators. The Agency for Healthcare Research and Quality (AHRQ, 2016) has listed a set of three broad desirable attributes of a quality indicator: (1) importance to stakeholders in the health care system; (2) scientific soundness, including clinical logic and measurement properties; and (3) feasibility of collection.

A variety of accreditation and regulatory bodies and a number of trade and professional associations—as well as health care quality assessment organizations (sometimes alliances of stakeholders)—have developed sets of standardized health care performance indicators for measuring outcomes (see Chapter 18). For example, a number of years ago the AHRQ developed a series of Patient Safety Indicators (PSIs) that include 18 preventable adverse events and complications that patients may experience in their contacts with the health care system. A recent study explored using the AHRQ's PSIs to identify nursing-specific opportunities to improve care (Zrelak et al., 2012). It is interesting to note, however, that quality measurement sets in health care have been critiqued for an excessive focus on processes rather than patient outcomes (Porter, 2010).

To assist in quantifying nursing's contribution to quality and safety, there have been long-standing efforts to develop indicator sets addressing outcomes of care that are believed to be especially nursing specific or nursing sensitive (Doran et al., 2011; Jeffs et al., 2015b; Loan et al., 2011). Widely used so-called nursing-sensitive measures include institutionally acquired pressure injuries (formerly pressure ulcers) and falls with injuries. These indicators are called nurse sensitive because there is some evidence that they reflect nursing availability, attention, and nurses' clinical judgment. The National Quality Forum (NQF) endorsed (and later re-endorsed and validated) a set of voluntary consensus standards for nursing-sensitive care that quantify the contribution of nursing to patient safety, health care outcomes, and the professional work environment. These standards have been very influential (Frith et al., 2010; Naylor, 2007; NQF, 2004). Identifying a set of measures potentially linked with nursing may help clinicians and administrators focus on areas of performance possibly tied to the organization of nursing services and processes of care. However, although no one questions the need to track these indicators, some have questioned the label "nursing sensitive" because of the status of proof that specific nursing interventions strongly predict these outcomes, as well as the strong role that patient characteristics and the efforts of other clinicians and workers play in them.

Common data elements (CDEs) are defined as variables that are operationalized and measured in identical ways in similar settings and contexts to enable comparison of data across datasets or studies in ways that would otherwise be impossible (National Institutes of Health [NIH], 2016; Redeker et al., 2015). Although CDEs are currently thought of primarily as a research tool, experts have recognized the potential for CDEs to inform standardized formats for electronic health records and eventually contribute comparison data for quality improvement initiatives.

Outcomes management, as originally described by Ellwood (1988), is a process used to assist managers and others make rational patient care–oriented decisions based on what is known about the effect of those choices on patient outcomes. To understand outcomes, the entire care process needs to be carefully examined, and variations must be analyzed. **Outcomes management** is defined as "a multidisciplinary process designed to provide quality health care, decrease fragmentation, enhance outcomes, and constrain costs. The core idea of outcomes management is the use of care process activities to improve outcomes" (Huber & Oermann, 1998, p. 4).

Outcomes management is a five-step process:
1. Data are collected about outcomes.
2. Trends are identified from data analysis.
3. Variances are investigated.
4. Potential service delivery changes are explored and selected.
5. Changes are implemented and their impacts evaluated.

In outcomes management, information about client experiences or other endpoints of care are assembled, trends are identified, departures from expectations are examined, and needed modifications are identified.

Potential changes in care delivery or the management of care are intended to improve care or reduce undesirable *variances* in care for a group of patients or a larger population. Goals of the overall process include quality improvement and risk reduction. For nurses, variations of interest may mean departures from anticipated clinical trajectories for some or all patients. Variances may be positive or negative, but identifying them is critical.

Outcomes research is a subfield of health services research that "seeks to understand the end results of particular health care practices and interventions" (AHRQ, 2000) or the extent to which services achieve the goals of health care. What makes outcomes research distinct from other bodies of research that examine endpoints in patients (i.e., much clinically oriented research) is that outcomes researchers seek to tease out the effects of patient-level care and systems-level environments from the background demographic, psychosocial, and clinical characteristics of patients as influences on endpoints. The goal is to understand which patients or clients fare well and which do not in relation to treatments selected and/or the organizational context of care delivery (Kane, 2006). Examples of variables that might be investigated as a predictor of patient outcomes might be the provider's professional background (e.g., physicians versus advanced practice nurses, registered nurses [RNs] versus licensed practical or vocational nurses [LPNs/LVNs]) or the characteristics of care settings.

A broadening of outcomes research has been **comparative effectiveness research (CER)** and patient-centered outcomes studies, which include the effects of treatment on health outcomes in different patient populations and settings of care. The goal is to produce new knowledge and reduce uncertainty about the effects on patient health outcomes of treatments, prevention, or other interventions.

> "CER is still a relatively new field of inquiry that has its origins across multiple disciplines, including health technology assessment, clinical research, epidemiology, economics, and health services research. Although the definition of CER and the body of work it represents is likely to evolve and be refined over time, a central focus that has emerged is the development of better scientific evidence on the effects of treatment on patient-centered health outcomes" (Velentgas, 2013, p. 3).

Nursing outcomes research is a subspecialty within the larger field of health outcomes research that focuses on determining the effect of different contexts and conditions that are related specifically to nurses and nursing care on the health status of patients. Nursing outcomes researchers are often interested in the structures or management strategies for nursing care delivery and the mix of health care workers best equipped to care for them or the types of patients who benefit most from certain nursing interventions. Outcomes research can help identify interventions that may be the most useful in improving clients' health status, sometimes leading to changes not only in care in the clinic or hospital but also in preparation and coaching of patients for self-management.

Ideally clinical care or the management of health services is at least partially guided by research evidence. Although outcomes research has a great deal in common with other forms of research, it involves some special elements. In particular, outcomes researchers are especially concerned about understanding "real" (clinically or practically important) differences between expected and observed outcomes and between outcomes on different units, in different institutions, or at different points in time. Outcomes research can provide key data for managerial decision making to improve quality of care. Data derived from outcomes research can be used to answer the following types of questions:

- What mix of staff types (including education levels among RNs) is most likely to achieve optimal outcomes for a clinical population with a particular level of services?
- Which technologies and blends of technology and staff achieve the best outcomes for high-risk patients?
- What are the optimal organizational structures to maintain efficiency, safety, and patient satisfaction at institutions that provide high volumes of services?

Although the answers to each of these questions depend on individual and institutional contexts and economic considerations, data from outcomes research can be used to inform decision making. For example, nurse practitioners may be interested in accomplishing outcomes for patients that improve their health yet also reduce costs. Thus they may investigate interventions such as pharmacogenetics testing and profiling to identify the best metabolized pain medication versus which ones provide an individual little benefit at a given dose.

INFLUENCES ON OUTCOMES

It is critical that consumers of outcomes data, including nurses and managers, understand how to interpret outcomes measures. Kane (2006) summarized the factors influencing outcomes and expressed this in the form of a mathematical "function" as follows:

Outcomes = f(patient clinical characteristics and risk factors, patient demographics, organizational characteristics of the setting, treatment, random chance)

Outcomes research tends to focus on aspects other than the impacts of treatment alone, especially variations across care settings. For example, variation in patient outcomes in long-term care (residents' pain level, catheter use, and pressure injuries) has been linked to nursing home managers' education and certification (Trinkoff et al., 2015). On a similar note, researchers have found that the severity of adverse events in care (in terms of lasting impacts) appears to be higher in intensive care unit (ICU) compared with non-ICU settings (Latif et al., 2013).

Nurses and nurse leaders are obviously most interested in the effects of treatment on patient and population health outcomes. For nurses, the focus is usually the care delivered by nurses and nursing personnel on outcomes, but it often encompasses the actions of the entire multidisciplinary health team. However, correctly interpreting health outcomes data across settings or providers (whether in practice or in research) and attributing differences and outcomes to the right causes or sources require attention to two major challenges. The first lies in ensuring that consistent definitions and data collection processes have been used in all cases, and accurate measures of the phenomena of interest are used. This includes the outcomes, treatment, and any other risk factors thought to influence outcomes. The second challenge, shared with all research dealing with dependent variables influenced by many factors, is that of risk adjustment (Iezzoni, 2013).

MEASUREMENT OF OUTCOMES

Jennings and colleagues (1999) presented a framework classifying outcome indicators in three categories by stakeholder perspective: patient focused, provider focused, and organization focused. Patient-focused outcomes can include such indicators as disease status, symptom experience, or pain. Other outcomes indicators incorporate a broader impact of disease and its management on clients' lives. These outcomes, often measured through surveys of patient perceptions and experiences, include quality of life, functional status, health status, and patient satisfaction. There are also provider and organizational outcomes. Provider-focused outcomes can include measures of processes and outcomes of care for individual professionals as well as health care work as experienced by workers in such phenomena as nurse burnout, turnover, job satisfaction, and occupational injuries. Organization-focused outcomes may include patient or provider outcomes that are aggregated to the organizational level, such as rates of hospital-wide inpatient or 30-day mortality, errors, and other adverse events; or they may examine aspects of performance of a system that are more of concern to managers than to clinicians or patients. For instance, cost of care indicators are commonly measured at the organizational (hospital-wide) or unit level. A number of health system level outcomes are also receiving increased attention and include measures of successful movements of patients across settings (i.e., care transitions) (Dusek et al., 2014) and readmission rates (Berkowitz et al., 2013).

ELEMENTS OF OUTCOMES RESEARCH

Indicators can highlight areas for improvement in structures and processes of nursing care and justify various investments in human and material resources needed to improve outcomes. Nurses can turn to research studies that have formally examined specific indicators for guidance to understand indicators, how they vary across settings, and the factors that most strongly influence them. Two areas to pay particular attention to in outcomes research include the choice of specific measures or variables to address quality and the role of risk adjustment.

Variable Selection

When reading outcomes research, nurses need to be aware that researchers face considerable challenges when selecting outcome measures. The specific measures used for an indicator (for instance whether staff, patients, or outside systems provide data about it) influence how managers interpret and apply study findings. For instance, outcomes can either be generic or broadly applicable to many patient groups or be condition-specific, but they must be clearly defined. An outcome that is not clearly operationalized (that is, for which there is no precise method for gathering and processing of data to measure it) is difficult to interpret, and any conclusions or decisions based on research results from those data may be flawed. Nurses also need to consider the sources of data used. For example, when evaluating a study examining the association of workload with nurse injuries, it would be important to know whether the injury data were gathered from nurse self-reports, an injury database, manager reports, insurance records, or some other source—and to be aware of the potential limitations or biases of each of these sources.

Risk Adjustment

Analyses of outcomes across groups are meaningful only if relevant individual differences in the patients examined are taken into consideration. Risk adjustment involves accounting for patient factors, such as the intrinsic risks that a patient brings to the health care encounter in the form of clinical and/or demographic factors, before drawing conclusions about the meaning of different values for indicators. Comparisons of outcomes across settings or time periods are meaningful only when potentially important differences in the characteristics of patients cared for are taken into account. Risk adjustment can be complicated, but is important because if key patient factors are not considered, differences across units, hospitals, or time periods may or may not be reflective of variations in quality of care. One caution is important. Certain types of outcomes are so dramatic and so closely tied to systems failures (e.g., transfusion errors, severe pressure injuries) that risk adjustment is unlikely to alter the interpretation of the relevant indicators. The literature contains some excellent references that discuss the state of the science in risk adjustment techniques (Iezzoni, 2013; Kane, 2006).

LEADERSHIP AND MANAGEMENT IMPLICATIONS

Health care leaders are accountable for ensuring high-quality services that achieve a variety of desired outcomes including the so-called "Triple Aim" of improving the patient experience of care, improving the health of populations, and reducing the per capita cost of health care (Institute for Healthcare Improvement [IHI], 2016).

Outcomes research can provide nurse leaders with evidence to guide decisions around resource allocation and ongoing monitoring of patient safety and quality care outcomes (NQF, 2015; Westra et al., 2015). Correctly analyzed and interpreted local outcomes data help leaders make evidence-informed decisions around creating healthier work environments and conditions for nurses to provide effective and efficient care resulting in positive outcomes and experiences for all.

Managers and executives today have a wealth of information available to them, and they are charged with determining which data indicate a need for action. A significant body of literature in nursing outcomes research continues to grow and is a valuable resource and reference point. This is seen in the large body of literature suggesting that lower staffing levels and skill mix in acute care hospitals are associated with increased risk of negative outcomes. For example, the RN4CAST study that involved nine European countries extended earlier findings and reported that an increase in a nurses' workload by one patient increased the likelihood of an inpatient dying within 30 days of admission by 7% (Aiken et al., 2014). This study also reported that every 10% increase in the proportion of RNs holding bachelor's degrees was associated with a decrease in the likelihood of an inpatient dying within 30 days of admission by 7%. Other unfavorable outcomes associated with lower nurse staffing levels include increased surgical mortality, failure to rescue, and rates of complications due to errors in care such as urinary tract infections, intravenous line infections, decubitus ulcers, and patient falls (Griffiths et al., 2016).

However, the specific context of the care environment and the patient population of interest call for continual monitoring of outcomes against internal and external benchmarks. Several data systems support the monitoring of nursing-sensitive outcomes. For example, the American Nurses Association (ANA) has developed a proprietary national database of quality indicators and measures called the National Database for Nursing Quality Indicators (NDNQI). NDNQI participants contribute unit-specific data on nursing-sensitive indicators that are then benchmarked across peer units elsewhere (Gallagher & Rowell, 2003). Beginning in 2014, NDNQI has been owned and administered by Press Ganey, a private patient experience and quality of care consultancy company. Similar databases were established for the military and veterans' health systems (MilNOD and VANOD), and a similar initiative that began in California (CalNOC) continues to recruit participants from across the United States and internationally. Also, agencies as diverse as the Centers for Medicare & Medicaid Services (CMS), The Joint Commission, and the Magnet Recognition Program® of the American Nurses Credentialing Center all now have outcome-based reporting requirements. Many believe that mandated quality reporting has greater potential to improve quality than voluntary reporting (Mukamel et al., 2015).

Nurses need to ensure that data drive patient care improvement strategies and are used as a vehicle for transforming their organizations (Jeffs et al., 2015b; Murphy et al., 2013; Reichert & Furlong, 2014). Specifically, nurse leaders need to steer how nursing data are captured and used for (1) improving nursing operations and advance nursing practice, (2) improving patient and population health outcomes, and (3) ensuring that data regarding processes and outcomes of nursing care find their way into Big Data architecture and translating Big Data into actionable information (Garcia et al., 2015). Nurse leaders have a pivotal role in ensuring that nursing perspectives and priorities are represented in collecting, understanding, interpreting, and using performance measures (Murphy et al., 2013). Nurse leaders are well positioned to develop infrastructure to ensure data are being used to inform decisions about care delivery in health care organizations and pivotal to achieving higher level quality and safety outcomes (Murphy et al., 2013). As Big Data initiatives become a greater and greater force in health care, nursing leaders need to lead development of systems for collecting, posting, and housing clinical documentation work flows, clinical decision system support tools, maps of nursing documentation and terminologies to national standards, and data queries and reports (Westra et al., 2015). Although the increasingly widespread use of electronic medical records (EMR) can be leveraged to gather outcomes data (Lin et al., 2013), nurse leaders should be aware of the limitations and inaccuracies of data from these systems and collaborate with health care informatics specialists to produce the most valid and relevant data possible (Morris et al., 2014).

Managers and executives often struggle to find a manageable number of data elements and indicators to collect and track to satisfy payers and regulators as well as meet the needs for managing quality. In terms of a guide or framework for selecting groups of outcomes for tracking purposes, balanced scorecard and dashboard approaches are gaining popularity (Jeffs et al., 2011). Metrics (specific measurement standards like operating room start time), key performance indicators (a metric with a performance indicator such as revenue by year end), and benchmarks (the gold standard or best practices such as the pulse should be between 50–80 beats per minute) are the specific elements for collecting, monitoring, and analyzing quality improvement and decision making data (Baker, 2015). Dashboards present the key indicators a nurse manager needs to monitor frequently to manage quality and costs (Jeffs et al., 2014). Scorecards and dashboards are visual display mechanisms that show critical information at a glance. They provide tools for monitoring operational performance and, coupled with internal and external best-practice benchmarks, provide a framework for targeting improvement opportunities and evoking improvement changes (Baker, 2015). For example, nurse-sensitive indicators could be arrayed on a dashboard then tracked and analyzed for continual, real-time improvements.

CURRENT ISSUES AND TRENDS

More than ever, decisions involving nursing services need to be justified in terms of their impact on organizational outcomes. Evidence-informed decision making based on reliable outcome data is of paramount importance, especially under financial constraints (Jeffs et al., 2009). Cost-containment strategies sometimes involve targeting personnel expenditures by dropping staff coverage or reducing the proportion of RNs in staff mixes without forethought to the potential consequences for patient outcomes. Outcomes research will be vital for understanding the consequences of deploying various configurations of staff in different circumstances, especially if circumstances arise where traditional models of care are no longer viable because sufficient numbers of the certain types of nursing staff are no longer available or affordable. Again, it is vital that management decision making be evidence based wherever possible in order to optimize quality of care, as called for by the Institute of Medicine.

Outcomes research can shape the policy environment and can ultimately influence constraints under which managers operate. Since 1999, when California Governor Gray Davis signed Assembly Bill 394 (AB 394) into law, requiring the California Department of Health Care Services to adopt regulations establishing minimum nurse-to-patient ratios, there has been widespread discussion of similar legislation at both the state and federal levels across the United States and elsewhere. The legislative intent behind the California initiative was to improve quality of care, patient safety, and nurse retention. Then and now, proposals to regulate nurse staffing in some way (requiring the reporting of staffing levels, submission of staffing plans, or mandating specific ratios) cite the body of evidence from outcomes research demonstrating links between low nurse staffing and poor outcomes. Evaluation of the impacts of the California experiment continues, and results in terms of net benefits to patients and the state's health care system have been decidedly mixed (Serratt, 2013a, b). Nonetheless, the continued dialogue reflects widespread interest in tracking and perhaps regulating structural elements in health care settings (like hospital nurse staffing) because of the potential impacts on safety outcomes.

Another trend is heightened interest in measuring and managing outcomes in the rapidly growing pool of aging patients in the health care system coping with multiple conditions and chronic disease. These patients account for a high proportion of health care costs and adverse events (e.g., medication errors, increased length of stay in hospital, unplanned readmissions). Poor outcomes in this group of patients are frequently associated with badly executed transfers of patients from inpatient settings to and from the community and from specialist to primary care and back (also known as care transitions) (Naylor, 2012; Naylor et al., 2011).

Innovative solutions aimed at improving integration and continuity across episodes of care include the Transitional Care Model (TCM). TCM is a delivery system innovation that is designed to increase alignment of the care system with the preferences, needs, and values of high-risk individuals and their family caregivers and achieve higher quality outcomes while reducing health care costs, notably (1) reductions in preventable hospital readmissions; (2) short-term improvements in physical health, functional status, and quality of life; (3) increased overall satisfaction with the care experience; and (4) reductions in total health care costs (Naylor, 2012).

Another continuing trend is the move toward pay-for-performance and value-based purchasing reimbursement systems that tie a preestablished portion of payment of services to achieving specific levels of measurable, targeted outcomes or attaining the highest scores on specific measures. Managers and institutions have clear incentives for altering organizational structures and practices to achieve better outcomes when particular nursing services and interventions are linked to improvements and consistency in pay-for-performance indicators (Kohlbrenner et al., 2011). However, there are continuing concerns that pay-for-performance initiatives in health care and in other sectors such as education may produce serious unintended consequences while not ultimately improving patient outcomes (Jha et al., 2012; Markovitz & Ryan, 2016; Naci & Soumerai, 2016).

As consumers, regulators, and payers increase their focus on outcomes, nurses need to proactively manage outcomes and participate in the ongoing development and implementation of indicators related to nursing care and services. Awareness of advances in outcomes measurement and familiarity with outcomes research findings are essential and will continue to be critical for effective nursing leadership.

Outcomes research findings offer insights and challenges for managers to use evidence in shaping practice environments to ensure best practices and positive patient outcomes. A wealth of research-based and research-informed measures and databases are available to managers to assist in databased decision making and outcomes management. As health care systems become more outcomes driven, nurse managers and leaders must be involved and spearhead the development of outcomes tracking and management systems where appropriate.

Big Data and Outcomes

Over the past 10 years the concept of Big Data has come to refer to the large amounts of data gathered using sensors, novel research techniques, and ever-present information technologies (IT). Big Data in health care includes information about patients, the environment, and administrative and claims data, using sources ranging from electronic health records (EHRs) to devices such as intravenous pumps or electrocardiographic monitors and from gene sequencing to patient-generated data elements (Westra et al., 2015). The integration of Big Data from EHRs and other information systems provides opportunities to predict patient outcomes and resource utilization that can be used to guide improvements in patient safety and other outcomes and control of costs (Westra et al., 2015). Further, Big Data offers a more comprehensive and synthesized understanding of health data across populations that can lead to discovering new knowledge that positively affects nurses and the people and populations they serve with improved health care (Healthcare Information and Management Systems Society [HIMSS], 2015; Westra et al., 2015).

Big Data refers to datasets that are too massive or too complex to manipulate or analyze with standard methods (Brennan & Bakken, 2015; Corwin et al., 2014). The data involved are considered "big" not only because of the size of the datasets being generated (the "volume") but also because of the other characteristics: variety, velocity, and questions of veracity, all of which are described in Table 19.1.

Nurses and nurse leaders need to participate in the development of Big Data initiatives to ensure that the databases constructed and explorations of the data that are carried out are informed by the profession's unique understanding of the patient experience and are meaningful and useful to nurses (Brennan & Bakken, 2015). Specifically, the profession and its leadership need to contribute to Big Data initiatives by (1) offering definitions and context for data elements, (2) providing expertise in

TABLE 19.1	**Big Data Characteristics**
Big Data Characteristic	**Description**
Volume	Large quantities of data accompanied by challenges in separating valuable information from "noise"
Variety	Potentially wide-ranging differences in collection and recording of information that must be overcome through standardization and normalization to allow for meaningful comparisons or application
Velocity	The speed at which data are generated and accumulate, creating large-scale challenges for timely analysis
Veracity	Wide-ranging issues around uncertainties in data that may have been collected under unanticipated or untraceable conditions

Data from Brennan, P.F., & Bakken, S. (2015). Nursing needs Big Data and Big Data needs nursing. *Journal of Nursing Scholarship, 47*(5), 477.

the use of theories to organize variables and interpret analysis results, and (3) creating interventions that assist patients in interpreting and acting on the information afforded through data science investigations (Brennan & Bakken, 2015). This is crucial to the measurement and management of outcomes.

There is growing interest in using common data elements (CDEs), measures, and data collection procedures. The National Institutes of Health (NIH) developed the Patient-Reported Outcomes Measurement Information System (PROMIS) system. PROMIS provides clinicians and researchers with access to validated, standardized, and common tools for measuring patient-reported health status, including symptoms of mental, physical, and social well-being (Corwin et al., 2014). Widespread use of CDEs and measures provides opportunities to compare results across studies and enhance the ability to disseminate and translate information into practice (Cohen et al., 2015).

Symptoms are an important focus of nursing care, and people with a broad range of acute and chronic conditions, developmental stages, and ethnic backgrounds often experience symptoms in common (e.g., anxiety, depression, fatigue, pain, sleep disturbance) (Redeker et al., 2015). Using common measures across studies could be possible to examine how symptoms (e.g., pain, fatigue, nausea) might vary in intensity, trajectory, or management across different conditions (e.g., cancer, congestive heart failure), across the life span, or between men and women (Corwin et al., 2014). Comparing and contrasting dimensions of symptoms across common conditions, between populations, and over time could enable nurses to tailor interventions to detect and manage symptoms more appropriately and improve quality of care for their patients.

Patient Experiences and Outcomes

For many reasons, outcomes measurement has emphasized health care processes and outcomes that reflect health professionals', researchers', and administrators' values and priorities. Over the past 5 years there has been an important movement by health care thought leaders toward measuring outcomes from the patient's standpoint (especially experiences in receiving health care and quality of life issues) (Porter et al., 2016). This has meant measuring variables in ways that directly consider patient preferences and choices and the potential trade-offs between various short- and long-term outcomes. Researchers and health care leaders are now being pushed to collect data about health care that can enhance decision making by health care leaders and policymakers as well as provide patients and families (and the clinicians who work with them) with data to make informed treatment choices.

The logistics of data collection have frequently played a big role in what has been measured historically, and until recently there has been relatively limited development of measures and measure sets related to patient experience and engagement (Black, 2013; Coulter et al., 2014). Patient-reported outcomes measures (PROMs) and patient-reported experience measures (PREMs) evaluate patients' health status and outcomes as well as their experiences receiving health care (Black, 2013; Coulter et al., 2014; Nilsson et al., 2016). In the 2015 CMS Quality Measure Development Plan, patient and caregiver experience was identified as one of the five quality domains along with clinical care, safety, care coordination, and population health and prevention to be targeted in quality-oriented reforms to payment structures (CMS, 2015). See Table 19.2 for examples of measures in each of the domains. It is notable that nursing databases (e.g., NDNQI and CALNOC) and nursing-oriented standard measure sets do not currently include performance measures related to patient and family engagement (Pelletier & Stichler, 2013).

Institutional leaders and the profession at large still hope to develop data repositories that can answer questions about how nursing-related structures and processes contribute to patient outcomes. The challenges remain considerable even with the remarkable progress in health care IT (Garcia et al., 2015). Variations in terminologies and data architecture persist. There are very limited widely adopted standards, and adoption of compatible systems across institutions on a wide scale is

TABLE 19.2 Centers for Medicare & Medicaid Services Quality Measure Domains

Quality Domain	Examples of Structures/Processes/Outcomes in the Domain
Clinical care	• "clinical care processes closely linked to outcomes, based on evidence and practice guidelines from professional clinical societies" [process] • "measures of patient-centered outcomes of disease conditions, including PROMs and measures of functional status" [outcomes]
Safety	• "structure[s] or process[es] . . . designed to reduce risk of harm or the occurrence of an untoward outcome in the delivery of healthcare, such as an adverse event" • "complications of procedures, treatments, or similar interventions during healthcare delivery" [outcomes] • "measures of inappropriate use [of treatments or procedures] that has the potential to harm a patient" [process]
Patient and caregiver experience	• "organizational structures or processes that foster the inclusion of persons and family members as active members of the healthcare team and collaborative partners with providers and provider organizations" • "involvement of persons and families in the care process" [process] • "knowledge, skill, and confidence to self-manage healthcare" [outcomes]
Care coordination	• "appropriate and timely sharing of information with patients, caregivers, and families" [process] • "coordination of services among health professionals" [process] • "admissions and readmissions to the hospital" [outcomes]
Population health and prevention	• "use of clinical and preventive services" [process] • "improvements in the health of the population served" [outcomes] • "process measures that focus on the primary prevention of disease or screening for early detection of disease that is unrelated to a current or prior condition"

PROMs, Patient-reported outcome measures.
Data from Centers for Medicare & Medicaid Services (CMS). (2015, December 18). *CMS Quality Measure Development Plan: Supporting the Transition to the Merit-based Incentive Payment System (MIPS) and Alternative Payment Models (APMs).* Retrieved from https://www.cms.gov/Medicare/Quality-Initiatives-Patient-Assessment-Instruments/Value-Based-Programs/MACRA-MIPS-and-APMs/Draft-CMS-Quality-Measure-Development-Plan-MDP.pdf pp. 30–34.

uncommon (HIMSS, 2015). Further, barriers to linking disparate data sources at the community level, individual patient level, and at different levels of the health care system persist (NQF, 2015). Although new types and sources of data have the potential to revolutionize the provision and management of health care, opinion leaders continue to comment on the distance still remaining before nurses achieve functional data systems that improve outcomes at the point of care (Kerfoot 2015; NQF, 2015).

RESEARCH NOTE

Source
Jeffs, L., Doran, D., Hayes, L., Mainville, C., VanDeVelde-Coke, S., Lamont, L., & Boal, A.S. (2015a). Implementation of the National Nursing Quality Report initiative in Canada: Insights from pilot participants. *Journal of Nursing Care Quality, 30*(4), E9–16.

Purpose
Around the world, data repositories containing standardized sets of quality indicators have been developed to help health care organizations benchmark their performance over time against other organizations. From 2012 to 2014, eight Canadian health care organizations participated in the pilot test of a national nursing database (National Nursing Quality Report Initiative in Canada [NNQR-C]). This study examined the perceptions and experiences of nurse leaders associated with their participation in the pilot testing of the program and their early attempts to use benchmarking in their work.

Discussion
Interviews with 18 nurse leaders participating in the NNQR-C were conducted and analyzed using a direct content analysis approach. Three themes emerged: (1) selecting, accessing, and uploading indicators; (2) using indicators and monitoring tools for improvement; and (3) perceiving involvement as a catalyst. This study revealed how participating sites overcame initial barriers associated with selecting and accessing the NNQR-C indicators to leverage the indicators to guide frontline staff and manager engagement in quality improvement (QI) efforts. At one organization the NNQR-C indicators on falls were used to develop a QI project on falls prevention that included an hourly rounding project. Based on data that had been collected, changes to staff mix were made on another unit to increase the number of RNs available to care for more complex patients after using benchmarking data. Furthermore, nurse leaders were able to align their selected NNQR-C indicators with required accreditation standards and criteria for best practice organization designation.

Application to Practice
Nurse leaders seeking to involve their organizations in indicator benchmarking by participating in data-sharing initiatives need to arrange for meaningful and accessible data and tie participation to quality improvement efforts and other organizational priorities.

CASE STUDY

Nurse Mary Pritchard works on a general medicine floor where she has noticed that more falls have been occurring recently. A few years earlier, the unit had been involved in a corporate falls prevention program, and additional resources were provided by the facility-wide nursing education and practice development department to ensure that accreditation standards were met and that mandatory reporting practices were in place. This program ended last year. Mary and her staff nurse colleagues are interested in reducing the number of falls on their unit and discussed developing a quality improvement (QI) project on the evening shift. Their unit manager suggested that they examine local data and previous falls prevention initiatives on their unit before starting a new project.

Nurse Pritchard wants to move forward on a QI project, but in addition to what has been recommended by the unit manager, several questions remain:
1. What are the implications of patients falling? (Why is it a problem?)
2. What data would Mary and her colleagues need, where would they find their information, and how would they use it in their planning?
3. What indicators and benchmarks are associated with falls?
4. What interventions are possible, and what logistical considerations are involved (e.g., cost and personnel)?
5. What is Mary and her colleagues' best first course of action?
6. What relevant outcome measures should be used to monitor ongoing QI efforts to prevent falls on the unit?

CRITICAL THINKING EXERCISE

Nancy is an advanced practice nurse with expertise in wound, ostomy, and continence care in the surgical division of Mt. St. Elsewhere Hospital. She has been asked by her clinical director and the quality improvement director for the hospital to develop a strategy to address the increase in pressure injuries (formerly known as pressure ulcers) reported on the hospital's recent quality scorecard. Data on pressure injuries are captured in what is abstracted from the patients' charts, analyzed in an aggregate format, and displayed on a dashboard. In addition to hospital reporting, the hospital's pressure injury rates are publicly reported and benchmarked with other hospitals in their state. Patients on Nancy's units had a very high number of injuries, many of which were not documented on admission, suggesting that they occurred during the patients' hospital stays. This finding is concerning from a quality of care perspective and financially because added hospital days and costs related to nosocomial pressure injuries are not billable to the Medicare program and other health insurance carriers. When determining the indicators to be measured to evaluate the impact of a targeted pressure injury intervention, Nancy needs to consider the following questions:

1. Using the AHRQ criteria, how could Nancy be sure that the indicators selected to measure the impact of the pressure injury intervention are sound measures? In answering this question consider drawing up a list of potential explanations that reflect a real decline in quality of care related to pressure injury prevention on the surgical service or related to something other than quality of care.

2. What are the structure, process, and outcomes elements associated with pressure injury incidence?

3. What would Nancy want to clarify about these data and how they were collected before getting too far into a discussion about next action steps?

4. If Nancy or her colleagues wanted to compare the division's rates of pressure ulcers with those of other units or hospitals (or even to last year's figures), what cautions should be applied? Where would they go to find benchmarks?

5. Drawing on your background and/or a search of the Internet, what investment of resources could be allocated to change this situation?

6. How would Nancy and her colleagues know if the approaches in question 5 worked? What kinds of data would you suggest they gather?

Prevention of Workplace Violence

Gregory O. Ginn, L. Jean Henry, Teresa Kathleen Sparks

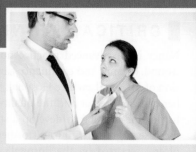

@http://evolve.elsevier.com/Huber/leadership

A study by the US Census Bureau found that although most workers felt safe at work, 7% of workers worried about being attacked at work, 4% experienced victimization, and 6% carried some type of self-protection while at work (Jenkins et al., 2012). Health care workers face significant risks for workplace violence. "From 2002 to 2013, incidents of serious workplace violence (those requiring days off for the injured worker to recuperate) were four times more common in healthcare than in private industry on average" (Occupational Safety and Health Administration [OSHA], 2015a, p. 1).

Nurses work in settings where they are exposed to both verbal and physical assaults. The Bureau of Labor Statistics (BLS) reports that 27 of the 100 fatalities in health care and social services that occurred in 2013 were due to assaults and violent acts. Although health care workers incur less than 20% of all workplace injuries, health care workers nevertheless suffer 50% of all assaults in the workplace. BLS data show that the majority of injuries that occur from assaults at work that resulted in days missed from work occurred in the health care and social services settings. Between 2011 and 2013, assaults in the health care and social services settings ranged from 70% to 74% of all workplace assaults annually (OSHA, 2015b, pp. 2–3).

Nurses are harmed by workplace violence. Some of the harm is difficult to measure in monetary terms. For example, researchers conducting a meta-analysis on verbal assaults violence (verbal abuse, which creates emotional pain and mental anguish) reported symptoms of posttraumatic stress, burnout, intentions to leave, reduced job satisfaction, and reduced organizational commitment (Nielsen & Einarsen, 2012). A systematic literature review of workplace violence against nurses found that psychological and emotional consequences and their impact on work functioning were the most frequent and important effects of workplace violence (Lanctot & Guay, 2014). In contrast, the damages from physical assaults are more amenable to measurement in financial terms. A survey of emergency room nurses who had reported physical assaults found that annual workplace violence charges for the 2.1% of nurses reporting injuries were $94,156. Of this amount, $78,924 was for treatment and $15,232 for indemnity (Speroni et al., 2014).

DEFINITIONS

Violence is narrowly defined as assault, battery, manslaughter, or homicide. Broadly, it is defined as a range of actions from verbal abuse, threats, and unwanted sexual advances to physical assault and homicide. **Workplace violence** is defined as violent acts, including physical assaults and threats of assault, directed toward persons at work or on duty (OSHA, 2015a, p. 1) and may be conceptualized as a spectrum. One end is aggressive behavior such as verbal abuse, threats, harassment, and menacing behavior that may cause psychological harm. The other end is behavior that causes harm such as battery, manslaughter, or homicide. It is important to define workplace violence as a spectrum, because people often manifest aggressive psychological behavior as a precursor to violent physical behavior

---

Photo used with permission from So-CoAddict/Getty Images.

(National Institute for Occupation Safety and Health, 2012). By using a broad definition of violence, workplace violence prevention policies can respond to the psychological precursors of violence in order to preempt physical violence.

Workplace bullying is defined as "a situation in which one or several individuals persistently, and over a period of time, perceive themselves as being on the receiving end of negative actions from superiors or coworkers, and where the target of the bullying finds it difficult to defend him- or herself against these actions" (Nielsen & Einarsen, 2012, p. 309). It is a gradually evolving process characterized by systematic and prolonged exposure to repeated negative and aggressive behavior of a primarily psychological nature, including nonbehavior and acts of social exclusion. This aggression can be from superiors, subordinates, or coworkers. Bullying mainly involves exposure to verbal hostility in one of seven categories: work-related bullying, social isolation, attacking the private sphere, verbal aggression, the spreading of rumors, physical intimidation, and attacking personal attitudes and values (Nielsen & Einarsen, 2012). It is the accumulated pattern of behavior that is the greatest threat, and it is related to the health and well-being of targeted employees.

BACKGROUND

The prevalence of violence in hospitals is partly a function of patient, client, and work setting factors. Nurses work with clients who have a history of violence, substance abuse, and criminal activity. They often work alone, either in a facility or in the home of a patient. They frequently work in facilities with features that are not conducive to the physical safety of workers in that they have poorly lit corridors or parking lots, visual obstructions, and limited means to call for assistance. Last, nurses often work in facilities that are located in areas where people carry weapons (OSHA, 2015b, p. 4).

The prevalence of violence in hospitals is also a function of organizational risk factors. Some health care organizations have weak or poorly enforced policies to prevent assaultive behavior. Nurses desire better implementation and enforcement of policies to prevent workplace violence as well as more visible and immediate support from managers (Christie, 2015). Health care organizations that have inadequate clinical staff,

insufficient security forces, high worker turnover, and allow unrestricted movement of the public are at higher risk for assaults (OSHA, 2015b, pp. 4–5). Finally, a major source of violence against nurses is bullying from other nurses, also referred to as **lateral or horizontal violence**. There is much speculation as to why this occurs. Analysis of data from nurses in hospitals found that incidents are often sparked by unprofessional behavior resulting from disagreement over responsibilities for work tasks or methods of patient care and dissatisfaction with a co-worker's performance. Incidents also result from conflicts or aggression arising from failure to follow protocol, patient assignments, limited resources, and high workload (Hamblin et al., 2015). A survey of health care workers in a public health care unit found that job strain and lack of social support were predictors of the occurrence of nonphysical aggression during the ensuing year. It further concluded that the relationship between work-related distress and workplace violence is recursive, in that stress causes violence, and violence causes more stress (Magnavita, 2014). The prevalence of bullying in nursing may be attributed to the work environment, as nursing is often high-strain work in a setting with little autonomy. In this framework, bullying can be seen as a tactic to gain power or control when one is threatened by events either downstream or upstream in the hierarchy. There are many reasons that bullying is common in nursing. The relationships among the factors are complex, but the bottom line is that bullying is prevalent in nursing (Branch et al., 2013).

From the perspective of an organization, the connection between workplace violence prevention and the attainment of broader organizational objectives such as financial performance may seem very tenuous. However, from a public health perspective or a socioecological perspective, it makes sense to approach workplace violence prevention in much the same way as other types of illnesses or injuries. The organization is uniquely situated to exert a powerful influence over the environment of the workplace and because of its position has far more ability to effectively reduce both the incidence and severity of incidents of workplace violence.

Policies to prevent workplace violence can make a difference (Foley & Rauser, 2012). Policies set the tone for an organizational climate that can be measured. A stronger workplace violence prevention climate can have

(1) a significant positive correlation with job satisfaction, (2) a significant negative correlation with employee depression, and (3) a negative correlation with stress (Aytaç & Dursun, 2012). At the organizational level, self-assessment using an accountability grid can help an organization determine whether it has a permissive or disciplined culture in response to aggression (Frederickson & McCorkle, 2013). Used to locate where accountability mechanisms fail to function properly, the accountability grid has four areas of accountability control: hierarchical, social/professional, legal/articulated, and political/community. Analyzing these pathways helps organizations understand how they do or do not permit interpersonal aggression.

On an individual level, cognitive rehearsal training can help nurses avoid bullying behavior. It can also teach nurses how to intervene in situations where they see others bullying (Stagg et al., 2013). In short, clear organizational policies, prompt responses to both verbal and physical assaults, and making safety a priority contribute positively to prevention behaviors through reduced strains and increased motivation (Chang et al., 2012).

A content analysis of reports of workplace violence concluded that evidence-based research by health care organizations that identified catalysts and situations involved in patient violence in hospitals can inform administrators about potential targets for intervention. Hospital staff can be trained to recognize these specific risk factors for patient violence and can be educated in how to best mitigate or prevent the most common forms of violent behavior (Ametz et al., 2015). Thus the issue is to convince organizations that they can (1) be effective using a socioecological approach to accomplish a public health objective such as prevention of workplace violence, and (2) attain broader organizational objectives such as acceptable operational and financial performance by successfully implementing workplace violence prevention programs.

PARAMETERS OF VIOLENCE

Sources of violence vary. One can logically conclude that in any workplace there are four sources of violence: (1) people who have no connection with the workplace but who intend to commit a crime or an act of terrorism; (2) people who have some connection with the workplace such as customers, clients, or patients; (3) people whose connection is that they are current or former employees; and (4) people whose only connection with the workplace is that they come to the workplace as a spillover of domestic violence (ASIS International and the Society for Human Resource Management [ASIS/SHRM], 2011, pp. 11–12).

Risk factors for violence in health care organizations include patient, client, and setting-related risk factors such as (1) working with people who have a history of violence, (2) transporting patients, (3) working alone with patients, (4) unsafe building and parking lot design, (5) lack of means of emergency communication, and (6) availability of items that can be used as weapons. Other risk factors are organizational, such as (1) lack of facility policies and training, (2) working when understaffed, (3) high worker turnover, (4) inadequate security personnel, (5) long waits for patients and clients in overcrowded waiting rooms, (6) unrestricted access by the public, and (7) a perception that violence is tolerated (OSHA, 2015b, pp. 3–5).

REGULATORY BACKGROUND

General Duty to Protect Workers Under the Occupational Safety and Health Administration

The Occupational Safety and Health Act of 1970 created the Occupational Safety and Health Administration (OSHA) in the US Department of Labor. This legislation declared that employers had a general duty to provide safe and healthy working conditions. OSHA followed up on the general duty requirement in 1989 with voluntary generic safety and health program management guidelines for all employers to use as a foundation for their safety and health programs. However, the guidelines were not regulations. Nevertheless, under the OSHA Act, employers face fines if an incident of workplace violence occurs. OSHA made it clear that safety and health programs could be construed to include workplace violence prevention programs. In 1998 OSHA built on the 1989 generic workplace safety and health guidelines by announcing guidelines designed to identify common risk factors. They also included policy recommendations and practical corrective methods to help prevent and mitigate the effects of workplace violence in the health care industry (OSHA, 2015b, p. 1). The Occupational Safety and Health Act of 1970 also created the National Institute for Occupation Safety and

Health (NIOSH), located within the Centers for Disease Control and Prevention (CDC) in the Department of Health and Human Services. Through this act, NIOSH was charged with drafting and recommending occupational safety and health standards (NIOSH, 2015).

Recommendations From the National Institute for Occupation Safety and Health

NIOSH recognizes that workplace violence is a particular issue in the health care industry and recommends the following violence prevention strategies for employers: environmental designs, administrative controls, and behavior modifications. Environmental designs include signaling systems, alarm systems, monitoring systems, security devices, security escorts, lighting, and architectural and furniture modifications to improve worker safety. Administrative controls include (1) adequate staffing patterns to prevent personnel from working alone and to reduce waiting times, (2) controlled access, and (3) development of systems to alert security personnel when violence is threatened. Behavior modifications provide all workers with training in recognizing and managing assaults, resolving conflicts, and maintaining hazard awareness (OSHA, 2015b, pp. 4–5). NIOSH (2013) has produced a free course on workplace violence prevention that earns three continuing education unit credits for nurses *(http://www.cdc.gov/niosh/topics/violence/training_nurses.html)*.

Recommendations From the Occupational Safety and Health Administration

OSHA suggests that all organizations have a violence prevention program. Ideally, violence prevention programs are available to all employees, track progress in reducing work-related assaults, reduce severity of injuries sustained by employees, decrease the threat to worker safety, and reflect the level and nature of threat faced by employees. The main components in a violence prevention program are (1) management commitment and worker participation, (2) worksite analysis and hazard identification, (3) hazard prevention and control, (4) safety and health training, and (5) record keeping and program evaluation. Violence prevention written plans demonstrate management commitment by disseminating a policy that violence will not be tolerated, ensuring that no reprisals are taken against employees who report or experience workplace violence, encouraging prompt reporting of all violent incidents, and establishing a plan for maintaining security in the workplace.

Worksite analysis is a common-sense but purposeful look at the workplace to find existing or potential hazards for workplace violence. Hazard prevention and control implement work practices to prevent and control identified hazards. Safety and health training makes all staff aware of security hazards and how to protect themselves through established policies, procedures, and training. Record keeping and evaluation of programs provide the data to track progress in reducing work-related assaults (OSHA, 2015b, pp. 5–27).

The Joint Commission

The Joint Commission (TJC) is an independent, not-for-profit organization that accredits and certifies nearly 21,000 health care organizations and programs in the United States. The mission of TJC is "to continuously improve health care for the public, in collaboration with other stakeholders, by evaluating health care organizations and inspiring them to excel in providing safe and effective care of the highest quality and value." Toward this end, TJC requires the reporting of incidents and causes of workplace violence in the Sentinel Event Database (TJC, 2017).

In summary, regulatory guidelines for the prevention of workplace violence derive from OSHA, NIOSH, and TJC. OSHA establishes that all managers have a general legal duty to prevent workplace violence, and it issues generic guidelines to promote safety and health. NIOSH makes recommendations for standards to protect workers from violence. TJC continuously collects data on failures of quality in many areas, including incidents of workplace violence, in the Sentinel Event Database. Thus a combination of regulation by several entities ensures that care managers are obligated to protect the safety of workers. Further, given the significant economic costs of workplace violence and the potential legal liability, managers of health care organizations also have a fiscal responsibility to prevent workplace violence.

Management of Workplace Violence

The implications for management of the threat of workplace violence vary depending somewhat on the source of violence. With regard to violence from persons with no connection to the employer, a risk management approach is appropriate. With regard to patients or their families, deescalation techniques and related employee training may be effective. Concerning violence from current or former workers, good human resource management policies and threat assessment teams are essential. In dealing with the violence from someone who has a personal relationship with an employee, employee assistance programs can be helpful.

Risk Management

Risk management is an integrated effort across all disciplines and functional areas to protect the financial assets of an organization from loss by focusing on the prevention of problems that can lead to untoward events and lawsuits. A wide variety of measures are appropriate to prevent violence from criminal activity. Among these measures are training employees in the recognition and prevention of criminal activity, posting security guards or hospital police, restricting access to the general public, adequate lighting, escort services for those coming or going from parking lots, and installing alarm systems and equipment to call for emergency assistance. All of these actions can help prevent or mitigate losses from actions by criminals with no connection to the workplace (Chang et al., 2012; Spector et al., 2015). Box 20.1 displays a checklist for risk factors for workplace violence.

Deescalation and Training

Deescalation is a long-standing mental health nursing tool. **Deescalation** is defined as "a gradual resolution of a potentially violent and/or aggressive situation through the use of verbal and physical expressions of empathy, alliance and non-confrontational limit setting that is based on respect" (Cowin et al., 2003, p. 65). Effective elements of deescalation are maintaining autonomy and dignity for the patient/person, using self-knowledge to achieve goals, being self-aware, intervening early, providing options and choice, and avoiding physical confrontations. The following tactics are used: finding a calmer personal space, avoidance of escalation, identification and reduction of possible stressors and triggers, provision of alternatives to escalation, providing a safe environment, and keeping other persons safe. Deescalation is a skill that can be taught and used with agitated patients (Richmond et al., 2012) and in conflict situations such as with lateral violence (Paccione, n.d.).

BOX 20.1 Risk Factors for Workplace Violence Checklist

- Do employees have contact with the public?
- Do they exchange money with the public?
- Do they work alone?
- Do they work late at night or during early morning hours?
- Is the workplace often understaffed?
- Is the workplace located in an area with a high crime rate?
- Do employees enter areas with a high crime rate?
- Do they have a mobile workplace (patrol vehicle, work van, etc.)?
- Do they deliver passengers or goods?
- Do employees perform jobs that might put them in conflict with others?
- Do they ever perform duties that could upset people (denying benefits, confiscating property, terminating child custody, etc.)?
- Do they deal with people known or suspected of having a history of violence?
- Do any employees or supervisors have a history of assault, verbal abuse, harassment, or other threatening behavior?
- Do you have any other risk factors not described above?

Modified from Occupational Safety and Health Administration (OSHA) US Department of Labor. (2015b). *Guidelines for preventing workplace violence for healthcare and social service workers.* OSHA publication 3148-04R 2015. Retrieved from https://www.osha.gov/Publications/osha3148.pdf

---

To promote a safety climate, all levels of the organization are expected to be involved in decision making and employee training. Training could include such topics as violence prevention policy, risk factors, procedures for documenting changes in behavior, operation of safety devices, understanding what constitutes violence, recognition of warning signs of impending violence, methods to diffuse violent situations, ways to take shelter, standard response plans, self-defense, buddy systems, policies for record keeping and reporting, and policies for obtaining medical care and counseling (OSHA, 2015b, p. 26). Essential to establishing a safety climate is developing systems for reporting and documenting incidents of assaults and acts of aggression, as well as taking prompt action when a report is made. The reporting system should include the creation of special forms to report violent incidents and the establishment of a hotline and confidential procedures for employees to encourage timely and accurate reporting of all forms of violence (OSHA, 2015b, pp. 27–30).

Human Resources Management Policies.

Human resources management (HRM) policies are essential for the prevention of violence from current or former workers in health care organizations. Policies on hiring, discipline, counseling, training, threat assessment, threat management, and reporting can prevent or mitigate loss caused by violence from co-workers. HRM is directly involved in creating a safety climate in the following ways:

- HRM develops workplace violence prevention policies and procedures to guide prevention efforts.
- HRM prepares the organization by organizing and conducting training to recognize, respond to, and report violence.
- HRM also participates in incident management and enforces workplace violence prevention programs designed to lower the risk of violence, contain the violence, and mitigate the effects of violence by providing assistance after the fact.
- HRM is the location where employees often make their complaints about threats of workplace violence (ASIS/SHRM, 2011, pp. 7–8).

HRM can also indirectly affect the safety climate in the following ways:

- HRM commitment to providing procedural fairness concerning layoffs, performance, and conflict resolution would logically lessen the likelihood of violence from current or former workers.
- HRM attention to the screening of applicants for positions could possibly be effective in deselecting those who may have a propensity for violence. For example, HRM could possibly screen applicants using public records to identify applicants with a history of involvement in domestic violence (ASIS/SHRM, 2011, p. 19).

HRM is tasked with the difficult job of collecting data on violent incidents (ASIS/SHRM, 2011). Like many other employees, nurses are often reluctant to report assaults for the obvious reasons. First, it takes time to fill out a report. Second, the ultimate use of the information in the report is unknown. Employees may have reason to fear that it can be held against them in future job searches. Third, nurses may feel that the level of violence is below the threshold that they consider reasonable for reporting. Nevertheless, incidents that seem insignificant in isolation may provide data that are meaningful to a team who is charged with promulgating a safety climate. The American Organization of Nurse Executives (AONE) partnered with the Emergency Room Nurses Association (ENA) and has a toolkit to address both violence from co-workers and violence from patients and their families (*http://www.aone.org/resources/final_toolkit.pdf*).

Threat Assessment Teams

Because perpetrators of targeted acts of violence engage in both covert and overt behaviors preceding their attacks, multidisciplinary assessment teams can be very useful in establishing a safety climate in health care organizations. A threat assessment team (TAT) with diverse representation can serve as a central convening body to make sure that independently observed warning signs are not overlooked. The Federal Bureau of Investigation (FBI) has sample questions for a TAT to ask (*https://www.fbi.gov/stats-services/publications/workplace-violence*). The TAT reviews troubling or threatening behavior of patients or workers. The TAT makes a holistic assessment of the threat itself and an evaluation of the person making the threats. The TAT assessment may also identify the most likely targets of the violence. Last, the TAT assessment will recommend an appropriate course of action such as referral to law enforcement, admonishment, counseling, termination, or whatever action might seem appropriate (Farkas & Tsukayama, 2012; FBI, 2015). Still another procedural approach for the TAT would be to circulate generalized information such as typical profiles of perpetrators of extreme workplace violence, characteristics of disgruntled employees, motivations for violent actions, and factors that contribute to the problem.

Employment Assistance Programs

Employee assistance programs (EAPs) provide a range of services to help employees cope with stressors that occur at home and at work. Family counseling might be useful in reducing domestic violence that can spill over into the workplace. Programs that counsel both the victim and the abuser could be instrumental in initiating needed interventions to defuse domestic violence situations that could affect the worksite. Furthermore, individual counseling can help employees cope with personal stressors that might contribute to unpredictable or violent behaviors. EAPs can be very useful in preventing or mitigating loss caused by domestic violence that extends to the workplace (ASIS/SHRM 2011, p. 10).

LEADERSHIP AND MANAGEMENT IMPLICATIONS

Data from The Joint Commission's Sentinel Event Database indicate that a failure of leadership was a causal factor of violence in 62% of reported events—notably policy and procedures development and implementation (TJC, 2010). Thus it is important to establish and maintain a corporate culture that is serious about protecting employees from violence. In contrast, a perception by workers that violence will be tolerated by the organization frequently correlates to the prevalence of both physical and verbal aggression. Depending on the choices that are made, organizations can create a violent or nonviolent climate. Employees often perceive the failure of management to prevent violent incidents—or the failure to respond quickly and appropriately when incidents do occur—as lack of organizational commitment and loyalty. Ensuring a nonviolent workplace may require culture change, and alterations in practice may be necessary in such areas as labor relations, injury management, and other human resource procedures. Consistent with the principles of quality improvement, leadership for such tasks as worksite analysis, threat assessment, and development of organizational policies and procedures should be provided by multidisciplinary teams composed of representatives of all aspects of the organization (Chang et al., 2012; Spector et al., 2015).

Legal Implications

Workplace bullying is legally problematic for both the employer and employee. Currently there is no federal law prohibiting workplace bullying, and few state laws address the issue. Employees seeking legal relief related to workplace bullying have filed causes of action based on the following legal theories (Bible, 2012; Mao, 2013; Sanders et al., 2012, pp. 5–11; Yamada, 2010):

- Assault
- Intentional infliction of emotional distress
- Tortious interference with a contract or business relationship
- Harassment/hostile environment

- Constructive discharge
- Statutes such as the Americans with Disabilities Act, Fair Labor Standards Act, Occupational Safety and Health Act, Employee Retirement Income Security Act, Family and Medical Leave Act, and False Claims Act, to name a few.

To date, 29 states have introduced legislation related to workplace bullying, often referred to as the Healthy Workplace Bill (HWB) or some version thereof (HWB, 2016; Mao, 2013). Basic provisions of the model HWB legislation, developed and introduced by Yamada in 2000, include a clear definition of an "abusive work environment," a legal right for those harmed by workplace bullying to seek recourse, and decreased employer liability when prevention and corrective policies and plans are implemented (Mao, 2013).

Employers should consider the following policy goals to proactively develop and implement policies and procedures that lend themselves to an organizational culture in opposition to workplace bullying (Sanders et al., 2012):

- Prevention—Employers are encouraged to develop zero tolerance policies that clearly define bullying and establish workplace bullying education and training.
- Protection—Employers should respond to employee claims of workplace bullying promptly, having processes in place to deal with any allegations efficiently and effectively.
- Enforcement—Developing an organizational culture in which workplace bullying is not tolerated requires follow through at all levels of an organization.

In general, court decisions—and the Equal Employment Opportunity Commission (EEOC)—have supported employer actions aimed at preventing acts of workplace violence despite legal claims brought forth by the affected employee, specifically related to employee claims of discrimination based upon the Americans with Disabilities Act (ADA). In *Mayo v. PCC Structurals Inc.* (2015), the plaintiff employee presented a claim of discrimination in violation of Oregon disability law. Timothy Mayo, who had been diagnosed with a major depressive disorder in 1999, was terminated from his employment with PCC after he made public statements to three different co-workers threatening to kill his supervisor and a manager. Mr. Mayo argued that job-related stress caused him to make the threatening statements and that the statements were a symptom—and a direct cause—of his disability. The US Court of Appeals for the 9th Circuit upheld the district court decision, granting summary judgment in favor of PCC Structurals Inc., recognizing that Mr. Mayo was not a "qualified individual" under the Oregon law. Mr. Mayo's disproportionate reaction to stress established that he could not perform the essential functions of his job, a requirement under both the ADA and the Oregon disability law (*Mayo v. PCC Structurals, Inc.*, 2015).

On June 22, 2015, an Occupational Safety and Health Review Commission (OSHRC) judge affirmed two OSHA citations against Integra Health Management, Inc. that were issued in response to a fatality-related safety and health inspection that was initiated after OSHA received an anonymous telephone call reporting a work-related death (*Secretary of Labor v. Integra Health Management Inc.*, OSHRC No. 13–1124, June 22, 2015). The citations alleged violation of Section 5(a)(1), the general duty clause of the OSH Act, and violation of OSHA's reporting standard. The employee, a service coordinator for Integra's home case management program, was fatally stabbed nine times by a known mentally ill client, known as a "service member," during a home visit. Although Integra argued that it did not violate the general duty clause, stating "existing procedures meet or exceed the general industry standards concerning the events that lead to the events referenced in the citations," the investigation conducted by OSHA's field office found differently (*Secretary of Labor v. Integra Health Management Inc.*, 2015, p. 10). The investigation revealed that Integra failed to adequately warn service coordinators of service member's propensity for violence based on known diagnoses and/or past criminal behavior and failed to protect its employees from this potential danger. Integra also failed to appropriately respond to a concern by the service coordinator written in the service member's progress notes, citing a need for an additional person to accompany the coordinator on home visits based on disturbing statements made by the service member. Additionally, Integra failed to develop policies to prevent violence in the workplace and failed to offer substantive training to employees despite the known risk of violence related to the service coordinator duties.

The Mayo and Integra cases illustrate the need for nurse leaders and care managers to be proactive in their commitment to prevent violence in the workplace. Developing workplace violence policies, implementing employee training, and executing timely follow-up procedures in the aftermath of threats or acts of violence in the workplace can avoid or mitigate legal action.

CURRENT ISSUES AND TRENDS

Bullying

The prevalence of nonfatal incidents of violence in the health care industry greatly exceeds the prevalence of violence in private industry (OSHA, 2015a). Much of this violence is the result of bullying and lateral or horizontal violence. The effects of both verbal and physical violence as a result of bullying have generated significant economic cost for health care organizations. In spite of the fact that most assaults in the health care industry do not result in fatalities, the economic costs—both direct and indirect—have spurred a sharper focus on the issue of bullying.

Environmental Design

Health care organizations should consider investing more funds in the environmental design of health care structures, as there is growing emphasis on evaluation of the contribution of the physical environment and institutional/organizational factors. Clearly, physical aspects of a facility could enable or contribute to the perpetration of violent incidents. OSHA presented a variety of suggestions for designing a safe work environment, including emergency signaling alarms and monitoring systems, metal detectors at entrances and security cameras in hallways, appropriate design of waiting areas for patients and families, adequate lighting and security escorts in parking lots, and design of triage and other public areas to minimize risk for assault (OSHA, 2015b, pp. 13–17). Box 20.2 displays a handy facility design checklist.

In a systems approach, organizational culture is also considered an aspect of environment. A worksite analysis conducted by a TAT or similar taskforce is among the recommendations by OSHA and is consistent with a total quality management approach. Such an effort analyzes records, trends, workplace security, physical characteristics, operating policies, and screening surveys of staff to provide an overview of the work environment. Based on the results of this assessment, direct action

BOX 20.2   Facility Design Checklist

- Are there enough exits and adequate routes of escape?
- Can exit doors be opened only from the inside to prevent unauthorized entry?
- Is the lighting adequate to see clearly in indoor areas?
- Are there employee-only work areas that are separate from public areas?
- Is access to work areas only through a reception area?
- Are reception and work areas designed to prevent unauthorized entry?
- Could someone hear a worker call for help?
- Can workers observe patients or clients in waiting areas?
- Do areas used for patient or client interviews allow co-workers to observe any problems?
- Are waiting and work areas free of objects that could be used as weapons?
- Are chairs and furniture secured to prevent their use as weapons?
- Is furniture in waiting and work areas arranged to prevent workers from becoming trapped?
- Are patient or client areas designed to maximize comfort and minimize stress?
- Is a secure place available for workers to store their personal belongings?
- Are private, locked restrooms available for staff?

Modified from Occupational Safety and Health Administration (OSHA) US Department of Labor. (2015b). *Guidelines for preventing workplace violence for healthcare and social service workers.* OSHA publication 3148-04R 2015. Retrieved from https://www.osha.gov/Publications/osha3148.pdf

BOX 20.3   Security Measures Checklist

Does the workplace have:
- Physical barriers (Plexiglas partitions, elevated counters to prevent people from jumping over them, bullet-resistant customer windows, etc.)?
- Security cameras or closed-circuit TV in high-risk areas?
- Panic buttons (portable or fixed)?
- Alarm systems?
- Metal detectors?
- X-ray machines for contraband?
- Door locks?
- Internal phone system to activate emergency assistance?
- Phones with an outside line programmed to call 911?
- Security mirrors (convex mirrors)?
- Secured entry (buzzers)?
- Personal alarm devices?

Modified from Occupational Safety and Health Administration (OSHA) US Department of Labor. (2015b). *Guidelines for preventing workplace violence for healthcare and social service workers.* OSHA publication 3148-04R 2015. Retrieved from https://www.osha.gov/Publications/osha3148.pdf

should be taken to resolve any identified areas of concern (OSHA, 2015b). In short, environmental design offers promise in addressing the threats from (1) patients or their families, and (2) individuals having no business with the organization, such as criminals in the neighborhood or terrorists. Box 20.3 presents a security measures checklist.

Terrorism

Although workplace violence against nurses is predominantly verbal assault or simple physical assault, there is some risk of fatalities due to truculent assaults carried out with weapons and explosives in an act of terrorism. Since September 11, 2001, it has been unclear whether terrorism would remain a significant theme in the literature on workplace violence prevention. On December 2, 2015, the terrorist attack on the San

Bernardino County Department of Public Health made it clear that terrorism would remain a significant theme for the foreseeable future. Although the death toll from this act was small compared with the death toll in 2001, the threat of terrorism is a significant theme in workplace violence prevention because of the amount of coordinated attention it requires across many organizational boundaries to devise plans that will prevent or mitigate workplace violence on a large regional or national scale. All nurses need to be cognizant of the high level of collaboration that the threat of terrorism demands.

Collaboration

The Department of Homeland Security (DHS) relies on public–private collaboration to carry out its mission of protecting the critical infrastructure of the United States. The Office of Infrastructure Protection (OIP) within the DHS prepares threat and vulnerability analyses of critical infrastructure, and the OIP coordinates on national and local levels with government and business organizations. The Critical Infrastructure Partnership Advisory Council (CIPAC) complements the OIP. CIPAC provides the organizational framework for the exchange of information between the government and business organizations that is essential to provide the collaboration necessary to safeguard our critical infrastructure against threats from both natural disasters and terrorism. Examples of public–private collaboration can be seen in (1) the response to the Deepwater Horizon drilling disaster, and (2) the response to Hurricane Katrina. Private contractors were engaged to do much of the containment and cleanup associated with the Deepwater Horizon drilling disaster, and Walmart used its worldwide logistics expertise to provide significant material relief after Katrina (Busch & Givens, 2012).

Violence against nurses is not only a matter of interest on the organizational level but also on the societal level. This is the case because part of the mission of the DHS is to protect health care organizations. The health care, chemical, commercial facilities, critical manufacturing, dams, and nuclear reactor sectors of the economy are designated as critical infrastructure to be protected by the DHS (Busch & Givens, 2012). Thus public–private partnerships between the DHS and health care organizations are needed to develop workplace violence prevention programs to protect nurses and other health care workers.

Active Shooter

A specific example of the collaboration called for by the DHS is found in their literature on dealing with an active shooter. Active shooter events present special challenges in a health care setting because of the large and vulnerable patient population, the presence of infections and hazardous materials, and imaging equipment such as magnetic resonance imaging machines that can produce strong magnetic forces. Although generic advice for schools and government organizations has been available since 2008, in 2014 the Healthcare and Public Health (HPH) sector of the Critical Infrastructure Protection (CIP) Partnership produced protocols for dealing with an active shooter in a health care setting (FBI, 2015). Box 20.4 has an abbreviated version of the protocols. The document is approximately 100 pages of guidelines for evacuating or protecting patients, dealing with the active shooter, dealing with the law enforcement agencies, dealing with the TAT, and more. An active shooting situation in a health care setting poses significant challenges. The event occurs infrequently, is often from an external source, can easily result in large numbers of fatalities and severe injuries, poses complex problems, and requires intense collaboration with armed responders who have

---

BOX 20.4 Active Shooter Procedures

In the event active shooters come into the facility:
A. **Run** if there is an accessible escape path, and attempt to evacuate the premises.
 - Have an escape route and plan in mind.
 - Evacuate regardless of whether others agree to follow.
 - Leave your belongings behind.
 - Help others escape, if possible.
 - Prevent individuals from entering an area where the active shooter may be.
 - Keep your hands visible.
 - Follow the instructions of any police officers.
 - Do not attempt to move wounded people.
 - Call 911 when you are safe.
B. **Hide** if evacuation is not possible.
 - Keep out of view.
 - Do not restrict your options for movement.
 - Lock the door.
 - Blockade the door.
 - Silence your cell phone.
 - Hide behind large barriers.
 If you cannot run or hide:
 - Be quiet.
 - Dial 911 to alert police and leave the line open for the dispatcher to listen if you cannot speak.
C. **Fight** as a last resort when your life is in imminent danger.
 - Disrupt and/or incapacitate the active shooter by:
   - Acting aggressively
   - Throwing items and use improvised weapons
   - Yelling
   - Committing fully to your actions

Adapted from Healthcare & Public Health Sector Coordinating Council (2017). *Active shooter planning and response in a healthcare setting* 3rd ed. Retrieved from https://www.fbi.gov/file-repository/active_shooter_planning_and_response_in_a_healthcare_setting.pdf/view

---

the weapons and training to counter an active shooter. In short, much planning and collaboration are required to deal with an active shooter in a health care organization.

CONCLUSION

Workplace violence against nurses can occur across a very broad spectrum. Regardless of whether the violence is from a terrorist attack, domestic violence spillover, patients or their families, or workplace bullying, the economic and emotional costs can be significant.

Clearly violence in the workplace has an impact that goes beyond a particular victim. It damages trust, community, and the sense of security that every employee has a right to feel while at work. Employing agencies need to show a commitment to safety for nurses, providing protection against acts of violence in all clinical areas and especially in high-risk settings. Educational institutions and employers need to share responsibility for properly preparing nurses to deal with potentially violent situations.

RESEARCH NOTE

Source
Branch, S., Ramsay, S., & Barker, M. (2013). Workplace bullying, mobbing, and general harassment: A review. *International Journal of Management Reviews, 15,* 280–299.

Purpose
This literature review concludes that a new conceptual model of bullying based on affective events theory (AET) would advance research. It concludes that bullying occurs due to the complex interaction of individual, interpersonal, group, and organizational factors. Use of this fine-grained model can serve as a useful guide for organization policies to mitigate the effects of workplace violence.

Discussion of Theory
First, the definition of bullying matters. Without a consensus about the appropriate definition of a phenomenon, it is difficult to develop any theory, and the lack of a theoretical foundation frustrates the gathering of data. Second, consensus about the application of an appropriate theoretical model such as AET to describe and explain the phenomenon of workplace bullying can provide insight into prevention and management, the processes involved such as interactions between targets and perpetrators, its escalation, and how the accumulation of bullying events can lead to increasingly negative outcomes for targets, bystanders, and organizations. Greater understanding of the affective elements of bullying may provide insight into how and why bullying occurs and thereby disclose the best paths of intervention by the organization. Examination of the way bullying escalates should provide insight into the way communication skills can be used to defuse bullying. Third, although the literature has focused on characteristics of the target, perpetrator, work group, and organization, there is room for examination of the effect of bystanders in the escalation or deescalation of bullying. Fourth, much research is needed on the efficacy of interventions. For example, organizations can conduct their own evidence-based research on the effectiveness of certain types of policies, punishments, rewards, mediations, and training.

Application to Practice
Rigorous empirical studies tell us what contributes to a safety climate and what works against it. On the one hand, clear organizational policies, prompt management responses to assaults, and making safety a priority contributed positively to prevention behaviors through reduced strain and increased motivation. On the other hand, prior experiences of being attacked were related to more strains and lower motivation, which were related to lower prevention compliance (Chang et al., 2012). Further, hierarchical linear modeling analyses show that incivility is positively associated with burnout. However, when organizations provide informational justice, nurses experience less burnout (Campana & Hammond, 2015).

CASE STUDY

Pat, RN, a nurse of 3 years, is a 7P-7A charge nurse for 6 Med-Surg, a 24-bed medical–surgical overflow unit in a large metropolitan hospital. Located on the sixth floor in the "old" hospital building, 6 Med-Surg is a busy—but often overlooked—unit in the hospital. It is accessible only through a set of elevators on one end of the circular hallway or a set of stairs on the other end, and employees often joke that once they get to work, they are trapped for 12 hours with nowhere to go. Pat arrives to work at 6:15 PM on a Saturday, and after putting a lunch box in the employee breakroom proceeds to go down the hallway to the nurses' station. Halfway down the hallway, Pat hears a loud noise and overhears a nurse saying in a loud voice, "please put down the chair, sir." In response to the nurse, Pat hears a man yell, "I NEED MY PAIN MEDICINE NOW!"

Afraid to proceed, Pat slips inside the center hallway dirty utility room, heart racing. While seeking refuge in the utility room, Pat looks out through the small window on the door and sees a shirtless man in soiled ripped jean shorts, Foley catheter bag hanging from his side pocket, holding a wooden chair overhead. The man continues to yell and is pacing back and forth in front of the nurses' station waving the wooden chair in the air. Pat

CASE STUDY—cont'd

decides to leave the utility room and walks toward the nurses' station. As Pat approaches the nurses' station, the man looks Pat in the eyes, yells an expletive, then turns and enters a patient room near the station. The day shift charge nurse sees Pat approaching the nurses' station and says, "What a mess, I sure feel sorry for you tonight!"

1. How would you feel if you were Pat?
2. At this point, what should Pat do? Is there any cause or potential cause for concern that you can identify?

3. Are there any resources Pat should seek before beginning the shift? If so, what resources?
4. What could the day shift charge nurse do differently, if anything?
5. Review the Risk Factors for Workplace Violence in Box 20.1, Facility Design Checklist in Box 20.2, and Security Measures Checklist in Box 20.3, as well as standards from The Joint Commission at *http://www.joint commission.org/assets/1/18/SEA_45.PDF*. How should the nurse manager respond to this incident?

CRITICAL THINKING EXERCISE

Terry is the nurse manager for a 30-bed, 24-hour observation unit located at Community Hospital, a large metropolitan teaching hospital. Because of its central location in the state, Community Hospital treats patients from the immediate vicinity and patients traveling from underserved areas. Positioned on the first floor of the hospital, the 24-hour observation unit can be accessed via two separate entrances: an electronic door that is located off of the main hospital hallway and a set of double doors adjoining the patient care area of the emergency department. The unit layout resembles an "H," with one main nursing station in the center. All patient rooms are private, with a curtain partition separating the room from the unit hallway. The unit follows a 12-hour shift schedule, with six registered nurses and two unlicensed assistants scheduled each shift. The unit evidence-based practice team (UEBPT) has come to Terry with concerns regarding some recent patient and family incidents on the unit and a growing concern over escalating violent acts across the nation in various health care facilities. Some of the concerns the UEBPT identified include:

- Vocalized patient dissatisfaction. Several patients have yelled at their assigned nurses when they received discharge instructions, believing they should be admitted to the hospital instead of discharged.

- Family members staying with patients in patient rooms for the duration of the 24-hour observation period. Depending on the patient's cultural heritage, often the number is as great as 10 family members.
- Emergency department patients and their family members getting lost and walking through the 24-hour observation unit.

Terry affirms the UEBPT's concerns and agrees to meet with the team at their next meeting in 5 days.

1. If you were Terry, what additional information would you want to gather before attending the UEBPT meeting?
2. What are some areas of concern related to violence in the workplace for the 24-hour observation unit at Community Hospital?
3. What resources would be helpful to the UEBPT in assessing their unit's risk for workplace violence?
4. What resources would be helpful to the UEBPT in developing a plan to manage the risk of workplace violence on the unit?
5. When the UEBPT implements unit training, what should be included and how should the training be executed?

Confronting the Nursing Shortage

Julie A. Holt

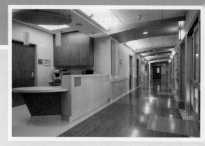

http://evolve.elsevier.com/Huber/leadership

DEFINITIONS

A nursing shortage is a condition in which the delicate balance of nurse supply and nurse demand is not at equilibrium. A **nursing shortage** is defined as a situation in which the demand for employment of nurses (how many nurses employers would *like* to employ) exceeds the available supply of nurses willing to be employed at a given salary. A nursing shortage is not just a matter of understaffing; in fact, understaffing can occur in conditions of shortage, equilibrium, or surplus, depending on local factors such as tight budgets or poor working conditions. The hallmark of a nursing shortage is the discrepancy between the supply and demand for registered nurses (RNs).

A nursing shortage can be identified by opinions of nurses, the public, or experts. Nurses or the public may believe there is a shortage based on a variety of factors. Experts generally use indicators such as employer reports, vacancy rates, turnover, recruitment difficulty, staffing levels, RN supply per population, or forecasting models to determine a nursing shortage.

Issues surrounding the nursing shortage have highlighted the important leadership and management interventions related to recruitment and retention of nursing personnel. **Civility** is authentic respect for others requiring time, presence, engagement, and intention to seek common ground. **Incivility** is low-intensity deviant behavior with ambiguous intent to harm the target, characteristically rude, discourteous, and displaying a lack of respect for others.

Missed care is defined by nine areas of routinely missed nursing care: "ambulation, turning, delayed or missed feedings, patient teaching, discharge planning, emotional support, hygiene, intake and output documentation, and surveillance" (Kalish & Xie, 2014, p. 876). This care is mainly missed due to one or more of seven reasons: too few staff, time required for the intervention, poor use of resources, "not my job" syndrome, ineffective delegation, habit, and denial (Kalish & Xie, 2014, p. 876).

Recruitment, defined as replenishment, is the process used by organizations to seek out or identify applicants for potential employment. The impact is to ensure that an adequate number of qualified workers are available for selection and employment.

Retention is the ability to continue the employment of qualified individuals, that is, nurses and/or other health care providers/associates who might otherwise leave the organization. The impact of this action is to maintain stability and enhance quality of care while reducing cost to the organization.

Selection is defined as the job of determining the most qualified candidate for a job. This process includes reviewing, sorting, ranking, and offering of candidates recruited for a job.

Staff vacancy is defined as an employee position, either full-time or part-time equivalent, that is budgeted but not filled.

Turnover is defined as the loss of an employee because of transfer, termination, or resignation. The turnover rate is derived by dividing the total number of

---

nurses who left a work unit in 1 year by the total number of nurses employed on that unit.

Transfer is the movement of an employee whose performance is satisfactory from one area to another within the same institution or corporation.

Termination is the discharge of an employee who is performing at a less-than-satisfactory level or is not a good match for the organization.

Resignation/voluntary turnover is the failure to retain an employee who is performing at or above satisfactory level. Although all turnovers have an associated cost to the organization, the most costly are those dealing with termination and resignations.

BACKGROUND

Historically, the nursing shortage has been cyclical, vacillating between a supply shortage and a demand glut as noted in the nursing timeline discussed later. However, never before has the problem reached the magnitude that is presented by the United States Registered Nurse Workforce Report Card and Shortage Forecast, published in the January 2012 issue of the *American Journal of Medical Quality* (Juraschek et al., 2012), predicted to last through 2030. Cycles of nursing shortages and surpluses have been the focus of study and discussion for many decades. Multiple factors contribute to these phenomena. Just as numerous factors contribute to the nursing shortage, multiple possible solutions are needed to resolve it. An analysis of these factors will highlight the nursing shortage as a current and future issue, and leadership and management implications will be discussed.

In 2010, the American Hospital Association (AHA) published the paper *Workforce 2015: Strategy Trumps Shortage* in an effort to formally address and explain not only the current shortage of health care workers/nurses but also to recommend best practices for engagement and retention. The AHA's corresponding *Workforce Strategy Map* (2002) is a comprehensive summary of both the causes and possible solutions for the nursing shortage (Fig. 21.1).

The nursing shortage cycles over the past few decades have been primarily driven by the following five factors:
- Aging of current nurses in the workforce and their preparation for retirement
- Lower numbers of students entering nursing as a career and a shift in need for both bachelor of science

in nursing (BSN) and master of science in nursing (MSN)/doctor of nursing practice (DNP) prepared nurses
- Aging of nursing faculty and inability of schools of nursing to meet education demands
- Aging of the American population and struggles to expand capacity to meet demand for care
- Significant changes in health care delivery system as the nation moves into health care reform

Figs. 21.2 and 21.3 show nursing supply and demand models.

The nursing shortage is now an increasing concern within the general public. Uncertainties about the Affordable Care Act (ACA) of 2010 implementation have captured newspaper headlines. An article published in *The Atlantic* represents the public's increasing concern that the United States is "running out of nurses" (Grant, 2016).

The Registered Nurse Workforce: Shortage and Surplus

The 2.9 million US RNs make up the largest health care occupation in the United States, holding about 2.8 million jobs in 2014, with about 61% of jobs in hospitals (American Nurses Association [ANA], 2014; Bureau of Health Workforce [BHW], 2014; Bureau of Labor Statistics [BLS], 2014). Despite large numbers, the supply of RNs has not been in balance with demand, nor has it been stable over time. Since the early 1900s, the US nursing shortage versus surplus has gone through phases. Although the length of each phase varies, clearly the alteration between shortage and surplus has been more frequent since the mid-1960s. Shortage phases have lasted longer, with only brief periods of surplus. Fig. 21.4 shows the cycles of nursing shortages and surpluses from 1901 to 2014. However, the game changed in 2007 with the onset of the second recession in the new millennium that lasted longer than all previous recessions since World War II and resulted in high unemployment (Buerhaus et al., 2009a). These cycles are interrelated with social and economic forces, shifts, and changes. For example, the nursing shortage from about 1915 to 1920 resulted from the inability to recruit qualified and suitable students, because students provided most of the service on hospital wards (King, 1989). A little more than a decade later, in the context of the Great Depression (1929 to 1932), a surplus prevailed (Carlson et al., 1992). The 20 years after World War II

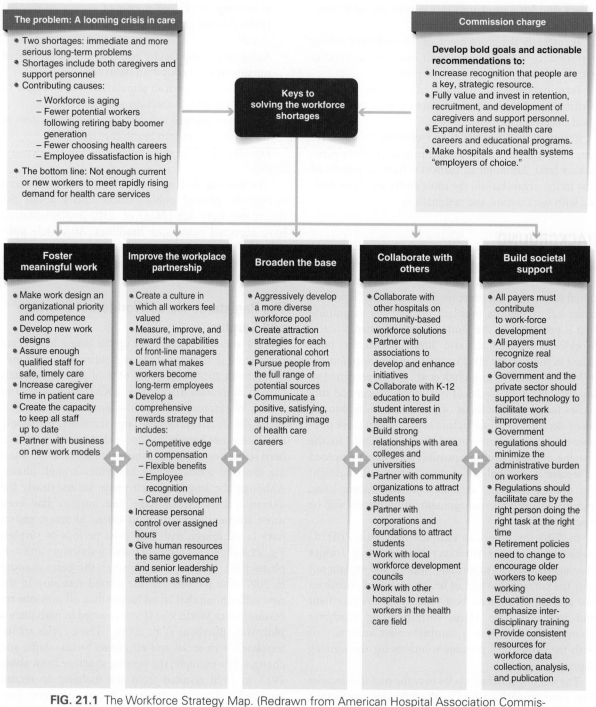

The problem: A looming crisis in care

- Two shortages: immediate and more serious long-term problems
- Shortages include both caregivers and support personnel
- Contributing causes:
  - Workforce is aging
  - Fewer potential workers following retiring baby boomer generation
  - Fewer choosing health careers
  - Employee dissatisfaction is high
- The bottom line: Not enough current or new workers to meet rapidly rising demand for health care services

Keys to solving the workforce shortages

Commission charge

Develop bold goals and actionable recommendations to:

- Increase recognition that people are a key, strategic resource.
- Fully value and invest in retention, recruitment, and development of caregivers and support personnel.
- Expand interest in health care careers and educational programs.
- Make hospitals and health systems "employers of choice."

Foster meaningful work

- Make work design an organizational priority and competence
- Develop new work designs
- Assure enough qualified staff for safe, timely care
- Increase caregiver time in patient care
- Create the capacity to keep all staff up to date
- Partner with business on new work models

Improve the workplace partnership

- Create a culture in which all workers feel valued
- Measure, improve, and reward the capabilities of front-line managers
- Learn what makes workers become long-term employees
- Develop a comprehensive rewards strategy that includes:
  - Competitive edge in compensation
  - Flexible benefits
  - Employee recognition
  - Career development
- Increase personal control over assigned hours
- Give human resources the same governance and senior leadership attention as finance

Broaden the base

- Aggressively develop a more diverse workforce pool
- Create attraction strategies for each generational cohort
- Pursue people from the full range of potential sources
- Communicate a positive, satisfying, and inspiring image of health care careers

Collaborate with others

- Collaborate with other hospitals on community-based workforce solutions
- Partner with associations to develop and enhance initiatives
- Collaborate with K-12 education to build student interest in health careers
- Build strong relationships with area colleges and universities
- Partner with community organizations to attract students
- Partner with corporations and foundations to attract students
- Work with local workforce development councils
- Work with other hospitals to retain workers in the health care field

Build societal support

- All payers must contribute to work-force development
- All payers must recognize real labor costs
- Government and the private sector should support technology to facilitate work improvement
- Government regulations should minimize the administrative burden on workers
- Regulations should facilitate care by the right person doing the right task at the right time
- Retirement policies need to change to encourage older workers to keep working
- Education needs to emphasize inter-disciplinary training
- Provide consistent resources for workforce data collection, analysis, and publication

FIG. 21.1 The Workforce Strategy Map. (Redrawn from American Hospital Association Commission on Workforce for Hospitals and Health Systems. [2002]. *The workforce strategy map in our hands: How hospital leaders can build a thriving workforce.* Retrieved from http://www.aha.org/content/00-10/loh11Map.pdf)

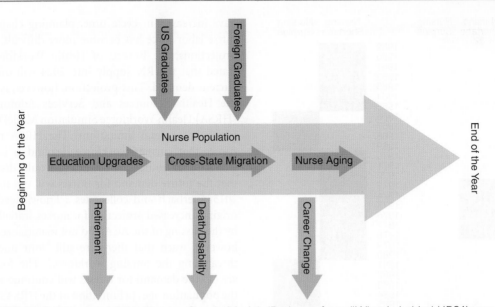

FIG. 21.2 Overview of the Nursing Supply Model. (Redrawn from "What is behind HRSA's projected supply, demand, and shortage of registered nurses?" [2004]. Retrieved from http://www .ohiocenterfornursing.org/PDFS/nursingworkforce/HRSAbehindshortage.pdf)

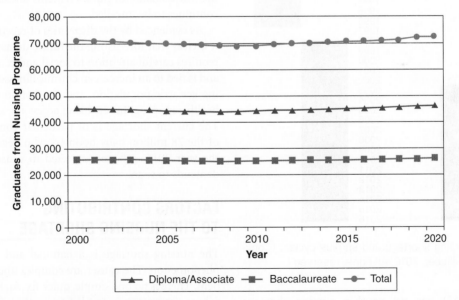

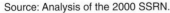
Source: Analysis of the 2000 SSRN.

FIG. 21.3 National baseline projections of annual nursing school graduates. (Redrawn from "What is behind HRSA's projected supply, demand, and shortage of registered nurses?" [2004]. Retrieved from http://www.ohiocenterfornursing.org/PDFS/nursingworkforce/HRSAbehindshortage.pdf)

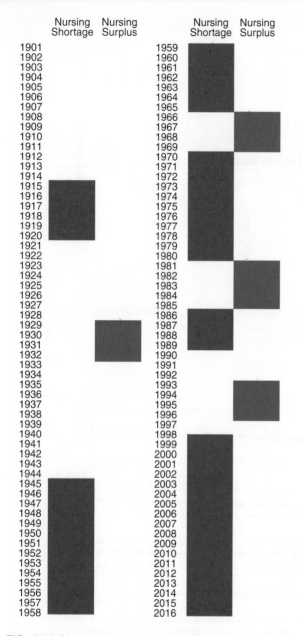

	Nursing Shortage	Nursing Surplus		Nursing Shortage	Nursing Surplus
1901			1959		
1902			1960		
1903			1961		
1904			1962		
1905			1963		
1906			1964		
1907			1965		
1908			1966		
1909			1967		
1910			1968		
1911			1969		
1912			1970		
1913			1971		
1914			1972		
1915			1973		
1916			1974		
1917			1975		
1918			1976		
1919			1977		
1920			1978		
1921			1979		
1922			1980		
1923			1981		
1924			1982		
1925			1983		
1926			1984		
1927			1985		
1928			1986		
1929			1987		
1930			1988		
1931			1989		
1932			1990		
1933			1991		
1934			1992		
1935			1993		
1936			1994		
1937			1995		
1938			1996		
1939			1997		
1940			1998		
1941			1999		
1942			2000		
1943			2001		
1944			2002		
1945			2003		
1946			2004		
1947			2005		
1948			2006		
1949			2007		
1950			2008		
1951			2009		
1952			2010		
1953			2011		
1954			2012		
1955			2013		
1956			2014		
1957			2015		
1958			2016		

FIG. 21.4 Nursing shortage and surplus cycles. (Copyright Diane L. Huber, 2016. All rights reserved.)

have increased in cycle time, planning change in the nurse labor force has become more difficult. In recent projections, the Bureau of Health Workforce (2014) stated that the RN supply into 2024 will outpace the current demand. This projection, however, is based on the Health Resources and Services Administration's (HRSA) Health Workforce Simulation Model (HWSM), which has several limitations. The HRSA model assumes that current workforce demand is in balance, which other sources (BLS, 2014) would dispute, and that the future demand for nurses will not increase. In 2013 Auerbach and colleagues acknowledged that the original increased projection for nurses, initially spurred by the passing of the ACA, did not materialize. They do, however, warn that there are still "four uncertainties threatening the nursing workforce." The four threats are (1) the demand for nurses will continue to grow as the population ages (a limitation of the HRSA's HWSM); (2) that the populations in need of nursing care and the population of nurses may not be matched, resulting in substantial community-level nurse shortages; (3) that the national recession continues to linger, causing the current labor market to swell artificially; and (4) that the true demand for nurses remains unclear as the ACA continues to be unveiled.

As evidenced by the disparities of recent projections, it is clear that forecasting the future demand for nurses requires careful attention to social and economic forces and is tied to an increase in chronic illnesses, an expanding geriatric population, and promotion of a national health care program ensuring access for all Americans. The current shortage is of particular concern because of the 78 million baby boomers who began retiring in the year 2015, a factor expected to cause health care demands to soar.

FACTORS CONTRIBUTING TO THE NURSING SHORTAGE

The nursing shortage is a national and international phenomenon. The causes are complex and interdependent. There is no one simple, quick fix. An informed and robust perspective is needed to understand which options to pursue to alleviate a shortage. For an analysis of the causes of the nursing shortage, it is best to examine and understand the factors that contribute: those affecting nursing supply and those influencing demand for nursing services into the future.

(1945 to 1965) saw yet another nursing shortage (Grando, 1998). Box 21.1 displays a timeline of nursing shortage cycles since 1964.

Clearly, the cycling through shortages and surpluses increased in frequency in the last quarter of the twentieth century. No doubt, as the shortage/surplus cycles

BOX 21.1   Nursing Shortage Time Line of Events and Predictions

1964 – Nurse Training Act financial aid program increases nursing enrollment and lowers job vacancy rates for next 6 years

1970 – Job vacancy rate steadily climbs through 1980, sparking the next shortage (Carlson et al., 1992)

1981 – Recession converts the vacancy rate to a surplus

1985 – Implementation of diagnosis-related groups (DRGs) passes and more patients are housed in hospitals, prompting the next decline

1986 –Through 1992, hospital RN vacancy rate at national level of 11% (Buerhaus et al., 2005)

1992 – Managed care, capped reimbursements, cost containment, and downsizing hit the hospital industry again, boosting a nursing surplus

1998 – Cycle again shows evidence of reversal into shortage and marks the beginning of the shortage lasting into 2008

2000 – Average age of registered nurses is 45.2 years, with only 9% younger than 30 years

2001 – Recession: hospital RN vacancy rate at a national average of 13%, ranging up to 20%

2001 – 126,000 full-time equivalent (FTE) RN positions unfilled (Bureau of Health Professions [BHPr], 2006)

2001 – American Nurses Association/American Organization of Nurse Executives (ANA/AONE) hold Nursing Professional Summit to analyze shortage and develop strategic plan for future

2001 – Institute of Medicine (IOM) releases Crossing the Quality Chasm: A New Health System for the 21st Century

2002 – The number of new licenses in nursing is projected to be 17% lower in 2020 than in 2002 (BHPr, 2002)

2002 – ANA releases *Nursing's Agenda for the Future: A Call to the Nation* report addressing shortage through education and workforce policy

2003 – Nursing shortage predictions continue

2004 – Average age of registered nurses is 46.8 years, and now only 8% report being under age 30; BHPr predicted that by the year 2015 all 48 contiguous states will experience a nursing shortage

2005 – The average age of nurse educators is 55 years (Davidhizar, 2005)

2006 – In April the BHPr's Health Resources and Services Administration (HRSA) releases projections of shortfall of more than 1 million nurses by 2020 (BHPr, 2006)

2006 – International Council of Nurses (ICN, 2007) report indicates that an aging population is a worldwide issue through first quarter of the twenty-first century, projecting more than 1 billion people over age 60 years; Japan, Italy, Greece, and Switzerland are at highest risk with 31% older than 60 years

2007 – Great recession hits and lasts into 2012. According to the US government (BHPr, 2006; BLS, 2007) more than 1 million nurses will be needed by 2016. Projected shortage growth:
- 405,800 in 2010
- 683,700 in 2015
- 1,016,900 in 2020

2007 – The American Association of Colleges of Nursing (AACN, 2008) reports a national nurse faculty vacancy rate of 8.8%, which equates to approximately 2.2 faculty vacancies per school.

2007 – 71.4% of US nursing schools turning away 40,285 qualified applicants to baccalaureate and graduate nursing programs because of faculty shortages

2008 – Recession results in unprecedented rise in hospital employment of nurses, with estimates at 243,000 FTEs and more than 100,000 RNs older than age 50 years (Staiger et al., 2012), with average age of 46 years

2009 – Buerhaus and colleagues (2008, 2009a) revise and reduce their prediction of shortage for 2020 from 1 million to 800,000

2009 – Since 2002, RN FTEs increase 62% for nurses ages 23 to 26 years to approximately 165,000 (Auerbach et al., 2011)

2010 – 12.7% of US population currently age 65 years or older

2010 – Enactment of the Patient Protection and Affordable Care Act to transform health care delivery

2011 – Enrollments in entry-level baccalaureate programs in nursing increase by 5.1% (American Association of Colleges of Nursing, 2011)

2011 – Institute of Medicine (IOM) releases *The Future of Nursing: Leading Change, Advancing Health,* calling for increased numbers of advanced-degree educated nurses to promote patient safety and quality of care (IOM, 2011)

2012 – American Association of Colleges of Nursing's 2011–2012 survey (AACN, 2011-2012) reports that 75,587 qualified applicants from baccalaureate and graduate nursing are turned away because of insufficient number of faculty, clinical sites, classroom space, and clinical preceptors and budget constraints

2012 – Current nursing workforce average age is now 44.2 years (Auerbach et al., 2011)

2012 – Nursing workforce now projected to grow at roughly the same rate as the population through 2030 (Auerbach et al., 2011)

2012 – Bureau of Labor Statistics (BLS) identifies registered nursing as one of the leading occupations in terms of job growth through 2020 (American Association of Colleges of Nursing, 2012a, b)

Continued

BOX 21.1   Nursing Shortage Time Line of Events and Predictions—cont'd

2013 – Nursing workforce growth outpaces the growth of the US population. A strong growth of new nurses in the field increased the number of RNs younger than 30. Despite this new influx of young nurses, one-third of the workforce remains older than 50 (BHPr, 2013)

2013 – The nursing workforce has grown by more than 24.1% in the 2000s. The nursing pipeline growth continues, with "the number of bachelor's prepared RN candidates taking the NCLEX-RN examination for the first time more than doubled from 24,832 individuals in 2001 to 58,246 in 2011" (BHPr, 2013)

2014 – Bureau of Labor Statistics (BLS) reports that the demand for nurses will continue to grow by 16% between 2014 and 2024, much faster than the average job growth (7%) (BLS, 2014)

2014 – The Bureau of Health Workforce (2014) reports that the national RN supply between 2012 and 2025 will outpace demand. There will be substantial variation of supply and demand at the individual state levels

2017 – AACN notes that the nurse shortage is predicted to spread across the nation between 2009 and 2030 and intensify. The Bureau of Health Workforce's 2014 report is the most recent government data available

---

Supply

Factors that affect nursing supply include:

- *Nursing education:* Those affecting the number of new nursing graduates
- *Demographics:* Those affecting the nature of the current RN workforce, thus the number of practitioners who can continue to work
- *Work environment:* Those influencing the ability of the workplace to recruit and retain nurses

Nursing Education

The ability of the educational system to produce new graduates is affected by many factors, including limited enrollment, a shift from associate degree– to baccalaureate-prepared RNs, and a shortage of nursing school faculty. These issues are compounded by an insufficient number of clinical sites, classroom space, and clinical preceptors, as well as budget constraints (American Association of Colleges of Nursing [AACN], 2012–2013). Adding complexity, the average age of nurse faculty (72% age 50+ years; ANA, 2014) suggests a probable large surge of retirements in the near future. The American Association of Colleges of Nursing's (AACN, 2013–2014) report *2013-2014 Salaries of Instructional and Administrative Nursing Faculty in Baccalaureate and Graduate Programs in Nursing* shows the following average ages of doctorally prepared and master's-prepared nurse faculty:

- Professors: 61.6 years (PhD); 57.1 years (master's)
- Associate professors: 57.6 years (PhD); 56.8 (master's)
- Assistant professors: 51.4 years (PhD); 51.2 years (master's)

Although overall nursing school enrollments continue to grow, there continues to be speculation about whether this growth will satisfy current and future demands. Even though the AACN (2014) reported a significantly higher percentage of increase (2.6%) in enrollments for entry-level baccalaureate nursing programs in 2013, the increase is not sufficient considering the implementation of the ACA and the increase of more than 32 million Americans accessing heath care services.

Clearly there is strong interest among new nursing students and across the RN workforce in advancing education. The question now becomes what is the ability of higher learning institutions to handle the high number of applicants? Over the past decade this issue has been of extreme concern. Although concern continues, in the 2014–2015 academic year, the data indicated that 44.9% of applicants were accepted for entry, whereas 68,938 qualified applicants were turned away (AACN, 2015a). This is an improvement from 2010, when only 39.5% of applications were accepted for entry and 53,667 qualified applicants were turned away. Although there has been improvement in overall numbers of enrollment and acceptance, "the top reasons reported by nursing schools for not accepting all qualified students include insufficient clinical teaching sites, a lack of qualified faculty, limited classroom space, insufficient preceptors, and budget cuts" (AACN, 2015a).

The AACN's 2014 fall survey noted an across-the-board increase in enrollment for both graduate and baccalaureate nursing programs. The survey reported a "4.2% increase in students in entry-level baccalaureate programs (BSN) and a 10.4% increase in 'RN-to-BSN' programs" (AACN, 2015a). For "graduate schools, student enrollment increased by 6.6% in master's programs and by 3.2% and 26.2% in research-focused and practice-focused doctoral programs, respectively" (AACN, 2015a). In 2015 the AACN reported that 111,634 students graduated from baccalaureate programs the previous year. "Certainly, the market for the BSN nurse has been stimulated by demand from employers who recognize the important role baccalaureate nurses play in achieving both individual and population health outcomes" (AACN, 2015a). Concurrently, Buerhaus and colleagues (2016, p. 46) concluded that the recent changes in nurses graduating is positive for the profession and will increase "the readiness of nursing professionals to capitalize on new opportunities, overcome challenges, and take on new roles and responsibilities as the nation's health care delivery and payments system evolve."

Demographic Factors

The Bureau of Health Workforce (BHW, 2014) had projected that the number of licensed RNs would remain relatively constant (2.9 million) between 2012 and 2025, yet the number of licensed RNs was projected to increase by 33% by 2025. This new projection was made using the HRSA Health Workforce Simulation Model. The model assumed that the RN supply and demand are equal in the year of forecasting (2012) and that the need progresses at the same steady rate as it has in the past. Using this limited methodology, the BHW calculated that the nationwide need for RNs would only increase by 21%, predicting that nursing supply will outpace demand in the next decade (BHW, 2014). Although nursing school graduations and the December 2014 BHW report indicated that the nursing shortage may be slowing, many experts continue to predict shortages into the next decade. Factors such as the increasing age of the baby boomers, improving economy, retiring nurses, expanding outpatient/community needs, regional/rural specific community shortages, and increasing turnover still suggest that nurse leaders plan for limited and/or decreasing numbers of nurses in the workforce (Auerbach et al., 2013; Staiger et al., 2012).

Aging of the registered nurse workforce. Understanding the demographic nature of the RN workforce requires an examination of the factors affecting the number of practitioners who may continue to work,

that is, the aging and the changing composition of the RN workforce.

The current nursing shortage may last longer because of the large number of RNs approaching retirement age and the growth and aging of the US population. Over the past two decades the average age of the nurse has continued to climb. According to the Bureau of Health Professions' (BHPr, 2013) report *The U.S. Nursing Workforce: Trends in Supply and Education,* the average age of the RN has increased by almost 2 years, moving from 42.7 years in 2000 to 44.6 (2010). More recently the number of nurses under the age of 36 is increasing, but as the entire RN workforce has grown, it has grown both in the younger and older ends and not in the middle. The growth in the number of nurses under the age of 35 is a very positive finding, although as was noted by Buerhaus and colleagues (2009a), most surveyed RNs continue to be white women working in hospitals located in urban and suburban areas, where the average nursing age only decreased by 2 years in 2008 compared with 2006. In 2013 the US Department of Health and Human Services reported that 23.4% of RNs were under age 35 years (an increase), 56.8% of nurses are between the ages 35 and 55, and 19.8% of nurses were over the age of 55 (Fig. 21.5).

The aging of the RN workforce is affected by two factors: the higher average age of recent graduates and the aging of the existing pool of licensed nurses.

- The "graying" factor makes the nursing shortage an even greater issue, as the RN loss is projected to be 128% higher in 2020 than in 2002. The graying of the existing licensed pool is evident in the following data. According to the 2008 National Sample Survey of Registered Nurses released in September 2010 by the federal BHPr (2010), the average age of the RN population in 2008 was 46 years, up from 45.2 years in 2000.
- With the average age of the RN at 50 in 2014, nurses in their 50s are expected to become the largest segment of the nursing workforce (53%) (ANA, 2014), accounting for almost one-quarter of the RN population (Buerhaus et al., 2009c).
- Within the next 8 years, the Bureau of Labor Statistics (BLS) projects the need for 439,300 additional nurses to fill new positions and replace those retiring from the profession (16% growth, 2014 to 2024) (BLS, 2014).

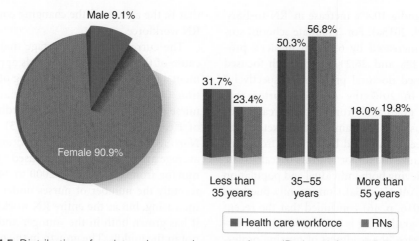

Male 9.1%

Female 90.9%

56.8%
50.3%
31.7%
23.4%
18.0% 19.8%

Less than 35 years
35–55 years
More than 55 years

■ Health care workforce   ■ RNs

FIG. 21.5 Distribution of registered nurses by sex and age. (Redrawn from US Department of Health and Human Services, Health Resources and Services Administration, National Center for Health Workforce Analysis. [2013]. *The U.S. Health Workforce Chartbook Part I: Clinicians.* Retrieved from https://bhw.hrsa.gov/sites/default/files/bhw/nchwa/chartbookpart1.pdf)

Historically, when the unemployment rate was high, the RN workforce tended to be larger than predicted, and when unemployment was low, the RN supply decreased more than expected. An increase of 1 percentage point in the unemployment rate was associated with 1.2% increase in the size of the RN workforce (Staiger et al., 2012).

Changing composition of the registered nurse workforce: age, diversity, and gender. As the nursing shortage is studied further, it has become apparent that the composition of the RN workforce must be analyzed, considered, and expanded. In an attempt to mitigate the nursing shortage, nursing needs to develop strategies to retain aging nurses and strategies to recruit men and minorities.

Age. As the nursing profession continues to age, it is important to understand the demographics and to create strategies to retain nurses as they age. Strategies need to be developed to keep the experienced nurse "brain" at the bedside when the experienced "back" may no longer be able to provide heavy patient care. Older RNs (above age 50) comprised 53.7% of the total RN population in 2014. The percentage of RNs who were 55 years and older increased from 15.5% in 2008 to 19.8% in 2013, and the average age of the RN population in 2014 was 50 years of age compared with 46 in 2008 (ANA, 2014; BHPr, 2010).

Between the years of 2001 and 2014, employment of older nurses in hospital settings fluctuated with the economy from boom to bust. From 2001 to 2008, 59% of the total increase in RN employment occurred in the hospital setting. During this same period, the nonhospital employment settings accounted for 18% of RN employment growth as well, but all growth in this period was represented by the older RN group over age 50 years (Buerhaus et al., 2009b). During this same period, the growth of middle-aged nurses (ages 35 to 49 years) was negative, with a substantial loss in nonhospital settings, thus overwhelming the hospital employment segment. Organizations reported that this shortage, which continues in many communities today, had a serious impact on nurse staffing, including increased overtime usage, higher stress, restricted expansion, changes in recruiting and hiring practices, decreased quality of care, and increased difficulty in scheduling coordination (May et al., 2006).

Today, as the need for nurses continues to grow (BLS, 2014) and as the current workforce continues to age, there is more of a need than ever to expand the recruitment base for nurses. Nurses today continue to be 90.8% female and 9.2% male, although the number of men in the field has expanded significantly in the past decade (US Department of Health & Human Services, 2015) (see Fig. 21.5). Significantly, the majority of RNs continue to be white at a percentage higher than that of

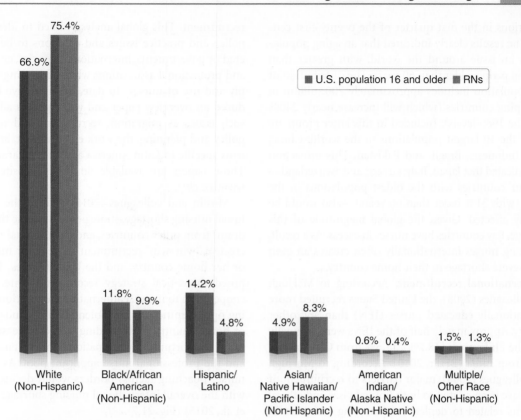

FIG. 21.6 Distribution of registered nurses by race/ethnicity, relative to the working-age population. (Redrawn from US Department of Health and Human Services, Health Resources and Services Administration, National Center for Health Workforce Analysis. [2013]. *The U.S. Health Workforce Chartbook Part I: Clinicians.* Retrieved from https://bhw.hrsa.gov/sites/default/files/bhw/nchwa/chartbookpart1.pdf)

the national working-age population (78.6%) (US Department of Health & Human Services, 2015). The RN workforce, although changing faster in recent years, remains extremely homogenous (Fig. 21.6). The opportunity exists for nursing to reach out to recruit more men and additional races/ethnicities in order to meet the predicted demand.

Diversity and inclusion. In an effort to address the nursing shortage, it is imperative to expand the diversity of students recruited beyond just white women. To provide quality, culturally competent patient care, the nursing workforce needs to expand to better reflect the population served (AACN, 2015b). In 2014 ethnic and racial minority groups accounted for 37.8% of the general US population (Colby & Ortman, 2015). Nurses from a minority background, however, accounted for just 19% of the total nursing workforce. In the AACN's

report *2014–2015 Enrollment and Graduations in Baccalaureate and Graduate Programs in Nursing,* minority nursing students represented 30.1% of students enrolling in baccalaureate programs. "Besides adding new clinicians to the RN workforce, a diverse nursing workforce will be better equipped to service a diverse patient population" (AACN, 2015a). Increasing the diversity of nursing faculty is also an opportunity to recruit a more diverse body of students.

The lack of an ethnically diverse nursing pool is further being fueled by the international demand for nurses. According to Daniel and colleagues (2000), international recruitment of nurses once again surfaced as a way of addressing the nursing shortage, specifically in the United States, United Kingdom, Canada, and Western Europe. The International Council of Nurses (ICN) (2007) reported worldwide population aging projections in the first quarter of the twenty-first century. The results clearly indicated that an aging population is an issue around the world, with greater than 1 billion people older than 60 years. The distribution of this population includes approximately 700 million in developing countries (which will increase nearly 240% from the 1980 levels). Included in this latter group are five of the 10 largest populations in the world: China, India, Indonesia, Brazil, and Pakistan. This projection also indicated that Japan, Italy, Greece, and Switzerland—the four countries with the oldest populations in the world (with 31% older than 60 years)—also would be severely affected. Given the global magnitude of this shortage, few countries have nurses in excess. As a result, recruiting nurses internationally often creates an even more severe shortage in their home country.

International recruitment. According to McHugh and colleagues (2008), the United States recruited more internationally educated nurses (IEN) than any other country. Approximately half of the IENs were originally from the Philippines (48.7%), 11.5% from Canada, and 9.3% from India (BHPr, 2010). According to McHugh and colleagues (2008), major barriers to recruitment of IENs have been related to both limited visas and ethical concerns related to depletion of nursing resources in other countries.

In 2004, the ICN and its sister organization, the Florence Nightingale International Foundation, investigated global nursing shortage issues related to international recruitment. This global analysis aimed to identify the policy and practice issues and solutions to be considered by governments, international agencies, employers, and professional associations when addressing the supply and use of nurses. To date, this initiative has produced an overview paper and white papers addressing such issues as migration, recruitment and retention, policy and planning, the work environment, and problems specific to Latin America and sub-Saharan Africa. Those papers are available on ICN's website *(http://www.icn.ch/)*.

Muslin and colleagues (2015) studied the international nursing shortage, strategies to decrease the "brain drain" from other countries, and a conceptual model to create a "win–win" recruitment strategy for nurses, his or her home country, and the United States. The proposed theoretical strategy recommends international cooperation to increase international educational funding opportunities for any potential nurse, independent of home country. This funding would increase educational opportunities, international nurse enrollment, and the professional nurse applicant pool. As a result, nurse "poaching" across borders would decrease along with the overall international nursing shortage (Muslin et al., 2015) (Fig. 21.7).

Men. Today's nurse workforce is approximately 9% male. In order to address the current and future nursing shortage, it is imperative that males are both recruited and retained in the profession. To achieve this goal it is

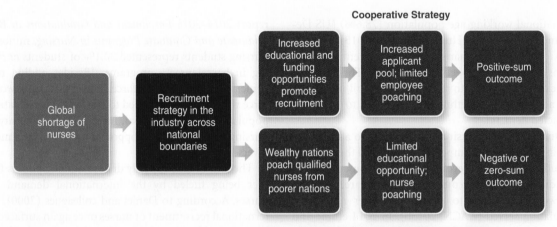

FIG. 21.7 A conceptual model of international nursing recruitment. (From Muslin, I., Willis, W.K., McInerney, M., & Deslich, S. [2015]. Global worker migration: Crisis and opportunity in the nursing profession. *Journal of Health Management, 17*[1], 1–10.)

BOX 21.2   Potential Barriers to Gender Diversity in Nursing

- Female language references (e.g., "she")
- Little or no reference to men's historical contribution to nursing
- Gender-related bias in obstetrical rotations
- Men's fear of suspect touch when providing care for female patients
- Lack of career choice support by significant people in the male student's lives
- Antimale remarks by nursing faculty, patients, and peers
- Nursing programs' failure to prepare men to work primarily with women
- Lack of mentorship
- No proactive male nurse recruitment strategies
- Limited numbers of male faculty and practicing male nurses
- No course content on communication differences between sexes
- Exclusive use of teaching techniques known to be more effective in women than men

Adapted from MacWilliams, B.R., Schmidt, B., & Bleich, M.R. (2013). Men in nursing. *American Journal of Nursing, 113*(1), 38–44.

important to understand the experience of the male nurse and remove barriers to practice. Research on these subjects is both recent and rare. Findings suggest that men are more likely to experience isolation and loneliness in the primarily female workplace (MacWilliams et al., 2013). In addition, many males report consistent barriers to both entry into practice and to inclusion (Box 21.2).

Despite the overwhelming historical dominance of women as nurses and the minority of men in the nursing workforce, male nurses have overall higher salaries than female nurses in both the inpatient and outpatient settings. On average, male ambulatory nurses made $7678 more than female nurses annually. In hospital settings, male nurses made $3873 more than female nurses (Muench et al., 2015).

The Image of Nursing

Following work with the American Organization of Nurse Executives (AONE) and AACN, Johnson & Johnson (J&J, 2016) launched a multiyear nursing initiative, *The Campaign for Nursing's Future,* in February 2002. This campaign grew out of J&J's concern over the nursing shortage, both current and future, and was designed to enhance the image of the nursing profession, recruit new nurses and nurse faculty, and help retain nurses. The goal of the *Campaign* was to increase population interest in nursing by promoting a thorough and accurate image of nursing. The *Campaign* maintains a comprehensive website *(https://www.discovernursing.com/)* for individuals interested in pursuing a nursing career. Since 2010, the *Campaign* has produced a Facebook fan page, television commercials, podcasts, the "Thank a Nurse" campaign, and a training program titled "Your Future in Nursing." The campaign was international and covered a broad spectrum of activities that were directed at enhancing the image of nursing as a profession, such as fundraising for student and faculty scholarships; research, awards, and support to nursing schools' program expansions; national television, print, and interactive advertising; development and maintenance of a website; and production and distribution of recruitment and retention materials. These activities clearly put nursing forward in public arenas and raised the status of nursing as a profession. According to Donelan and colleagues (2010), this campaign has had a positive effect on nursing recruitment and enrollment in schools of nursing. The campaign was a major initiative in the private corporate sector and has provided valuable insights into ways to examine challenges confronting the nursing workforce.

Unfortunately the image of nursing has not always been so positive. Literary and media references as far back as Charles Dickens' character Sairey Gamp (Summers, 1997) have often depicted nurses as unprofessional, unkempt, or uninterested in the patient. Representations of the female nurse in film and television have included stereotypical figures such as the battle-ax, handmaiden, and sex-craved vixen. In 2005 Suzanne Gordon further examined the effect of media on the image of nursing in her book *Nursing Against the Odds*. Gordon explored historical media portrayals of the nurse from childhood books, television, and film. It is Gordon's position that these representations have influenced what "many people believe: nurses are people, mainly women, who don't have the patience, stamina, ambition, curiosity, or intelligence to make it through medical school, and who work in a field wholly owned and operated by doctors" (p. 148).

One study examined the portrayal of male nurses in television and film dramas including *Nurse Jackie, Grey's Anatomy,* and *Private Practice.* Findings verified that male nurses are often portrayed as homosexual, feminine, or inappropriate. In several situations, the male nurse character represented not only the nursing minority but also ethnic minorities. Male nurses were not found to be main characters in any of the dramas (Stanley, 2012).

Other research has been conducted regarding the disparity between how nurses see themselves and the views of the general public. A study in London found that nurses identify three themes for their profession: diversity, fulfillment, and privilege (Morris-Thompson et al., 2011). The general public, however, did not agree with the nurses, and although they had an overall positive image of nurses, statistically they declared they would not recommend nursing as a career choice.

Today additional research is being conducted on the "brand image" of nursing. As a result of the unfavorable, inaccurate, and stereotypical images of nurses in the media, nurses have experienced a disconnect between the image they have of themselves and the profession and that of the general public. Hayes and Godsey (2016) conducted a study comparing the perceptions of the brand image of nursing in both a sample of nursing faculty (n = 264) and the American public (n = 801). The study found that nurses ranked their profession significantly higher than the American public on the following brand image descriptors: advocates, diverse career options, holistic approach, collaborators/facilitators, teachers/educators, critical thinkers, communicators, and empathetic. The public ranked the nursing professing significantly higher than the nursing faculty on the following descriptors: physician's assistant, white cap/uniform, subservient, task oriented, and nurturing/mothering. The study found that two gaps in nursing brand image exist: how nurses perceive their profession versus how they would like it to be perceived and how nurses perceive their profession versus the perception of the general public. Implications for the profession include the need for a large-scale strategic management of the profession's brand identity, similar to that of *The Campaign for Nursing's Future* (J&J, 2016), in order to enhance the overall image of nursing and encourage individuals to join the nursing workforce.

Work Environment Factors

RN employment overall has risen from 2 million in 2001 to 2.35 million in 2007, 2.6 million in 2008, and 2.9 million in 2014, with the majority of this increase occurring in hospitals. The continued increases in the number of nurses in the United States are the combined result of nurses working longer and retiring later, the increasing enrollments of nurses into recently expanding nursing programs, and the use of non–US-born nurses (Buerhaus, 2008; Buerhaus et al., 2016).

In general terms, a nursing shortage has been shown to have adverse effects, including decreased access to care, decreased job satisfaction, and increased turnover. For example, an inadequate number of nurses to staff the operating room (OR) results in decreased OR capacity, which in turn increases wait time for surgical procedures. The concern about the effect of RN shortages on the quality of patient care is growing. A meta-analysis conducted by Kane and colleagues (2007) found that the shortage of RNs and the increased workload can negatively affect the quality of patient care. Duffield and colleagues (2007) found that stabilizing the work environment—whether by low nurse turnover, stable nurse leadership, or adequate competent staff—enhances patient outcomes.

Nurse vacancy and turnover rates are predictors of nursing shortages as well. Nurse turnover rates from 2008 to 2010 slowly decreased to 11.2% in 2011 (NSI Nursing Solutions, Inc., 2016). In 2015 the national nurse turnover rate was reported at 16.4%. This rate is especially concerning as it relates to first-year nurses. In 2007, during an era when overall turnover was decreasing, one survey reported 27.1% turnover (PricewaterhouseCoopers, 2007) with another noting that 37% of first-year nurses reported they felt "ready to change jobs" (Kovner et al., 2007). This trend continues in this new era of increasing overall turnover. Several work environment factors have been cited as reasons for increased turnover (Buerhaus et al., 2000; Tri-Council for Nursing, 2004), including workload, autonomy, relations with managers, and compensation. Such factors influence job stress, in turn leading to job satisfaction or dissatisfaction (Hayhurst et al., 2005) and ultimately turnover and intent to stay.

One remedy is the healthy work environment initiative (see Chapters 3, 4, and 8). The American Association of Critical-Care Nurses (2016) published *AACN Standards for Establishing and Sustaining Healthy Work*

Environments and developed six tenets to promote a healthy work environment that will in turn improve nurse retention. They are skilled communication, true collaboration, effective decision making, appropriate staffing (workload), meaningful recognition, and authentic leadership.

Workload and Staffing

Inappropriate or inadequate staffing can negatively affect patient safety and nurses' well-being (American Association of Critical-Care Nurses, 2016). In 2012 the American Nurses Association (ANA) published *Principles of Staffing,* linking optimal nurse staffing levels with an optimal practice environment. In an early study on this subject, Aiken and colleagues (2002) found that nurses with the highest nurse-to-patient ratios (fewer nurses for the number of patients) were more likely to describe feelings of burnout, emotional exhaustion, and job dissatisfaction than nurses with lower ratios (more RNs for the number of patients). In addition, 43% of nurses who reported high levels of burnout and dissatisfaction intended to leave their jobs within a year. In contrast, only 11% of nurses who did not complain of burnout or dissatisfaction expressed intent to leave their current jobs. Buerhaus and colleagues (2005) found that insufficient staffing raises the stress level of nurses, affecting job satisfaction and causing nurses to leave the nursing profession. Another study found similar results noting that "improving job satisfaction among nurses will be a key factor in retaining experienced nurses at the bedside ... the study suggests a relationship between job satisfaction and an appropriate patient assignment" (Hairr et al., 2014, p. 146).

Stam and colleagues (2013) found that new graduates viewed "staffing adequacy" as an important predictor of job satisfaction. In addition to the relationship between staffing levels and nurse satisfaction, there is also a growing body of literature demonstrating a correlation between nurse staffing levels and patient outcomes. It can be inferred that nurses who do not believe they are able to provide optimal patient care may be more likely to change jobs or professions. To further explore why patient outcomes are influenced by nurse staffing levels, Kalish and Lee (2014) reported that nursing hours per patient day are a "significant positive predictor for registered nurse satisfaction" (p. 465). Kalish and Xie (2014) have further searched for a cause between nurse staffing levels and patient outcomes.

They propose the concept of "missed care," explaining that "the higher the staffing levels, the fewer occurrences of missed nursing care" (p. 875). Kalish and Xie (2014, p. 875) reported that "Magnet status and higher level of teamwork are associated with less missed nursing care, and more missed care leads to lower levels of staff (RN) satisfaction."

Critical elements to ensure appropriate staffing need to be established to ensure manageable workloads and high levels of nurse retention. The elements include staffing policies that are based on evidence and ethical principles, nursing input in staffing decisions from the frontline staff, appropriate definition and application of competencies, methods to evaluate staffing levels and patient outcomes (nurse-sensitive indicators), adequate support services, and appropriate equipment and technologies to support patient care (American Association of Critical-Care Nurses, 2016).

Compensation

An increase in salary for nurses relative to the salary in other occupations increases the attractiveness of nursing as a profession. An increase in salary now correlates more to the education level, expertise, and/or higher certification of the nurse as an individual. The impact of the recessionary decade (2007 to 2017) resulted in an increase in the supply of nurses through several mechanisms. Part-time RNs were motivated to work more hours or go full time, and older RNs delayed retirement or returned to work from retirement. Licensed RNs working in non-nursing jobs returned to nursing, and young people decided to enroll in nursing programs, a demand occupation with future stability (Staiger et al., 2012). As seen in the law of supply and demand, during shortages—whether local or national—market pressures to increase nurse salary levels result. In 2014 the RN national salary was $68,910 annually (ANA, 2014).

Demand

The recent increase in demand for RNs is projected to continue as a result of accelerating demand for health care services. This demand is affected by population growth, a rising proportion of people older than 65 years—with Americans 65 years and older representing nearly 20% of the population by 2030 (IOM, 2011), socioeconomic and cultural shifts, and advances in technology.

Changing Demographic Nature of the Population

Population growth and aging baby boomers are the major factors changing the demographic nature of the population, which in turn are affecting the demand for RNs. According to the Bureau of Health Professions (2004), the US population will grow 18% between 2000 and 2020, which equates to an additional 50 million people requiring health care. Increased life expectancy resulting from advances in science and medicine accounts for most of this population growth, as well as the increase in the proportion of the population older than 65 years. A rapid increase in the elderly population began around 2010, when those at the top end of the baby boom generation reached age 65 years. The subgroup of people 65 years and older will grow 54% between 2000 and 2020, which equates to an additional 19 million people in this age group. This is equivalent to a tsunami wave that cannot be stopped yet has huge implications for health care delivery and financing.

Individuals older than 65 years, particularly those ages 85 years and older, have the greatest per capita demand for health care and thus the greatest need for the services of RNs. These individuals tend to have (1) a higher incidence of chronic conditions such as arthritis (50%), hypertension (36%), and heart disease (32%); and (2) a higher occurrence of multiple conditions requiring more regular care. Thus with living longer and current rates of obesity comes the increased prevalence of chronic medical conditions. As a result, this population uses a larger portion of the available health care services and resources. They visit physicians twice as often as those younger than 65 years, account for 38% of hospital discharges (they represent 13% of the population), and have annual per capita health care expenditures of $5400 compared with $1500 for those younger than 65 years.

Health Delivery System

Health delivery systems form the structure around how care is delivered, where it is delivered, and how it is paid for. For example, Medicare and Medicaid reimbursement, the Patient Protection and Affordable Care Act, and regional and local customs and cultures influence the demand for nursing services. It is commonly known that socioeconomic determinants such as culture, income, educational level, and age affect an individual's health practices, which in turn affect the person's health status and subsequent use of and access to health care services.

Increased acuity of patients puts more demand on critical care services such as emergency and intensive care areas, thereby increasing the need for nurses. A combination of decreased supply and increasing demand creates a potential nursing shortage situation that varies by geographical region. Urban and suburban hospitals have reported higher vacancy rates than rural hospitals, and individual and multihospital systems have reported higher average RN vacancy rates than integrated delivery systems.

AMERICAN NURSES ASSOCIATION'S CALL TO ACTION

In September 2001, the American Nurses Association (ANA), in conjunction with AONE, Sigma Theta Tau International (STTI), 60 other professional nursing organizations, and 19 steering committee organizations, held a summit meeting to begin to analyze the nursing shortage problem and to develop a strategic plan called *Nursing's Agenda for the Future: A Call to the Nation* (ANA, 2002). The outcome of this meeting was a vision statement and 10 domains for action.

The 10 domains that emerged from this summit were derived from the research literature and the Institute of Medicine's study *Crossing the Quality Chasm: A New Health System for the 21st Century,* published in 2001. The domains are as follows (Institute of Medicine, 2001, p. 7):

1. Leadership and planning
2. Delivery systems
3. Legislative/regulatory/policy
4. Professional/nursing culture
5. Recruitment/retention
6. Economic value
7. Work environment
8. Public relations/communication
9. Education
10. Diversity

As part of *Nursing's Agenda for the Future: A Call to the Nation* (2002), the ANA developed a "Desired Future Statement (Vision)" for each of the 10 domains. The statement for the domain of "Recruitment and Retention" clearly delineated the comprehensiveness of the undertaking (ANA, 2002, p. 17): "Nursing is comprised of a diverse body of individuals committed to promoting and sustaining the profession through addressing diversity, image, education, funding, practice models and environments, and professional development."

Five strategies were formulated to achieve this vision. The strategies also addressed the two-pronged recruitment issue of the shortage (supply side economics) and recruitment of (1) students for nursing education programs, and (2) qualified nurses for health care agencies. The strategies also targeted retention issues to be addressed within health care agencies and academic programs focusing on the development of career-based opportunities within health care, development and funding of creative educational initiatives, creation of a desirable and appealing image for nursing as a career choice, formulation and implementation of professional practice models, work environments that ensure career satisfaction, and development of comprehensive recruitment and retention strategies that will appeal to a diverse customer group/population (ANA, 2002). The ANA also identified strategies that could be used to enhance student and faculty recruitment and/or retention (Table 21.1). In addition, Erickson and colleagues (2004) identified the following nine strategies for promoting nursing as a career (Erickson et al., 2004, p. 86):

1. Classroom ambassadors program
2. Job-shadowing experiences
3. Bring-your-child-to-work day
4. Volunteer health care settings opportunities for students and adults
5. Part-time employment opportunities for students and adults
6. Presentation to clubs/organizations regarding nursing
7. Participation at community health fairs
8. Advertising campaigns directed at job satisfaction, making a difference in people's lives, flexible scheduling, and competitive salary and benefits
9. Advertising that directs people to dynamic, comprehensive websites that offer positive, motivating information about nursing and its rewards

THE FUTURE OF NURSING: LEADING CHANGE, ADVANCING HEALTH

In the fall of 2010, the Institute of Medicine (IOM, now called the National Academies of Science, Engineering, and Medicine, Health and Medicine Division) published an online draft of the *Future of Nursing (FON): Leading Change and Advancing Health* report. The later-published report offered four key messages and eight recommendations with the purpose of establishing a professional and political agenda for nursing in the United

TABLE 21.1 Student-Related and Faculty-Related Strategies for Recruitment and Retention

Recruitment and Retention Strategies	Students	Faculty
Develop professional mentoring models	X	
Create a specific curriculum to address diversity	X	X
Obtain funding to support minority enrollment	X	
Develop and distribute promotional and recruitment materials to attract individuals from diverse backgrounds into nursing	X	
Recruit retired nurses to form professional mentoring corps	X	
Provide joint educational and service standardized internships and residencies	X	X
Co-op program/student clinical assistant (SCA) program	X	
Negotiate professional paid development opportunities with employers	X	
Create a website for leadership development that can be used by education, service, and professional organization members	X	X

States (IOM, 2011). Each key message calls for a specific research agenda. The four key messages establish the need (1) to transform practice, (2) to transform education, (3) to transform leadership, and (4) to better collect data on the health care workforce (IOM, 2011). Another key theme that is emphasized throughout the report is the importance of increased diversity in nursing. In addition to the IOM publication, the Robert Wood Johnson Foundation (RWJF) in partnership with the AARP launched the Future of Nursing: Campaign for Action (*The Campaign*) (*http://campaignforaction.org/*). *The Campaign's* main function is to oversee the implementation of the IOM recommendations at both the national and state levels.

The report's eight recommendations further outline an implementation plan and call to action. The eight recommendations were (IOM, 2011): "(1) Remove scope-of-practice barriers, (2) expand opportunities for nurses to lead and diffuse collaborate improvement efforts, (3) implement nurse residency programs, (4) increase the proportion of nurses with a baccalaureate degree to 80% by 2020, (5) double the number of nurses with a doctorate by 2020, (6) ensure that nurses engage in lifelong learning, (7) prepare and enable nurses to lead change to advance health, and (8) build an infrastructure for the collection and analysis of the interprofessional health care workforce." The IOM *FON* report affected the nursing workforce by calling for increasing diversity, advancing education, and recommending standardization and structure around health care workforce data collection.

In 2016, the IOM published *Assessing Progress on the Institute of Medicine Report: The Future of Nursing*. This publication not only evaluated movement on the original report's recommendations, but it also created additional recommendations designed to further move *The Campaign* forward. Significant progress has been made in three IOM recommendations: (1) raising the number of RNs with a baccalaureate degree; (2) increased numbers of nurse residency programs; and (3) increased opportunities for continuing nurse education (Pittman et al.,

2015). In areas where opportunity continues to exist, 10 new recommendations have been published (Table 21.2). The new and enhanced recommendations around diversity in the workforce and workforce data collection are designed to directly influence state implementation plans and initiatives. Thus the IOM *FON* report affects the nursing shortage by formally calling for increased workforce diversity and improved workforce data collection.

RECRUITMENT

Recruitment is about the replacement of non-retained staff and the hiring of staff to fill newly created and/or expanded positions. With the changes that have occurred in health care over the past two decades, the concept of recruitment has begun to focus more and more on the identification and development of pre-employment hires. If employers move to increase the diversity of nurses at the bedside (IOM, 2016), pre-employment relationships with nursing colleges are critical. This means marketing the health care agency to potentially diverse pre-nursing students and active nursing students. Recruitment therefore has become more complex and more linked to partnerships than ever before. These partnerships are not only with schools of nursing but also with elementary and secondary schools and other community agencies. Co-op programs and/or student clinical assistant (SCA) programs

TABLE 21.2 Assessing Progress on the Institute of Medicine Report: The Future of Nursing New Recommendations	
2011 Recommendation	**2016 Progress Recommendation**
Remove barriers to practice and care.	1. Build common ground around scope of practice and other issues in policy and practice.
Achieve higher levels of education.	2. Continue pathways toward increasing the percentage of nurses with a baccalaureate degree.
	3. Create and fund transition-to-practice residency programs.
	4. Promote nurses' pursuit of doctoral degrees.
	5. Promote nurses' inter-professional and lifelong learning.
Promote diversity.	6. Make diversity in the nursing workforce a priority.
Collaborate and lead in care delivery and redesign.	7. Expand efforts and opportunities for inter-professional collaboration and leadership development for nurses.
	8. Promote the involvement of nurses in the redesign of care delivery and payment systems.
	9. Communicate with a wider and more diverse audience to gain broad support for campaign objectives.
Improve workforce data infrastructure.	10. Improve workforce data collection.

Adapted from Institute of Medicine (IOM). (2016). *Assessing progress on the Institute of Medicine Report: The future of nursing.* Washington, DC: National Academies Press.

(Henriksen et al., 2003) and other related preceptor programs create a model for attracting and retaining new graduates. These and other student-related activities blend the student-employee role, thus changing recruitment to a retention strategy once the student gets linked to the health care facility in a nursing capacity.

To be effective, employers and hiring managers should establish measurable goals to drive toward success. Goals need to include monitoring the number of positons posted (reduction in vacancy rates and turnover, the number of candidates interviewed per position, the number of diverse candidates interviewed and recruited, and days to fill). For national diversity goals (IOM, 2016), the American Hospital Association Career Center (2015) reported only 48% of hospitals with formal plans to recruit and retain diverse workers. Furthermore, only 22% of hiring managers had a diversity goal for performance (AHA, 2015). Collecting these data is also consistent with the profession's need to improve and standardize workforce metrics (IOM, 2016).

Clearly, recruitment needs both long-term and short-term strategies. Although the long-term plan is extremely important, most of the organization's resources tend to go to short-term initiatives such as filling vacant and/or newly created positions. The recruitment focus of this chapter is directed at short-term strategies.

Recruitment of Professional Nurses: The Evidence-Based Magnet Recognition Program®

The evidence-based Magnet Recognition Program® has a long history of research behind its recognition criteria. In 1983 a study was conducted (1) to identify variables in hospital organizations and their nursing services that create a magnetism that attracts and retains professional nurse staff, and (2) to identify particular combinations of variables that produce nursing practice models within hospitals in which nurses receive professional and personal satisfaction to the degree that recruitment and retention of qualified staff are achieved (McClure et al., 1983). The results of the study clearly showed that the three major variables of administration, professional practice, and professional development—with related attributes—positively affect hospitals' ability to recruit and retain registered nurse staff.

This study was one of the first to describe organizational and leadership factors that are important to the recruitment and retention of nurses in the workplace.

Nurses specifically wanted a leadership and organizational structure that supported participatory involvement, as well as flexibility for work scheduling and personal/professional development. In addition, nurses wanted to work in an institution that had a clearly defined professional practice model that used the skills and knowledge of the professional nurse. Nurses were also interested in working in an organization that allowed them to be able to practice nursing as they defined it. Managerial visibility and support were viewed as strengths in promoting autonomy. Nurses also wanted to have control over their practice (autonomy) and collaborative relationships with physicians relative to care management. This study and the follow-up study conducted by Kramer and Hafner (1989) 5 years later were the basis for the ANA'S Magnet Recognition Program®.

Human Resources, Managerial, and Staff Roles Associated With Recruitment

Recruitment initiatives have used strategies targeted at nurse satisfiers as reported in the nursing and health care literature. Satisfiers have included strategies such as professional practice model usage, preceptor/mentorship opportunities, increased flexibility in work scheduling, low patient-to-RN ratios, a collaborative practice environment, Magnet Recognition status, an environment of respect and value, and a competitive compensation model. Strategies commonly used that are related to nurse recruitment of new and experienced nurses are identified in Box 21.3.

In the context of a nurse shortage, recruitment is a major human resources (HR) strategy. Because the organization needs to find and hire the best qualified nurses who also "fit" with the culture and are willing to work for a specific salary and work conditions, both recruitment and retention are important. Both managers and staff contribute to successful recruitment and retention. A complex and detailed process is followed for effective recruitment and retention. The nine major processes or phases of recruitment are position posting, advertising, screening, interviewing, selecting, orienting, counseling/coaching, evaluating performance, and developing staff.

Position Posting

Position posting for recruitment begins after determination of vacancies based on position controls developed for each of the clinical/service areas. The vacancies are identified based on the full-time equivalent (FTE) status

BOX 21.3   Recruitment Strategies

- Flexible hours
- Competitive salaries
- Bonus pay
- Relocation pay
- Fixed shifts
- Weekend option program
- Part-time pay with bonus hours
- Flexible benefits packages
- Scholarships for bachelor of science in nursing or graduate studies
- Tuition benefit plan
- Educational loan repayment
- Residency programs and registered nurse (RN) specialty internships
- Onboarding
- Refresher courses—return to work
- Professional development opportunities
- Career opportunities
- Specialty certification reimbursement
- Low nurse-to-patient ratios; higher numbers of RNs for the patient load (workload staffing)
- Shared governance/leadership models
- Care delivery model that promotes professional care at the bedside
- Clinical ladder/career ladder
- Free parking
- Magnet Recognition Program®
- Culture of safety: zero tolerance for incivility
- Research/evidence-based practice
- NCLEX review course
- Qualified managerial support
- Clinical support: staff educators, clinical nurse specialists
- Workforce diversity
- Interdisciplinary collaboration opportunities

for each of the positions. Once the positions have been identified and the shift/holiday schedules are determined, the first step is to post them internally for staff review and selection. The length of this posting time is determined by each organization and/or respective collective bargaining contracts. Positions not filled within a defined period are then posted externally to the organization. Based on the need and/or limited number of nurses in a given specialty, recruitment agencies may be contacted at this time to conduct a regional, statewide, or national search for the position.

Advertising

Advertising includes the development of an institutional advertisement outlining the positions or job opportunities within an organization. The advertisement addresses the area of need and specific information that would be likely to attract an employee (RN) to the position. The HR department determines distribution sites with input from the specific departments. Sites may include professional journals or newspapers, local or regional newspapers, radio, or the organization's website. An advantage of online advertisement is that the application process can be made available at the same time, making it a one-stop process for the person seeking employment.

If the recruiter is planning to attend special events, information about the position will be taken for posting along with the application forms and/or directions. In addition, information about the organization and related benefits and specialty strengths will be highlighted. A shortcoming that needs to be addressed related to advertising is that organizations often spend a considerable amount of money on advertising only to miss the most important aspect—that of a quick, effective, courteous follow-up with potential candidates (Curran, 2003). Positive results from expensive advertising and recruiting efforts can be lost depending on how the institution follows up with candidates. For example, if potential candidates for a position have been encouraged to apply through advertising and recruitment efforts and then log on to an institution's website and find that they cannot complete an application for the job, they may become frustrated and decide not to pursue the job (Curran, 2003). In addition, if candidates cannot obtain a response about the status of their application after submitting it, they may decide that they do not want to work for this type of institution. If recruitment and advertising efforts are to be productive, these kinds of flaws in the system need to be avoided or engineered out of the system.

Screening

Screening is the process in which the application is reviewed before determining whether the nurse meets the preestablished criteria for the position. During this activity, the reviewer selects whom should be interviewed. According to Nall (2012), all applicants should be reviewed for gaps in employment and skill experiences, as well as for a match with the job description for the position under review. It is important to remember that if an organization is classified as an *equal opportunity employer,* the reviewers are required to follow the guidelines established by the federal government. Most application processes are currently completed and reviewed online, thus increasing the pool of applicants, which in turn requires more recruitment time in screening. Review of large applicant pools may result in delays in responding to the applicants unless auto-responses are generated. Electronic applications are easier to file and sort relative to identified areas of interest by the applicant.

Interviewing

Interviewing is the time for clarification of information presented in the application and dossier submitted by the applicant. The job description is the basis for a hiring interview. The interview can be conducted in person or over the telephone, in a group/committee or one-on-one meeting. For best results, predefined questions should be used to interview all candidates for the position. Also, questions should be directed at the work expectations outlined in the position description and/or practices. Open-ended and follow-up questions are recommended. For example, the following questions or discussion points can be posed:

- Tell me about your current position.
- What do you like least about it?
- What do you like best about it?

Questions can be framed as follows to get more in-depth responses and to determine behavior-specific examples:

- Think of a time in your experience when X was needed, and describe how you did X.
- How did you handle X?

It is appropriate to ask the candidate about aspects of his or her actions and decisions related to the job, such as the following:

- Given the varied work hour requirements, how would you handle this?
- What problems do you see the work hour requirements presenting?
- Based on the work requirements relative to lifting, how would you go about transferring a patient whose body weight is more than 350 pounds?

The information obtained through this process will help the committee or manager assigned to the recruitment process determine the applicant's "fit" with the unit and/or organizational culture, and it will provide consistent data for comparison of candidates. Use of formalized questions is often referred to as a *structured interview* or *targeted selection process* (Lipsey, 2004). The targeted selection process is built on analysis of work per job, organizational values, clear identification of competencies for key positions, and development of interview skills and confidence of the interviewers. The targeted interview ensures that all candidates are interviewed based on the same criteria. In addition, during the targeted interview process, the interviewer asks questions that are directed at having the candidates describe typical situations that they have encountered in previous jobs. Use of the targeted interview method allows the interviewers to gain data from the candidates to more fully evaluate their values and practice patterns. It further allows for objective comparison of candidates based on their responses, and it decreases personal biases and assumptions. It prevents interviewers from veering off target and/or asking questions that may be inappropriate or illegal. Questions that should be avoided during the interview relate specifically to personal information about the candidate such as age, marital status, living arrangements, children, limitations or disabilities, religion, substance abuse, and membership in professional organizations.

Selecting

Selecting is the determination of who will be offered an opportunity for employment (termination of the recruitment process). A committee or manager may complete the selection process. For best results, data from the screening and interviewing phases should be used when comparing candidate responses and other related data. The selection process also involves the formal activity of making an offer to the candidate. Who performs this activity varies according to institutional policy, but it usually involves either the manager or HR personnel. At the time the job offer is made, the employee is informed of the position/job being offered, the FTE allocation (full time [FT] or part time [PT]) for the position, and the salary offer and benefits. Regardless of who makes the final offer, HR plays a role in determining the salary range.

Selection of an employee who is a match with the core values of an organization has been shown to have important implications. It facilitates ease of employee transition into the new role and fit with staff in the unit and organization. Employee fit and related retention have also been shown to have an impact on cost savings within the organization. According to Lipsey (2004), return on investment of hiring the right versus the wrong person (poor performer) is more significant than just the costs of simple replacement of an employee. The costs of hiring the wrong person are associated not only with recruitment, replacement, and hiring expenses, but also the secondary costs. Secondary costs of hiring a poor performer include increased dollars wasted on training and development, decreased productivity and increased errors, lost opportunities to improve processes and/or outcomes, decreased or poor staff morale that results from staff struggling to pick up slack from the poor performer, and dissatisfied customers. The secondary costs have a significant impact on the organization and workers and are often much greater than those associated with the initial recruitment process.

Orienting

Orienting is an important activity for bringing new employees into the organization, department, and unit. It is the employee's introduction to the culture and values of the organization and discipline. Changes in orientation format and content have occurred as a result of study outcomes that have shown the relationship between job satisfaction and staff retention. An important approach to orienting is referred to as "onboarding" (Lee, 2008). The approach is directed at fully engaging and integrating the employee in the organization by focusing on how to assist him or her in successfully preparing for the job. Onboarding expands the orientation beyond the employee's initial introduction to the organization and role expectations by providing ongoing coaching and mentorship through a defined program (Lee, 2008). These programs usually last from 3 months to 1 year. A prime example is new graduate nurse residency programs. This approach is consistent with expectations expressed by the new nurse graduate (Pine & Tart, 2007), especially those in the Generation Y group (Hart, 2006). Onboarding, including new graduate residency programs, is consistent with a Magnet culture (Halfer, 2007). Onboarding has also brought about a change in learning; it has moved from a fairly passive, didactic experience to an interactive process built around self-learning and renewal.

As recommended by the IOM *Future of Nursing* report (2011), many hospitals have adopted residency and/or internship programs with RN preceptors working one on one with the new graduate (Park & Jones, 2010). In addition to the IOM (2011) recommendations, the American Organization of Nurse Executives (AONE, 2016)—building on the research of the National Council of State Boards of Nursing's (NCSBN) Transition to Practice (TTP)—established the *AONE Guiding Principles for the Newly Licensed Nurse's Transition Into Practice.* All of these programs strive to better prepare the new graduate RN to be successful in his or her chosen work environment. Residencies, internships, and transition to practice programs teach new RNs about not only the clinical environment but also effective communication, problem solving, stress management, hospital-specific information technology, and performance/quality improvement. The success of these programs has been closely tied with retention. Halfer (2007) reported a 17.2% increase in retention with $707,608 cost savings. Pine and Tart (2007) reported that residency programs have been shown to have a positive return on investment (ROI). For example, over a 1-year period the program decreased turnover by 37%, and ROI was 325.5%. Mills and Mullins (2008) reported a 15% increase in retention over 3 years. Intangible benefits associated with these programs include improved morale, increased nursing and health team satisfaction, increased confidence, and improved quality of care (Halfer, 2007; Mills & Mullins, 2008).

Counseling and Coaching

Counseling and coaching are strategies used to promote a sense of community for new and ongoing employees. These strategies create a professional and social network for new employees, an attribute identified in Magnet-recognized institutions. Use of these strategies also creates a sense of a non-punitive culture in which staff can learn and grow. Graduate nurses have indicated the need for positive support and timely verbal feedback from preceptors to gain the confidence and competence needed during their transition into the RN role, although this is not always received (Duchscher, 2009; Park & Jones, 2010). According to VanWyngeeren and Stuart (n.d.), healthy working relationships and group cohesion enhance retention for both new and experienced employees.

Performance Evaluation

Performance evaluation is a mechanism for giving feedback to both new and experienced employees. In addition to receiving ongoing evaluation during their onboarding by an assigned preceptor/coach, new employees are expected to receive an initial performance evaluation within the first 60 to 120 days, depending on the policies of the organization. This feedback is directed at the individual employee's progress relative to their onboarding program (formative evaluation). During this evaluation, the employee and managerial staff also need to take the time to evaluate the employee's "fit" with the organizational and departmental culture (summative evaluation). Strategies to address further needs and/or employment status should be decided at this time. A full performance evaluation then occurs at the end of the orientation period and annually thereafter. Feedback regarding ongoing performance needs to be provided to employees on a regular basis. Performance evaluation needs to focus on the employee's achievement toward defined goals, with feedback directed at the individual's contribution to the development of peers and clinical and/or leadership practices. The meeting can be conducted using a formal or informal process, one on one or in a group. According to Hall and colleagues (2011) and Palumbo and colleagues (2009), performance feedback/evaluation has been tied to staff satisfaction and intent to stay.

Staff Development

Staff development has been identified in the literature as an important factor in job satisfaction. It provides employees with an opportunity to improve their practice, level of competency, or other areas of self-interest. Programs for staff development are typically determined based on annual staff surveys. Programs are usually posted for staff selection, and the institution provides scheduling flexibility and funding for employees to participate.

Staff development, as defined in the Magnet studies (Halfer, 2007; Kramer & Hafner, 1989; McClure et al., 1983), was identified as having four areas of professional development beyond orientation. The four areas included in-service education, continuing education, formal education, and career development. Professional development was valued for its economic potential. However, other attributes identified were personal and professional growth opportunities, career advancement opportunities, and preceptor skill development. Nurses in these institutions viewed education as being valued. Administrative support was provided and available, as were clinical and managerial resources. Professional development opportunities overall were shown to have a positive influence on nurse satisfaction. Ongoing staff development at all levels of employment has been shown to increase retention and enhance staff entry into clinical ladder programs (Halfer, 2007; Pierson et al., 2010). Clinical ladder programs have also been shown to encourage further formal education and to result in formal promotion and leadership opportunities (Ko & Yu, 2014).

RETENTION: NEW GRADUATES AND EXPERIENCED REGISTERED NURSES

Renewed attention has been directed at retention of nurses in a multigenerational workforce (Palumbo et al., 2009). In 2010 the American Hospital Association (AHA) published the paper *Workforce 2015: Strategy Trumps Shortage* in an effort to formally address and explain not only a shortage of health care workers/nurses but also to recommend best practices for engagement and retention. The turnover rate of new graduates ranges from 22.6% to 60% in the first year (vanWyngeeren & Stuart, n.d.). Nursing has begun to focus attention on expanding retention programs beyond the promotion of job satisfaction, safety, respect, and financial security (e.g., 401[k] plans, gain sharing, individual retirement accounts) to the development of an infrastructure to improve the work environment to meet the diverse needs of current employees. The primary focus of these changes is to promote nurse autonomy and the nurse role on the interdisciplinary team while providing services that will enhance the work environment and life of the nurse both inside and outside of the organization. Today more than ever it is imperative that nurses and other health care workers experience a sense of community and teamwork in the workplace because many spend more time at work than at any other single place.

With four generational groups now in the workplace, it is important that managers and staff consider differences when developing strategies for change or rewards. Each generation has its own perspective, and diversity exists even within each generation. Therefore it is imperative that generational groups have representation or

BOX 21.4   Retention Strategies Used to Retain New Graduates and Experienced Nurses

Positive Work Environment and Organizational Culture
- Values driven
- Culture of safety
- Streamlined processes
- Physician–nurse collaborative partnership
- Creation of community culture
- Magnet culture/designation
- Volunteer opportunities, inside and outside of organization
- Diverse workforce
- Authentic and transformational leaders
- Appropriate staffing levels
- Meaningful recognition programs
- Clinician relaxation and meditation rooms

Onboarding Supports
- Mentoring/precepting
- Social supports
- Internship/residency program
- Support services: discussion groups and social networking opportunities

Compensation/Financial Incentives
- Competitive salaries
- Financial support associated with credentialing and professional development opportunities
- Part-time pay with bonus hours
- Bonus pay
- Bonus pay for recruitment of employees
- Profit/gains sharing
- Child/elder care
- Phased retirement

- Increased vacation/paid time off (PTO) offerings
- Wellness plans
- Free meal programs

Professional Development Opportunities
- Career/clinical advancement programs
- Ongoing educational offerings/opportunities
- Scholarships for bachelor of science in nursing/graduate programs
- Provisions for sabbatical
- Specialty training opportunities

Flexibility in Work Opportunities
- Flexible hours/schedules
- Fixed shifts
- Shift bidding
- Weekend options

Leadership Opportunities
- Creation of autonomous self-managed units
- Shared governance/leadership model
- Succession planning/development
- Precepting roles: staff and students

Technology
- Specialty equipment for use in care delivery
- Initialization of new technology into practice
- Technology/skill development support and training as integral part of roles

Miscellaneous Services
- Free parking
- Concierge services

opportunity for input in planning and decision making. In addition, it is important to develop a variety of alternatives from which employees can select rather than targeting a single approach. General strategies commonly used for nurse retention of new and experienced nurses are identified in Box 21.4.

According to a study conducted by Palumbo and colleagues (2009), although common retention expectations have been identified as important to nurses of all ages, some differences were noted related to the perceived significance of various retention strategies reported by generational groups (Table 21.3). There often were inconsistencies between what the nurses saw as important retention factors and HR/institutional

offerings provided by the various organization. Although the study by Palumbo and colleagues (2009) was specifically related to a 12-institution sample in a small rural state, it has implications for consideration on a broader scale, given that all institutions/agencies are currently working with generationally diverse groups. In addition, Leiter and colleagues (2010) have shown a difference in Generation X's and boomers' perceptions related to negative encounters (incivility) in the workplace. Although both generations reported significant levels of exhaustion, cynicism, turnover intention, and physical symptoms related to the incivility by supervisors, co-workers, and teams, the greatest distress was found in Generation X. Exhaustion and

TABLE 21.3 Retention Factors Related to Retaining Multigenerational Workforce

Retention Factors	SIGNIFICANCE BY AGE		
	<35–40	40–54	≥55
Recognition and respect	X	X	X
Having a voice	X	X	X
Receiving ongoing feedback about performance	X	X	X
Compensation	X	X	X
Employee health and safety	X	X	X
Job design	X	X	X
Training and development	X	X	X
Flexible work options	X	X	X
Retirement options	X	X	X
Recruitment of older nurses			X

From Palumbo, M.V., McIntosh, B., Rambur, B., & Naud, S. (2009). Retaining an aging nurse workforce: Perceptions of human resource practices. *Nursing Economic$, 27*(4), 221–232.

- Practice models—using specialty roles (e.g., wound nurse, audit nurse, admission and/or discharge nurse, telephone triage)
- Technology usage—lifting equipment, ergonomic computers and electrical devices, soften hard floor surfaces, cell phones, tracking systems, improved lighting
- Streamline processes—revised documentation systems, bed utilization programs, online continuing education, computer training, multisite computer access
- Communication and recognition opportunities—membership on unit-based and organizational committees, participation in shared governance activities, volunteer roles as institutional representatives, ambassador programs
- Educational opportunities—ongoing development, tuition reimbursement, scholarships

These and other changes are important if experienced nurses are to be retained at the bedside.

Another important factor in retention of nurses is managerial leadership (Acree, 2006; Kleinman, 2004). The two leadership styles that predominate in the literature are *transformational* and *transactional.* Managerial use of transformational leadership has been shown to have the greatest impact on nurse job satisfaction. This is no surprise given the need for ongoing support, recognition, and life balance expressed by both new graduates and experienced nurses. To provide this level of leadership, organizations will need to commit to the ongoing development of nurse managers and direct-care nurses as leaders and promote the cultural changes needed by them to actualize this level of leadership. Decreased cost has also been associated with effective recruitment strategies, consistent with the Magnet Recognition Program® (Halfer, 2007; Pine & Tart, 2007; vanWyngeeren & Stuart, n.d.).

Although retention has been shown to be affected by selection, orientation, and leadership, new and emerging research suggests that the nurse's practice environment is the most predictive of retention (American Nurses Credentialing Center, 2016; Kenny et al., 2016; Kramer et al., 2012; Press Ganey, 2016). In addition, the physical space of the work environment can also have an impact on the overall practice. Inherently high stress environments can lead to job dissatisfaction and burnout. Opportunities to reduce stress and workplace fatigue through clinician-reserved relaxation and meditation

turnover were strongly associated with supervisor incivility, whereas cynicism was strongly associated with supervisor and co-worker incivility. Greater incivility from co-workers and supervisors was found for Generation X than for boomers.

Although significant efforts have been directed at the recruitment and retention of new graduates, in the past few years, equal effort has been directed at the retention of experienced older nurses because of their depth of knowledge relative to the organization and their clinical expertise. Retention factors related to the older nurse have been shown to vary significantly from that of the new graduate, as older nurses find it harder to manage the physical demands of hospital work and are focusing on establishing financial security for retirement. To meet the needs of the older nurse, organizations have had to rethink the rules and roles that have been in place. According to Mion and colleagues (2006), a number of changes to be made in the area of retention include the following (Park & Jones, 2010; Pierson et al., 2010):

- Scheduling—decreasing frequency of rotations, reducing length of shifts, using sabbaticals
- Assignment requirements—geographical location, assignment consistency, work with preceptor

spaces can promote a healthier work environment (Sanders et al., 2013).

Although there is a large amount of evidence to support the concept that healthy work environments support not only nurse retention but also positive patient outcomes, work still remains. For example, the overall health of critical care nurse work environments has declined since 2008, along with nurses' perceptions of quality of care (Ulrich et al., 2014).

LEADERSHIP AND MANAGEMENT IMPLICATIONS

Turnover: Cost and Management Strategies

Managing turnover is a joint responsibility shared between nurses and nurse managers. Turnover of qualified staff is not only disruptive to the care community in which the nurse works (Atencio et al., 2003; Hunt, 2009; Kuhar et al., 2004; Manion & Bartholomew, 2004) but also is extremely costly to the organization (Jones, 2004a, b). According to Hunt (2009), the literature indicates that the total/real costs associated with nurse turnover have been evaluated using various approaches such as direct and indirect, visible and invisible, and pre-hire and post-hire. The most common factors used in determining nurse turnover costs include (Hunt, 2009):

- Advertising and recruitment
- Vacancy costs
- Hiring
- Orientation and training
- Decreased productivity
- Termination
- Potential patient errors/decreased quality of care
- Poor work environment and culture
- Loss of organizational knowledge
- Increased accident and absenteeism rates
- Increased nurse and medical staff turnover

According to Hunt (2009, p. 2), "the average hospital is estimated to lose about $300,000 per year for each percentage increase in annual nurse turnover." Hunt further cited one 9000-person health care organization that lost over $15 million per year because of nursing turnover. Other figures for the average cost for a medical/surgical RN are reported to be $42,000, but it can be as high as $85,000 for specialty RNs. Often agency/traveler nurses are used as temporary coverage. Although this practice appears to meet institutional needs and comes at an estimated cost of 1.5 times the salary of a permanent employee, the practice often further perpetuates turnover. Residency programs for new graduates, however, have been shown to have a positive impact on retention and cost.

In order to better understand RN turnover over time, in accordance with the IOM (2016) recommendations, the Robert Wood Johnson Foundation (RWJF) has initiated *The RN Work Project*, which is a 10-year panel study of the RN workforce (Kovner et al., 2014). New RNs, unfortunately have the highest overall turnover by year of employment. The 1-year turnover of new RNs in 2014 was 17.5%, with the 3-year turnover rising to 33.5% (Kovner et al., 2014). It is important to note that like the nursing shortage, nurse turnover is not a problem limited to just the United States (Duffield et al., 2014).

The average rate of all RN turnovers remains around 15%, or approximately 195,000 RNs, at an estimated yearly cost of $9.75 billion (AONE, 2016). Clearly, money spent for replacement could have been used by the organization to improve their competitive advantage, nurse satisfaction, and consumer perception of workforce quality and expansion of services. Fig. 21.8 shows the cost per RN hire. Fig. 21.9 displays a formula for calculating turnover.

Managing the Shortage

Auerbach and colleagues (2011) concluded that the nursing shortage remains but has stabilized somewhat with the addition of both online and campus-based nursing programs, offering traditional BSN, accelerated BSN, MSN, DNP, and PhD. Although it should be noted that the nurses and nurse educators are moving into retirement faster than they can be replaced, it is imperative that academic programs redesign their programs

$$\frac{\text{Total cost (e.g., recruitment, training, coverage)}}{\text{Total RNs hired}} = \text{Cost per RN hired}$$

FIG. 21.8 Cost per RN hired. (Derived from Hoffman, P.M. [1984]. *Financial management for nurse managers*. Norwalk, CT: Appleton-Century-Crofts.)

$$\frac{\text{Number of terminations per year}}{\text{Average workforce per year}} \times 100 = \%\ \text{Turnover}$$

FIG. 21.9 Turnover formula. (Derived from Hoffman, P.M. [1984]. *Financial management for nurse managers.* Norwalk, CT: Appleton-Century-Crofts.)

and offerings, find ways to move students through each of the programs more quickly, and find ways to increase the number of students who enter programs. Partnerships with health care delivery organizations are essential.

It is difficult to predict the extent of the nursing shortage moving forward, but this issue needs to be further monitored and addressed. Although nursing and health care organizations are moving forward to address the current shortage, efforts also need to be directed at the development of new practice models and changes in organizational systems, processes, and practices that enhance nurses' ability to successfully perform their work. Changes in health care and nurse reimbursement systems will also need to be addressed.

According to the literature, to truly address and effectively manage the changes needed relative to this current nurse shortage, partnerships will have to be formed among health care organizations, educational programs, professional organizations, and collective bargaining groups. To achieve the desired outcomes, extensive data analysis, strategy design, and policy changes will be required (Buerhaus et al., 2009a; IOM, 2011, 2016).

Current Issues and Trends

Nursing has led the way in navigating a serious nursing shortage through commitment to quality of care. Quality of care is predicated on a stable complement of prepared registered nurses. The frontline nurse manager is the linchpin for ongoing recruitment and retention of both new graduates and career nurses. Although it has been reported in numerous studies that frontline managers are key to successful recruitment and retention of staff and quality of care at the point of service (Leiter et al., 2010), this role is currently more important than ever given that for the first time in history there are four generations of workers at the point of care. According to Kleinman (2004), research studies have consistently indicated leadership behaviors that positively influence staff nurse retention. These behaviors include support

and consideration of staff, high visibility, and willingness to share leadership responsibility. Additional behaviors noted by Laschinger and colleagues (2009) and Leiter and colleagues (2010) include civility and structural empowerment. According to the *AONE Guiding Principles for the Newly Licensed Nurse's Transition Into Practice* (AONE, 2016), nurse managers are identified as the key driver for ensuring the experience of the newly licensed nurse is successful. The success of nurse managers is related to understanding and using transformational leadership skills (Weberg, 2010).

Given the nurse manager's pivotal role, it is imperative that additional focus be given to the role of the nurse manager. Although this role is crucial to staff retention, staff satisfaction, quality of patient care, and achievement of organizational goals, the number of qualified nurse managers in acute care institutions is decreasing (Zastock & Holly, 2010). Factors shown to affect nurse manager retention include aging and retirement, demands related to span of control (number of direct reports), decreased resources, decreased clinical involvement, increased staff diversity, increased coordination across differing nursing units, issues with assistive personnel, changing regulatory requirements, and need for new management skills coupled with increasing complexity of hospitalized patients and widespread use of personal communication devices. Enabling constant communication through cell phones, e-mail, and pagers leads to a sense of being "on" 24 hours a day, 7 days a week (Zastock & Holly, 2010). Clearly these issues need to be addressed to retain the number of nurse managers needed within health care institutions. Mackoff and Triolo (2008a, b) have developed a model of manager engagement that looks at both work entry into the organization and into the nurse manager position as ways to enhance effective communication and organizational support.

The current nursing shortage is driven by a number of factors, such as inadequate supply of students, increased aging of the registered nurse workforce, increased demand for nurses within and outside of health care, and generational differences in nurses related to their intention to stay in nursing (Palumbo et al., 2009). In addition to the shortage of nurses, health care is facing a reduction in all health care workers, both professional and nonprofessional. Nursing care has been strongly linked to both quality and cost, yet organizations are struggling to establish an environment and culture that promotes job satisfaction and retention of nurses (Aiken, 2008). Onboarding of new graduates and experienced staff is a major factor in enhancing staff satisfaction and intent to stay (Park & Jones, 2010). Strategies that improve the work life of older experienced nurses will facilitate them staying in the workforce longer (Palumbo et al., 2009).

It is clear from the literature that considerable work needs to be done within nursing services and health care administration to establish a community/culture of caring and safety/security for nurses and other health care providers. For the most part, people want to be able to go to work each day with a sense of pride and respect for their contributions. In return, they expect to be treated with respect and have a sense of security within the job and work environment. It is projected that this area of study and the application of related strategies will be a major thrust in the future. This approach is consistent with the Magnet Recognition Program® of the ANA, the AHA (2002) report *In Our Hands,* and the IOM (2001) report *Crossing the Quality Chasm.*

It appears that market and political forces have begun to create pressure in an attempt to help mitigate the nursing shortage and its impact on health care. These actions have been directed at the supply end, through funding availability for students who choose nursing as a career, nursing program expansion, and faculty funding. In addition, more efforts are being directed at the retention of experienced bedside nurses and managerial staff. As the full impact of the ACA plays out in the future, demand for unmet health care needs from the 30 to 40 million uninsured Americans may become the more predominant market force. Nurses—and the health care delivery system—will feel the impact.

RESEARCH NOTE

Source
Lartey, S., Cummings, G., & Profetto-McGrath, J. (2014). Interventions that promote retention of experienced registered nurses in health care settings: A systematic review. *Journal of Nursing Management, 22,* 1027–1041.

Purpose
Given the reported nursing shortage at the time of the study, as well as the projected future shortage and the cost associated with recruitment of staff, the authors believed it was important and timely to begin to scientifically evaluate factors that might promote the retention of staff. The aim of the study was to share the effectiveness of strategies for retaining experienced RNs. The study is a systematic review of multiple research studies measuring the effect of nurse retention factors identified in the literature.

Discussion
Nurse retention has been studied over the past several decades as an important strategy to combat the nursing shortage. High turnover of nurses at the organizational level has proven to be costly, adding to the overall cost of health care delivery. Additional research has shown that high nurse turnover may negatively affect patient satisfaction and patient outcomes (Kleinman, 2004). Nurse retention strategies, therefore, need to be further examined as possible solutions to nurse turnover and the nursing shortage.

A systematic review methodology was used to evaluate the effectiveness of specific retention strategies identified in the literature. Criteria for inclusion were also developed. Research included in the review had to be quantitative with clearly defined terms and retention strategies. Studies exploring the retention of new graduate nurses were not considered. Six electronic databases were searched. Website and manual searches of article reference lists were also conducted. Article abstracts were reviewed to further refine inclusion in one of two categories: those that described clear interventions associated with measured retention (Yes) and those that did not (No). Yes articles were further reviewed to ensure inclusion criteria utilizing a specific screening tool (adopted from Estabrooks et al., 2003). At the conclusion of the review, 12 quantitative studies were included for the final analysis. All studies were published after 1988, with the majority published after 2005. Studies were then rated for quality using a Quality Assessment and Validity Tool for Correlational Studies (adapted from Estabrooks et al., 2003).

After rigorous screening and review, the effectiveness of study interventions was explored, finding that 58% of the studies reported an improvement in retention as a direct result of the intervention studied. Five categories of interventions were created: nursing practice modes, teamwork approach, leadership practice, organizational factors, and individual nurse strategies.

RESEARCH NOTE—cont'd

This systematic review found little evidence of the effectiveness of any specific intervention targeting the retention of experienced RNs. It is the position of Lartey and colleagues that retention is influenced by many factors and that the best strategy to improve retention of experienced nurses is a combination of interventions.

Application to Practice

Although this review did not find one specific intervention that significantly improves experienced nurse retention, it is important for nurses and nurse leaders to explore and implement a combination of strategies shown in the literature to correlate with either improved retention or a decrease in turnover. In addition, "this review reveals that a limited number of quality quantitative studies exist that have examined interventions that could be adopted by healthcare settings to help retain highly trained and experienced nurses in the workforce." The authors also recommended that experienced nurses become more articulate and assertive in expressing their needs, which could result in improved retention. Additional research should be conducted that is initiated by and/or includes experienced staff RNs.

It is critical that nursing leaders discover, implement, and share evidence-based solutions for the nursing shortage. As the literature in this review suggests, organizational solutions and models of practice may play a larger role in overall experienced RN retention than individual unit or leader characteristics. The programs explored in the literature of this review need to be considered as part of a package for experienced RN retention. This systematic review adds to the evidence relating to nurse retention and the overall goal to impede the nurse shortage.

CASE STUDY

What are the challenges of nurse retention? A 28-bed telemetry medical surgical unit has recently started to experience turnover on the night shift. At first it was just two nurses over a period of about 3 months, but recently a total of seven nurses have resigned in a 6-month period. In the past few weeks, two resigned and one announced she did not want to come back from maternity leave.

Patient care is reported as good by staff, patients, and physicians. Patient experience scores are stable and good but have room for improvement. Nurse-sensitive patient outcomes are consistently better than the national mean but not yet consistently at the seventy-fifth percentile of the National Database for Nursing Quality Indicators (NDNQI). Other patient outcomes are consistently positive, and the unit was successful in achieving two third-party program accreditations. The hospital overall received Magnet designation in 2010 and maintained that designation to the present time.

Not long after the rash of resignations, employee exit interview data were reviewed by human resources and nursing leadership. Nurses who were leaving were not specific but did comment that they did not feel valued. The new graduates all reported on exit interview that the unit was "not the right fit." The clinical manager was asked for her interpretation. She stated that she did have a nurse or two who could occasionally be "hard on new hires." Nursing leadership also reviewed 90-day probationary performance appraisal data and found that few of the new hire evaluations had been completed over the past several years. Nursing leadership and the clinical manager met to discuss this, and she reported she was "too busy" and would try to do better. The next week the clinical manager resigned, giving 1 month's notice.

The nursing department has a robust succession planning program. Deborah is an experienced nurse, clinical shift supervisor, and critical care assistant nurse manager. She is next in line for a promotion and is quickly selected as the new clinical manager of the unit. She then moves her office to the unit and spends approximately 3 weeks orienting with the departing clinical manager. The chief nursing officer (CNO) immediately begins to receive positive feedback on Deborah's performance from the staff, physicians, and clinical shift supervisors. Deborah meets with her clinical director weekly and formulates her first 90-day plan. Without hesitation, Deborah has determined that nurse retention is the most serious issue facing the unit. Deborah is asked to assess the unit workplace environment and to develop a plan to both recruit new nurses and retain the experienced nurses.

CRITICAL THINKING EXERCISE

Assume that you are placed in Deborah's situation (see Case Study). You are a new manager with great experience behind you. You have the full support of your mentor, your clinical director, and the CNO. HR is a well-developed department with a strong HR business partner. Although you have many pressing priorities, you know that retention is a priority. Analyze the case study by reviewing the processes that might be affecting the retention of the nurses on this unit and what actions you would take in the future. Address the following questions:

1. How would you begin to assess the work environment?
    a. Could one of the following components of the American Association of Critical-Care Nurses' Healthy Work Environment (2016) be deficient?
        i. **Skilled communication** between nurses, leadership, and the interdisciplinary team?
        ii. **True collaboration** between team members?
        iii. **Effective shared decision making**?
        iv. **Appropriate staffing levels**?
        v. **Meaningful recognition** of performance?
        vi. **Authentic leadership**? What role did the previous clinical manager play in the culture of the unit? Who are the formal and informal leaders on the unit?
    b. How would you conduct your assessment? The unit overall? What about each shift?
    c. Do the clinical shift supervisors have any input or ideas about the unit work environment? What other stakeholders would you interview to get more information?
2. How would you assess the nurse staffing levels? Is acuity included and considered? Has there been any new or drastic change?
3. What staff demographic data would you want to obtain and assess, especially as you work to recruit new nurses to fill the vacant positions?
4. When you hire new nurses, what management practices will you put in place to improve the likeliness of retaining them?
5. How would you measure your success? How often will you review metrics and evaluate the plan of action?

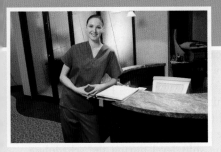

Staffing and Scheduling

M. Lindell Joseph

http://evolve.elsevier.com/Huber/leadership

Staffing and scheduling are perennial concerns for nurses. Nursing is essential in the delivery of health care to society. The American Nurses Association's (ANA) *Nursing's Social Policy Statement* reflects the societal contract for the provision of safe and quality nursing care and services for all people in every health care setting (ANA, 2010). Therefore staffing management is a critical contributor to achieving the societal contract. Staffing management is one of the most crucial yet highly complex and time-consuming activities for nurses and nurse leaders at every level of the health care organization today.

Although nursing's goals remain focused on providing patients the right nursing resources in an effort to achieve the best clinical outcomes for a reasonable cost, the environment in which leaders contend has becoming increasingly complex and chaotic (T.A. Fitzpatrick, personal communication, August 31, 2016). The seminal work of Aydelotte (1973) stated that the aim of staffing is to provide, at a reasonable cost, a standard of nursing care acceptable to its clientele and the nursing staff serving it. This continues and remains as a critical issue affecting the quality, safety, and cost of health care (Aiken et al., 2002, 2003, 2014, 2016; Blegen et al., 1998; Kane et al., 2007a, b; Litvak et al., 2005; Mensik, 2014; Needleman et al., 2002, 2006, 2011; Unruh, 2008). Emerging knowledge suggests that we begin to examine staffing as a complex adaptive system. What is needed is the means to measure and manage the confluence of competing and dynamic interests using a

system of staffing influenced by a changing external environment, data, many interacting agents (work rules, work load, work flow, and financial targets), and individual factors such as schedules, communications, and policies. These forces all influence how one staffs optimally (Gavigan et al., 2016). In addition, the nursing workforce is undergoing transformation and is being affected by generational differences, diversity, new lifestyles, family lives, cultural differences, technological skills, and the need for greater integration of work life into personal life. These traditions, emerging knowledge, and workforce transformations call for the profession of nursing to fulfill its societal contract and envision staffing methodologies to inform the future (Flanders & Carr, 2016; Joseph & Fowler, 2016; National Council of State Boards of Nursing [NCSBN], 2016).

The major goal of staffing management is to provide the right number of nursing staff with the right qualifications to deliver safe, high-quality, and cost-effective nursing care to a group of patients and their families as evidenced by positive clinical outcomes, satisfaction with care, and progression across the care continuum (Eck Birmingham, 2010; T.A. Fitzpatrick, personal communication, August 31, 2016). ANA (2016a) noted that nurses are the largest clinical subgroup in hospitals and a common target for cost containment by reduced nurse hours. However, "appropriate safe nurse staffing and skill mix levels are essential to optimize quality of care" (ANA, 2016a), and this determination is challenging yet essential.

Staffing management is one of the most critical yet highly complex and time-consuming activities for nurse leaders at every level of the health care organization. How well or poorly nursing leaders execute staff management affects the safety and quality of patient care, financial results, and organizational outcomes, such as job satisfaction and retention of registered nurses (RNs). The purpose of this chapter is to assist students, nurses, and nursing leaders at all levels to understand the complex issues associated with staffing management in patient care. A framework for staffing management is presented, and critical components of the staffing management plan are described. New evidence that fosters an understanding of just-in-time data, technology, and algorithmically driven applications are presented for optimal and effective staffing.

DEFINITIONS

Staffing terminology in nursing is multifaceted and often confusing, with a specific set of terms used.

Human resources staffing strategy: A process that determines human resource needs, links to the strategic plan, recruits and selects qualified applicants, and meets the needs of the organization by ensuring that there is appropriate, sufficient, qualified, and competent staff.

Optimizing a staffing strategy: The planning of staffing is predicted by predicting the future state of a system and this is highly dependent on describing its current state. The ability to analyze demand is a powerful means to describe and understand the behavior of the system, and the results of these analyses form the basis of an optimal strategy.

Nurse staffing management plan: A structured approach to the process of identifying and allocating unit-based personnel resources to optimize care needs, quality outcomes, and effectiveness.

Nurse staffing: Nurse staffing refers to the process of identifying and allocating nursing staff on a shift to a patient care area. It typically is a daily operations function. "Appropriate nurse staffing is a match of registered nurse expertise with the needs of the recipient of nursing care services in the context of the practice setting and situation. The provision of appropriate nurse staffing is necessary to reach safe, quality outcomes; it is achieved by dynamic, multifaceted decision-making processes that must take into account a wide range of variables" (ANA, 2012, p. 6).

Skill mix: The range of types and levels of ability and preparation in the workforce. In nursing it is the proportion of direct-care RNs to total direct-care nursing staff; expressed as a percentage of RNs to total nursing staff. For example, a medical surgical patient care unit may have a skill mix of 60% RNs and 40% unlicensed assistive personnel (UAP). A skill mix ratio is typically budgeted for at the patient care unit level but must also be examined at the shift level during the scheduling process.

Staffing pattern: A staffing pattern lists the total number of direct-care staff by skill level scheduled for each day and each shift. For example, for a 12-hour day shift for a pediatric unit on Mondays, there may be six RNs and two UAP for direct care. An additional RN assigned to care for children being admitted or discharged may be scheduled from 3 to 6 PM, during this peak time where children are returning from the operating room or going home.

Scheduling: The process of determining a set number and type of staff for a future time period by assigning individual personnel to work specific hours, days, or shifts and in a specific unit or area over a specified period of time.

Staffing effectiveness: An evaluation of the effect of nurse staffing on quality, patient, financial, and organizational outcomes.

Nurse-to-patient ratio: The RN-to-patient ratio reflects the actual patient care assignment or a state-mandated regulatory requirement for an RN-to-patient assignment. The number of RNs assigned to care for a certain number of patients is stated as a ratio. For example, 1:2 is a common ratio for one RN to care for two patients in an intensive care unit and may be changed based on the condition of the patients.

Skill level: A function of education and competency for the job. In nursing, it is measured by the licensure (e.g., RN, LPN, LVN) or certification (e.g., UAP, NA) of a staff member.

Nursing workload: The patient care plus non-patient care activities (direct and indirect) performed by a nurse and includes the time, complexity of skill mix, patient dependency, and severity of illness (intensity in terms of effort required) of the work a nurse performs within a given period (Morris et al., 2007). It is typically measured by units of service.

Nursing direct-care hours: Direct-care hours are the number of nursing staff hours that are assigned to provide direct care to a patient or groups of patients for a specified period; the most common direct-care staff include the RN, LPN/LVN, and UAP. The hours are typically calculated per patient day or nursing hours per patient day (NHPPD).

Average daily census (ACD): The average number of inpatients on any given day, calculated by dividing the number of patients cared for per day over a certain period by the number of days in a period. It may be an actual ADC or a budgeted ADC.

Admissions, discharges, and transfers (ADT): Refers to the patients who are admitted, discharged, and transferred. The ADT factor has also been referred to as a churn or turnover of patients. ADT is associated with increased care or workload to meet the standard of care for the patient and with safe and effective RN-to-RN communication or handoff regarding the patient's condition and plan of care.

Average length of stay (ALOS): The average number of days each patient is in the hospital. It is determined by dividing the total number of patient days by the total number of admissions (Finkler et al., 2013; Fitzpatrick & Brooks, 2010).

Staffing strategies reflect the organization's mission and annual strategic goals and are executed to meet the staffing management plan of an organization. In hospitals, chief nursing officers are accountable to establish and translate staffing management strategies for the overall patient care areas. The nurse manager who is accountable for a patient care unit or area executes staffing management strategies to yield an optimal health experience and clinical outcomes for patients and their families; a healthy, satisfying work environment; and cost-effective staffing model for the organization. Nursing leaders at all levels are challenged to fairly balance staffing management and adopt technologies that provide the real-time tools to execute, measure, and achieve desired outcomes. Direct-care nurses are involved in the responsibility for coverage of patient care needs, determining patient acuity and intensity, and making patient assignments.

FRAMEWORK FOR STAFFING MANAGEMENT

Nurse staffing can be determined in multiple ways. The three main models of nurse staffing are (1) budget based: Nurse staff are allocated according to nursing

hours per patient day (NHPPD), which is a financial metric; (2) nurse–patient ratio: This is the number of nurses per number of patients or patient days, which is a mathematical workload balancing; and (3) patient acuity (or intensity): Patient characteristics are used to determine staffing needs, which is a determination of the need for care and not based on raw numbers of patients (Mensik, 2014). Staffing management is complex and challenging because of the numerous dependencies and interrelated organizational processes. A conceptual framework provides logic and order to complex processes for administrators and scientists to consider (Edwardson, 2007). A conceptual framework for staffing management is proposed and illustrated in Fig. 22.1.

This conceptual framework is adapted from Donabedian's (1966) framework for the evaluation of quality of care, relating various structures (e.g., hospital characteristics) that affect various processes (e.g., actual staffing) and subsequently influence various outcomes (e.g., patient quality, patient satisfaction, and staff satisfaction). Multiple staffing studies have adapted this framework to organize the variables of interest (Edwardson, 2007; Kane et al., 2007a, b; Mark et al., 2007). In the proposed framework, structures represent the various nursing strategies—both internal and external to the organization—that directly influence an organization's ability to effectively manage processes for staffing. The processes are a series of defined stages with outputs that directly affect subsequent stages of staffing. Finally, the outcomes of staffing management are multidimensional and measured in terms of organizational outcomes including patient, fiscal, and staff outcomes. The staffing management framework is not intended to address all possible variables, but instead is intended to provide a guide for nursing leaders to assess staffing management in their organizations.

STRATEGIES INFLUENCING STAFFING MANAGEMENT

It is important for all nursing leaders to remain current on both the internal and external influences affecting staffing management. Some major influences are (1) professional resources and recommendations, (2) patient acuity and intensity, (3) nursing care delivery models, (4) The Joint Commission regulations, and (5) nurse union agreements.

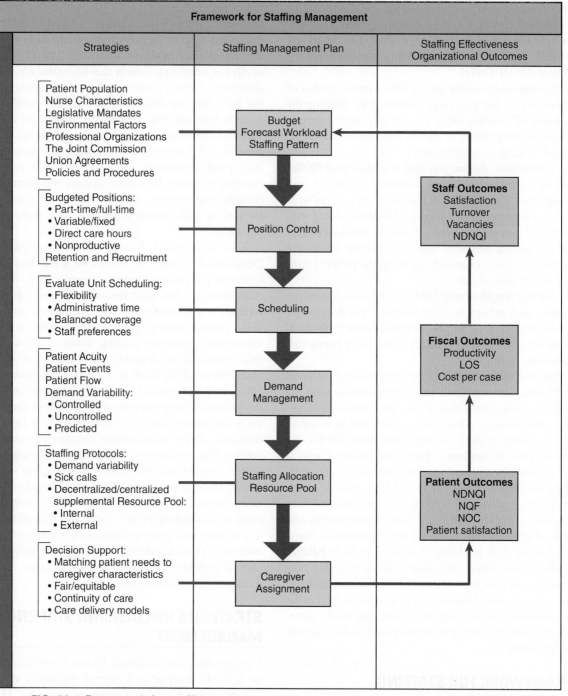

FIG. 22.1 Framework for staffing management. *LOS,* Length of stay; *NDNQI,* National Database of Nursing Quality Indicators; *NOC,* nursing outcomes classification; *NQF,* National Quality Forum.

American Nurses Association's Principles for Nurse Staffing

The ANA is the professional organization that speaks for the profession of nursing and develops and maintains scope and standards of practice and ethics. ANA has published guiding documents that serve as resources to understand the complex staffing issues associated with creating a nursing unit schedule, doing an organization-wide staffing plan, or meeting staffing legislation. *ANA's Principles for Nurse Staffing* (ANA, 2012) identify the major elements needed for achieving optimal nurse staffing. After the document defines appropriate nurse staffing and presents the core components of nurse staffing, it groups the principles in the five areas of (1) the health care consumer, (2) RNs and other staff, (3) organization and workplace culture, (4) the practice environment, and (5) staffing evaluation. ANA emphasized their use of evidence to drive the development of the principles, which serve as guidelines for RN staffing solutions.

In its second edition, ANA (2012) noted that since the initial publication of the original *Principles for Nurse Staffing*, the evidence has grown supporting the link between adequate nurse staffing and better patient outcomes. Under principles related to the practice environment, ANA (2012, p. 10) stated, "Registered nurses should be provided a professional nursing practice environment in which they have control over nursing practice and autonomy in their workplace," and "routine mandatory overtime is an unacceptable solution to achieve appropriate nurse staffing. Policies on length of shifts; management of meal and rest periods; and overtime should be in place to ensure the health and stamina of nurses and prevent fatigue-related errors."

ANA's Principles for Nurse Staffing (ANA, 2012) has been augmented by ANA's advocacy for the proposed Registered Nurse Safe Staffing Act, which would require Medicare-participating hospitals to establish and publically report unit-by-unit staffing plans. These plans would establish adjustable minimum numbers of RNs; have input from RNs; be based on patient numbers and variable intensity of care needed; consider elements such as education, training, and experience levels of RNs and staffing recommendations from professional organizations; ensure RNs are not forced to float to areas where they have no experience; have whistleblower protections; and require public reporting (ANA, n.d.).

American Organization of Nurse Executives

The American Organization of Nurse Executives (AONE), a subsidiary of the American Hospital Association, is a national organization whose mission is to represent nurse leaders. This key leadership group published *Staffing Management and Methods: Tools and Techniques for Nurse Leaders* (AONE, 2000), which presents an introduction to evolving staffing measures. It has a chapter dedicated to staffing management approaches in each of four hospital types: the large academic medical center, an integrated health care system, a small community hospital, and a rural hospital setting. The final chapter discusses how various innovations in information systems support nurse staffing. AONE continues to be involved in advocacy, policy, and issues around nurse staffing.

Staffing Recommendations by Professional Organizations

Adoption of staffing recommendations in clinical settings by relevant professional organizations is endorsed in the *Principles of Nurse Staffing* (ANA, 2012) and frequently seen written into staffing plans. Nursing leaders in specialty practice need to encourage identification and discussion of the position statement or guidelines promulgated by the relevant specialty professional organization during the annual staffing plan review. A number of professional nursing specialty organizations have published position statements for nurse staffing to offer evidence-based guidelines for specialty practice. For example, the National Association of Neonatal Nurses (2014) has a staffing position statement. Recommended staffing ratios are also described in the *Guidelines for Perinatal Care* (American Academy of Pediatrics [AAP] and the American College of Obstetricians and Gynecologists [ACOG], 2012). The ratios delineate care provided for women and newborns in the antepartum, intrapartum, and postpartum settings, as well as the newborn nursery. The Association of Women's Health, Obstetric and Neonatal Nurses (AWHONN, 2010) described the specific staffing recommendations for women in the various stages of normal labor and labor with complications.

Similarly, the Association of periOperative Registered Nurses (AORN, 2014) has a position paper addressing key staffing issues in the operating room (OR), and the Emergency Nurses Association (ENA, 2015) has published recommendations for staffing in emergency departments. The American Academy of Ambulatory

Care Nursing (AAACN, 2005) published an annotated bibliography summarizing the ambulatory nurse staffing literature. Although they do not offer a position paper or guidelines, research continues in staffing models in ambulatory care, where staffing needs to be highly related to the problems, complexity, and needs of patient populations (Haas et al., 2016).

Patient Acuity and Nursing Intensity

Patient acuity is a concept commonly referenced but without specificity or consistency (Habesevich, 2012). In a concept analysis, Brennan and Daly (2008) defined acuity as the severity of the physical and psychological status of the patient, while the intensity attribute of acuity indicates the nursing care needs and the corresponding workload required. Essentially, patient acuity is a measure of the severity of illness of the patient, whereas nursing intensity is the number of nursing hours with associated costs and total time and staff mix of nursing personnel resources consumed by an individual patient during the episode of care under review (Thompson & Diers, 1985; Welton & Dismuke, 2008). According to Unruh and Fottler (2004), estimation of staffing should be considered based on work intensity. The authors defined two indicators for nurse intensity: patient acuity and patient turnover. Because nursing accounts for the highest expenditures in hospitals, Welton and Dismuke (2008) called for a nursing billing model. A billing model based on the intensity of care allows appropriate reimbursement and thus allows for appropriate staffing and a way to capture the direct value of nursing. Despite changes in health care reimbursement structures, nurses still need to demonstrate value, which is determined by a fair and accurate method that shows nurses' work.

Patient classification systems aimed at adjusting staffing for acuity have been plagued with an inability to accurately and reliably measure patient care variability. Further, they have lacked organizational credibility and added documentation burden to the direct-care nurse. The Health Information Technology for Economic and Clinical Health (HITECH) Act, enacted as part of the American Recovery and Reinvestment Act of 2009, was signed into law on February 17, 2009, to promote the adoption and meaningful use of health information technology. This health care reform and meaningful use legislation has catapulted the advancement of health information technology into widespread adoption of electronic medical records (EMR) in the

United States (http://www.hipaasurvivalguide.com/hitech-act-summary.php). These advances additionally offer nursing leaders technologies that leverage the automated patient assessment information entered in the patient EMR by nurses to generate accurate measurements of patient acuity (Eck Birmingham et al., 2011). The electronic patient assessment information is translated not only into workload information at the patient level but also standardized outcomes of care that may assist the nurse and care team in tracking patient progression to the Medicare Severity Diagnosis Related Groups (MS-DRGs) and length of stay (Eck Birmingham, 2010). The objective patient acuity information generated as a by-product of routine clinical documentation allows frontline charge nurses to make informed patient care assignment decisions. From the chief nurse's perspective, new acuity technologies help build the business case for acuity-adjusted staffing for both improved quality and cost outcomes (Dent & Bradshaw, 2012).

Nursing Care Delivery Models

Nursing care delivery models significantly influence staffing management. Care delivery models are the operational mechanisms by which care is actually provided to patients and families. Specific nursing care delivery models are discussed in Chapter 15.

Person (2004) described the four fundamental elements of any nursing care delivery model as follows: (1) nurse/patient relationship and decision making, (2) work allocation and patient assignments, (3) communication among members of the health team, and (4) management of the unit or environment of care. Translating the nursing care delivery model's elements and inherent values to staffing management is a key role for nursing leaders. One common element among care models is the value of the nurse and patient/family relationship. Patient assignment technology offers charge nurses access to real-time data in order to match the right nurse (i.e., competency, expertise) with the right patient and provide continuity of care during an episode of care. A second common trend is the evolving role of the charge nurse as a hospital's frontline leader with responsibility to coordinate patient flow with expert communication among health care team members. Increasingly a charge nurse is appointed as a resource, managing patient flow and supporting novice nurses, and thus does not assume a direct-care assignment.

Three nursing care delivery models of relationship-based care influence staffing management: the synergy model, case management, and the clinical nurse leader (CNL). Relationship-based care (RBC) is a common model used in care delivery (Koloroutis, 2004) that supports achieving recognition by the Magnet Recognition Program® (Guanci & Felgen, 2016).

The Synergy Model for Patient Care was developed by the American Association of Critical-Care Nurses (2016) and is a patient-centered model focused on the needs of the patient, the competencies of the nurse, and the synergy created when the needs and competencies match. Synergy—or optimum patient outcomes—results when the needs and characteristics of the patient and clinical unit or system are matched with a nurse's competencies. Patient assignment technology may assist in defining—and thereby aligning—patient needs with the nurse's abilities, a concept that is central to the model.

Case management is defined by the Case Management Society of America (CMSA) as "a collaborative process of assessment, planning, facilitation, care coordination, evaluation, and advocacy for options and services to meet an individual's and family's comprehensive health needs through communication and available resources to promote quality, cost-effective outcomes" (CMSA, 2016). Case management can be coupled with demand management to best coordinate care and resources to achieve positive patient outcomes, transitions of care coordination, and hospital reimbursement (Pickard & Warner, 2007).

Complementing these models, the American Association of Colleges of Nursing (AACN, 2007) has introduced a new professional nurse role, the clinical nurse leader (CNL), in current care delivery models. The CNL role integrates various aspects of previous roles in nursing, such as the case manager and clinical nurse specialist. The CNL vision statement notes that the CNL champions innovations to improve patient outcomes, ensure quality care, and reduce health care costs. The CNL leads this effort to enhance patient care. The CNL is an advocate for putting best practices into action (AACN, 2007). CNLs are master's prepared and are being used at the unit level to provide knowledge, clinical expertise, and skill in evidence-based practice implementation.

The staffing management plan should reflect the values and roles established in the care delivery model that will ultimately influence patient and organizational outcomes. Both the care delivery model and staffing plan within the context of patient populations in the health care organization are critical to the overall annual strategic plan for nursing.

The Joint Commission Staffing Regulation

Private regulatory agencies such as The Joint Commission (TJC) are widely used by hospitals today to conduct external reviews for quality of care and patient safety. TJC standards include the human resources function of verifying that nurses are qualified and competent to ensure that the hospital determines the qualifications and competencies for staff positions based on its mission, populations, care, treatment, and services. Hospitals must also provide the right number of competent staff members to meet the patients' needs (TJC, 2016). TJC human resources standards clearly outline the complex requirements associated with staffing management and include, but are not limited to, the adequacy of staff numbers, mix of staff levels, licensure, education, certification, experience, and continuing education.

Collective Bargaining Agreements and Staffing Management

Provisions in the ANA Code of Ethics articulate the rights of nurses to address work conditions through collective action (ANA, 2015a). The two largest nursing and health care unions are (1) National Nurses United, a branch of the ANA; and (2) the Service Employees International Union (SEIU) District 1199. Nursing unions are organizations that represent nurses for the purpose of collective bargaining, which has been defined as "the performance of the mutual obligations of the employer and the representative of the employees to meet at reasonable times and confer in good faith with respect to wages, hours, and other terms and conditions of employment . . . such obligation does not compel either party to agree to a proposal or require the making of a concession" (National Labor Relations Board, 2016, Section 8b, paragraph 7d).

In nursing, there is a process of negotiation between the health care employer and the union representatives of nurse employees to reach a written agreement regarding certain terms of employment. The mandatory terms of employment vary widely, but they include subjects such as, but not limited to, wages, hours, overtime, low census call-off procedures, recall, floating, use of UAP, seniority, sick leave, discharges, and leaves of absence. These employment subjects have significant implications for staffing management and vary in their specificity regarding nurse staffing and scheduling. Nursing leaders working in settings with collective bargaining units need to have detailed knowledge of the relevant contractual implications for staffing management and incorporate them into the staffing technologies for compliance monitoring. Collective bargaining environments are compatible with professional nursing practice. Porter (2010) described a successful model of professional practice labor partnerships. Lawson and colleagues (2011) described a program to recognize nurse professional growth and development and its implementation in a collective bargaining environment.

LEADERSHIP AND MANAGEMENT IMPLICATIONS

Legislative Impact on Staffing Management

Evidence has accumulated over the years to indicate that low nurse staffing levels have an adverse effect on patient outcomes and that there is an association between higher levels of experienced RN staffing and lower rates of adverse patient outcomes (ANA, 2016b). This is seen, for example, in the work of Kane and colleagues (2007a, b) and multiple studies by Aiken and colleagues (e.g., Aiken et al., 2002, 2003, 2007, 2014, 2016). At issue are safety, attainment of outcomes, and patient and nurse satisfaction.

Nurse dissatisfaction and concern for adequate staffing to provide quality nursing care to patients and their families arose from hospital cost-reduction initiatives throughout the 1990s. Armed with quality-of-care concerns, nurses began to organize and craft proposed staffing legislation in many states. The historical context that led to quality-of-care concerns continues to affect legislation today. Throughout the 1990s, hospital administrators relied on consultants to implement work redesign to promote patient-focused care as a method of cost reduction. The central labor reduction approach in patient-focused care was reducing the number of RNs and increasing the number of UAP. This approach for decreasing nursing RN skill mix was implemented in a "one size fits all" approach across organizations and often lacked evaluation of the skill mix change and other changes on the quality of care and nurse job satisfaction and retention (Norrish & Rundall, 2001). This was most apparent in California, where a leaner RN skill mix was

tried by Kaiser Permanente Northern California in the early 1990s. Skill mix was reduced from 55% RNs to 30% RNs in 1995 (Robertson & Samuelson, 1996). The changes in skill mix led to widespread real and perceived increases in RN workload, patient safety concerns, and nurse and consumer complaints (Norrish & Rundall, 2001; Seago et al., 2003). This is partially because the workload element of supervision responsibility of the RN for UAPs was not accounted for.

Despite patient complaints and reports of nurse dissatisfaction, little was done until 1999. Only then did the California legislature pass Assembly Bill 394 (AB 394) to mandate minimum nurse staffing ratios and acuity-adjusted staffing. The mandating of minimum nurse-to-patient ratios legislated in California ignited great debate, controversy, and study. Nurse scientists and policy experts have presented compelling arguments against mandated ratios and note that local nursing leaders are in the best position to determine the actual staffing required by the particular patient population (Clarke, 2005). However, the bold action of the California state legislative mandate stimulated focused attention on addressing nurse staffing issues.

Since the late 1990s, state legislation regarding nurse staffing issues has been commonplace, and 14 states have various regulations (ANA, 2016b). There are three general models of state staffing laws: (1) require a nurse-driven staffing committee to create staffing plans, (2) mandate specific nurse-to-patient ratios (California is the only one, but Massachusetts passed a law specific to intensive care units), or (3) require disclosure of staffing levels to the public and/or a regulatory body (ANA, 2016b). ANA supports the first model (nurse-driven staffing plans). Primary areas of focus for state legislation include limiting or precluding mandatory overtime, requiring staffing committees with direct-care nurse input, whistleblower protection, mandated public access to staffing information, and a requirement that implementation of patient acuity methodologies must adjust for staffing workload. State nurse staffing legislation has a significant impact on staffing management through regulation. The economic downturn in 2008 following the end of the George W. Bush administration shifted political attention to jobs and the economy and stalled further legislative nurse staffing mandates. However, the reductions in nursing budgets and challenges of the nurse shortage have resulted in fewer nurses and longer hours of work under the burden of care for sicker patients. The result is compromise to care and exacerbation of the nurse shortage due to the environment of care. ANA (2015b) urged passage of the Registered Nurse Safe Staffing Act (H.R. 2083/S. 1132), national legislation to require all Medicare-participating hospitals to establish RN staffing plans using a committee.

THE STAFFING MANAGEMENT PLAN

The staffing management plan provides the structured processes to identify patient needs and then to deliver the staff resources as efficiently and effectively as possible. An effective plan first focuses on stabilizing the unit core staffing. A staffing pattern, or core coverage, is determined through a forecasted workload and a recommended care standard (e.g., HPPD). Hiring to the associated position complement and developing balanced and filled schedules without holes are essential building blocks for efficient and cost-effective daily resource allocation. Daily staffing allocation requires managing a variable staffing plan, measuring and predicting demand, and then providing balanced workload assignments to ensure that the correct caregivers are best matched to patient needs (ANA, 2012). A successful staffing management plan incorporates the policies of the organization, patient care unit, and nurse population including union and contracting affiliations. Kane and colleagues (2007a, b) suggested that nurse staffing policies should address both patient care units and organizations, such as shift rotation, overtime, full-time/part-time mix, and weekend staffing. The traditional emphasis in staffing planning has been on hospital settings. However, with shifts to primary care as the predominant site of care delivery, staffing planning is equally critical there and in all settings where nurses practice.

Forecasted Workload and Staffing Pattern (Core Coverage)

Forecasting nursing workload for each patient care area is typically carried out at least once a year and as part of the annual budgeting process or when the patient characteristics, services, and/or volume changes. The amount of work performed by a unit is referred to as its *workload*, and workload volume is measured in terms of units of service. The unit of service is specific to the type of unit, such as the number of patients, patient days, deliveries, clinic or home visits, treatments, encounters, or procedures.

Once the unit of service is determined, the number of units of service that will be provided in the coming year must be forecasted. Total patient days are commonly used in inpatient hospital areas. This is calculated by multiplying the average length of stay (ALOS) and the average daily census (ADC). The workload standard commonly used is nursing hours per patient day (NHPPD), although the validity of this measure is disputed. In outpatient settings, balanced workload, patient waiting times, and staff overtime are measures used. There are intensity/acuity tools in ambulatory settings to establish appropriate staffing levels (Liang & Turkcan, 2016).

However, not all patients require the same number of care hours, and the total number of patient days may be inadequate for planning purposes. Finkler and colleagues (2013) suggested using adjusted units of service. For example, a nursing unit can be adjusted using a system for classifying patients, such as a patient acuity system, based on the resources each classification category is expected to use. Segregating patients into acuity classifications allows the staffing pattern to be developed based on the resource requirements of the specific mix of patients forecasted for the unit. Similar calculations can be made in ambulatory and primary care by using a method to classify patients into different categories to estimate the average resource required for patients in each category (Finkler et al., 2013). Nursing's work is complex, and measuring nursing care requires sophisticated methods. Malloch (2015) presented a nursing workforce staffing model that aimed for accurate and reliable determination of the required time for care needs aligned with the appropriate nurse competencies and available time. Clear identification of care needs leads to required staff for nurse interventions, which leads to a matching process and then to value-based outcomes. High variability and intensity (or acuity) are complex patient scheduling and nurse assignment factors in clinic settings (Liang & Turkcan, 2016).

In addition to workload adjustment based on acuity, patient turnover on the unit is an important factor in patient care workload measurement. Reduced length of stay in hospitals or higher patient turnover require intensive periods of higher resources for patient admissions, transfer, discharge, and other 1:1 activities that will affect overall workload, such as when the RN with an unstable patient is off the patient care unit for a test or procedure.

Outside of state-mandated nurse staffing ratios, there is no one gold care standard or recommended process to determine nursing workload. Inconsistent operational definitions and methods of measuring care have been a challenge both for benchmarking resources across organizations and for research analysis related to adequate nursing care (Kane et al., 2007a, b). Therefore each organization must document and provide rationale regarding how staffing standards are determined within each patient care area. Once the annual workload is forecasted, the skill mix required on each shift is determined.

There are two general staffing methods: (1) with *fixed staffing*, staffing is built around a fixed projected maximum workload requirement, and the staffing pattern is based on maximum workload conditions; (2) with *variable staffing*, units are staffed below maximum workload conditions and staff is then supplemented when needed. An effective staffing pattern requires clear definitions for productive time, non-patient care or "nonproductive" time (i.e., benefits time, work for the organization, knowledge-related projects), worked time, paid full-time equivalents (FTEs), and hours per unit of service. In addition, staff roles must be clearly defined as to whether they are fixed or variable. The necessary number of FTEs to yield the desired care standard for the forecasted number of patients in each department must be calculated. In addition, the number of FTEs to replace staff members when they use non-patient care, such as benefit time, must be accounted for in the model. Finkler

and colleagues (2013) described the method for calculating a staffing pattern as follows:

1. Determine the number of paid hours per FTE.
2. Determine the percentage of productive hours to total paid hours.
3. Multiply the number of paid hours per FTE by the percentage of productive hours to find the number of productive hours per FTE.
4. Divide the required care hours by productive hours per FTE to find the required number of FTEs.
5. Divide the required care hours by the number of days per year that the unit has patients to find care hours/day.
6. Divide that result by hours per shift to find the number of person shifts needed per working day.
7. Assign staff by employee type and among required shifts per day.

Box 22.1 refers to an example of variable staff calculation. Table 22.1 provides a sample staffing pattern that

BOX 22.1   Variable Staff Calculation

2080 paid hours per full-time equivalent (FTE)
80% productive hours to total paid hours
2080 × 0.8 = 1664 productive hours per FTE
71,830 care hours ÷ 1664 = 43.17 FTEs
71,830 care hours ÷ 365 days per year = 197 hours of care per day
197 hours of care per day ÷ 8-hour shifts = 24.6 person shifts

TABLE 22.1   Sample Staffing Pattern for a Wednesday for an Intermediate Care Nursery (40 Beds)

Staff Type	7 AM–7 PM Shift	7 PM–7 AM Shift	Skill Mix	Total
Fixed 8-hour day staff				
Nurse manager	1			1
Nurse educator—shared	0.5			0.5
Lactation specialist	1			1
Variable staff				
Charge nurse	1*			1
RN	8	7	75% RN	15
LPN/LVN	0	1	5% LPN	1
UAP	2	2	20% UAP	4
HUC	1	1		2

*Charge nurse on day shift without a direct-care assignment.
HUC, Health unit coordinator; *LPN/LVN*, licensed practical nurse/licensed vocational nurse; *RN*, registered nurse; *UAP*, unlicensed assistive personnel.

includes the final step of allocating total FTEs across shifts and by skill mix. In many patient care areas, the staffing pattern may be different by day of week. For example, a post-surgical unit may have a lower patient census on weekends because of the lack of a surgical schedule, thus a different staffing pattern may apply (McKinley & Cavouras, 2000).

Position Control

Once the staffing pattern for each unit has been established, the next step for safe staffing coverage is to provide a structured measurement and evaluation of position control. Future schedule coverage and adequate staffing first require that unit staff are available to work the needed shifts. Therefore the hours of care requirement on a unit must be converted to the correct number of FTE positions. Position control is the process of providing and measuring the correct FTE, or complement, to adequately staff a given area. Full-time and part-time mix, shift lengths, weekend commitments, and available contingency, or flex staff, are components to be analyzed to produce the ideal complement. The correct complement of full-time and part-time employees requires an understanding of the institution's non-patient care time and other budgeted activities (e.g., new staff orientation, continuing education) that are not included in the direct patient care hours required for the staffing pattern. An ideal measure of nursing staff adequacy considers intensity. A staffing adequacy measure needs to indicate the volume of nurses of a certain skill level needed for a given volume of patients and the given intensity of nursing care required for those patients.

Once position control is established to support the staffing patterns, vacancy and turnover rates need to be managed. A strategy for covering future vacant positions needs to be identified to prevent the use of costly, last-minute staff resources. For example, one organization reported actual cost savings by over-recruiting by 1.0 FTE in the intensive care unit (ICU) area, which resulted in lower use of more expensive contingency and external staff resources (Cipriano & Cutruzzula, 2007). With fiscal and human resources support, managers need to recruit and retain the FTE complement of the full-time and part-time mix needed for each staffing level. This will then increase the available resource pool to respond to higher-than-budgeted patient volume. Filled positions are the foundation for adequate, balanced work schedules.

Scheduling

Best practice for scheduling is a system that is automated, provides data driven targets for core coverage, and engages staff members to participate in working specific shifts, hours, and days in their clinical area. The schedule typically spans a period of 4 to 6 weeks into the future. Staff members are usually hired by the organization with a commitment to work a particular number and type of hours (e.g., 36 hours, rotating day and night shifts). Balanced, flexible, and predictable work schedules are powerful human resource strategies for recruitment and retention, because, for nurses, choice over work schedules is one of the most important aspects of a healthy work environment (MacPhee & Borra, 2012). There is some controversy over the advantages of flexible self-scheduling versus fixed scheduling. Koning (2014) advocated for the freedom to organize shifts worked around nonwork commitments using self-scheduling; Kullberg and colleagues (2016) advocated for fixed scheduling because it lowered overtime.

An assessment of scheduling procedures should include the manager's role and time spent in scheduling. A recent strategy to better align the nurse manager's role to the accountabilities of the role included providing support through technology, staffing office assistants, and having staff members on scheduling committees. The manager's role is accountable for the oversight of the scheduling process and approval of the final complete schedule. The final schedule then needs to be accessible electronically to all staff members, whether at work or remotely from home or on their cell phone. Maintaining a consistent annual schedule of the precise dates for each scheduling request period and for when the final schedule is available is a best practice for staff satisfaction and work–life balance. The managerial role shifts from time-consuming scheduling tasks to a role approving a complete schedule that meets the guidelines of the organization and *ANA's Principles for Nurse Staffing* (ANA, 2012).

The definition or perception of a "complete" schedule is likely as variable as nursing staff member satisfaction with staffing. Direct-care nurses, however, expect when a schedule is electronically submitted to their home computer or cell phone that is it complete. Specifically, the staff expects that RNs, licensed practical nurses/licensed vocational nurses (LPNs/LVNs), UAP, unit secretaries, and key staff are scheduled to their target number for every shift of the schedule. Sharing the patient census and acuity trends by month, day of week, and time of day with the staff will foster mutual understanding in how targets are established. Dialogue about nurse staffing for patient care is credible when it is data driven. Direct-care nurses expect that there will be a clinical expert on every shift and that new graduates are distributed across shifts with their preceptors. These are a few examples of how nursing leaders at all levels may engage staff to develop value statements and data-driven guidelines that serve to explicitly and transparently articulate the organization's scheduling process. Many scheduling committees have developed such documents to reflect values such as a shared commitment to safe and excellent nursing care for all patients and families, support for staff members' pursuit of education leading to a bachelor of science in nursing, fairness in scheduling the major holidays (e.g., Thanksgiving, Christmas, and New Year's), fiscal stewardship to not pre-schedule overtime, guidelines for numbers of staff vacations at one time by role, clarity in self-service dates for scheduling and communication, fatigue management guidelines, and a fair on-call schedule.

Demand Management

Demand management as a discipline focuses on (1) measuring, predicting, and understanding demand for an institution's products and services; and (2) deploying resources and management to ensure that demand is met in the way the consumer's wants and needs are satisfied. For hospitals, a key component of the "product and service" equation is high-quality, safe patient care, with the goal of having the patient leave the hospital with the best care experience, in the shortest amount of time and at the lowest cost care (Pickard & Warner, 2007). McDonough (2013) described an evidence-based optimum staffing method based on patient demand with a focus on work activities. Time observations determined nursing work activities and were then matched to patient demand by hour of day and day of the week.

An often overlooked strategy for creating predictable and cost-effective staffing is the need to staff according to real-time patient information or to make staffing decisions that facilitate individual patients moving through their stay as quickly as possible with high-quality, safe care (throughput or patient flow initiatives). Because most staffing plans staff to average forecasted care levels, periods of higher patient volume and/or acuity levels or peaks may create serious stressors for both patients and nurses. Severe stress occurs with sustained peaks of volume or acuity. Litvak and colleagues (2005) described the following three types of stress intrinsic to daily operations:

- Flow stress, representing the rapid rate of patients presenting for hospital care
- Clinical stress, which is expressed in the variability in type and severity of disease
- Stress caused by competing responsibilities of health care providers

System stress introduced by demand for nurses to care for more or sicker patients has been shown to be a leading cause of adverse patient outcomes (Litvak et al., 2005). When variability is minimized and/or better predicted, a hospital has greater resources for the remaining patient-driven peaks in demand over which it has no control. Effective staffing requires an assessment of demand variability or the required hourly nursing care for each day on each unit. Ways to control variability (and hence decrease peaks and valleys) include better planning for scheduled events such as elective OR procedures, physician vacations or major conferences, seasonal variations, integration to patient flow and bed management systems, better control over bed assignments based on current unit workload, and improved planning for discharges—all of which decrease the demand and stress for nursing resources.

Computer technologies that continuously track and predict demand assist managers with variability analysis and prospective planning for predicted variability. These data support managerial decisions for non-traditional shorter shifts for the care areas that have high requirements at select predictable portions of the day. Predictive modeling can forecast unplanned patient and staff events, such as admissions by day of week and unplanned sick calls. Several examples driven by data include higher cesarean section rates in a labor and delivery unit may necessitate two RNs in the OR; infant births that are higher in the evening than during the day may require a shift of resources from days to evenings; or late-afternoon patient transfers from the recovery room after neurosurgery on Tuesdays and Thursdays may require an increase in RN staff for those days and specific hours in a neurosurgical ICU.

Pickard and Warner (2007) outlined the essential components for effective demand management as the following 10 principles:

1. Being based on patient outcomes (how well he or she is progressing)
2. Being focused on the individual patient
3. Incorporating progress goals for each patient throughout his or her stay with which actual progress may be compared
4. Continuously measuring progress in real time so that decisions can be made as the patient's needs change (rather than once a shift or once a day, which inherently bases decisions on information that is typically 8 to 16 hours old)
5. Being projected into the near future (several days ahead) to allow time for optimal staffing decisions to be made while there is still time for numerous choices among available caregivers and cost-effective options
6. Being able to be embedded in a decision support system
7. Being acceptable to all stakeholders, especially administration and finance, to avoid organizational polarity
8. Producing a need for care in terms of not only quantity and skill but also the caregiver attributes necessary to provide optimal care for the patient
9. Using outcomes-driven acuity system based on an established taxonomy for assessing and documenting patient care on outcomes
10. Incorporating all presently and planned electronically available data to reduce nursing time in data gathering and provide as much real-time, valid data as possible.

"Incorporating these elements is not a simple task, but doing so offers significant advantages and benefits. By focusing on the individual patient, with individual outcome progress goals for each patient, hospitals can achieve results not previously addressed with traditional models" (Pickard & Warner, 2007, p. 3). In addition, this allows organizations to be informed and responsive when a select population of patients typically cared for in one location is housed in a new location. These results include (1) best-practice staffing protocols based on what is called "true (outcomes-oriented) demand" and the optimal staffing levels to move a patient through each phase of his or her stay as quickly as possible, (2) early identification of patients who are not moving through their hospital stay as planned, and (3) improved near-term projection and prediction of staffing needs.

Staffing Allocation and Resource Pool

Even with the best planning and most accurate prediction of supply and demand, uncontrolled events such as unexpected high demand and sick calls are intrinsic to the health care environment. Key to effective staffing are protocols and processes for daily staffing decision support that are aligned with a budget-sensitive variable staffing plan. In a decentralized model, individual department managers and directors are responsible for daily staffing allocation. Units with decentralized staffing are typically units in which volume and/or acuity may be most unpredictable and the nursing competencies are unique to that area (e.g., emergency department, labor and delivery, critical care). However, a decentralized model places a higher level of staffing responsibility on managers, which may take them away from other more strategic responsibilities.

In contrast, centralized staffing is filtered through a central staffing office, which maintains responsibility for ensuring adequate staffing for multiple units. Centralized staffing offers the benefit of being able to view supply and demand from an enterprise perspective. With patient acuity, nursing competencies, and available staff viewed across multiple units, staffing resources can be optimized by increasing staff in one area and reducing staff in another to accommodate variable patient demand. Staffing protocols for obtaining supplemental staff can be standardized, such as procedures for using internal staff, per diems, and external sources (e.g., travelers and agency). The staffing office can relieve nurse managers and/or charges nurses of the time-consuming administrative task of responding to sick calls and obtaining supplemental staff. In addition, the central staffing office provides a command center with protocols and information to manage disasters in which staff must be quickly obtained and deployed.

The downside to relying solely on a centralized staffing office is that it can become too remote from the unit, thus losing some of the intelligence that may be considered when making staffing decisions (Lauw & Gares, 2005). Policies and procedures clearly define the roles and responsibilities and communication among areas. But as with any of these staffing models, the key to eliminating chaotic, last-minute staffing decisions is to adopt predictive tools and move more of the staffing decisions to the near future or the next 2 to 4 days (Pickard & Warner, 2007). Assessment and analysis of staffing needs in the near future provide more available options, including more competent staff, at optimal costs.

Computerized staffing systems play a pivotal role in providing what is described as a "single version of the truth" and offering decision support such as staffing variances across units, workload indicators, employee competencies, and decision costs. Information for staffing decisions must be readily available and accurate. Staffing systems serve as a communication tool for all staffing "stakeholders," including employees, unit managers, centralized staffing office, and executives. Staffing systems also offer automated open-shift management, which posts open shifts electronically to qualified staff. Protocols direct which personnel are the best qualified and the most cost effective to fill needed shifts. The staffing system measures and reports the staffing management performance at both unit and organization levels, providing staffing effectiveness data for the organization.

Access to nurses outside the unit to cover transient shortages is critical to meet last-minute, unplanned nurse shortages, such as sick calls, and high patient demand. Supplemental staffing resources—frequently referred to as the *staffing pool*—are defined as a group of nurses who supplement the core unit staffing. This includes per diem nurses, float pool nurses, part-time nurses desiring additional hours, seasonal nurses, agency nurses, and traveling nurses. The scope of clinical competency, pay rates, and contractual arrangements varies among these internal and external pools of nurses as well. For example, select nurses may be competent to work on all of the adult medical–surgical units, whereas other specialty nurses may be competent to work in several areas, such as perioperative practice sites, or only one area, such as labor and delivery, the emergency department, or the dialysis unit.

Supplemental staffing resource guidelines need to be established to direct the use of additional resources detailing the data for decision making and algorithms for staffing. These guidelines are designed to prevent depletion of supplemental resources for core staff coverage and instead to reserve them for unexpected intervals of high acuity or transient shortages. For example, a guideline may direct the use of a part-time nurse who has signed up to work extra shifts to fill a sick call, then to use a supplemental float pool nurse, and finally to use an external agency nurse if previous resources are unavailable. The option for overtime is also a consideration based on policy regarding the fatigue associated with excessive hours in a day or days worked in a row and cost. The costs associated with each resource progression are then inherently built into the staffing decision model. Additional strategies for covering long-term family medical leaves are also needed to meet core coverage. Strategies for covering these longer-term shortages are critical, otherwise a manager is depleting the resource pools intended for last-minute and transient shortages.

Operational metrics for the supplemental resource pool are not only defined for daily staffing allocation but also may be defined during the scheduling stage. The operational total nurse vacancy rate for scheduling purposes is defined as all budgeted nurse positions that are vacant during the scheduling period, including the unfilled or vacant positions and positions for which nurses are on short-term or long-term leaves of absence (e.g., Family and Medical Leave Act [FMLA], workers' compensation). For example, if a unit has an operational RN vacancy rate of 5% to 10%, it may be approved to cover the shortage with part-time nurses working additional shifts and possibly overtime but would not be approved for agency nurses. Alternatively, a unit with a 22% operational RN vacancy rate may be approved for longer-term contracted higher labor expense (e.g., travelers). Defining operational vacancy rates and incremental resource actions are important aspects of consistently managing staff shortages and ensuring a standard of care delivery. As such, protocols driven by operational vacancy rates generate consistency in how higher labor costs are aligned with the greatest need. In addition, wages, benefits, transfers, and work policies of supplemental internal float pools should be carefully designed so that the stability of unit-based core nursing staff is not compromised.

Fitzpatrick and Brooks (2010) and Gavigan and colleagues (2016) called for the optimization of human capital as a staffing consideration. These authors believe that there is a need to build a scaffolding structure to allow for optimal mathematical optimization for best staffing solutions. Box 22.2 lists criteria to optimize modeling of staffing for best solutions.

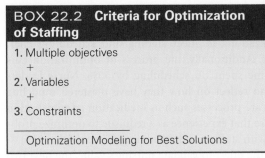

From Fitzpatrick, T., & Brooks, B. (2010). The nurse leader as a logistician: Optimizing human capital. *Journal of Nursing Administration, 40*(2), 69–74.

Patient Assignments

Nurse managers are responsible not only for forthcoming schedules and immediate staffing but also for ensuring that the patient care assignments reflect appropriate use of personnel considering scope of practice, competencies, patient needs, and complexity of care. Patient assignment in hospitals is defined as the task of assigning the scheduled staff to specific patients for the shift duration. Nurse managers in hospitals typically delegate assignment making to the charge nurse in the patient care area. The charge nurse is responsible for matching the qualified caregivers to meet the patients' needs and for providing a balanced workload across caregivers. Often the nursing care delivery model articulates the value of nurse-to-patient continuity across time. A balanced workload enables nurses to provide reasonable equity in nursing care delivery to patients and their families. In addition, the staff members expect the charge nurse to create equitable assignments as a valued measure of fairness in workload distribution. Many organizations require an annual charge nurse competency review and peer feedback demonstrating effective assignment making.

In the staffing management framework, the patient assignment is the point at which individual patients are linked with individual nurses. Welton (2010) identified this as a critical new level of analysis to examine the relationship between staffing and clinical quality and cost that may better inform operational decision making.

ORGANIZATIONAL OUTCOMES

Staffing Effectiveness

ANA says that identifying and maintaining the appropriate number and mix of nursing staff are central to the provision of quality care (ANA, 2016b). Optimal nurse staffing is appropriate to patients' needs. Hospital organizations examine the relationships between staffing and nurse-sensitive outcomes to meet TJC staffing effectiveness requirements showing that there is the appropriate number, competency, and skill mix of staff in relation to the provision of needed care and treatment. However, staffing for effectiveness, including cost effectiveness, is highly complex and a critical issue for nurse leaders.

The Staffing Evidence on Quality

The link between nurse staffing and quality of care is evidence based and long-standing. Better RN staffing has been shown to reduce patient mortality, enhance outcomes, and improve nurse satisfaction (Mensik, 2014). Over a decade of rigorous studies and a summary of current research conducted by the Ruckelshaus Center at the University of Washington concluded that "fewer patients per nurse or more nursing hours per patient day is associated with fewer adverse outcomes—in particular mortality, failure to rescue, and some specific adverse events among surgical patients" (Mitchell, 2008, p. 30). Comprehensive reviews of staffing evidence and sentinel works are available (Aiken et al., 2002, 2003, 2014; Blegen et al., 1998; Needleman et al., 2002, 2006, 2011; Unruh, 2008). These studies and a meta-analysis by Kane and colleagues (2007a, b) demonstrated the strong evidence linking inadequate staffing with adverse events and failure to rescue. Frith and colleagues (2010) found that higher RN staffing was associated with a reduced length of stay (LOS) among community hospitals. These findings suggest the direct fiscal impact that nurses have on hospital margin today (Bogue, 2012). A body of research over at least the past decade has shown that sufficient nurse staffing levels and favorable work environments function to facilitate nurses' effectiveness as a surveillance system. Sufficient numbers of RNs are necessary to manage complex patient care needs and identify and intervene when something goes wrong (McHugh et al., 2016). Because research continues to confirm the many associations of nurse staffing with outcomes, innovative and technology-based strategies are being employed to more precisely manage staffing for quality outcomes.

Hospitals routinely employ supplemental nurses to provide additional resources to cover transient shortages. However, little is known about this nurse workforce and its relationship to quality of care. Aiken and colleagues (2007) examined the characteristics of supplemental nurses and the relationships of the supplemental staff to nurse outcomes and adverse events. Their findings suggested that widely held negative perceptions of temporary nurses may be unfounded. However, the effect on the organization's culture is unknown but suspected to be disruptive. The employment patterns of nurses and their effect on cost and quality is an important area needing further study.

Nurse leaders at all levels are called to action to incorporate relevant scientific findings in staffing administrative policy and practice and to lead the evaluation of all innovations in care delivery. Balancing these decisions with organizational fiscal constraints and conducting cost-effectiveness analyses are the current challenges for organizations and nurse leaders.

CURRENT ISSUES AND TRENDS

There is an increasing call to use technology and innovate with scheduling. Fitzpatrick (2015) suggested nurses reflect on the airline industry and how they have managed to coordinate flights, maintenance, staggering across different time zones, and weather conditions. These industries use logistics science and a form of mathematical modeling called optimization to solve scheduling problems. Logistic science offers new insights in planning and deployment of clinical workers because it recognizes the complexities and interconnectedness of the systems and processes involved in scheduling and deploying nurses (Joseph & Fowler, 2016).

Fitzpatrick (2015) illustrated how the field of nursing has started to transition from standardized, computerized scheduling to the use of sophisticated, algorithmically driven applications like how the airline industry used logistics science and a form of mathematical modeling called optimization to solve scheduling problems. To ensure optimization of staffing modeling, the author calls for three key variables: (1) business objectives such as staffing costs and ensuring adequate coverage, (2) decision variables such as skill mix and cost differences, and (3) business constraints such as vacancy rates, work rules (e.g., weekend requirement), and cultural issues such as being off for Mother's Day. The use of optimization can move decision making from "what-if" to "what is the best" solution. When all these factors are considered, there is more precise modeling of staffing to actual demands, allowing health care organizations to meet staffing and scheduling challenges. Additionally, the process of optimization cuts the time spent on scheduling by 50%. Nurse leaders need to reflect on how they have mastered modeling with care processes such as medication administration and use that experience as a requisite to optimize problems with staffing and scheduling (Fitzpatrick, 2015).

In the quest to validate nursing's value, the next two discussions illustrate good examples of how the appropriate data can guide administrators with appropriate decision making for staffing. Pappas and colleagues (2015) called for greater precision with staffing. The authors demonstrated that approaches to minimize patient risks are needed to avoid unwanted clinical and subsequent negative financial outcome. The authors advocated for staffing models that are based on unit-specific data that incorporate the nurse's view of the amount of surveillance to prevent hospital-acquired harm and the associated costs.

Pruinelli and colleagues (2016) stated that the emergence of Big Data for data analytics is poised to influence the value of nurses' work. Their recent article advocates for the use of the nursing management minimum data set (NMMDS) in conjunction with staffing systems in electronic health systems. The NMMDS is an evidence-based tool that defines and measures the context of care within and across all enterprise settings. Use of the NMMDS provides data about variables affecting the delivery of timely, cost-effective care. This knowledge is critical to maintain clinical and operational excellence. The authors advocated for integration of data from multiple sources because this helps nurse leaders to balance workloads, thus improving patient outcomes and nurse satisfaction. Technology that integrates elements of the NMMDS for staffing or other complex management decisions can return valuable hours to the nurse leaders. This is the emergence of Big Data for data analytics.

A health care system in Oregon underwent a transformation to define and implement staffing and scheduling by using software to optimize scheduling. The criteria included a simple and easy-to-use network, remote and mobile access, integration of personal calendars, and time and attendance. Intelligence included definitions, predictive staffing, acuity-based scheduling, and patient acuity. Customization included staffing based on skill mix, with customization of reports, shifts, and dashboards. Bonus features were ease of build, maintenance, upgrades, and successful integration.

The Magnet Recognition Program® continues to be a driver of current staffing trends. For more than 20 years, Magnet designation has been associated with healthier work environments (better staffing—excluding California, where there is a state-mandated ratio; lower burnout; lower turnover; and improved RN–MD collaboration) (Kelly et al., 2011) and higher-quality patient care. Achieving Magnet designation has been increasingly associated with quality. It is now incorporated in the scoring for *U.S. News & World Report*'s Best Hospitals in America Honor Roll and earns full credit for Safe Practice Standard #9 Nursing Workforce in the Leapfrog Hospital Survey, which scores hospitals on their commitment to staffing with highly trained nurses. Given the advent of value-based purchasing (VBP) and the Centers for Medicare & Medicaid Services (CMS) provision 1533-F, health care leaders have been incentivized to focus on improving care processes. CMS provides health care coverage for 80 million Americans via Medicaid, Medicare, and state children's programs and represents the largest payer in the world, administering more than $800 billion in benefits annually. Many of the clinical processes and patient satisfaction measures under VBP are directly affected by the quality and quantity of nursing care, and the outcomes will have a significant impact on the key metrics that will drive hospital reimbursements (Bogue, 2012).

Since CMS provision 1533-F became effective on October 1, 2008, hospitals are not being reimbursed for hospital-acquired conditions (HACs). These are conditions such as skin pressure ulcers, urinary tract infections, ventilator-acquired pneumonia, and falls with injury that occurred within the hospital stay and were not present on admission (POA). Among the 14 HACs in the provision, at least nine of the conditions are sensitive to nursing care intervention. Thus hospitals have new financial incentives to support both nursing education and appropriate staffing to prevent HACs, reduce costs, and increase reimbursement. In addition, the Patient Protection and Affordable Care Act (ACA) mandates 2% of hospitals' Medicare payment will be at risk under value-based payments in 2017. Penalties for certain 30-day admissions began in 2012. The LOS and readmissions financial penalties are the most compelling incentives for hospitals to support the appropriate amount of nursing care that is of high quality because of the known positive effect of nursing care and coordination on patients' transitions of care and acute care LOS (Frith et al., 2010). The nurse's inherent role in discharge planning with the interdisciplinary team, linkages to community services, and effective medication, symptom, and disease management teaching in all care settings is becoming increasingly important to organizational outcomes.

There are national policy initiatives to identify and make visible nursing care in the US health care reimbursement system. It has long been known that nursing care historically has been bundled within the "room and board" hospital charges, which do not capture the variability in nursing care costs. Given the variability in nursing care intensity and cost of nurse staffing, this traditional costing system has resulted in cost compression and distortion in the inpatient prospective payment system (Dalton, 2007). A proposed solution separates nursing care from the room and board charges and accounts for this care as a variable, direct cost within the billing system based on actual nursing time delivered to patients (Welton & Harris, 2007; Welton et al., 2006). Finkler and colleagues (2013) describe this as nursing as a revenue center and explain the use of variable billing. Even in a bundled payment system, nurses need both cost and productivity data to better manage care for both efficiency and effectiveness. Welton (2010) suggested a new value-based nursing care model, including (1) allocating nursing cost and intensity to each patient, (2) new metrics that link nursing-specific outcomes to individual patients, and (3) moving the focus from staffing to the assignment of caregivers to individual patients. Simpson (2012) further called to action the adoption of technology at the point of care to achieve value-based nursing care.

These current issues in health care policy raise the visibility and importance of nursing care in society and create a climate to advocate for safe, cost-effective, high-quality nursing care for all. Current issues and trends in staffing and scheduling demonstrate that nursing has transformed its thinking and approaches based on the evolving science of systems theory, technology, advanced mathematics, and logistics science—as well as human capital and social theory—to optimize its staffing needs.

RESEARCH NOTE

Source
Maloney, S., Fencl, J.L., & Hardin, S.R. (2015). Is nursing care missed? A comparative study of three North Carolina hospitals. *MEDSURG Nursing, 24*(4), 229–235.

Purpose
The purpose of this article is to describe and discuss the results of survey measuring frequency, types, and reasons for missed care at three acute care hospitals in North Carolina. The results were compared with the findings of the 10-hospital MISSCARE survey done in the Midwest.

Discussion
Previous research identified that increased RN staffing improved patient outcomes and quality of care. Conversely, inadequate RN staffing had adverse effects such as increased absenteeism and turnover. Lower patient satisfaction scores and increased falls and infections were associated with missed care, which is nursing care that is omitted or delayed. One study in the Midwest showed the significance and prevalence of missed care. Legislation of staffing ratios, staffing levels, and overtime varies among states. The MISSCARE study was done in the Midwest, revealing frequencies, types, and reasons for missed care and providing data for quality improvement efforts. The researchers conducted the study in a state not previously included in studies. Nursing staff from 16 inpatient units of three North Carolina acute care hospitals (205 of 750; 27.3%) completed the MISSCARE survey. Response choices were coded as care missed or care not missed. Of 24 types of missed care, the five most frequent were unexpected rise in volume or acuity, inadequate number of staff, inadequate assistive/clerical help, heavy admission/discharges, and medications not available. Reasons, types, and frequencies were similar among hospitals and consistent with the Midwest study. Percentages of missed care were quite high for several types, such as ambulation (missed frequently or occasionally at 76.7%).

Application to Practice
Certain types of care are missed frequently. Consistent findings occurred across both a previous study and the present study, making missed care a significant and prevalent finding. There is a potential for serious ramification for patients. Because the negative impact of missed care has been documented in the literature, the findings can be applied to practice by targeting interventions to reduce missed care. Developing patient care improvement strategies can be based on identifying problem areas using the MISSCARE survey. Patient satisfaction may also improve with targeted interventions, such as timely response to call lights.

CASE STUDY

Behavioral health services are scarce in many places, and nurses face the challenge of managing patients with dual physical health and behavioral health issues. Often this occurs within medical–surgical units. In response to staff feedback and escalating workplace violence events, an inter-professional team developed and implemented a pilot model of care where medical patients who were exhibiting specific disruptive behaviors would be cohorted on one unit, 4 Wellness.

Baseline data included increased calls to security for assistance and number of staff injuries. Included in this pilot was extensive education and training, environmental safety initiatives including the presence of security 24/7, and a new staffing model to support the challenges of caring for this population. This unit also contained a medical stabilization unit for alcohol and opiate withdrawal (STEPS Program). Keeping both of these populations in mind, the nursing leaders developed a staffing plan that ensured the delivery of safe patient care. The inter-professional team—composed of nursing, process management, psychiatry, security, and finance—created a continuous cycle of improvement for this population. Incorporating a PDSA (Plan, Do, Study, Act) approach and a structural tension model, a common vison was created and a greater goal for the unit was established: "To create an environment to safely provide care to medical patients who are exhibiting inappropriate behaviors, by staff who have demonstrated competency in this patient population."

Upon review of the literature there were a few similar models to provide a framework for replication. They served as a guide to develop this unique medical model for patients with enhanced psychosocial needs. There was a blended staffing ratio dependent on the number of STEPS patients and behavioral patients assigned to each nurse. No nurse would ever have more than two behavioral patients at any given time. Based on the number of nurses needed to safely staff this unit, recommended hours per patient day were developed with nursing

CASE STUDY—cont'd

finance partners. Appropriate staffing levels were reviewed on a daily basis, taking into consideration the number of STEPS patients, the number and acuity of medical/behavioral patients, and the need for 1:1 behavioral observation.

A core staffing grid was developed along with a staffing matrix to support the unique staffing needs on this pilot unit based on budgeted average daily census, historical data, and skill mix. When the budget was built with the finance team, established benchmark data were used consistent with the overall nursing budgetary processes. Rather than select staff to work on this unit,

nurses were asked to self-select if they had an interest in caring for this patient population. Financial incentives and increased educational support were offered to nursing and nursing support staff. An online self-scheduling program was used that factored in appropriate staffing levels and skill mix. To ensure safe staffing, the manager has the ability to post opportunities and use supplemental staffing.

Source
AtlantiCare Regional Medical Center (used with permission Dr. Robyn Begely and Ms. Elizabeth Readeau).

CRITICAL THINKING EXERCISE

Geneva Guadalupe is a new manager on the busiest medical and surgical unit in a tertiary hospital. There are 39 beds on 9 Tower, which has a high volume of diabetes patients. She is excited to improve the quality and outcomes on this unit. During her interview, she learned that under the previous leadership the quality was deteriorating, as reflected in Hospital Consumer Assessment of Healthcare Providers and Systems (HCHAPS) scores and absenteeism and turnover rates. It was costing the unit between $42,000 to $65,000 to replace a nurse.

While making rounds, Nurse Guadalupe observed complaints about missed nursing care from all shifts and decided to make staff accountable for ensuring that patient care is completed. She asked a CNL to monitor the types of patient care activities that were being omitted. After 1 week, the CNL stated that it was difficult to

make that determination because everyone had a different opinion on which interventions were being omitted. Additionally, staffing was an issue. The manager's initial response was, "What's wrong with staffing? Why would you blame staffing for omitting patient care?"

1. What is your first approach to showing a link between missed nursing care and staffing?
2. What questions could you pose to frontline nurses to understand how their staffing experience related to missed care?
3. Whom will you engage institutionally to understand the issue fully? Why them?
4. Which data elements may be required to build a case for staffing and missed nursing care?
5. What ideas would you propose to administration to reverse the financial effects and improve HCHAPS scores?

Budgeting, Productivity, and Costing Out Nursing

Linda B. Talley, Diane H. Thorgrimson

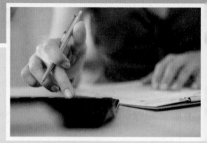

ℯ http://evolve.elsevier.com/Huber/leadership

National Health Expenditures (NHEs) are a measure of spending for health care in the United States. In 1998 NHEs exceeded $1 trillion for the first time. By 2020, NHEs are projected to increase to $4.6 trillion (Keehan et al., 2011). Considered from another perspective, this amount of money in 1998 represented 13.1% of the gross domestic product (GDP), the value of all the goods and services produced in the United States in 1 year. In 2014 NHEs represented 17.5% of the GDP. Health care spending is projected to increase at a rate of 5.8% per year for the next 10 years. By 2024, NHEs are projected to represent 19.6% of the GDP (Centers for Medicare & Medicaid Services [CMS], 2015).

The magnitude of these expenditure increases—along with the changes in practice related to the Affordable Care Act—emphasizes that nurses, as members of the largest health care profession, need to understand the implications of these data for clinical practice. Understanding budgeting, productivity, and costing out nursing and relating that knowledge to the management of professional nursing is a leadership skill that will serve the nursing profession in an era of accelerating health care expenditures.

BACKGROUND

All nurses will be involved in budgeting for nursing services in different ways and to different degrees. Staff nurses in particular often report, "I just want to take

care of patients—don't bother me with money matters." Some nurse administrators have said, "Show me your budget, and I will tell you your values." Nurses at all levels need to understand that "finance is not a dirty word" (Sorbello, 2008). Given that health care resources are limited, nurses do compete for these resources and need to understand how to manage financial resources responsibly. In many organizations, staff nurses are expected to be aware of their unit's financial performance and use this knowledge to guide their decision making in terms of resource allocation. Staff nurses' involvement is essential to the ability to contain costs at the unit level because they make many decisions about supply and resource use.

Budgeting is a major aspect of an organization's or unit's planning processes. A budget is a plan that is specified in dollar amounts. This plan becomes a guiding framework for organizational activities. It conveys management's intentions and financial expectations regarding revenues and expenditures. An organization-level budget compares expected revenues with expected expenses to forecast profit (margin) or loss (deficit). Budgeting is a cyclical process of planning, implementing, and evaluating.

Budgets are designed to be planning documents, but one often hears the statement "we don't have the budget for that" or "the budget won't allow it." It is crucial to understand that the budget is a tool created by humans. To be useful, it must be flexible and have processes in place to modify it when necessary. Individuals and organizations should not become so constrained by the approved budget that they hesitate to take appropriate

Photo used with permission from Dutko/Getty Images.

actions or make appropriate decisions that vary from, or were unanticipated in, the budget process.

DEFINITIONS

A **budget** is defined as a written financial plan aimed at controlling the allocation of resources. It functions as both a planning instrument and an evaluation tool useful for financial management. A budget is used to manage programs, plan for goal accomplishment, measure change, and control costs.

Expenses are defined as the costs or prices of activities undertaken in the organization's operations.

Revenue is defined as income or amounts owed for purchased services or goods. *Total operating expenses* are the result of summing the costs of all resources (e.g., labor, patient consumable supplies, small medical equipment, utilities, office supplies, and other related miscellaneous fees and materials) used to produce services.

Total operating revenues are the result of multiplying the volume of services provided by the charges (rate) for the services.

Income (or profit) is the excess of revenues over expenses, or revenues minus expenses.

A **variance** is the difference between the budgeted and the actual amounts. A variance may be favorable or unfavorable relative to the budget amount. A budget developed to provide resources for direct patient care, such as nursing budgets, will use actual volumes (units of service) to interpret favorable or unfavorable variances.

There are three main types of organizational budgets, as follows:

1. *Capital budget:* This budget is the plan for the purchase of major equipment or assets. Each organization will define its own capital dollar threshold limits.
2. *Operating budget:* The operating budget is the annual plan for the unit's or organization's daily functioning revenue and expenses for a single year. For nursing units, this is a plan that lays out what it is going to cost to run the unit in the coming year. It includes such things as consumable and nonconsumable supplies, small medical equipment, telephones, postage, paper, personal electronic devices for staff, printers, and copy machines. In addition, there may be a cost allocation for such things as heat, light, and housekeeping. Inflation projections for goods need to be factored into each year's budget.
3. *Personnel budget:* This is the staffing budget of the cost center (department or unit). It may be developed as part of the operating budget, or it may stand alone. Personnel budgets must include expenses related to productive and nonproductive time as well as projected replacement time. Use of premium pay—to include but not be limited to overtime and shift differential—is to be included in all personnel budgets. A good personnel budget contains fiscal resources to flex up staffing during periods of high inpatient census and/or patient volumes.

THE BUDGET PROCESS

Each institution establishes standard budgetary formats and processes. Because employees of a cost center will have to implement the budget decision, it is imperative that they have input in the process. This is often done in staff meetings where the manager uses the opportunity to teach about the process, present financial and volume data, and solicit staff input. Nursing and administrative leadership rounds also provide a forum for staff nurses to share their observations and recommendations regarding the many factors that affect resource use related to direct patient care on their unit and/or across the organization. Such factors may include quality and safety concerns, patient acuity, volumes, staffing, patient throughput, average length of stay, and patient experience.

The annual budgeting cycle process is complex and requires the completion of several related documents. It may be compared with income tax preparation, where an individual gathers all the necessary data and receipts, completes all of the required forms, and submits them to the Internal Revenue Service. Like tax preparation, the budget process may require multiple revisions.

A typical budget process follows the priorities identified in the organization's strategic plan and supports the organization's mission and vision. This is done to ensure that resources are appropriately aligned with key organizational initiatives. The budget process consists of three periods:

1. *Preparation:* As a beginning point, the manager reviews the organization's strategic plan and the last year's budget for the cost center (including budget and current year projected). The strategic plan will aid in writing budget justifications and links requests to organizational priorities. The prior year's budget for the cost center will help the manager to identify

volume projections and changes in the past year and potential changes in the coming year. In concert with nursing leadership, the organization's finance staff and other members of the leadership team will often establish the next year's budgeted volumes through analysis of relative internal and external environmental factors and activity. Such analysis includes input from key departments such as strategy, managed care, case management, and reimbursement. Hospitals that employ physicians will also include physicians in budget volume projection work. In the hospital, patient days and adjusted patient days are the usual volume measurement. For example, if the manager of a surgical unit knows that two general surgeons are being recruited to the organization, it is reasonable to project an increase in patient days. With a review of the previous year's data, an informed projection can be made about the increase that can be anticipated. Similarly, the manager may be aware of factors that will decrease the volume of patient days, such as a new hospital being built nearby. In ambulatory care, the volume unit of measurement is clinic visits. If a new nurse practitioner is being hired, how will that affect the volume of visits projected? Volume measurements, or units of service, are determined by the type of service provided. For example, in the operating room (OR), budgets are based on resources required for OR minutes; in an outpatient setting, budgets are based on resources required for a patient visit.

2. *Completing the forms:* Typically, the manager will have access to sophisticated budget software for use in preparing the cost center budget. The software includes embedded formulas that compute differential pay, premium pay, productivity, and other summary statistics, thereby reducing human error. Firm due dates are assigned for the completion of this first draft of the budget. Typically, a margin target is assigned to each cost center to guide managers in preparing their first draft. The finance department then "rolls up" the unit budget into the organizational budget.

3. *Revise and resubmit:* As budget documents go through review by senior management, requests tend to exceed the available resources. This necessitates review, adjustment, and appeal. This is when competition for available resources enters the process. Managers may be asked to reduce their unit budget by a dollar

percentage, leaving the question of where to cut as the manager's decision. At other times, a manager may be directed to reduce the personnel budget by a number of full-time equivalents (FTEs), thereby reducing labor expenses and addressing productivity. This is the point at which the nurse manager needs to skillfully advocate for patient care to ensure safety and quality. The nurse manager's knowledge of clinical care processes may be in conflict with directives of a financial administrator who lacks clinical expertise. This is when nurses need to be prepared to "speak finance" to effectively respond to budget challenges. The nurse manager must be able to speak to the variable needs of a patient care budget, for example, the ability to flex up direct-care nursing (variable) staff when patient volumes surge and/or patient acuity increases and the ability to flex down nursing staff when patient volumes and acuity decrease. The nurse manager needs to be sure that budgets include adequate expenses for reasonable productive and nonproductive paid hours for all staff. Nonproductive hours include sick, vacation, holiday, family leave, jury duty, and other types of leave as well as time spent away from the patient care area in education programs or working on administrative assignments and meetings. "Nonproductive" is an accounting term. When referring to knowledge work such as education, training, and shared governance activities, "nonproductive" can be called "non-patient care" hours. Failure to ensure that nonproductive labor expenses are budgeted appropriately will lead to a budget bust as well as staffing difficulties and other issues related to patient care, patient outcomes, patient experience, and employee relations. An often overlooked aspect of the labor budget is anticipated turnover. Turnover will typically generate additional labor expenses through replacement of exiting staff with premium pay labor. In addition, expenses related to training new staff can extend through several months to a year. To this end, those areas that experience significant turnover need to focus on staying ahead of the turnover through an "overhired" or "rightsizing" strategy. There may be multiple iterations of rebudgeting before the final budget is approved.

Capital Budget Development

Capital budget preparation is usually the first step in the annual budget cycle. The organization will define a capital expense in terms of a dollar amount and the anticipated life span of the purchase. For example, capital expenditures may be "items costing over $10,000 and having a life span of 5 years." Items of this magnitude are not placed in the operating budget.

The specific process used to create a capital budget will vary from organization to organization, but most organizations require extensive background material to support capital budget requests. The background or supporting material required will probably include vendor quotes for costs of purchase, installation, staff education and training, and a justification or explanation of the reasons that the capital expenditure is needed. The justification must relate the expenditure to the organization's strategic goals or objective. For capital construction projects, architectural plans, regulatory considerations, and other supporting materials may also be required as part of the capital budget preparation process.

After each unit submits the capital expenditure list to the finance department, a compiled list is generated and typically prioritized by senior management. This is a period of intense negotiation. Given that there are rarely enough financial and/or labor resources to meet all of the requests, difficult decisions must be made.

Operating Budget Development

The *operating* budget covers a specific period, called a *fiscal year*. The fiscal year may begin July 1, may correspond to the calendar year beginning January 1, or may follow the federal government year that starts on October 1. Either way, it is the budget plan for day-to-day service delivery operations. It has at least two parts: the labor budget and the expense budget for costs other than labor. Expense budgets typically include consumable and nonconsumable patient supplies, office supplies, pharmacy, and nutrition expenses. Use of budget software easily allows for the sharing of information regarding historical or trend data, expenses, and revenues. Typically, the revenue associated with a nursing unit reflects charges for room and board services. Room and board charges represent a bundling of hospital expenses related to patient care that are not individually billed elsewhere. Such expenses may include nursing and non-nursing labor, utilities, housekeeping, linen, and miscellaneous administrative services. All nursing service areas will adopt a unit of service measure that reflects the type of service provided. Inpatient nursing units measure volume activity using patient days. The OR measures volumes in

terms of OR minutes, and ambulatory settings measure volume in terms of patient visits. Use of units of service measures comes into play when productivity analyses are conducted for budgeting, trending, benchmarking, regulatory reporting, and other purposes. The nurse manager who conducts his or her budget performance analysis referencing units of service can better represent his or her budget performance to hospital administration and finance. An astute manager will look for multiple ways to interpret budget performance.

The specific process used to develop operating budgets will vary considerably from one organization to another. The nurse manager's and/or nurse executive's role in developing operating budgets for nursing units and services will typically include input on or determination of volume projections, development of associated expense projections (including supplies, equipment, and salary/labor expenses), and some form of revenue projection. Many organizations develop and disseminate a set of budget assumptions that are to be used by managers and leaders in developing the operating budget. These assumptions may include such items as preestablished increases in labor or salary expenses based on contractual obligations, adjustments that must be made based on economic forecasts for supply charge changes (e.g., increased utility rates, increased cost of pharmaceuticals), or factors that will affect patient volume, such as the addition of a new service line. The nurse manager who can share benchmark comparisons, both internal and external, demonstrates greater knowledge of the impact of required resources throughout the budget process.

Projected Volume

The foundation of the development of the operating budget at the unit level is based on the projected volume of work for the coming year. The workload aspect often is measured in units of service. Key units of service need to be identified, the number of units predicted, and expenses and staffing calculated accordingly. Activity reports such as historical census and average length of stay identify trends related to volume of activity. The unit of service often needs to be adjusted to the case or patient mix, which is a proxy for severity of illness or need (Finkler et al., 2013). Given that a budget is a plan prepared several months before implementation, budget assumptions can be proven wrong throughout the budget year. In this event, budget variances—the measure between actual and budget—are often demonstrated. The successful nurse manager will know when and why budget assumptions have been incorrect and can speak to the related impact and possible adjustments required for the following budget year.

Tables 23.1 and 23.2 show sample volume budget flow sheets. Historical trend data are needed (e.g., occupancy percentages by time frames such as weekly or monthly) to determine growth projections and any impact of seasonality. Table 23.1 displays volume changes on Unit X by month for 1 fiscal year, with variances clearly demonstrated. Table 23.2 shows volume changes on Unit X over 4 fiscal years, with variances rolled up to yearly values for comparison purposes. The volume of services delivered for a year may be expressed as patient days, visits, procedures, or other units of service. Effects on volume are environmental effects such as reimbursement changes, new programs, process improvements, new technology, and marketing. If volume projections depend on another service or department, it is important for the two departments to communicate closely so that similar assumptions are used in establishing volume projections.

Staffing Calculation

Once the volume projection has been completed, the manager can determine the *personnel services* (or *staffing/labor budget*) portion of the expense budget. Calculation of staffing in a variable environment is complex, and given that staffing expenses generally are the largest portion of the nursing operating budget, nurse managers and nurse executives need to have a consistent and well-defined approach to estimating staffing expenses. The methodology and/or terminology used will likely vary from organization to organization.

Rundio (2016) described the following method that may be used to estimate staffing expenses. For inpatient nursing units, the first step in budgeting variable staffing expenses is to know the number of planned patient days. This number can be presented on an annual basis or daily basis, known as average daily census (ADC). The next step is to determine the number of required hours, by discipline, for each patient day. For instance, based on projected patient acuity for Unit X, it is determined that each patient will require an average of 9.0 direct nursing care hours each day. This is stated as 9.0 direct RN hours per patient day (HPPD). Note that this is a calculated average, not actual needs. To determine the number of FTEs required on Unit X, the nurse manager will multiply 9 hours by the projected number of patient days (8021) and find that 72,189 hours of direct RN care are required for patient care. Dividing the 72,189 hours by 2080 hours (1 FTE) the nurse manager will conclude that 34.71 direct-care RN FTEs are required to deliver safe patient care. The unit manager will next add in nonproductive time to determine the number of required budgeted RNs for Unit X. Should the manager determine that nonproductive time equals 13% per each RN FTE, the total number of "replacement" RNs equals 4.51 FTEs. Therefore Unit X needs to budget for a total of 39.22 RN FTEs for direct patient care.

TABLE 23.1   Volume Budget Flow Sheet

Fiscal Year Y; Volumes for Unit X

Month	Patient Days Budgeted	Patient Days Actual	Variance	% Variance
July	650	667	17	2.6%
August	668	652	−16	−2.4%
September	652	680	28	4.3%
October	667	692	25	3.7%
November	700	665	−35	−5.0%
December	752	721	−31	−4.1%
January	691	682	−9	−1.3%
February	683	692	9	1.3%
March	667	671	4	0.6%
April	665	652	−13	−2.0%
May	667	674	7	1.0%
June	673	685	12	1.8%
TOTAL	**8135**	**8133**	**−2**	**0.0%**

TABLE 23.2   Volume Budget Flow Sheet

Fiscal Year Trends; Volumes for Unit X

Fiscal Year	Patient Days Budgeted	Patient Days Actual	Variance	% Variance
FY A	8021	8650	629	7.8%
FY B	8210	8689	479	5.8%
FY C	7658	7789	131	1.7%
FY D	7432	7652	220	3.0%
TOTAL	**31,321**	**32,780**	**1459**	**4.7%**

TABLE 23.3 Budgeted Salary Expense Flow Sheet

Salaries and Wages: Unit X for Fiscal Year Y

	Budget	Actual	Variance	% Variance
Regular				
Overtime				
Differential				
Holiday				
Vacation				
Sick				
Education				
Administrative				
Other				
TOTAL				

Salary Calculations

Table 23.3 displays a sample budget expense sheet for salaries based on the total unit. Similar tables can be created for subgroups, such as direct-care RNs. Table 23.4 demonstrates how personnel budgets might be displayed. Salary increases might also be included as another column. These are examples to show how data might easily be displayed as a report. Today's sophisticated budget software has reduced the effort once required for these calculations. The software will calculate salary expenses in an expeditious manner, working from historical data related to pay rates, use of premium pay, and differentials.

Supply and Revenue Budgets

Supply budgets are a major component of the operating budget. Similar to labor, many supply items are variable (the amount used will vary based on the volume of

TABLE 23.4 Personnel Budget Flow Sheet

Fiscal Year Y; Personnel Budget for Unit X

Position	FTE	Average Hourly Rate	Annual Salary
Unit Manager	1.0	40.00	83,200
Direct-Care RN	22.3	37.00	1,716,208
RN Education	1.0	34.00	70,720
Patient Care Tech	4.7	19.00	185,744
Unit Clerk	5.2	17.00	183,872
	34.2	31.49	2,239,744

FTE, Full-time equivalent.

service provided). Other supply costs are fixed and will be incurred at the same level no matter the volume of service that is provided. Items such as office supplies, intravenous (IV) solutions, instruments, linens, gloves and other personal protective equipment, medical/surgical supplies, and drugs are examples of supplies that would vary with a higher volume of patient days. Leases, maintenance contracts, staff education funds for travel to conferences or meetings, and books and subscriptions are all examples of supply items that would not vary with a higher volume of patient days. Dollar amounts are assigned based on historical projections and any known or anticipated adjustments resulting from inflation, contractual increases, or other factors as specified in the organization's budgetary assumptions. The operating budget will also need to include expenses for overhead, depreciation, utilities, telecommunications services, and other related facility expenses. Finance will typically guide nurse managers in budgeting for these overhead expenses.

Revenue budgets are based on a set of calculations that determine expected receipts that will result from charging patients and payers for services. Nursing services are often not viewed as revenue-generating departments, but in many organizations the patient days and related charges are used as a proxy for revenue. Revenue projections are based on volume projections. Factors such as payer mix and contractual rates will affect the overall revenue that is received. Contractual allowances (discounts), bad debt, and indigent care all become reductions of gross revenue and generally are not under the nurse manager's control (Finkler et al., 2013).

TRACKING AND MONITORING OF BUDGETS

The budget process is continual. It is not an event that occurs once a year and then ends until the next budget development process begins. Although "formal" budget development may occur once a year, the budget sets the stage for ongoing monitoring and evaluation of the organization's financial performance related to the budget projection (plan) as well as external benchmarking. Regular budget analyses (e.g., quarterly or monthly) are used for monitoring, feedback, and managerial control. The variance (difference) between budgeted and actual revenue and expenses is determined to identify problem areas, enhance control, and ensure timely adjustments.

Variances between actual and budgeted (planned) performance need to be analyzed to determine the cause so that nurses and managers can take the appropriate action. Variances can be favorable or unfavorable. Most organizations now use electronic reporting formats that automatically calculate variance rates, but it is important that nurses understand the reasons for the variances. Variances can result from a single cause (e.g., volume of patients or a rate change such as salary, usage, or price) or from a combination of causes.

Nurse executives often require nurse managers to document their analysis of budget variances on a monthly basis. Many nurse managers also find it is useful to share variance reports and the reasons for budget variances at unit meetings with their nursing staff. If, for example, the overtime was 4% over the budget rate, staff can engage in discussing the reasons for this expense and perhaps how it may be managed differently in the future. It may be that acuity was very high or that there were sick calls that required nurses to "work short," resulting in overtime. This will enhance the nursing staff's awareness of the unit's financial performance. Engaging unit staff in discussions about the unit's financial performance will also provide nursing staff the opportunity to suggest cost-saving strategies to control costs at the unit level. Some managers post and present unit financial data monthly. This way, all nurses and staff better understand and can be a part of generating solutions to financial issues. Use of a dashboard tool to review monthly financial performance measures is helpful to the manager and staff. In addition to tracking of expenses and revenues, related workforce measures such as premium pay, vacancy rate, turnover, and absenteeism assist the manager in telling his or her story. Working together as a team, nurse managers can better understand and guide activities that influence budget development and fiscal performance.

LEADERSHIP AND MANAGEMENT IMPLICATIONS

Nursing services make up the single largest aggregate expense in most health care organizations because they represent a large personnel component and control a large share of supplies and equipment. This is both an advantage and a vulnerability. It is a strength and advantage because nurses clearly manage the organization and system, especially at the operational unit level. With powerful and accurate data and analysis support, unit-level management becomes effective and efficient. However, many organizations simply do not provide a nurse-friendly support structure.

It is a vulnerability to be the largest aggregate expense because quick, short-term economic gains can be made by ratcheting down resources allocated to nursing services. This often occurs at the expense of strategy, long-term gains, staff satisfaction, group cohesion, patient experience, quality, and safety. Because health care generally faces strict fiscal constraints, both staff nurses and nurse managers need to be knowledgeable and skilled in anticipating financial fluctuations and trends and in making bold decisions based on rapid analysis of information. Staff nurses often will be handling day-to-day budgetary decisions; thus they must be aware of the unit's budget, the financial status of the unit and the organization, and the impact of their decisions about supply and resource (staff) utilization on the financial performance of the unit. Nurse leaders are more involved with strategic or long-range financial planning and decision making, but they may track unit productivity carefully.

The budgeting process requires a broad range of leadership and management skills. Resources are limited. This fact is difficult for some nurses, especially if they believe they should be able to do everything for every patient under every circumstance. Some professionals think that their job is to provide the maximum quantity and quality of service and that cost consciousness should not be a concern of direct-care providers. Nurses are familiar with managing clinical care delivery. These skills can be transferred to the management of money as a necessary component of providing care. However, the management of any scarce resource such as money includes balancing competing interests and making difficult decisions.

Leadership is involved in influencing others to achieve the group's goals within the constraints of scarce resources. Leaders need to be actively involved in setting the vision for how to accomplish goals through budget planning. Ethical considerations such as fairness, transparency, and reasonable targets are part of leadership decision making. Leaders can influence employee morale and organizational culture through role modeling and the decision-making process. Organizational culture can be engaged to diminish negative aspects of budgeting and financial management. There is an opportunity for innovation to occur in a way that eases financial pressures. For example, with the use of data, a better schedule may be devised that deploys the same RN and assistive personnel in a new configuration that better addresses peaks and flows and the needs of patients for nursing care.

Fiscal Responsibility for Clinical Practice

Continuous change in the health care delivery and reimbursement systems has created a challenge to controlling costs while continually improving the quality of care. One nurse author has advocated that nurses assume fiscal responsibility for their clinical practice (Murray, 2012). Fiscal responsibility is defined as using the resources of the patient to maximize health benefit while simultaneously using the resources of the institution to maximize cost effectiveness. Fiscal responsibility is essential when trying to improve client care by improving managerial and clinical decisions in nursing. The cost to clients from health care services is a social and professional concern. Cost and quality remain two major themes for nursing practice. The questions that will be asked are: What is the cost? What if the cost of the intervention is unaffordable but produces superior quality? What will the cost be (to the patient and to the institution and ultimately to society) if the care is not provided or is not of high quality? Cost variables are one consideration to use in decision making.

Being fiscally responsible means that the nurse manager makes responsible resource allocation decisions. Some decisions a nurse manager might need to make include the following:

- Staff time: Are there sufficient budgeted hours per patient day to provide quality care?
- Staff assignments: Which member of the patient care team can care for the patient in a cost-effective manner?
- Discharge planning: Is there a process in place to avoid delays in discharges to nursing homes?
- Costs of human resources: How can you evaluate workforce metrics and track the impact of turnover, onboarding, and orientation as related to the budget?
- Professional growth and development: How do you support continual growth and professional development of nursing staff across the continuum in equitable and diverse ways?

There are also multiple opportunities for staff nurse nurses to demonstrate fiscal responsibility. For a client

with poor skin integrity, perhaps the most expensive tape should be used because the tape needs to stick and be waterproof. However, in a routine situation, can a lower-cost item be substituted with equal results? Nurses cannot help reduce costs unless they know the per-item cost of the supplies they use and then use this information to evaluate substitutions. Even small cost reductions can be significant if they are applied to high-volume items. Immediately apparent is the costliness of inappropriate use of items (e.g., wiping up spills with a sterile pad; opening a sterile pack in the OR "to be ready just in case" or to use only one of the instruments). Convenience versus cost trade-off must be considered (e.g., bag baths may be convenient or necessary in a staffing shortage but are an expensive supply cost).

Evaluation of Budget Expenditures

The public is becoming increasingly knowledgeable regarding the quality and safety of health care. Health care consumers and payers expect that money for new initiatives will result in added value in terms of improved quality, safety of care, and patient experience. Business plans must include specific metrics that will be used to measure the impact of expenditures on clinical outcomes, quality, safety, and patient experience, as well as on cost. Metrics should specify the impact on nurse-sensitive indicators when feasible to further validate the significant role that nurses play in improving the health status of patients.

Costing Out Nursing Services

Accurately determining the costs of providing nursing service is an important budgetary function. Nurses need to know their costs to plan better and negotiate more effectively. Nursing has historically been seen as a cost center but not a revenue generator. One strategy proposed to compensate for nursing's revenue disparity was to cost out nursing services. This idea became popular for a while but lost attraction as capitated reimbursement systems gained prominence. With a "per member per month" flat payment structure, many felt that efforts to cost out for purposes of charging a fee for service were useless. Therefore costing out nursing services was abandoned by some. However, the unintended consequence was that the value of knowing precisely what it costs to deliver nursing services was lost.

Costing out nursing services is defined as the determination of the costs of the services provided by nurses. By identifying the specific costs related to the delivery of nursing care to each client, nurses have data to identify the actual amount of services received. In reviews of the literature related to costing out nursing services, a variety of variables were examined, such as length of stay, nursing care costs, direct-care costs, patient acuity, and diagnosis-related group (DRG) reimbursements. Analyses of cost data continue to expand in correlation with increasing sophistication of related software products. Cost data can be linked to patient severity, scheduling and staffing, care delivery decisions, and other benchmarking metrics (Jenkins & Welton, 2014).

The process of costing out nursing services provides data for productivity comparisons. Activity-based costing (ABC) is one approach to service costing that may be useful in multiple settings. The key advantage of ABC is that it reflects what it costs to provide services and identifies why costs were incurred. The first step in ABC is to identify all the cost drivers associated with a specific service. For example, if the service is a preschool physical examination provided by a nurse practitioner, here are some potential costs associated with the service:

- Nursing assistant (NA): 5 minutes to room the patient and 5 minutes to clean the room after the visit. The nursing assistant is paid $15 per hour with a 35% benefit rate and works 52 weeks per year, 40 hours per week. The cost of the NA time is $31,200 + $10,920 = $42,120/2080 (number of hours in a year), for an hourly cost of $20.25, or $20.25/60, $0.3375 per minute or $1.69 cost per visit.
- One-half hour of nurse practitioner (NP) time: The nurse is paid $86,000 per year and associated benefits at 35% ($30,100); the NP works 52 weeks (40 hours per week) per year. The cost of the time of the NP is ($116,100/2080) = $55.86 cost per hour or $27.91 cost per NP time.
- All other costs are identified in the same manner: equipment, such as stethoscope, tongue depressor, and linens on examination table; cost of electronic health record (EHR); costs of a billing clerk.

Once this process is completed, the costs are aggregated, yielding what it costs to provide one unit of one nursing service—providing a preschool physical examination. The next step is to assign activities to cost centers, service lines, or programs. In the previous example, the cost of the service may be placed in a pediatric well-child clinic program.

A more sophisticated and rapidly expanding approach to collecting nursing's cost data is using *acuity*, or patient classification systems. The premise is that nursing care needs to be based on patients' actual needs for care, not on historical allocation of nursing time. *Acuity* is defined as a measure of the severity of illness of an individual patient or the aggregate patient population on a unit. The acuity of patients has increased dramatically in the past 10 to 15 years. Formerly, patients were admitted for diagnostic tests and for additional preparation before surgery. They typically remained in the hospital until they were able to care for themselves, often through a lengthy convalescence. A nurse was able to provide care to larger numbers of these patients because they required less care, assessment, and monitoring. Today, these patients are receiving care in other settings and only very ill patients remain in the hospital. Utilization review experts have stated that the only reason a patient is in the hospital is because he or she needs monitoring and assessment by a registered nurse. If these skills are not needed, patients can probably be safely cared for in a less expensive setting. The increased acuity seen today decreases the number of patients for whom a nurse may safely provide care. This results in what might look like (on paper) a decrease in productivity. Any measure of the productivity of nursing staff that does not consider the acuity level of patients is seriously flawed and would probably result in a gross underestimation of the output. Nurse executives reflect that patient acuity increases year after year, creating increased demand for additional direct-care RNs.

Many of the classifications share a similar approach to the determination of the workload based on the required hours of nursing care. This is intuitively attractive because it can be assumed that a ventilator-dependent patient in an intensive care unit (ICU) will require more care than a patient who has had a total knee replacement. If the nurse manager uses a classification system whereby, for example, type 1 patients receive 2 to 4 hours of nursing care per day and type 2 patients receive 5 to 8 hours per day, these data can be used in constructing a personnel budget when it is linked to the volume indicator of patient days. If the nurse manager predicts that the unit will provide 800 days of type 1 patients, this information can be used to predict the staffing requirements for that patient group. Multiple commercial patient classifications systems are available for purchase. Some involve entering nurse-collected patient data in a software program, yet increasingly this information can be extracted from electronic medical records to calculate objective scores for acuity. One caveat to this process is that, when used to create staffing ratios, the judgment of an expert nurse clinician must override an empirical system and be based on patients' needs in real time.

Various approaches are used to determine this acuity level and then relate it to staffing needs. Patient classification software is available from vendors. These systems attempt to categorize the levels of nursing care required by patients and then project appropriate nursing and ancillary staff. Some of these may be expensive to purchase and then modify to meet the needs of a specific hospital; they may also be costly to install and maintain. Critics argue that such systems cannot capture the invisible knowledge work of nursing. The systems often inadequately adjust for the experience level and varied expertise of RNs, such as a new graduate versus an experienced senior nurse.

In general, too little effort has been devoted to isolating actual nursing costs and determining the costs of nursing and the provision of care. With actual data, nurses are in a better position to demonstrate the economic value of their service, and nurse managers will have appropriate information with which to accurately manage nursing services.

PRODUCTIVITY

Understanding the concept of productivity and relating it to the management of professional nursing is a leadership skill that will serve nursing in an era of accelerating health care expenditures. Based on this understanding, the nurse manager will be able to determine the costs associated with providing nursing care. Productivity is defined as the relationship between output and the goods and services used to produce them.

Measures of Productivity

Various measures of productivity exist, but all involve relationships between volume of inputs and cost. Nurses' time is the critical input in the production of nursing care. Home health agencies measure their productivity in patient home visits and hours of care, hospitals measure patient days, and clinics measure the number of patient visits. The cost measure is the cost of the nursing time required to produce this care. Table 23.5 displays some productivity measures that track and benchmark unit performance and assist the unit manager in presenting unit-related fiscal outcomes to nurse executives and hospital leadership.

The oldest method of measuring nursing productivity is the analysis of hours per patient day (HPPD). The input is the nursing hours worked. The number of hospitalized patient days is the output. This index is imprecise because of the wide variation in patient acuity, with the result that the measure of patient days is not equivalent across cases. Patient "churn" further complicates this calculation. The number of heads in a bed at midnight (midnight census) is often less than what is seen at noon or 4 PM.

A variety of data sources and productivity indices can also be considered. In nursing, productivity has been tightly linked to staffing numbers. For example, staffing—calculated as the total number of hours of a given staff for a given time period—can be compared with patient volume or census. Using this method, if the output (patient days) increased while staffing remained the same, then strictly speaking the productivity would be increased. This typically happens in hospitals, for example, when the influenza season is severe and a large number of geriatric patients are admitted to the hospital. In this short-term staffing crisis, the same numbers of staff are available to care for the high census, and productivity temporarily increases. However, the gains

TABLE 23.5 Measures of Productivity				
Fiscal Year Y; Productivity for Unit X				
	Budget	Actual	Variance	% Variance
Total productive hours/patient day	12.2	13.1	0.9	−7.4%
Total productive direct-care RN hours/patient day	9.0	9.2	0.2	−2.2%
Salaries and wages/patient day	621.2	643.2	21.9	−3.5%
Contract hours/day	12.0	36.0	24.0	−200.0%
Contract expenses/day	600.0	1980.0	1380.0	−230.0%
Total supplies/patient day	32.0	35.3	3.3	−10.3%

may be short lived in that the short-staffing situation may result in nurse burnout, overtime, and resignations. To this end, during the budget process, it is important that the nurse executive advocates for expenses to fund a flexible workforce (as needed, float pool, overtime, and contract staff). Some organizations track productivity and quickly adjust for when it is both too high and too low.

No one measure of productivity adequately captures the knowledge-based work of nursing. Productivity measurement is complex for several reasons. The causal linkages between nursing interventions and patient outcomes are not always well established. There is little research that addresses economic efficiency—that is, what is the least cost combination of inputs required to produce an outcome.

One solution has been to emphasize outcomes measurement. Research on outcomes measurement is accelerating and provides empirical data to support staffing decision making. Nurse researchers (Aiken et al., 2014) demonstrated a relationship between staffing and adverse patient outcomes. They found that an increase in 1 hour worked by RNs per patient day was associated with an 8.9% decrease in the odds of patients acquiring pneumonia. These researchers also found that the occurrence of all adverse events (pneumonia, pressure ulcers, and wound infections) was associated with a prolonged length of hospital stay, increased mortality, and increased hospital costs. This is an example of outcomes research that will aid managers' decision making in the future. Enhancing the productivity of nurses while protecting the quality of patient care will continue to be a major challenge for nurse leaders. As outcomes research continues, the nurse executive needs to share this information with hospital leadership to support increased nursing expenses.

CURRENT ISSUES AND TRENDS

Evaluation of Budget Expenditures

The public is becoming increasingly knowledgeable regarding the quality and safety of health care. Health care consumers and payers expect that money for new initiatives will be well invested and that a significant return on investment will be realized in terms of improved quality or safety of care. Business plans must include specific metrics that will be used to measure the impact of expenditures on clinical outcomes, quality, safety, and cost. Metrics should specify the impact on nurse-sensitive indicators when feasible to further validate the significant role that nurses play in improving the health status of patients.

Nurse Workforce Participation

The continuing nurse shortage and related nurse workforce participation issues carry ramifications for budgeting and financial management. Two trends to watch are nurses nearing retirement and the educational capacity available for the nurse workforce (see Chapters 1 and 21). The concern is with the number of projected nurses retiring, although to date the projections have not been realized, possibly due to economic pressures. However, it appears to be a matter of time.

For replacement prospects, the job of an RN is attractive for its employment potential. The Bureau of Labor Statistics (2015) noted the positive job outlook for RNs: "Employment of registered nurses is projected to grow 16 percent from 2014 to 2024, much faster than the average for all occupations. Growth will occur for a number of reasons, including an increased emphasis on preventive care; growing rates of chronic conditions, such as diabetes and obesity; and demand for health care services from the baby-boom population, as they live longer and more active lives."

Educational capacity is a concern due to the finite number of slots in schools and colleges of nursing plus an even more severe nurse faculty shortage, which limits student capacity (see Chapter 21). The age of nursing faculty is an acute issue due to impending retirements. Strategies are needed to address the nurse faculty shortage.

Clearly there is a need to maximize the productivity of professional nurses, but this productivity cannot be accomplished at the cost of nursing care quality. Lucero and colleagues (2009) conducted a study about patient care activities left undone by registered nurses in 168 hospitals. On average, 41% left developing or updating care plans undone, 12% left preparing patients and families for discharge undone, and 28.5% left patient teaching undone. The authors suggested that learning the consequences of unmet nursing care may influence nurse managers to develop evidence-based resource allocation.

It is possible that increased use of technology will be a partial solution to increasing nursing productivity. Computerized documentation and medication administration systems are widespread applications of technology that have resulted in time savings and subsequent increased productivity for nurses. Information technology is another enhancement to nurses' productivity. Medical records are easily accessed from multiple sites, results of diagnostics tests are communicated instantly, and monitoring devices detect deviations from normal limits and communicate these to the nurse as they occur. However, Abass and colleagues (2012) found "It is unclear to what extent any differences in nurse productivity can be attributed to the use of more EHR applications." Further they demonstrated that hospitals with advanced use of electronic medical records did not necessarily demonstrate improved productivity measures. It is suggested that the value of technology can more appropriately be assessed as it relates to the business case in terms of improved methods of demonstrating quality and value.

Another responsibility of nurse leaders related to productivity is ensuring a future workforce by participating in the recruitment of future nurses. One conference speaker reported that as a colleague leaves her home for work each day, she tells her young children, "Mom is going to go to the hospital to save lives today." Although nursing does not *always* offer that level of drama, it certainly speaks of the importance of the work that nurses do. That importance needs to be communicated to the pool of potential nurses.

Integration of Economics in Clinical Practice

The incorporation of economic evaluation in clinical practice is important to productivity because health care resources are limited and choices must—and will—be made. In the years preceding managed care, health care providers acted as if health care resources were infinite,

with the result that health care costs spun out of control. Today, providers are faced with difficult decisions about "who gets what." Although rationing health care is inherently unacceptable to most of the US population, it is true that rationing is occurring. Currently, rationing is done based on the ability to pay for health care, with the uninsured receiving less health care. Well-educated nurse leaders who understand economics and finance are in a unique position to bring the values of nursing to decision making about the allocation of health care resources.

Nurses are able to tap into their full skill set to assess, educate, intervene, and evaluate the care they provide to increasing numbers of patients. Care providers are evaluated in their ability to provide efficient and quality care, and their reimbursements are directly related to their ability to demonstrate best practices. Their results are compared with others, and performance that varies from agreed-on outcomes will not be reimbursed. This means nurses are encountering more patients than ever before, but the reimbursement for these services is negotiated and often times less than in the past.

Simply put, nurses need to commit to continued learning and professional development over the course of their careers, seek collaborative and productive partnerships with all members of the provider team and beyond with members of the community at large, and become increasingly comfortable using data to measure outcomes, demonstrate achievements, and drive improvements across the continuum.

RESEARCH NOTE

Source
Kovner, C.T., Brewer, C.S., Fatehi, F., & Jun, J. (2014). What does nurse turnover rate mean and what is the rate? *Policy, Politics & Nursing Practice, 15*(3/4), 64–71.

Purpose
To gain a better understanding of registered nurse (RN) turnover and develop improved ways of measuring RN turnover.

Method
The Robert Wood Johnson Foundation funded a 10-year panel study of new RNs, seeking to conduct longitudinal study of RNs in the United States to understand and describe the drivers for RN turnover. Data were collected through a mailed survey with $5 incentive and a maximum of five mailings for nonresponders.

Discussion
There is a difference in reported rates of turnover primarily driven by the fact that there are measurement differences in definitions, response rates, and sample. Hospitals have a net loss of 5.1% of new RNs. Direct surveys of nurses versus hospital-based surveys may provide the best source of data. Hospitals should study reasons for turnover to differentiate if the reasons are hospital based or driven by shortages in specific specialty or geographical areas.

Application to Practice
Researchers, nurse leaders, and policy makers should strive for a consistent and standardized way of measuring RN turnover so that measuring and reporting are used to drive improvements and strengthen the RN workforce. It is especially helpful to have solid data during budget planning and negotiations.

CASE STUDY

This hospital opened its first cardiac ICU 8 years ago. At the time of the opening it was an eight-bed unit. After demonstrating 100% capacity 2 years in a row, leadership approved a plan to open five additional beds, making it a 13-bed unit. Following 2 years of sustained growth, leadership once again approved a plan to double bed capacity and build a new unit with 26 beds.

Anne Stone, MSN, RN, the nurse leader for this ICU, has been leading an aggressive effort to support the growing volumes through continuous hiring and onboarding of new staff. The average time to hire and onboard for this unit is 9 months (including posting of the position, hiring, and onboarding). The first year after the new 26-bed ICU opened, the unit was budgeted for an average daily census (ADC) of 10, and their RN full-time equivalents (FTEs) were budgeted at 37. Patient volumes exceeded the budgeted ADC by 7, with year-end actual ADC running at 17. In year two, the budgeted ADC was 14. By the end of the first quarter of the fiscal year, ADC was running at 20. To make up for the gap in RN resources, the nurse leader was incurring significant costs in premium pay expenses, including overtime, bonus pay, and contractual nursing. The nurse leader has been asked to prepare a plan to decrease premium pay expenses while meeting the growing demand for nursing services.

1. What financial metrics would be helpful as Ms. Stone prepares her response for the chief nursing officer (CNO)?
2. What strategies might be deployed to decrease the expenses related to the positive variance in patient days?
3. Which trends and analyses does Ms. Stone need to best project future needs?
4. Prepare a timeline for decreasing the costs associated with premium pay.
5. With whom should Ms. Stone work to prepare her report to the CNO?

▌CRITICAL THINKING EXERCISE

Sue Black, RN, has been appointed manager of the new pain clinic at an academic medical center located in the southeastern United States. Due to a number of circumstances outside of Ms. Black's control, since the unit opened 2 years ago, actual patient volumes (infusions) in this new pain clinic have occupied less than 20% of the available space and steadily remain under budget by 65%. Ms. Black is keenly aware that hospital leadership is reviewing the performance and productivity of the pain clinic and that in all likelihood most of her staff is in jeopardy of being reassigned to other areas and/or the pain clinic may close.

As a strong advocate for those patients who stand to benefit from the expertise of a dedicated pain clinic, Ms. Black began to explore other disciplines that could share the same space, thereby gaining improved productivity metrics. To this end, Ms. Black was aware of patients requiring Remicade and pamidronate infusions who were put on a wait list. Working with her chief nursing officer (CNO), Ms. Black began a series of meetings with respective physicians to determine how the pain clinic could better serve their infusion patients. As this concept gained support from prospective users, Ms. Black's CNO asked her to prepare an infusion center business plan for presentation to hospital leadership.

1. What are the key components that Ms. Black should address in the business plan?
2. What guiding principles should be addressed in the business plan?
3. What components should be referenced in preparing a high-level current state assessment of infusion services at this institution?
4. What financial outcomes/measures would interest the chief finance officer?

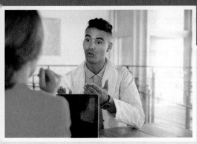

Performance Appraisal

Marie-Hélène Budworth

http://evolve.elsevier.com/Huber/leadership

Performance appraisals serve many different and often competing functions. Performance appraisal is part of a broader performance management system feeding into human resource management (HRM) systems. Although performance appraisal is examined as a distinct feature within management, it cannot be completely separated from its related processes. These purposes and connections are reviewed and discussed in this chapter.

The performance appraisal process is an opportunity for the manager to gain insight into staff. This is really a process of discovering each employee's perception of his or her job. Thus the leadership part of the manager's performance appraisal work includes the opportunity to identify what motivates staff members and gain awareness of their values and interests.

The prevailing purpose of performance appraisal is to improve and motivate the staff, which in turn will enhance organizational effectiveness. Thus the process of performance appraisal is a means to address both institutional needs and the needs and abilities of staff.

DEFINITIONS

Performance is defined as "the execution of an action"; "something accomplished"; and "the fulfillment of a claim, promise, or request" ("Performance," n.d.).

Performance appraisal means evaluating the work of others. It is "the process by which a manager or consultant (1) examines and evaluates an employee's work behavior by comparing it with preset standards, (2) documents the results of the comparison, and (3) uses

Photo used with permission from julief514/Getty Images.

the results to provide feedback to the employee to show where improvements are needed and why" ("Performance appraisal," 2016). The employee's work is measured against standards, much like in the quality improvement process. Standards, whether explicit or not, are applied to what ought to be or to what is superior, excellent, average, or unacceptable performance.

A **performance improvement plan (PIP)** is defined as a formal performance action plan that is used as a tool to facilitate conversation in the form of constructive discussion between a staff member and his or her manager/supervisor in order to clarify work performance and needed improvements (Heathfield, 2016). A PIP outlines specific goals to work toward and specific improvement steps to take.

Peer review in nursing is the process by which nurses systematically access, monitor, and make judgments about the quality of nursing care provided by peers as measured against professional standards of practice. Nursing care is evaluated by individuals at the same rank or standing and according to established standards of practice (American Nurse Today, 2011).

Self-evaluation is the aspect of performance appraisal whereby employees do self-assessments of their own perceptions about their performance compared with stated objectives and expectations.

PURPOSES OF PERFORMANCE APPRAISAL

Administrative

Performance appraisals provide data that are used to make a series of administrative and management decisions.

Individual ratings can be used to inform compensation, promotion, and layoff decisions. More broadly, evaluations provide information that is critical to human resources (HR) planning. Having a sense of the current skills of the workforce is critical to being prepared for future needs, including skill gaps, new areas of specialization, and treatment needs. For instance, nursing skills in geriatric care become increasingly important as the population continues to change and the percentage of persons over 65 grows. Performance appraisal can be used to understand who already has these skills and who might be able to either develop them or transfer an existing skill set to the area of need. Similarly, understanding the skills related to management and leadership that exist within the workforce gives the organization the information required to plan for future leadership needs and do succession planning.

In cases where performance is weak or problematic, appraisals provide the "paper trail" needed to support tough decisions such as remedial training or dismissal, in some cases. Appraisals provide documentation that allows the organization to track both employee and management's efforts in a way that is required for legal compliance in termination cases.

Measurement

Another purpose of the performance appraisal system is simply to measure performance. If the performance objectives are set well, then measurement gives us a sense of whether they are being achieved. Aligning performance objectives with the strategic goals of the organization helps to guide, direct, and evaluate the extent to which individual behaviors are linked to organizational objectives. For example, a hospital might hold excellent patient care as its core value. This might be operationalized as access to cutting-edge treatment as well as a responsive, patient-centered approach to care. To the extent that these organizational objectives inform the ways in which nurses are evaluated, the hospital is able to inform their own understanding of how well they are working collectively toward their strategic initiatives.

Development

A third reason for conducting performance appraisals is to develop the nurse. Opportunities for skill development can be identified by understanding both the strengths and the weaknesses of each employee. This might be through training, coaching, or some other learning opportunity.

Although the focus of performance appraisals has been on remedial learning or correcting weaknesses, researchers have more recently called for a reframing of performance development after feedback. A focus on building strengths has the potential to reorient the conversation, engage high-performing nurses, and motivate people toward even higher levels of performance. This will be discussed in greater detail in the section "The Manager as Coach."

Relationship Building

This is not typically included as one of the core purposes of the performance appraisal system, but it is increasingly being understood as central to the process. The performance appraisal process should not harm the relationship between nurse manager and staff nurse. In fact, it should be viewed as an opportunity to open the lines of communication. Effective nursing is predicated on being able to develop effective caring relationships with patients. Building effective relationships among all team members can only support this goal. Reviewing, planning, and rewarding positive performance should be viewed as an opportunity for the nurse manager to strengthen his or her relationship with the team.

ISSUES IN PERFORMANCE APPRAISAL

Researchers have long been concerned with what has been referred to as the criteria problem in HRM. The criteria problem is about measurement. What are we measuring when measuring performance? Can we measure it accurately? Both of these questions will be explored.

What Are We Measuring in Performance Appraisal?
The Criteria Used
At the core of evaluation is the question of performance. The methods used to measure performance have undergone a great deal of change in response to research, technical improvements, and legal requirements. A discussion of various criteria used to measure performance focuses on traits, behaviors, and results.

Traits

Under trait rating systems, workers are measured according to the extent to which they possess a given personal characteristic. Traits that could be measured include dependability, conscientiousness, responsibility, self-management, responsiveness, and decision-making ability. When using a trait method, a supervisor might be asked to rate to what extent an employee exhibits a certain trait. For example, the nurse manager might be asked to rate a nurse for whom she is responsible on a scale from 1, "not at all responsive," to 5, "exceptionally responsive."

There are a number of limitations to trait ratings. First, for most jobs, there is no reliable set of traits that predicts performance. Researchers have spent a great deal of time measuring the relationship between personality dimensions across various employment settings and have not found a consistent connection between constellations of traits and performance in various roles. For example, one might assume that an extrovert is better at outward-facing roles, but this is not necessarily the case. Introverted individuals can "extrovert" themselves quite well in order to complete the essential tasks of their employment.

Second, raters vary on how they define and perceive different traits. One rater might rate a nurse as a 5 on conscientiousness and another might give the same individual a 3. This discrepancy can be due to differences in personal definitions of conscientiousness rather than the individual being rated. Although the raters can be trained to develop common understandings of the personal dimensions, it can still be difficult to interpret observed performance in a rating on a trait scale. In sum, traits are vague and subjective and not clearly linked to performance on the job.

Behaviors

Behaviors are often measured in order to reduce bias and increase accuracy within performance ratings. Behaviors have an advantage over traits because they can be directly observed, thus reducing the subjectivity of the rating. On these scales, the rater is asked to assess the quality and/or quantity of a specific behavior such as "explains procedures accurately to patient," "responds to concerns in a timely manner," and "treats other members of the team respectfully." The scale itself can take a number of forms. On a behavioral checklist, the rater simply indicates with a check mark which behaviors have been observed. Alternatively, the rater can be asked to indicate on a numerical scale how often or with how much competence the individual being rated exhibits the indicated behaviors.

The behaviorally anchored scales are a significant improvement over trait scales. These have been found to be valid and reliable measurement tools. There are still drawbacks to this type of measurement. First, the rater does not see everything that the person being rated does on the job. For example, the nurse manager is not beside the nurse during every patient interaction. In fact, there are large amounts of time when the nurse works outside of her or his manager's presence, thus there are few opportunities to directly observe performance. Under these circumstances, it can be difficult to fully capture accurate performance metrics.

A second limitation of behavioral scales is that they are static. Tools and techniques are constantly changing in today's health care environment. There is a need to ensure that the measures are able to keep up with the pace of change. After spending a great deal of time and effort creating a behavioral rating scale, it would be easy to find oneself in a position where a number of the behaviors listed are obsolete. Due to this limitation, practitioners have developed competency-based models of evaluation.

Competencies

A competency is the ability to perform a skill successfully. Competencies are more adaptable than behaviors because they describe the capability that underlies the behaviors. Skills might not change, although tasks and the ensuing required behaviors change regularly. Some potential nursing competencies include developing a therapeutic relationship, identifying health care needs in a caring environment that facilitates achieving mutually agreed health outcomes, collaborating with all members of the health care team, and advocating for the patient.

Competency models are often linked to organizational objectives or professional standards. There are various professional organizations that have developed competency models for nurses. For example, the American Association of Colleges of Nursing (AACN, 2013) has developed competencies for clinical nurse leaders *(http://www.aacn.nche.edu/publications/white-papers/ cnl)*. Although there is still some subjectivity and bias in rating competencies, these types of scales have been shown to have acceptable levels of validity and reliability.

Results

In an effort to reduce as much bias as possible in performance ratings, some evaluators look to results-based measures of performance. This type of measurement asks the question "What will be the outcome of high performance?" As an example, in an emergency department, a triage nurse might be evaluated according to the accuracy of her assessments. In a family clinic, the nurse might be assessed relative to patient history completed at the beginning of the visit. Although these types of measurements allow for objectivity in the rating, there are some clear limitations.

First, the rating is deficient. This refers to the fact that results do not capture everything that is important to performance for a job well done. In an emergency, a triage nurse needs to make a patient feel safe and help reduce his or her anxiety. This cannot be captured easily in a results-based measure. Second, the measure is contaminated. This relates to the fact that results-based measures capture factors that affect performance but are beyond the control of the person being rated. For example, if an emergency department is understaffed on a given night, the nurse's ability to triage appropriately may be compromised but not due to his or her competence.

Which Performance Metric Should Be Used?

Clearly, there is no perfect performance metric. Each criterion has its strengths and weaknesses. The approach used should be based on the purpose of the system. An example from the private sector will help to illustrate this point.

At about the same time both Deloitte, a large professional services firm, and Adobe, a giant of the technology industry, decided to radically change their performance appraisal processes. They both had most recently used a version of competency models to assess their employees.

Deloitte started by asking what they wanted out of a performance management system. The leaders at Deloitte wanted to be able to track individual performance clearly and transparently. In recognizing the challenges of rating past performance, Deloitte found a way to ask managers to assess employees by looking toward the future. After each project, they asked the project leads to indicate what they would do with the employee in the future (e.g., work on a team with them again, give them a raise, or promote them). They found that these future-oriented questions were better predictors of past performance than the observationally based measures they had previously used. They also found that everyone in

the organization was much more satisfied with this system than the previous one.

In contrast, Adobe abolished ratings altogether. Their focus was on employee development. They wanted a system that would focus on providing useful, timely feedback, allowing their employees to grow and develop skills. They did not need numbers and metrics to accomplish learning. So instead of a system anchored in performance measurements, Adobe shifted to a flexible annual performance review process with periodic, ongoing check-ins that occurred throughout the year. The review and the check-ins are opportunities for goal setting, the tracking of expectations, ongoing feedback, and coaching.

Rating Accuracy: Can We Measure It Accurately?

Researchers spent decades trying to improve the ability to measure performance. Despite significant advancements, measurements continue to be imperfect. What gets in the way? The short answer is the rater. Accurately assessing and rating someone according to a predetermined scale is a challenging task. There is a tremendous amount of bias in a performance rating. Bias refers to inaccuracy in the measurement in favor of or against a person or group, typically in a way that is unfair. Bias occurs for a wide range of reasons. Some commons forms of bias are:

- Halo (or horns): An employee is rated positively (or negatively) based on one event or skill. The full spectrum of performance is not considered.
- Recency: The most recent events are the focus of the review.
- Leniency: All members of the team receive the same satisfactory rating.
- Similar-to-me: Individuals who are similar to the rater in some way are rated more favorably.
- Contrast: The employees are rated relative to one another rather than relative to some organizational standard.

Some of the biases described in this list are caused by rating inaccuracy. In other words, raters make mistakes because they are not able to accurately recall performance examples and observations (e.g., recency). Other forms of bias are due to the nature of how work is performed, especially in professional environments. Raters do not always have the opportunity to observe people in a range of tasks. In fact, raters might see subordinates performing the essential tasks of their job only on rare occasions. Once off orientation or a residency, how often do you expect that your supervisor will be in the room with you while you care for a patient?

Finally, it could also be that the tool itself is flawed. It might not describe performance accurately or might be easy to misinterpret. For these reasons, it is important to understand that there is likely to be some bias in performance appraisals. In 2000 Scullen and colleagues found that 62% of the variance in the ratings in performance appraisals could be explained by differences in the perceptions of the individual raters.

Political Motivations

It is important to highlight that there is the potential for deliberate inaccuracy in a performance appraisal. Tziner (1999) found that managers often considered opportunities, resources, and relationships with subordinates when completing appraisals. Managers admitted that they used promotions as a way to move out an employee with whom they were not getting along. When bonuses or other rewards are scarce, appraisals are sometimes "gamed" to ensure that a favored employee receives the reward or perhaps a reward is shared among a team by coordinating appraisals given to team members. These types of political issues are especially problematic when resources are scarce and evaluation is tightly linked to compensation. It is worth remembering that inaccuracies in appraisal occur for all kinds of reasons.

Who Should Do the Rating?

Historically, the manager has been at the center of the employment review process. Although this is still the case today, others are often involved in providing feedback. This can be an important part of the process. Anyone who has the opportunity to observe the individual under review has something to offer. This might include peers, physicians, and patients. In team environments, it is useful to have team members provide feedback.

In a 360-degree feedback review, managers, peers, subordinates, and patients all provide feedback. In these circumstances, it is not expected that all of the feedback will converge. In fact, discrepancies between the sources might be expected. Each source offers a unique perspective because they are able to observe the individual in unique circumstances under varied conditions. The 360-degree process is intended to give the reviewer a fuller and more robust picture of the individual's performance.

When multisource rating systems, such as 360-degree feedback, are used, there is a need to balance competing demands. If subordinates or peers are asked to rate a boss or colleagues, they might be hesitant to be direct and honest, especially if that feedback is constructive or negative. At the same time, individuals are more critical when providing feedback anonymously than they would be if their name were known. Because of these factors, there must be a balance between the need for anonymity and the need for accountability.

A self-report rating is often part of a 360-degree feedback process, in which the individual being rated is given an opportunity to speak to his or her own self-perception of performance. This can be quite useful for two key reasons. First, the rater then has an opportunity to reflect on the disagreement between his or her self-rating and the ratings given by others. These discrepancies have been shown to heighten awareness of performance deficits and motivate performance change. Second, self-reports increase perceptions of fairness on the part of the person being reviewed. If employees have an opportunity to have input in the process, then they feel that they have a voice and are actively participating in the process. This influences perceptions of justice and fairness. When persons feel as though they have had some input in the process, the process itself is perceived as more fair.

Developing Employees Through Performance Appraisal and Review

The measurement of performance is such a significant challenge that it often occupies much of the organization's and the manager's efforts. However, consider the core reasons for conducting reviews. Employee development is a critical focus of this system yet is often overlooked in practice. When developing a review process, it is important to avoid getting bogged down with measurement. Following through to the end of the review cycle by putting just as much effort into the development of performance as into its evaluation is the key.

One of the most important principles of the performance review is that there should not be any surprises during the review meeting. Although the formal review is the appropriate time for problem solving and goal setting, it is not the appropriate time to revisit negative feedback on issues that arose months before the meeting. A seminal study of feedback by Kluger and DeNisi (1996) found that feedback has the potential to improve performance, do nothing at all, and even decrease performance.

These findings highlight the need for managers to deliver performance feedback in ways that can support behavior change and performance improvement.

A nurse manager needs to provide ongoing regular feedback about performance. If something is amiss, it should be dealt with immediately. Regular and timely feedback has a greater potential to be helpful to the employee. When the lines of communication are open between nurse manager and nurse, there is an opportunity for ongoing, regular coaching and support.

The performance review meeting needs to be seen as an opportunity. In most organizations, both managers and employees are apprehensive about these meetings. Managers hate delivering bad news, and employees dislike the feeling of being under the microscope. A reframing of the performance review as a meeting where the manager and the nurse can collaboratively set goals, make developmental plans, and talk about future prospects has the potential to shift the effectiveness of the entire performance review process. If performance corrections are given on the job as the need arises, then the review meeting can be refocused on meaningful development.

The Manager as Coach

Recently a team of researchers led by the author of this chapter tested a new orientation for the performance review conversation (Budworth et al., 2015). The technique itself was pioneered by Avi Kluger and is called feedforward. The technique asks the manager to guide the employee through a conversation about his or her past successes as a way of identifying strengths. The dyad then has a detailed discussion about how the employee can use the strengths to enhance future performance. In this way, the manager behaves as a coach rather than an evaluator, thus allowing for richer conversations about employee growth and development. The feedforward technique has been found to be effective for improving performance in a service-oriented professional equipment firm.

Performance Improvement Plans

Managers use the performance appraisal process as a method for translating organizational goals into concrete objectives for the individual employee to fulfill. This is a part of the managerial directing function. Through communication, coaching, and development, employees are provided with feedback regarding how their performance fits with the expectations for the organization and the manager's vision regarding the culture of the individual unit or microsystem. The manager identifies the strengths and weaknesses of the employee and provides recognition and support for positive behavior as well as encouragement and specific recommendations about opportunities for improvement. The appraisal needs to show both the employee and the manager what the employee's growth and development possibilities are. The developmental activities that a manager provides for the employee need to be aimed at helping the individual better use his or her skills and improve performance in the current position or develop toward desired future opportunities for advancement.

A performance improvement plan (PIP) is a formal action plan that addresses work performance and needed improvements using identified goals and specific improvement plans. A PIP can be used as a coaching device for personal professional improvement or as a way of tracking and monitoring the performance of a staff member who may be a cause for concern. As a positive action, for example, PIP can be used to encourage staff and a whole team to rise to being the best they can be. There may be team performance goals such as the percentage of RNs certified in their specialty.

A PIP can be seen as negative when a staff person underperforms and needs specific behavioral correction. In that case a formal PIP may be put in place. This occurs when an individual is not meeting targets, or perhaps it is in response to workplace behavior problems. This means the person's performance is not satisfactory and his or her future performance will be monitored. The PIP may be associated with a sense of personal or professional failure.

In the case of a poor performance appraisal, the nurse needs to look for a formal PIP with goals, strategies, expected outcomes, and deadlines. The nurse needs to be involved in the conversation around the PIP, discussing areas of failure, suggesting steps for improvement, and setting goals and action steps that are reasonable and achievable in the time frame. A plan for monitoring and check-ins needs to be clear and agreed to, including set dates to review the progress. The reasons for the PIP need to be clear and all questions answered. The optimum outcome is that the PIP becomes an opportunity to educate the employee, provide support in making improvements, and promote successful performance that benefits the employee and the organization. "Crucial conversations" (see Chapter 7) is one helpful tool. Training in crucial conversations or other interpersonal communication techniques can be most helpful in preparing nurses for participating in peer review as a part of performance appraisal.

When preparing for any performance appraisal—with or without a PIP—the nurse is advised to continually compile a personal and professional portfolio or dossier of performance and accomplishments. For example, further graduate courses taken, certifications, work on quality improvement projects, or shared governance committee work provide evidence of accomplishments that advantage both the nurse and the organization. Continually compiling the elements of the portfolio positions the nurse for being ready more quickly for an annual performance appraisal but also may help in applying for awards, promotions, clinical ladder steps, or other opportunities that arise.

LEADERSHIP AND MANAGEMENT IMPLICATIONS

Elements of a Successful Performance Review System

Performance review processes are an important part of the HRM systems within an organization and are connected to all other aspects of HRM. In order to ensure that the review system is being executed effectively, the following objectives need to be kept in mind.

First, the performance review process needs to be in line with the organization's strategic objectives. For example, if the nurse is working in a hospital where cutting-edge research and treatment is a core initiative, then ongoing learning and development should be a key factor in how people are reviewed and coached. If quality and safety are core strategic priorities, then nurses need to be rewarded for leading quality and safety initiatives.

Second, an effective review system should be fair, transparent, and perceived as just by both those who administer the process and those who are evaluated. Justice is an important factor in other attitudinal outcomes for employees such as satisfaction with one's job and commitment to the work. Performance appraisal systems play a role in whether everyone believes there are fair processes in place and whether rewards are equitably distributed.

Third, the review system needs to be administratively practical. If the system is too onerous, too time consuming, or too taxing on anyone, it can easily fall apart. That is not to say that it cannot require an investment of time and effort. It certainly can and does. However, managers will need to see the connection between their efforts and potential desired outcomes. In other words, it needs to be worth it.

Finally, a review system that is well constructed and effectively administered has the potential to support employee development. One of the ways in which this is accomplished is by creating meaningful, effective relationships between the manager and the employee. In these high-quality relationships, the manager is seen as a coach, someone who is able to support the setting of goals and the planning of future development. Nurse leaders and managers face the challenge of effective performance appraisal as part of their work role. Addressing the known issues and structuring the performance appraisal forms, ratings scales, and processes for maximum effectiveness can be done with thoughtful deliberation.

CURRENT ISSUES AND TRENDS

One of the primary purposes of performance appraisal is to support the development of employees. Researchers have investigated the effects of managerial feedback interventions on subordinates' task performance for decades. The basic premise of this research is that feedback helps to increase employee learning and knowledge of results. Employees need knowledge about their performance, especially if their performance is not up to standard, to be able to take corrective action and improve.

In 1996, Kluger and Denisi conducted a seminal study in which they found that feedback improves performance only one-third of the time. Another third of the time, performance does not change following feedback, and feedback leads to performance decrements in the other third of the time. Subsequent research supported the idea that feedback on its own is generally ineffective, demotivational, and counterproductive (Coens & Jenkins, 2000; Smither et al., 2005). There is also a great deal of dissatisfaction with performance management systems. Managers find them frustrating, and employees find them unhelpful, even when they receive good or outstanding ratings. A current issue for both research and practice is finding ways to ensure that performance reviews support performance improvement.

The most common problems associated with the traditional appraisal interview are a lack of strategic focus, too much subjectivity, and heavy emphasis on past performance rather than future potential. In order to address these drawbacks, decades of research has focused on either the appraisal or the rater's ability to perform an unbiased evaluation. In practice, the managers conducting the appraisals continue to feel that they are not adequately trained in how to appraise performance and feel uncomfortable judging others.

DeNisi and Sonesh (2011) have argued that it is more important for the feedback to be perceived as accurate than it is for accuracy to be the focus of the appraisal process. This argument is a result of the acknowledgment that complex appraisal processes that both the appraiser and the employee find difficult to understand can undermine the ultimate goal of feedback, namely to improve performance. They have encouraged movement away from concerns around increasing accuracy toward research that addresses the procedural concerns with evaluative processes.

This conversation has affected how practitioners roll out performance appraisal systems within organizations. The technology giant Adobe made a big splash in their industry when they abolished performance appraisals entirely in favor of regular, ongoing check-in conversations. The shift has been away from evaluation and toward genuine conversations wherein feedback is shared using an approach similar to coaching. As a result, Adobe has enjoyed a decrease in turnover and a significant savings in managerial time.

The professional services firm Deloitte also overhauled their performance appraisal system. They traded in the traditional 1-year review for a faster, more agile system that reflected the fast pace of change in their business. After conducting a carefully controlled study of their organization, they found that employees thrived when they were able to use their strengths every day. The revised system involved asking team leaders a series of questions at the completion of each project rather than once per year. The questions focused on what they would do with each team member (promote, want him or her on my team, give a bonus or a raise) rather than what they thought of that individual. For a complete review of the Deloitte system, see Buckingham and Goodall (2015).

Organizations are moving away from traditional review, ranking, and feedback sessions because of current understanding that these systems do not consistently produce performance improvement. A focus on improving the conversations that take place when feedback is delivered has shown promise from both a research and practical perspective. It is unknown whether health care organizations will follow the lead of business and industry with regard to current trends in performance appraisal. It is intriguing to speculate how revised systems might meet accreditation and quality review standards such as those of The Joint Commission. For example, for the Magnet Recognition Program®, the nursing organization must have in place systematic peer-review practices, including formalized, systematic peer-review nursing practices to evaluate nursing care and nursing care providers. This is done to stimulate professionalism through increased accountability and to promote self-regulation of nursing practice by nurses (American Nurse Today, 2011). Although peer review processes need to be evident, the form and character are not specified and could be updated.

⚡ RESEARCH NOTE

Source
Decramer, A., Audenaert, M., Van Waeyenberg, T., Claeys, T., Laes, C., Vandevelde, S., et al. (2015). Does performance management affect nurses' well-being? *Evaluation and Program Planning, 49*, 98–105.

Purpose
This study aimed to investigate the relationship between performance management and attitudinal outcomes for nurses. The outcomes under investigation included job satisfaction and commitment to the organization.

Discussion
A questionnaire was completed by 140 Flemish nurses working in hospital settings. The researchers assessed job satisfaction and affective commitment (dependent variables) using valid and reliable survey tools. Data were also collected on the features of the performance management systems used to evaluate each respondent in his or her workplace. Specifically, respondents indicated whether they (1) were evaluated as part a performance evaluation system, (2) were evaluated relative to personal objectives, (3) set goals that were linked to organizational goals, and (4) were satisfied with the performance management system. Regression analysis was used to understand whether the characteristics of the performance management system affected the dependent variables.

The results indicated that some features of the performance management system predicted job satisfaction and affective commitment. In particular, the researchers found that when the goals set were aligned with the

RESEARCH NOTE—cont'd

organizational goals, the individual was more committed to the hospital. Goal alignment was not correlated with job satisfaction. Satisfaction with the performance management system was found to predict affective well-being.

Application to Practice

In recent years, health care organizations have faced periodic shortages in the nursing complement. As a result, there is a need to ensure that the management of nurses increases both in efficiency and in the engagement of the nurses on staff. Research in human resource management supports the notion that investing in employees yields improvements for the organization. The key findings in this study stress the importance of aligning individual goals with outcomes that are important to the organization. There is also a need to ensure that employees are satisfied with the performance management system, a task that requires alignment and communication.

CASE STUDY

There is a growing sense among the leadership team at this large rural hospital that the performance appraisal system is not working. Nurse manager Kathy Stewart, MSN, RN, reflects that "each year we chase down reviewers to submit their appraisals but it really feels like a futile exercise. I am not certain that our system is making us better in any way." A team of nurses, human resources professionals, and allied health care professionals speak with stakeholders within the hospital and come to a few clear conclusions. For nurses who have good relationships with their managers and who are performing well, the appraisals are a good opportunity to set goals and identify ways of advancing their career. For everyone else, the reviews cause stress and anxiety and do not really lead anywhere. Kathy identifies this as an opportunity to introduce some positive change.

After consulting with the broader management team, Kathy decides that the performance appraisal system needs to get back to basics. The core strategic value of the hospital is "health care service excellence." Yet the performance appraisal system is rooted in skill development and technical learning and advancement. Kathy has an epiphany when she recognizes that although professional development is critically important for patient care, the performance appraisal process has strayed too far away from the core mission. There is a need to move away from a system that is provider centric to a model that is patient focused. For Kathy's hospital this makes sense. By reframing the purpose of the performance appraisals, Kathy is able to align the goals of the hospital with the performance review and development experiences of the nursing staff.

CRITICAL THINKING EXERCISE

Julianne Hughes is a new nurse manager in the pediatric unit of her hospital. She has been told that one of her responsibilities will be to evaluate the nurses within her unit once yearly. As a new manager, she has been given direct supervisory responsibilities for 12 nurses. Her staff work on various shifts on a rotating 24-hour schedule. She sees some of them far more than others. Although she is nervous about providing performance feedback for the first time, she feels she has a good sense of everyone's performance levels. She completes her reviews, submits them, and sets up performance interviews with each of her staff. Her first meeting goes quite well. Rob is happy with his review, and both he and Julianne leave feeling as though they have had a positive interaction.

Julianne is nervous about her second interview. Lisa has worked mainly evenings over the past few months, and Julianne has found that some of the overnight duties are not complete when she returns in the morning. Julianne has some corrective feedback to deliver to Lisa. Lisa is shocked. She felt that she was doing a great job with patient care. Both individuals leave the meeting frustrated and dismayed.

1. What is the problem?
2. What should Julianne have done differently?
3. What might explain the discrepancy between Julianne's and Lisa's perspectives?
4. Would you make any recommendations for improving the performance review process more generally?

Emergency Management and Preparedness

Elizabeth T. Dugan, Lynn Christensen

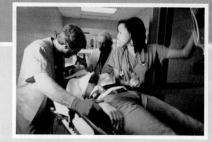

ℯ http://evolve.elsevier.com/Huber/leadership

TRANSITIONING THEORY INTO PRACTICE FOR ALL-HAZARDS PREPAREDNESS

September 11, 2001, was a tragic day that touched everyone's lives and forever changed Americans' perception of a "safe" world. As a result, people of all backgrounds have given thought to preparing themselves, their homes, and their work environments for the eventuality of a disaster. Most people are knowledgeable about how to prepare for potential natural disasters within their local regions, but many have not had to consider the devastation that can be caused by terrorism. A list of terrorism possibilities is endless: biological exposures, chemical spills, radiological exposures, nuclear blasts, conventional bombings, agricultural contamination, cyber viruses, and other unforeseen cataclysmic events. Thus developing a contingency plan for most types of disasters, including bioterrorism, is most appropriately termed **all-hazards disaster preparedness.**

Since the occurrence of major disasters such as the attack on the World Trade Center, Hurricane Sandy in 2012, and the devastating tornado in Joplin, Missouri, in 2011, key community stakeholders such as local government, fire and rescue workers, and hospitals have been focused on gathering information from a variety of resources, developing collaborative response plans, and preparing for a probable disaster. The Joint Commission (TJC) has advanced hospital efforts

through the development of six crucial areas for emergency preparedness: communication, safety and security, resources and assets, staff responsibilities, utilities management, and patient clinical and support activities (Joint Commission Resources, 2008, 2016). These crucial areas create a framework for all-hazards disaster preparedness planning in hospitals. So how does one go about preparing for an event in the workplace, and more specifically, the hospital environment? Traditionally the community hospital is a place of refuge for the sick and wounded. How is all of this affected in the event of a disaster?

Health care executives across the country understand the need to dedicate resources to support effective all-hazards preparedness. The Health Insurance Portability and Accountability Act (HIPAA) and TJC require all health care facilities to have detailed all-hazard preparedness plans. Nursing leaders are an integral part of the planning process and should have knowledge of the national response plan (NRP) promulgated by the Federal Emergency Management Agency (FEMA) and state and local disaster response plans *(http://www.fema.gov/media-library)*. Effective planning skills for all-hazards preparedness is an essential management competency for nurse executives.

This chapter describes how to orchestrate a multi-level plan for a health care facility. A comprehensive all-hazards preparedness plan will assist in establishing (1) an organized hospital-based plan for both internal and external disasters at the department/unit level, (2) an interhospital plan for effectively collaborating with other hospitals within a health care system and

---

within the vicinity, (3) a community plan that will integrate the hospital plan with other external community plans, and (4) a national plan that will guide nurse leaders in accessing financial assistance from federal and state all-hazards preparedness resources.

DEFINITIONS

From a health care perspective, a **disaster** is "a type of emergency that, due to its complexity, scope, or duration, threatens a health care center's capabilities . . . and requires outside assistance to sustain patient care, safety, or security functions" (TJC, 2008, p. 2). There are a wide variety of types and causes of disasters, including sudden onset (severe weather events or chemical spills) and slow-onset events (progressive disease outbreaks) (World Health Organization [WHO], 2013). Although often triggered by nature, disasters can be caused by human acts, including chemical, biological, radiological, nuclear, or explosives (CBRNE). Wars and civil disturbances that destroy homelands and displace people are included among man-made disasters. Causes of natural disasters include severe weather events such as blizzards, wildfires, floods, tsunamis, volcanic eruptions, earthquakes, tornadoes, hurricanes, and the devastation caused by Hurricane Sandy in 2012 or the earthquake and resulting tsunami in Japan in 2011. Disasters can be *internal,* such as a catastrophic event that occurs within a facility, making it difficult to maintain operations (TJC, 2012); or *external,* such as a catastrophic event that affects the community that may or may not affect the facility.

Other disaster-related definitions are:

- *All-hazards:* A general term that is descriptive of all types of natural and/or human terrorist events
- *All-hazards disaster preparedness:* An effective and consistent response to any disaster or emergency regardless of the cause (Wright State University, 2016)
- *Crisis standards of care:* "Substantial change in the usual healthcare operations and the level of care it is possible to deliver . . . in a public health emergency, justified by specific circumstances, declared by a state government in recognition that crisis operations will be in effect for a sustained period" (Institute of Medicine [IOM], 2012)
- *CBRNE:* Chemical, biological, radiological, nuclear, explosives (US Department of Defense, 2015)

- *Biological disaster:* Disease epidemics and insect/animal plagues or an incident occurring as a result of the deliberate or unintentional release of biological materials that may adversely affect the health of those exposed (International Federation of Red Cross and Red Crescent Societies [IFRC], 2016; US Department of Defense, 2015)
- *Chemical disaster:* The deliberate or unintentional release of poisonous vapors, liquids, or solids that have a toxic effect on people, plants, and animals (Ready.gov, 2016)
- *Radiological/nuclear disaster:* Radiological or nuclear emergencies may be intentional (caused by terrorists) or unintentional (accidents that may result from accidents within a facility, e.g., the departments of nuclear medicine and radiation oncology or from external sources involving vehicles transporting radioactive materials) (Centers for Disease Control and Prevention [CDC], 2014)
- *Explosives:* A catastrophic event caused by the use of weapons such as guns, bombs, missiles, or grenades
- *Cyber disaster:* A catastrophic event that results from an attack initiated from one computer against another computer with the purpose of compromising the information stored on it (Arnand, 2014)
- *Hazard vulnerability analysis:* An exercise that is a systematic approach to recognizing hazards and identifying an organization's potential emergencies, the likelihood of the event occurring, and the impact it would have on the organization. The risks associated with each hazard are analyzed to prioritize planning, mitigation, response, and recovery activities (California Hospital Association, 2011)
- *Mass casualty incident:* A natural or manmade event generating large numbers of patients requiring medical care and that overwhelms a health care facility and prevents it from delivering medical services that are consistent with accepted standards (Agency for Healthcare Research and Quality [AHRQ], 2012)

GETTING STARTED: FIRST STEPS

Starting any systems project can be complex and difficult. Beginning the work of establishing a comprehensive all-hazards preparedness plan is no exception. Historically, most hospitals have had some type of disaster plan in place. Evaluating the hospital's existing emergency operations plan (EOP) while focusing on maintaining a state of constant readiness can be a complicated process. One of the first steps to gaining participation from appropriate stakeholders and moving the evaluation process forward is the creation of an emergency management oversight committee, or an all-hazards preparedness task force. Based on the American Organization of Nurse Executive's (AONE, 2016) *Role of the Nurse Leader in Crisis Management,* the nurse executive—often called the *chief nursing officer (CNO)*—will play a pivotal role in facilitating the initial committee. The AONE guiding principles include:

- Nurse leaders are trained in media relations and understand the tenets of good communication.
- Leaders are skilled critical thinkers, collaborative, and able to manage ambiguity.
- Nurse leaders project calm, confidence, and authority in all situations. They also are empathetic to how people react to loss, challenges, and uncertainty.
- Nurse leaders are prepared to review and practice the organization's crisis readiness plan with nursing staff.
- The chief nursing officer is a member of the senior leadership team, whose role is clearly defined and sought by colleagues, particularly during a crisis.

Creating an Emergency Management Committee

As many nurses understand, effective projects start with the basic nursing process: assessment, planning, implementation, evaluation, and, if necessary, modification. The emergency management committee will follow a similar process when developing an emergency management plan. Developing an original plan is best accomplished by establishing a high-level administrative committee whose purpose will be oversight of the multilevel emergency management plan development. Whether the hospital is part of a larger health care system or is a freestanding, independent hospital, the committee will function similarly.

Health care systems with multiple facilities are very familiar with the complexity and intricacies of trying to establish a standardized system-wide approach to care needs. In organizations such as these, system-wide executive administrators need to be part of the committee. Having a senior executive administrator of the health care system serve as the chairperson of the committee will provide the leadership needed to communicate the importance of emergency preparedness as a system priority. A representative CNO and emergency medicine physician, serving as co-chairs with the senior executive administrator, can create a dynamic team that is uniquely prepared to tackle any issues that arise. A project facilitator is helpful in getting the committee started and operational. The project facilitator can also serve in a pivotal maintenance role, keeping the emergency management plan current and in the forefront of the administration's strategic planning over time.

Establishing the committee requires that all departments be committed to the tasks at hand and cognizant of the need for consensus building and standardization of processes. Bidirectional communication is imperative. The standing membership should be composed of stakeholders representing all areas of the organization. Because not all departments can logistically be on the committee, the members will have large areas of oversight and communication. Committee membership might typically look like that outlined in Table 25.1.

As the team evolves in its work, ad hoc members can be added as needed. Internal ad hoc members might include radiology, facility engineering, telecommunications, volunteer support, chaplain services, physician chairs, social work, case management, and dietary, respiratory, and laboratory services. External ad hoc members might include representatives from the local public health department, government liaison, police, fire and rescue, public school system, representatives from the faith community, community physicians, and even vendor representatives who can be contracted to provide such things as oxygen, ice, food, cots, and linens in the event of a disaster.

During the start-up, the system-wide committee will need to meet frequently. To begin, the committee should perform a hazard vulnerability analysis (HVA). The HVA will be used as a starting point to create an EOP that identifies risks and prioritizes likely emergencies in order to mitigate them when possible and develop strategies for preparedness (Joint Commission Resources, 2016). For specific details on the HVA process, there are several resources available, including the Federal Emergency Management Agency (FEMA) and Joint Commission Resources websites.

Performing an Effective Gap Analysis

There are many ways to perform an all-hazards preparedness gap analysis, and a multitude of online reference websites exist, including these examples:

- FEMA: *https://www.fema.gov/media-library/assets/documents/21635*

TABLE 25.1   **Emergency Management Committee Membership Responsibilities**

Responsibility Area(S)	Position Title	Detail of Area Covered
Executive owner (chair)	Executive administrator	Leads the emergency management committee as chair. If the hospital is part of a health care system, this person will be a system-wide senior administrator. If the hospital is a freestanding, independent facility, this person will be the hospital's chief operating officer.
Clinical operations (co-chair)	Chief nurse officer	Represents all nursing and clinical departments; co-chairs the emergency management committee.
Chemical, biological, radiological, nuclear, or explosives (CBRNE) threats (co-chair)	Emergency department/medical director	Represents all aspects of emergency medicine and physician needs related to all-hazards preparedness. This person also will co-chair the committee.
Physician liaison(s)	Department chiefs	Serve as spokespersons for physician needs with regard to disaster preparedness. Facilitate communication of timely information should an event occur. Have oversight for physician credentialing in times of a disaster. Assist in approval of medical standards established for various types of disasters.
Chief operating officers (COOs) from health care system facilities	Chief operating officer(s)	Represent the needs of their facilities in establishing an effective all-hazards preparedness plan. Facilitate system-wide collaboration in standardizing practices and communicate essential information to employees.
Security	Safety and security director	Serves as liaison for system-wide safety and security departments in the system. Coordinates and synchronizes efforts of all departments as related to all-hazards preparedness. Responsible for rapid "lockdown" of all entrances and flow of people in the event of a disaster.
Communications	Chief information technology officer	Oversees successful operation of the integrated information system, including telephones, radios, and computers and satellite technology, during times of instability. Creates and maintains redundant systems to ensure an ability to communicate within facilities, outside to other hospitals, and partners with community.
Messages/media	Marketing director/ information officer	Plays an active role in communicating the all-hazards preparedness message to all employees, patients, and community. Acts on behalf of the health care system or hospital in speaking with press about impending or actual disaster situations.
Human resources	Human resources director	Serves as the staff's voice in meeting the needs of employees during a disaster. Creates manuals to guide staff in preparing for and responding to a disaster. Manages the human resources pool when the incident command center is active.
Financial reimbursement	Chief financial officer	Leads efforts in monitoring financial expenses related to establishing an effective all-hazards preparedness plan. Seeks out state/federal reimbursement opportunities for planning.
Government funding	Government affairs director	Serves as a vital link to local, state, and federal boards representing the system financial and operational needs regarding all-hazards preparedness. Advocates for funding related to all-hazards preparedness.

Continued

TABLE 25.1 Emergency Management Committee Membership Responsibilities—cont'd

Responsibility Area(S)	Position Title	Detail of Area Covered
Biological threats	Infectious disease medical director	Serves as the liaison for all infection control (IC) departments in the system.
Infection control	Infection prevention and control practitioner	Coordinates and synchronizes efforts of all IC departments as related to all-hazards preparedness. Responsible for development, dissemination, and understanding of procedures related to biological events.
Legal	Executive attorney	Advises all-hazards preparedness task force in legal matters related to establishing an effective all-hazards preparedness plan.
Education planning	Education director	Has oversight for planning and implementing educational efforts for staff and patients. As needed, coordinates "just in time" training for any arising incident and is an integral partner in planning and implementing internal and external disaster drills.
Logistics	Pharmacy director	Serves as the liaison for all system pharmacies. Has oversight for stockpiling medications for use in a disaster. Establishes par levels of drugs for use in "patient surge" situations. Establishes contracts with pharmaceutical vendors to ensure adequate supply of medications in the event of a disaster. Has oversight for any medical supply trucks ready for deployment in times of a disaster (e.g., stocking par level of drugs used in a chemical disaster).
Logistics	Materials management director	Serves as an active participant on the task force. This liaison is the system representative for all materials management departments. Is very involved in setting par levels for supplies and equipment on the units at the time of a disaster. Establishes contracts with materials management vendors to ensure adequate supply of medications in the event of a disaster (e.g., stocking a supplemental supply truck for use in a disaster).
Logistics	Engineering	Directs any operational building redesign needed to prepare hospital for handling a disaster (e.g., decontamination showers).

NOTE: This assessment tool was developed by Inova Health System based on a bioterrorism preparedness survey created by a committee consisting of representatives from Baylor University's Graduate Program in Healthcare Administration, the US Army Center for Healthcare Education and Studies, and the University of Texas Health Science Center at San Antonio. (For more information, see Drenkard et al., 2002.) Courtesy Inova Health System, Falls Church, VA.

- Office of Emergency Management, US Department of Health and Human Services: *https://www.phe.gov/about/oem/Pages/default.aspx* and the American Hospital Association (AHA): *http://www.aha.org/*
- Centers for Disease Control and Prevention (CDC): *https://www.cdc.gov*
- Agency for Healthcare Research and Quality (AHRQ): *https://archive.ahrq.gov/research/epri/*

- CCHC (Clinics and Community Health Centers) Emergency Preparedness Gap Analysis: *http://www.cpca.org/cpca/assets/File/Emergency-Preparedness/Resources/2011-08-11-Gap-Analysis-Tool-Final.pdf*

The guiding principle for creating a hospital-specific all-hazards gap analysis is to keep it simple. One example of a simple way to assess the current state is to create an emergency preparedness survey that is easy to read and requires the department directors to answer in simple checklists one of two ways: (1) "Yes, we have it," or (2) "No, we don't have it." Survey questions need to be concise and clear. The goal is to begin by identifying the areas where there are gaps in the facility's preparedness plans. Questions should be addressed to appropriate departments who then assess the items and determine the current state. A review of the literature and online searches will assist the team in identifying the

areas of assessment (FEMA Emergency Management Institute, 2014; Joint Commission Resources, 2008, 2016). Examples of questions to ask in the survey might include those listed in Box 25.1.

Once the survey is created, it should be distributed to all stakeholders. Directors should be challenged to complete and return it within an appropriate deadline so that work can be initiated to address outstanding issues. The committee should review the survey results and

---

BOX 25.1 Hospital Gap Analysis Survey: Sample Questions

General

- Has your organization conducted a thorough hazard vulnerability analysis (HVA)?
- Does your organization have an emergency operations plan (EOP) that specifically addresses the four disaster phases?
- Does your EOP identify how to activate an emergency response and who is in charge of the command center in a disaster?
- Does your facility have an operational command center to coordinate the hospital's response to a disaster?
- Does your department staff know the chain of command in an emergency?
- Does your department know their role in each type of disaster?
- Does your hospital know their role in the community in an emergency situation?
- Are there specific plans for chemical, biological, radiological, nuclear, or explosives (CBRNE) emergencies?
- Is there a bed and staffing plan for surge capacity for 50 patients? 100 patients? 250 patients? Do you have the necessary supplies and equipment for use in a surge situation?

Human Resources

- Does your department staff know how to prepare themselves, their significant others, and pets in the event of a disaster?
- Is there a credentialing plan for health care professionals who come to the nearest facility in a disaster to volunteer their services?

Safety and Security

- Does your facility have the following during an emergency:
  - A lockdown plan?
  - A plan for facility traffic flow and staff entry?
  - Multi-language signage to direct people where to go?

Communication

- Does your hospital have emergency-powered phones in case of a disaster?
- Does your facility have a backup radio system and volunteer staff to run it?
- Does your facility have a tiered paging system that can reach multiple staff simultaneously?
- Does your department know the central command center telephone number (if there is one)?
- Is there an on-call procedure for notifying the administrator on-call and opening the command center in the event of a disaster?
- Are there established linkages to the external community (e.g., other hospitals in the region, fire department, police, emergency medical system, public schools, public health)?
- Is there a procedure for how to link patients and families both in your facility and in the community should a disaster occur?

Logistics

- Does your facility have:
  - Backup emergency supplies, pharmaceuticals, and equipment?
  - The ability to release and send pharmaceuticals, medical supplies, and equipment such as respirators to the areas in need in the event of a chemical or biological emergency?
  - Prearranged plans with physicians, ambulances, nearby churches, and nursing homes to clear beds in an emergency? (What sites can take patients?)
  - Contracts with vendors to bring in food, ice, oxygen, and other needed supplies?
- Is there an established written psychosocial role for social work, chaplains, psychiatry, employee health, and case management in the event of a disaster?
- Are there contingency plans for 4 to 5 days of no power, no water, no computers, and/or no food?

Continued

BOX 25.1   Hospital Gap Analysis Survey: Sample Questions—cont'd

- Are there contingency plans for staff to report to nearest facility to work?
- Are there contingency plans for childcare during an emergency so that parents can work?
- Is there common nomenclature used during an emergency so that everyone understands what is happening and who has what responsibility?

Clinical Operations
- Does your facility have:
  - Procedures established to maximize staff safety in the event of a disaster?
  - Procedures for respiratory mask fit testing and training for personal protective equipment for staff?
  - The ability to track patients until discharge, admission, or death using HIPAA guidelines?
  - Clear established policies and procedures to respond to CBRNE emergencies?
  - A decontamination area and detailed step-by-step procedures on how to work in this area?
  - A backup staff to assist with people/patients arriving to the hospital?
- Does your facility have procedures for how to:
  - Track available beds, arriving patients, and discharges?

- Track regular and volunteer staff and direct them to a designated area?
- Operate every department of the hospital during an emergency?
- Handle surge capacity situations including an understanding of crisis standards of care?
- Handle operating room cases in the event of an emergency?
- Track biological, chemical, or nuclear events and report them to authorities?

Financial
- Is there an established plan for tracking costs and submitting them for reimbursement or claims during an emergency?

Messages/Media
- Is there an established communication plan in case of an emergency?
- Is there an established communication script in the event of an emergency?
- Is there an alternative communication plan if power, telephones, and radios are not working?

Courtesy Inova Health System. From Drenkard, K., & Rigotti, G. (2002, updated 2016). *Inova Health System survey.* Falls Church, VA: Inova Health System.

---

start an issues list to address deficiencies. Nursing leaders will play key roles in creating aggressive timelines for resolving issues identified. Most resolutions will be modified and enhanced over time as the committee gains more knowledge about all-hazards planning.

From the gap analysis, the committee needs to establish high-level, multifaceted standards of practice and system-wide goals for all-hazards preparedness. These standards and goals will be implemented at the facility level and department level as directed by the chief operating officer (COO), CNO, and emergency department (ED) medical director. At this point, there is latitude for departments to design and implement the standards and goals based on the unique needs of the populations served. Annual review and evaluation of goals is an effective project management activity, with new goals being created based on the HVA, changing regulatory requirements, new threats, and the results of gaps identified during drills. Sustaining attention and focus on disaster preparedness efforts becomes a key role of the

nurse executive in ensuring a constant state of organizational readiness. The project facilitator assists the nurse executive in researching new and evolving initiatives in the discipline of all-hazards preparedness, determining the importance of new trends to the effective operations of the health care organization's all-hazard plan, and implementing relevant enhancements that support the strategic vision for preparedness within the organization.

Keeping the Momentum Going

Once the gap analysis is completed and the issues are identified, development of a comprehensive plan is a critical next step. The work can appear daunting, and it is hard to know where to start. It is at this point that nursing leadership has the opportunity to take charge of the process. Even though the gap analysis may show a multitude of areas for improvement, issues are solvable one step at a time. The CNO and nurse leaders can help focus the committee and department directors. Efforts should be directed toward creating a streamlined, comprehensive internal emergency management plan that will set the foundation for later steps when the hospital begins to work externally with the community.

Action Items List

Over the next phase, the development of an actions items list will become the working action plan used to prioritize and organize work to be done. Subgroups made up of members from the task force who are content experts can be assigned to lead efforts to resolve issues. Issues need to be constantly added and resolved as the facility refines the plan. Reports from subgroups on their progress should be regularly submitted to the committee. The committee needs to have oversight of the subgroups and should strive to clear the road for subgroup progress as needed. Hospitals may need to address common issues such as allocation of resources, including funds to educate staff. Educating the nursing workforce will be critical to promote an effective disaster response.

Establishing a Common Nomenclature, Structure, and Role Definition for Writing All-Hazards Preparedness Plans

When working with the community, using common language becomes especially important for promoting interagency communication in crisis situations. Therefore the National Incident Management System (NIMS) was created by the US Department of Homeland Security (2016) Secretary to further standardize and integrate response practices nationally.

The National Incident Management System (NIMS) is a systematic, proactive approach to guide departments and agencies at all levels of government, nongovernmental organizations, and the private sector to work together seamlessly and manage incidents involving all threats and hazards—regardless of cause, size, location, or complexity—in order to reduce loss of life, property and harm to the environment. The NIMS is the essential foundation to the National Preparedness System (NPS) and provides the template for the management of incidents and operations in support of all five National Planning Frameworks (Federal Emergency Management Agency [FEMA], 2016).

In the past, the limited focus of the disaster plan on file at a hospital usually related specifically to safety and security preparedness. Today the primary responsibility for the safety and security department, in conjunction with nursing leadership, is to develop or refine the hospital's EOP for incidents based on the HVA. The safety and security department needs to have assigned oversight for facility security, quick lockdown or controlled access, and management of people flowing into and out of the hospital.

Nursing leadership needs to ensure that all facility departments understand their role in a disaster situation. Nurse leaders are the coordinators in synchronizing department plans so that everything fits together to meet the essential needs of the staff, patients, hospital, and community. Once the comprehensive emergency management plans are complete, every department should understand its identified written role.

Creating Procedural Annexes to All-Hazards Preparedness Plans

In addition to overall all-hazards preparedness plans, the hospital will need to define procedures regarding what will be done in any CBRNE disaster and what the surge capacity needs will be related to any of these events. *Surge capacity* is a measurable representation of the ability to manage a sudden influx of patients (American College of Emergency Physicians [ACEP], 2011). These specific procedures are added separately to the plan and are called annexes. The committee can assign the creation of each of these procedures to a subgroup. These teams are often led by nursing leadership and the emergency medicine director, with appropriate ad hoc participation. For example, the infection prevention and control department, in partnership with public health, can co-lead the biological planning efforts; the radiology department can co-lead the nuclear/radiological efforts partnering closely with local authorities; and nursing, pharmacy, and emergency medicine can co-lead the explosives, chemical, and surge capacity efforts, partnering closely with police, fire, and rescue. The goal with these procedural annexes is to create easy, step-by-step action plans, fact sheets, and algorithms for identifying, intervening, and notifying the appropriate authorities. As with most all-hazards preparedness literature, the most current references will be online. Some essential websites to assist in writing specific hospital procedures include the Centers for Disease Control and Prevention

(CDC), the Department of Homeland Security (DHS), and the US Department of Labor's Occupational Safety and Health Administration (OSHA).

In establishing procedural annexes and the overall all-hazards disaster preparedness plan, The Joint Commission's (TJC) emergency management accreditation standards call for hospitals to sustain disaster operations for at least 96 hours should an external disaster occur that affects the local area or region (TJC, 2012). Lessons learned from Hurricane Katrina illustrate just how long it can take before assistance is available. Hospital leadership needs to make sure every operating unit and department is prepared. The following are only a few examples of what hospitals will need:

- A conservative stockpile of essential antibiotics for biological threats
- Antidotes for chemical exposures
- Basic food and bottled water surpluses for environmental contamination events
- Preplanned contracts with local supply companies and businesses for ice, oxygen and other gases, and emergency power
- Alternative communication methods and plans, both internal and external, in case of power outage
- Staff and volunteer credentialing and identification procedures
- Established entrances for staff during lockdowns or controlled access situations
- Patient identification and tracking systems for families in search of loved ones
- Downtime procedures for cyber threats (with the ability to function up to 5 days)
- Accommodations for staff to bring in their children for care while they are working

Creating a Planning Subgroup

Even with comprehensive emergency management plans and annexes, the unexpected will happen, such as in threats and incidents involving anthrax, severe acute respiratory syndrome (SARS), smallpox, potentially harmful H1N1 influenza, and most recently Ebola and Zika viruses. Initially no one will know whether these are true terrorist threats or isolated spontaneous incidents. The hospital must be ready to respond at all times. An ongoing emergency management planning group needs to be formed at the local level and chaired by a nurse executive who sits on the system emergency management committee along with key stakeholder

membership (including ED, employee health staff, and infection prevention and control). Based on the changing needs of the events, this planning group will enable the facility to respond quickly to the "just in time" educational needs of the staff, allow for rapid procedural planning for community needs, and ensure appropriate authority notification in the event of a disaster. For example, the staff will be expected to recognize the symptoms and presentation of Ebola and respond by critical thinking, as follows:

- Triaging and isolating the patient on admission to the ED and placing the patient in the hospital or facility's negative pressure room if available
- Obtaining and having the staff wear appropriate personal protective equipment (PPE)
- Controlling access to the ED and possibly the entire hospital
- Identifying (name, address, telephone number) all patient contacts, transport services (emergency medical services [EMS]), staff, and patients in the waiting room
- Notifying the infection prevention and control practitioner, hospital/facility infectious disease physician or epidemiologist, public health officials, and police

Biological and chemical terrorism are examples of unexpected severe events needing a strategic plan for preparedness and response. The CDC (2001) has provided recommendations for biological and chemical terrorism. They noted that:

Terrorist incidents in the United States and elsewhere involving bacterial pathogens (3), nerve gas (1), and a lethal plant toxin (i.e., ricin) (4), have demonstrated that the United States is vulnerable to biological and chemical threats as well as explosives. Recipes for preparing "homemade" agents are readily available (5), and reports of arsenals of military bioweapons (2) raise the possibility that terrorists might have access to highly dangerous agents, which have been engineered for mass dissemination as small-particle aerosols. Such agents as the variola virus, the causative agent of smallpox, are highly contagious and often fatal. Responding to large-scale outbreaks caused by these agents will require the rapid mobilization of public health workers, emergency responders, and private health-care providers. Large-scale outbreaks will also require rapid procurement and distribution of large quantities of drugs and vaccines, which must be available quickly.

There are numerous potential biological and chemical agents. Attacks with biological agents are more likely to be covert. There are three categories of biological agents, with the highest priority agents including emerging pathogens that could be engineered for mass dissemination in the future. Chemical agents that might be used by terrorists range from warfare agents to toxic chemicals commonly used in industry: nerve gas, blood agents, blister agents, heavy metals, volatile toxins, pulmonary agents, incapacitating agents, pesticides, polychlorinated biphenyls (PCBs), nitro compounds, flammable gasses and liquids, poisons, and corrosive acids and bases.

Managing causes of biological or chemical mass casualty or terrorism events includes strategies for preparedness and prevention, detection and surveillance, diagnosis and characterization of biological and chemical agents, and response and rapid deployment in the event of an overt attack. Communication is essential. For example, educational materials need to be prepared to inform the public during and after an attack. The initial detection of a covert biological or chemical attack will probably occur at the local level. Thus disease surveillance systems at state and local health agencies need to be capable of detecting unusual patterns of disease or injury, including those caused by unusual or unknown threat agents (CDC, 2001).

Despite the best PPE guidance by the CDC (*https://www.cdc.gov/vhf/ebola/healthcare-us/ppe/guidance.html*), the recent Ebola crisis highlighted serious issues in the health care delivery system, such as gaps in training, the cost of PPE, and a story reported by *60 Minutes* about a company accused of providing faulty surgical gowns to US hospitals and the US strategic national stockpile, although the company denied the allegations (CBS News, 2016). Because Ebola is so lethal, these gaps and the ways organizations responded to protect their employees came to the forefront. Nurses were directly affected.

Developing a Command Center

In the event of a disaster, the hospital would need a dedicated centralized command center where all department directors can report for instructions. The four essential elements of a command center, explained in more detail in later sections, are as follows:

1. Setting up the room
2. Developing processes in the command center
3. Establishing the hospital's role in the community
4. Testing the all-hazards preparedness plans and command center functionality

Setting Up the Command Center Room

The location of the incident command center will depend on the organization's physical layout, but it often is located near the safety and security department. It is commanded by the on-call administrator along with the CNO, the ED medical director, and the safety and security director. The following equipment should be available in the room:

- Multiple telephones/telephone lines with speed dial for frequently called numbers
- Computer access (with both intranet and Internet capabilities)
- Printing capability
- Batch fax and copying capabilities
- Alternative phone options (e.g., 800 MHz radio technology and/or Voice over Internet Protocol [VoIP] technology—a phone system that operates over Internet lines with functioning antenna) and people trained to use them
- Tiered paging capability
- Television access
- Office-related supplies such as paper, pens, easels, dry erase boards, work tables, phone books, and reference materials such as the all-hazards preparedness plans for each hospital area

The command center should be available at a moment's notice and fully functional within minutes. A common scenario is that the call comes into the ED, but many internal disasters, such as utility failures, may come from other sources. When an external disaster occurs, nursing leadership staff in the ED, along with medical staff, will determine the gravity of the situation and decide whether the incident can be handled in the ED or whether the hospital administrator needs to be contacted. If it is deemed appropriate to contact the hospital administrator, there will be dialogue among nursing leadership, medical leadership, and the administrator to decide whether the command center should be opened. If the command center is to be opened, the hospital administrator will start the process and call in the additional staff necessary to assist with incident command operations. In the event that the disaster involves the area where the command center is located, the hospital will have to have a predetermined plan to establish a backup command center in another location. In the case of a multifacility system, the alternate command center could be at another hospital.

Developing Processes in the Command Center

Because one of the rotating on-call administrators may be called on to open the command center, the creation of a simple, step-by-step, short document (one to two pages) of how to open, operate, and close down the command center is important. A more extensive manual can also be created, but in times of a disaster, the short "How to Open the Command Center" document is crucial. If the facility does not have an on-call administrator list, one should be established, and staff must know how to reach the on-call person(s). A clear decision matrix should be in place outlining when to open the command center and who needs to be notified. It may be helpful to create a communication tree identifying the process for quickly notifying the administrative team and emergency management committee members. Using a group paging function can be helpful for rapid notification of the leadership team.

To facilitate the incident command structure during a disaster, many hospitals have adopted the Hospital Incident Command System (HICS) for their all-hazards preparedness plans, because it allows logical standardization with common nomenclature that is understood both in the hospital environment and in the community setting (US Department of Health & Human Services, 2012). In addition, the HICS organizational chart provides a comprehensive structure that is scalable to the size of the event and has standardized role descriptions. Techniques such as using vests to identify people in charge during a disaster, with a one-page job action sheet in each vest pocket, are essential in a crisis situation. Color-coded vests may also be useful in identifying the role of each leader based on the incident command structure utilized. All hospital and department all-hazards preparedness plans must be on hand and clearly labeled in the command center, along with in-house phone and pager directories.

Testing the Emergency Management Plans and Command Center

The benefits of conducting biannual emergency drills, both announced and unannounced, includes being able to test the EOP, the command center, and staff roles and responsibilities. Announced drills have the added benefit of teaching opportunities. Tabletop exercises test a group's ability to cooperate and their readiness to respond to a disaster situation (FEMA, 2015a). There are many types of drills, including:

- *Internal drills* to test specific department and/or hospital responses. Examples include setting up and operating the command center, recognizing a biological event both in the ED and on the units, locking down the hospital entrances, simulating decontamination processes, using downtime procedures during a communications or cyber disaster event, and handling various surge capacity situations.
- *External drills* in collaboration with community agencies and departments involving patients (police, fire, and rescue; public health); tabletop drills simulating an unknown biological, nuclear/radiological, or chemical scenario and prioritizing the response by departments; and surge capacity drills testing a community's ability to respond to overwhelming demand.

All of these drills offer great insight into the merit of the all-hazards preparedness plan and allow facilities the opportunity to modify plans to improve processes.

Establishing the Hospital's Role in the Community

The hospital will play an important role in the community in the case of a disaster. Knowing how the hospital fits in the all-hazards disaster response plan from the perspective of such entities as the police and fire departments, EMS, public health department, and the local school system will be important in coordinating efforts. The emergency management committee will be instrumental in defining the hospital's role locally in the community and nationally to meet federal government expectations and regulatory compliance.

On a local level, the lead person of the committee (often this will be a designated hospital administrator) will partner with public health, local police, fire departments, EMS, community physicians, regional alliances with other health care facilities, and local emergency management agencies/councils. It will be important to define the hospital's and community's role in emergency situations. Testing of plans using local community disaster drills, often biannually, is essential to continually improve processes. The hospital should strive to test its internal all-hazards preparedness plans whenever there is a planned community drill in order to get a full picture of its ability to respond in a disaster in step with the community response.

Nationally, each hospital will play an important role in the political arena by helping local and federal government personnel understand that hospitals, like police and fire departments, are first responders in a disaster. The materials, equipment, and training required for hospitals to prepare adequately for their role in responding to disasters are very expensive. Capital expenditures will be required to create decontamination facilities; purchase PPE; train and educate staff on effective all-hazards preparedness; stockpile emergency equipment, supplies, and pharmaceuticals; ensure adequate isolation rooms; and outfit a hospital command center. Hospitals need financial assistance to do this well, and the committee members can be advocates for federal and state funding. It is helpful to establish a financial subgroup whose mission will be to develop a set plan for capturing costs related to the event as the disaster unfolds. This will enable the hospital to submit immediately for any reimbursement funding that becomes available after the event. This may include business disruption insurance. In addition, the subgroup can identify potential federal grants or public funding that might be available to support costly financial expenditures.

Helping Staff Overcome Fear Associated With Disaster and All-Hazards Preparedness

It is important to know that the first rule of disaster preparedness is to keep staff safe. In a disaster, the paradigm of keeping the patient safe first must be modified to focus on helping staff members (and their families) feel as safe as possible. This may be a shift in thinking, but the reality is that if staff members do not feel comfortable coming to work, then the patients' needs cannot be met.

Nursing leadership, in partnership with human resources and the education department, will need to develop educational tools to assist staff in creating personal disaster preparedness plans for themselves and their significant others. Many websites are available to assist in developing educational tools, such as the FEMA and America Red Cross websites. Tools such as personal disaster preparedness plans should be effectively communicated so that employees know that the organization's first priority in a disaster is to keep staff safe. Arrangements will need to be made for 24-hour childcare somewhere close to the hospital or on-site. Employee assistance programs need to be available at

all times to help employees cope with fear related to a disaster. It is important that nurse leaders understand the psychological impact of a disaster on the victims as well as the staff (Tillman, 2011), so that staff can positively influence victims of a disaster. This requires educating nurses about how to provide care during extreme conditions.

CRISIS STANDARDS OF CARE

During times of crisis in health care delivery, it may become necessary to make decisions about allocating resources. When the number of patients exceeds the available supplies, equipment, and medications, health care organizations may have to change the way they use their resources in order to deliver the best care to the most people. In 2012 the Institute of Medicine (IOM, now called the National Academies of Science, Engineering, and Medicine, Health and Medicine Division) developed *Crisis Standards of Care* to help with this decision-making process with the understanding that these decisions are complex and must be made using fair and equitable principles (Hodge et al., 2013). The framework for these decisions works to inspire fairness and trust and includes heightened ethical sensitivity, understanding what is at stake ethically, adequate planning and policy making, and flexibility (McLean, 2013). *Crisis Standards of Care* have specific applications based on changing situations. The decisions are often difficult for caregivers but are designed to be consistent in their execution across all disciplines. This type of framework allows for ethical decision making based on caring for the community as a whole in a disaster situation (McLean, 2013).

LEADERSHIP AND MANAGEMENT IMPLICATIONS
Moving Into the Future With Confidence

Nursing leaders can effect change and ensure that a fully functional emergency management plan for the hospital is developed within 6 to 12 months. Nursing leadership competencies in disaster planning and crisis management are invaluable, and fortunately they have been developed by a collaborative group led by the Department of Veterans Affairs, Office of Nursing Services. These disaster competencies are categorized into four domains: assessment of the disaster scene, technical skills, risk communication, and critical thinking (Coyle et al., 2007).

Clearly, nurse executives are in a position to take a greater role in planning and implementing a disaster response for their organizations. Nurse leaders are called on to take charge, make decisions, successfully implement protocols, and then modify their action plans based on routine evaluation. In addition, being willing to take risks is an important attribute of the nursing leader. Nurse executives are in a unique position to forge new pathways in the arena of emergency management because of their combination of clinical skills, strong organizational ability, networking expertise, and training in clinical crises. If the emergency management committee is not diligent in its efforts to keep everyone continually focused on preparedness, a sense of complacency about refining the emergency management plan may result. With strong nursing leadership at the managerial and executive level, the oversight of disaster planning can be proactively addressed, and a constant state of readiness can be achieved. Engagement of staff nurses—often through shared governance committees or organization-wide all-hazards disaster preparedness planning—is essential for keeping readiness high. Participation in disaster drills is one example of action learning.

CURRENT ISSUES AND TRENDS

Current nursing and medical literature is focused on specific departments and how they are establishing their unique roles and responsibilities in a disaster. Nurse leaders can use these benchmark articles to motivate units and departments to move forward in fully assessing and defining their roles in all-hazards preparedness. For instance, making decisions about consolidating care sites may require closing clinics, emergency care centers, and community health programs during a disaster to free up clinical staff to assist in a hospital's surge capacity planning in a disaster, provide staff for vaccination teams in a biological event, or help with decontamination in a chemical exposure event. Allocation of staff may be required to build capacity in outpatient and community arenas depending on the disaster threat. Decisions about alternate care sites should be considered well ahead of an event and often require regional collaboration across many disciplines and agencies. Clinical staff may need to flex up or assume roles not usual to their job assignment.

All-hazards preparedness has become a way of life, and knowledge about the level of alertness is an everyday expectation. Hospital staff and leadership have begun to settle in at a heightened state of preparedness. In April 2011, the federal government implemented a new alert system, the National Terrorism Advisory System (NTAS), which replaced the colored-coded system implemented by the Department of Homeland Security. The new two-level system will alert the American public about an "elevated threat" in the event of a credible terrorist threat or an "imminent threat," if a credible and specific terrorist threat is about to occur (US Department of Homeland Security, 2011).

One area of all-hazards preparedness that has not been fully developed, yet has great potential in disaster planning, is the role of various community resources such as outpatient centers, schools, and even churches. The nurse executive can facilitate the establishment of partnerships between the hospital and the community facilities. Once established, these partnerships can be used to set up communication centers where people can congregate to receive support and obtain information about the disaster situation or family and friends who may have been injured.

To effectively manage large-scale events, networking beyond the hospital will be critical to create partnerships with other facilities, hospitals, community agencies, and local, state, and federal departments. To assist in this process, it may be helpful to have a signed agreement or memorandum of understanding (MOU) with community organizations and businesses for assistance. A trend is underway, as evidenced by a growing alliance between regional hospitals and the community at large throughout the United States, to strategically plan for allocation and sharing of federal and state resources in the event of a disaster. As an example, in Virginia, a Regional Hospital Command Center (RHCC) has been established in which 14 northern Virginia hospitals have been networked to more effectively respond in a disaster. This is accomplished via radio communication and a shared web-based bed availability tracking system displaying each hospital's ability to take varying levels of patient acuities. These hospitals can directly link with hospitals in Washington, DC, to coordinate efforts during an event and communicate effectively with fire, police, EMS, public health, the emergency operating center (a local command center for overseeing the event), and the field incident commander in coordinating the disaster response. Similar to the Virginia RHCC just mentioned, cohorts of hospitals, firefighters, EMS, law enforcement, schools, public health, and businesses are joining together to form regional alliances and collaborations to leverage their capability to respond in a coordinated manner.

Under the direction of FEMA, incident management assistance teams (IMATs) were created to provide rapidly deployable (within 2 hours) supplemental assistance to the region affected by a disaster. These teams consist of trained personnel from different departments, organizations, agencies, and jurisdictions, activated to support incident management at major or complex emergency incidents. IMATS function as an initial interface with regional and state responders (FEMA, 2015a).

Building on the idea of partnering with the community to strengthen preparedness, in 2012 FEMA established a community-based assistance program called FEMA Corps. FEMA Corps is dedicated to disaster preparedness, response, and recovery. It is designed to help communities prepare for, respond to, and recover from disasters by supporting disaster recovery centers; assisting in logistics, community relations, and outreach; and performing other critical functions (Corporation for National & Community Service, n.d.). The FEMA Corps provides a pool of trained personnel and pays long-term dividends by adding depth to existing workforce reserves. Hospital executives need to stay abreast of these newly emerging resources and explore ways to partner with them. These types of programs will be pivotal in providing extra human resources and support services desperately needed for hospitals to function effectively in times of crisis.

One other emerging issue that challenges care during a disaster is allocation of scarce resources when the system is overwhelmed. This need was directly experienced in the United States during the Hurricane Katrina and Sandy events, was also witnessed with the Haiti earthquake, and with devastating tornadoes in Joplin, Missouri. As a result of these catastrophic events, both state and national disaster preparedness leaders examined planning needs for response requirements when resources are scarce. These efforts include substantial planning efforts to address immediate needs, including ethical considerations and planning assumptions, as well as management issues regarding responder protection, with the health care workforce as a primary concern. In recommendations of the Ethics Subcommittee of the

Advisory Committee to the Director, CDC, ethical guidelines were outlined for pandemic planning (CDC, 2007) and are a useful resource. To maximize the level of national and regional preparedness, these principles included the identification of clear overall goals, principles of transparency in decision making, public engagement and involvement in the process, use of sound scientific evidence for decision making, and thinking in a global context.

The guidelines recommended early planning efforts that balance utilitarian concepts with respect of persons, nonmaleficence, and justice. The recommendations gave examples of distribution criteria that will need to be considered well ahead of the time of an actual event. The development of triage criteria for allocation of scarce resources has been documented in several articles (Hick & O'Laughlin, 2006; Kraus et al., 2007). Further, adopting standards of care under altered conditions has been described and addressed in numerous documents from states and associations seeking to offer guidelines to care providers (American Nurses Association, 2008; New York State Department of Health Task Force on Life and the Law, 2007; Phillips & Knebel, 2007). Each nursing leader and team needs to understand these guidelines and begin the planning process at both the local and regional levels for developing protocols to allocate scarce resources and implementing triage criteria for care in overwhelming events. Implementing periodic tabletop discussions regarding how to allocate resources in a time of scarcity will prove to be a powerful tool in setting the stage for what to do if such an event occurs. Collaborative professional staff and hospital leadership discussions about scarce resource allocation will present ethical dilemmas that need to be thoughtfully considered in a planning time that is devoid of emotion. Questions to be discussed at the tabletop include: (1) Which hospital and/or clinical leader will make the final decision about ventilator allocation and other scarce resource distribution? (2) What are the criteria used to determine which patients receive aggressive treatment and which will receive palliative care, both imminently and long term, as other life-threatening complications ensue? and (3) How are prophylactic pharmaceutical dissemination plans going to be activated to protect staff and their families? Knowing the hospital's approach to handling these types of scenarios will be a critical precursor in implementing an effective plan in the event of a disaster that is compounded by a shortage of resources.

RESEARCH NOTE

Source
Powell, T., Christ, K.C., & Birkhead, G.S. (2008). Allocation of ventilators in a public health disaster. *Disaster Medicine and Public Health Preparedness, 2*(1), 20–26.

Purpose
In the event of a large-scale public health emergency such as a flu pandemic, a vast amount of resources would be required to treat the victims. This would include the need for mechanical ventilators to support the survival of patients who have respiratory compromise. Currently, many regions have created stockpiles of ventilators for this very purpose, but it would still require additional efforts to manage these scare resources. The purpose of this research was to plan for rationing of scarce resources through the development of an ethical and clinical guideline for a ventilator triage system.

Discussion
A panel of experts in medicine, policymaking, law, ethics, and representatives from medical facilities and various levels of governments were brought together to form a workgroup to discuss potential changes to standards of care during large-scale disasters or public health emergencies. An ethical framework was developed that included principles such as duty to care, duty to steward resources, duty to plan, distributive justice, and transparency. The ventilator allocation guidelines were based on ethical norms to be used during overwhelming circumstances to avoid making medical decisions while under tremendous pressure. A draft of the new guidelines was posted for public comment, and feedback was evaluated through a legal and critical care lens.

The clinical component of the ventilator allocation guidelines had eight components:
- Pretriage requirements
- Patient categories
- Acute versus chronic care facilities
- Clinical evaluation
- Triage decision makers
- Palliative care
- Review of triage decisions
- Communication

The scope of the emergency and its demand on the hospital needs to be communicated to regional emergency management networks along with requests for supplies. All patients, not just those presenting to the emergency department, will be categorized for ventilator allocation in the same manner, using the draft clinical guidelines.

Application to Practice
Implementing the guidelines for ventilator allocation should only be done in collaboration with public health authorities. Clinical evaluation incorporates the use of two systems: the Ontario Health Plan for an Influenza Pandemic (OHPIP) and the sequential organ failure assessment (SOFA) score. Only the clinical evaluation will be used to make allocation decisions and not a patient's age or existence of co-morbidities. All final allocation decisions will be made by the triage decision maker. Having a triage decision maker will assist clinical care providers with making allocation decisions that are based on data and will relieve the provider of the responsibility of making such decisions on their own. The guidelines require reassessment of ventilator use in 48 hours and then again in 120 hours. Implementation of these guidelines for allocation of ventilators requires advance planning and education. Clear lines of communication with local health department officials and other emergency management leadership are necessary to ensure the necessary support for altering normal standards of care during large-scale emergencies.

CASE STUDY

Day 1 (Wednesday)
A hurricane's projected path takes it north over mountainous regions near your area. It will be a tropical storm by the time it reaches you in 2 days. The winds are forecast to be in the 50 mph range with higher gusts in the 60 to 65 mph range. Conditions are such that tornado watches are predicted. Heavy rains are expected to reach 10 inches because the weather system is moving slowly. Your community hospital is 50 miles from the nearest health care facility, is not in a direct flood plain (it is located near the commercial area of your town), and has an average daily inpatient occupancy of 120. Your service line includes a small eight-bed pediatric wing; a 12-bed labor, delivery, and postpartum unit; an emergency department; four operating rooms; and a 10-bed medical–surgical intensive care unit.

Day 3 (Friday)
The tropical storm hits with the predicted high winds and heavy rain. Your ED is receiving an increase in motor

CASE STUDY—cont'd

vehicle accidents, some with severe injuries that potentially need transfer to a trauma center. No helicopters are flying because of the poor weather. Trees are down and multiple roads in the community are flooding. Staff are becoming concerned about their homes, and incoming staff on the evening shift are calling stating that roads are blocked and they are attempting to find alternate routes to the hospital. Electricity has been flickering off and on for the past hour. The outside temperatures are in the 70s with relative humidity at 100%.

Day 4 (Saturday, 7 AM)

Staff are now unable to get in to or go home from the hospital. You are holding 27 patients in the ED, some of whom have been discharged but have no transportation home. One patient is a trauma patient who needs surgery and blood transfusions, but there is no transport available because of the road conditions. The power failed around 5 AM, and you are running on 100% generator power. Local media are calling in to ask about your plans and if you have food and power. The tropical storm has stalled over the nearby mountains, causing flooding in the area. Residents in the community are arriving at the hospital looking for power, food, and clean water. The pharmacy tells you it is low on or out of many critical medications needed for treatment of infection and pain control.

Day 5 (Sunday, 7 AM)

The hospital has been sheltering in place for 2 days. There has been flooding in the community, but the public water system is operational and electricity has been restored. Roads are still blocked in some areas but most are passable, and the main roads have been cleared for emergency vehicles. You continue to use the emergency generator for power, but the storm has subsided to a steady rain and gusty winds.

Considerations

How do you plan for the following areas of potential impact on service given the weather forecast?

Communications	Day 1: Check and test redundant communications systems (telephone, radio, satellite, Internet). Communicate with hospital leadership and established community partners regarding the hospital's emergency plan.

Day 3: Open the incident command center and review action plans for the next 24 to 48 hours. Open the manpower pool to communicate with staff, including surgeons, to be prepared to stay at the hospital and work extra shifts if necessary. Notify community partners regarding the plan for the duration of the storm. Prepare spaces for housing staff and arrange for personnel to assign sleeping spaces and distribute bedding.

Day 4: The incident command center should be fully staffed and operational. Review internal surge plan specific to bed capacity, discharges, and staff and communicate the plans to physicians and leadership. The appointed media relations personnel will provide accommodations for media. Communicate with local, state, regional, and federal resources for support including supplies, personnel, and infrastructure. Provide frequent situational updates to staff and visitors. Receive frequent updates from department leadership for effective decision making. Request support from state and/or local authorities to help transport personnel to the hospital to relieve on-duty staff if possible.

Day 5: Connect with local and regional partners to update your situation, request help if needed, and offer assistance if possible.

Safety and security	Day 1: Complete a facility safety survey concerning the approaching storm including the possibility of high winds and flooding. Day 3: Do frequent facility surveys inside and outside to check for damage or potential problems.

Continued

Day 4: Prepare for an influx of patients in the emergency department. Set up a space for the "worried well" (community members who are not ill but are distressed about the storm). Monitor patients and visitors for stress-related behavioral problems.

Day 5: Monitor the exterior building and grounds for any safety hazards.

Resources and assets

Day 1: Inventory supplies including food, fuel, water, medical supplies, and staff. Order for any shortages from vendors.

Day 3: Organize emergency supplies for rapid deployment to units. Food service changes to surge-level meal planning.

Day 4: Consider allocating resources and medical supplies according to crisis standards of care. Request any needed supplies from the central warehouse if available.

Day 5: Inventory supplies, food, water, linens, and pharmaceuticals. Begin restocking units with available supplies.

Staff responsibilities

Day 1: Remind staff to prepare to be able to respond to the hospital's needs as essential personnel. This includes arranging for child, elder, or pet care; securing their homes against damage; and having adequate supplies for their families.

Day 3: Staff should be prepared for the possibility of working in an area other than their home unit. Prepare for "just in time" training.

Day 4: Alter the nurse/patient ratio to accommodate surge levels, train personnel who will work in a different area. Coordinate patient tracking with EMS.

Day 5: Work to arrange timely discharge for appropriate patients and receive new admits from the emergency department.

Utilities management

Day 1: Check and test redundant utilities systems including having a 96-hour supply of fuel.

Day 3: Transfer all essential equipment to emergency outlets. Continue to check utility operations frequently including outside the facility for infrastructure problems.

Day 4: Monitor fuel supply, equipment operations, and infrastructure. Respond to any internal or external damage.

Day 5: Restore equipment to main power source. Arrange generator fuel delivery, and test that systems are functioning adequately including air handlers, water, and lighting.

Patient clinical and support activities

Day 1: Consider discharging appropriate patients and canceling elective surgeries to increase bed capacity.

Day 3: Consider a discharge holding area for patients who are discharged but not able to go home.

Day 4: Incident commander orders surge capacity plan in effect. Open surge beds. Incident commander and medical director review *Crisis Standards of Care* for possible implementation. Monitor blood supply and storage capability. Inventory pharmaceutical supplies and consider using the emergency supply if necessary.

Day 5: Arrange for discharges to accommodate emergency department patients.

After Action

An after-action meeting is necessary to evaluate the hospital's response to the emergency event. Leaders will discuss what went well and what did not, what could have been done better, and how to plan for the next event. It is also an opportunity to evaluate and make needed updates or changes to the emergency operations plan. Some common questions for this meeting may include:

• Did your incident command team maintain planning using the six critical areas of preparedness (communications,

resources and assets, safety and security, staff responsibilities, utilities management, and patient clinical and support activities)?
- Did you document every action over the past 6 days, with time, date, and names?
- Were communications effective?

- Were you able to integrate your response with state, regional, and local authorities?
- How could you have improved your response to the surge situation?
- Were the crisis standards of care decisions consistent and decided using fair and equitable principles?

CRITICAL THINKING EXERCISE

It is a spring afternoon, and you have just been briefed on a school bus accident that occurred within two miles from the hospital involving 18 elementary school children. The bus driver succumbed to his injuries at the scene. The ED is staffed with three registered nurses, one ED physician provider, and two emergency medical technicians. The only information shared by EMS is that two children are on backboards, and seven children have at least one laceration. EMS is requesting that your ED take all 18 children, and the ED physician agrees. You think back to your training several years ago at a Level I trauma center and remember that in mass casualty events, the number of pediatric patients could easily overwhelm a minimally staffed emergency department. The ED team requests that assistance from other staff outside of the ED be assembled, and roles are assigned to help manage the influx of pediatric patients.

Planning Process: Mass casualty incident (MCI) preparation for managing pediatric patients.

Purpose: To prepare and educate all staff on their role during the MCI and how to manage a large number of children without the assistance of their parents or school personnel.

Background Information: You are the chief nursing officer or nursing supervisor in charge at a 150-bed acute care hospital with a 16-bed ED. The next closest hospital is 30 miles away. Your ED staff has done many MCI drills, but none of them involved more than a few pediatric patients. According to disaster preparedness literature, during a disaster, seriously injured children are often quickly transported to the hospital from the scene by EMS or the police. In addition, just because they are children, pediatric patients are often overtriaged to a higher triage category than the actual severity of their

injuries (Harvin et al., 2014). You are leading the effort to develop a plan to manage the MCI.

1. Should an emergency physician or pediatrician be brought to the scene of the accident because of the significant number of pediatric victims?
2. What triage and safety considerations need to be put in place for children who are not accompanied by an adult and are not carrying any emergency information?
3. What considerations will be included when determining where to treat the pediatric patients?
4. What is the process for obtaining staff from other departments to assist as needed?
5. What "just in time" training do the staff need to manage their pediatric patients? How will this training be delivered and by whom?
6. What provisions will be made for assessing and managing each pediatric patient's emotional status?
7. What should be done to secure the ED area to manage the arrival of parents and media?
8. What kind of pediatric equipment is available for elementary school–age children?
9. Is there an available Broselow tape or other weight-based measuring tape system designed to eliminate error by removing the need to estimate the child's weight?
10. Is there a pediatric formulary and assistance from a pharmacy available?
11. What if the staff finds on secondary triage that a pediatric victim is deteriorating and was undertriaged?
12. If the incident occurred during an off shift without adequate staffing on site, where would you get your help?

Data Management and Clinical Informatics

Jane M. Brokel

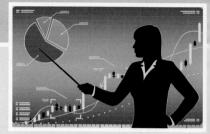

http://evolve.elsevier.com/Huber/leadership

Information and communication technologies and knowledge resources have changed the way people work, play, learn, manage their personal lives, and view the world. Consequently, information and evidence-based knowledge databases and applications have become a commodity to be bought, sold, and managed. The information and knowledge age has progressed decision support by storing and sharing more data and exchanging patient and population data. In the past 50 years, society has seen the widespread adoption of wireless personal computers, pads, smartphones with database and digital applications and multi-messaging capabilities, global positioning systems, and satellite and cable networks for real-time broadcasting and contiguous communication. More types of information can now be transmitted or exchanged across the world, immediately, in a variety of formats.

The business of health care information technologies is evolving rapidly in all settings where people spend time, including schools, work settings, homes, and where they shop. Management of the health care industry and care delivery relies extensively on not only the device capture, collection, and analysis of data but also on the workflow process for what, when, where, who, and how the data are captured. Data about the patient, provider, outcomes, and processes of care delivery are collected from many individuals practicing in different specialties and must be standardized, integrated, coordinated, and managed. Moreover, widespread demand to use these data for performance measurement and reporting to accountable care customers, regulators, and accrediting/certification bodies comes at a time when incentive payments to providers and health care institutions are linked with patient outcome measures (Centers for Medicare & Medicaid Services [CMS], 2011; Petersen et al., 2006). Reimbursement for health care services can be increased, decreased, or denied based on the patient's response to treatment, provider documentation, and the transition to International Classification of Diseases version 10, implemented in October 2015, which resulted in fewer claims rejected in last quarter of 2015 (CMS, 2016a).

In 2008, Medicare stopped paying for eight hospital-acquired patient conditions deemed preventable, including objects left in the patient during surgery, urinary tract infections, and pressure ulcers (Fuller et al., 2009). Today, 14 categories of hospital-acquired conditions affect reimbursement with the Inpatient Prospective Payment System for fiscal year 2013, which included Surgical Site Infection Following Cardiac Implantable Electronic Device (CIED) and Iatrogenic Pneumothorax With Venous Catheterization. Nothing was added in 2014 or 2015 (CMS, 2016b). Regulatory and governmental agencies require the collection of data to measure performance (e.g., The Joint Commission [TJC]); the organization of these data into specific formats for hospitals, long-term care, and home health care (e.g., Medicare/Medicaid, Outcomes and Assessment Information Sets [OASIS]); and adequate protections to ensure the confidentiality of these data (e.g., Health Insurance Portability and Accountability Act [HIPAA]). To meet these demands, administrators need data that can be compared across multiple settings, both geographically and clinically.

Photo used with permission from Photos.com.

DEFINITIONS

The language of data management and clinical informatics contains many acronyms and specific technical terminology.

Business intelligence is defined as a platform that enables and organization to build application capabilities for analysis such as online analytical processing (OLAP), information delivery such as reports and dashboards, and platform integration such as business intelligence metadata management and development environment with self-service analytics allowing professionals to perform queries and generate reports on their own. These tools are characterized by basic analytic capabilities and an underlying data model simplified for ease of understanding how to access the data.

Clinical decision support systems (CDS) provide clinicians, patients, or caregivers with clinical knowledge and patient-specific information to help them make decisions that enhance patient care (Das & Eichner, 2010). Das and Eichner (2010) explained how the patient's characteristics are matched to evidence-based parameters present in patient-specific assessments. Pursuing logic forces an action with recommendations communicated effectively at appropriate times during patient care when nurses or others interact with the electronic health record. CDS interventions include alerts, reminders, info-buttons with health/clinical protocol, workflow orchestration supports, displays of context-relevant data, topic-oriented documentation forms and orders sets, as well as other techniques for knowledge delivery, including reference information and education delivered with or without context sensitivity (Osheroff, 2009). Berner (2009) explained how CDS may be designed to (1) remind clinicians of things they intend to do but should not have to remember, (2) provide information when clinicians are unsure what to do, (3) correct errors clinicians have made, or (4) recommend that the clinicians change their plans. The first requirement for designing CDS is the evidence-based knowledge to support the clinical decision support.

Clinical information systems (CIS) capture clinical data from device download (e.g., monitors, ventilators), scanning (e.g., barcodes on medications or supplies), and electronic documentation of the patient's clinical assessments, preferences, planning, scheduling treatments, and direct-care interventions to support more efficient and effective decision making and clinical care delivery (Ward et al., 2006).

The National Institute of Standards and Testing (NIST) promotes a health information infrastructure that allows cross-enterprise document sharing, messaging profiles, medical device communication, nationwide health information exchange network, patient identification matching, and continuity of care document (CCD) specifications or sematic interoperability of patient data (NIST, 2011). Semantic interoperability can be described as the ability to automatically interpret the information exchanged meaningfully and accurately to produce useful results between two or more systems. Therefore the CCD exchanged will need to have common information structure so that when others receive the list of problems and treatments, the information includes necessary details on start and stop dates, indications, dose, frequency, route and instructions for nursing interventions, respiratory treatments, and medications. Not all systems today are capable of disseminating the information in an easily understood format, and the variation or duplication of information among documents creates even more confusion for nurse providers. More often, nursing problems, risks, and associated interventions are missing when CCDs are shared.

CIS help organize clinical data for display in multiple subsets for different specialties to view averages and ranges or last entered status and generate trend charts for clinical parameters and results. Safety features include checking medications for interactions and errors before administration, providing evidence-based knowledge resources for quick view, and summarizing the client's current story from nursing documentation for nurses to review when care is interrupted. Nursing documentation systems include structured entry using drop-down menus, checklists, and computerized ordering/planning for scheduled care interventions. When completed, the documentation is often used within clinical decision support logic to automate actions for communication, add problems or risk diagnoses to the problem list, or elicit intervention reminder messages for evidence-based practice (Brokel et al., 2011a). CIS also allow unstructured narrative documentation that is not included in the structured portion of the system (Moss et al., 2007).

Data warehouse is defined as data storage architecture designed to hold data extracted from transaction systems, operational data stores, and external sources. The warehouse then combines those data in an aggregate, summary form suitable for enterprise-wide data analysis and reporting for predefined business needs. The five components of a data warehouse are production data sources, data extraction and conversion, the data warehouse database management system, data warehouse administration, and business intelligence tools (Gartner, Inc., 2016). In the data warehouse the data are arranged in subject areas and classes with time-variant versions. Detail is associated with the data within that subject area and class.

Effectiveness research applies epidemiological methods to large databases to study relationships among health care problems, interventions, outcomes, and costs, and determine alternatives and their effects with different patient characteristics and intervening variables. With the prevalence of data warehouses, comparative effectiveness research is made possible to inform health care decisions by providing evidence on the effectiveness, benefits, and harms of different interventions (Agency for Healthcare Research and Quality [AHRQ], 2016). Evidence is generated from designed research studies using data to compare outcomes from different drugs, interventions, medical devices, tests, or work flows to deliver health care with specific diagnoses and patient characteristics. Researchers obtain the available evidence from the array of outcomes measured by standardized nursing assessments and laboratory values. These parameters are aligned with each intervention for different groups of people from existing electronic health records (EHRs). Nurse practitioners and researchers can also conduct integrated reviews that are systematic to find existing evidence and subsequently conduct designed studies or quality improvement projects that generate new evidence of effectiveness of nursing interventions or work flows. For comparative effectiveness research, the development, expansion, and use of a variety of data sources and methods are necessary to conduct timely and relevant research and disseminate the results in a form that is quickly usable by clinicians in the EHR, patients in their personal health records (PHR), and others.

Health information exchange (HIE) is defined as the electronic movement of health-related information among organizations according to nationally recognized standards that allows health care providers to access and securely share vital medical information electronically (HealthIT.gov, 2014a). The HIE is a process within either a state health information network or a regional health information organization (RHIO), often for a geographical area.

The Interoperable health information technology (HIT) ecosystem integrates the applications in nursing services to provide the intersection of three areas: nursing administration, clinical informatics, and effectiveness research on client outcomes. The infrastructure with technologies provides processes for downloading, collecting, organizing, analyzing vast amounts of complex data, and constructing clinical decision support. Having these data in an accessible interoperable format supports daily care and increases nursing leaders', managers', and administrators' ability to make informed decisions regarding the organization and delivery of patient care. Achieving interoperable data for health care is planned and executed through leadership and management and remains a current issue to achieve. The domain of technology and informatics combines the sciences of engineering, computers, and information with the cognitive health sciences.

Knowledge resources are described as a collection of clinical information on such things as diagnoses, drug interactions, and evidence-based guidelines. Content for the knowledge base can come from internal as well as external sources such as specialty societies, commercial knowledge vendors, and health care organizations. The development, time, and expertise taken to define and organize knowledge-based content are substantial. Health care providers usually depend on developers of clinical information systems for the knowledge base resources, and they often will obtain and incorporate commercial knowledge bases in their CDS products. Some examples available in the marketplace include drug databases (e.g., Micromedex, Medscape), order sets (e.g., Zynx Health order solution), nursing diagnoses (e.g., NANDA International knowledge), and guidelines for perioperative practice (e.g., Association of periOperative Registered Nurses).

Management information systems (MIS) describe a broad scope of activities that includes but are not limited to managing: decision support systems, resource and people management applications, project management, and database retrieval applications. Although the boundaries have become fuzzy over the years, typically MIS still cover systems that are critical to the health care organization and company's ability to sustain operations. Professionals in **health information management (HIM)** (management of the coded medical and health record electronic and paper content uses), **biomedical technicians** (manage the equipment, devices, and software upgrades), **clinical informatics**

(design, upgrade, and implement processes, data details, and knowledge resources for pharmacists, nurses, medicine, dentists, radiology, pathology, ophthalmology, etc.), and **data analyst** (design analysis, assimilate datasets, create report options) work with MIS to provide integrated services to automate and support clinicians' and managers' decision-making processes. These services include downloading from monitoring and screening devices and diagnostic equipment, electronic streamlined real-time scanning and collecting, storing in EHR or other data registries (e.g., cancer, immunization), retrieving from tables of data, and processing collective sets of data through the use of applications and networking technology to locate and aggregate the data from an integrated data repository. Today, MIS and HIM departments work with clinical informatics roles (i.e., nurse informaticians) to organize and process information and provide accessible knowledge resource databases (e.g., drug, medical, and nursing evidence-based databases) to guide and support decisions during patient care work flow; to monitor patient safety, satisfaction, and quality of care; and to manage human resources, physical resources, fiscal resources, and more recently evidence-based knowledge resources (Hannah et al., 2006; Osheroff, 2009; Sewell & Thede, 2013). A good MIS has 10 characteristics. It is (1) informative, (2) relevant, (3) sensitive, (4) unbiased, (5) comprehensive, (6) timely, (7) action oriented, (8) uniform, (9) performance targeted, and (10) cost effective (Austin, 1979).

An example of a component of an MIS is a nursing workload management system—also called a patient classification system (PCS). A PCS is designed to measure the average sum of patient acuity indicator weights, using electronic documentation, with the maximum and minimum total workload assigned to any nurse. This is done in conjuncton with a staffing model to ensure a more balanced workload with incoming patients (Malloch, 2015; Sir et al., 2015). These PCS are widely used to determine how many nursing hours a patient needs for his or her care and help managers to estimate the required number of nursing staff. Another example of a component of an HIM is generating a CCD for the HIE network. The HIM and MIS departments are capable of extracting nurses' documentation from the EHR repository to support reports for exchanging nursing data with other agencies or nurses responsible for ongoing care.

Nursing informatics is a "specialty that integrates nursing science with multiple information and analytical sciences to identify, define, manage and communicate data, information, knowledge, and wisdom in nursing practice" (American Nurses Association [ANA], 2015a, p. 1). Nursing informatics supports nurses, consumers, patients, the inter-professional health care team, and other stakeholders in their decision making in all roles and settings to achieve desired outcomes. This support is accomplished through the use of information structures, information processes, and information technology (IT). The management of information and communication technologies is designed to promote the health of people, families, and communities worldwide (IMIA Special Interest Group on Nursing Informatics, 2016).

NURSING'S DATA NEEDS

An organized approach to studying information needs is necessary at every level and with every service to make operational, tactical, and strategic decisions. This helps in the design and implementation of procedures, processes, and practices for nurses. MIS and nursing leadership continuously gather nursing's data needs from inside and outside an organization. The data, when known, are constantly updated and made available to all who have the authority to access it in formats that ease practice, management, research, and education. Examples are patient acuity data for nurse staffing and scheduling and number of falls for nurse-sensitive patient outcomes analysis.

Nursing's data needs fall in four domains: client care, provider competencies and staffing, administration of care and sustainability of the organization, and knowledge-based research for evidence-based practice. The first three are distinct areas for workflow processes, although the fourth domain, research, interacts with all of the other three. The four areas and the sources for the data are as follows:

1. *Client:* Longitudinal client care/clinical care data and its evaluation, clinical findings, and client outcomes. Source: the client's health care record, personal health record, patient–provider messages, and information from the HIE network.
2. *Provider:* Professional data, role responsibilities (i.e., competencies, skills), caregiver outcomes, and decision-maker variables. Source: personnel records, national data banks, and documentation links to client records.

3. *Administrative:* Management and resource oversight, organization statistics, system outcomes, contextual variables, and comparative targets. Source: administrative, fiscal, population, registry, and regulatory performance data.

4. *Research:* Knowledge base development and comparative effectiveness with phenotype data dictionaries (Pathak et al., 2011). Source: existing and newly gathered data, relational databases, and common data elements from emerging exchange networks.

Table 26.1 displays examples of outcomes and variables to be measured in relation to the three distinct domains of nursing's data needs. For example, in the client domain, the cost and continuity of care for the client are important because data are now shared among providers within the HIE to manage care. In the provider domain, professional skills/knowledge and intensity of nursing care are variables that may be measured to monitor variability and control workforce capacity. The quality and type of services are dependent on the competencies of the professional workforce. Nurse administrators need data to prepare a plan for strengthening the quality and capacity of not only the nursing workforce but also those of other services such as mental health services (Institute of Medicine [IOM], 2006, 2011).

TABLE 26.1	Outcomes and Variables in Three Domains of Nursing Data Needs	
Domain	**Outcomes**	**Variables**
Client	Client satisfaction	Attitudes/beliefs
	Achieved care outcomes	Diagnosis, gender, age
	Preferences for personal outcomes	Marital status
	Costs	Support system
	Access to care	Satisfaction
	Continuity of care	Level of dependency
	Access to personal health records	Severity of illness
	Medication reconciliation	Intensity of nursing care
		Nursing patient sensitive outcomes
		Provider–patient messaging
Provider	Job enrichment	Attitudes/beliefs
	Job/work satisfaction	Education level
	Physician/nurse satisfaction	Competency with care interventions
	Job stress	Years of experience
	Intent to leave	Age
	Certification	Work excitement
	Hours work	Position level with electronic health/medical records
	Access to information	Provider–provider messaging
	Skill set/competency with health	Health information exchange network
	information technology	Clinical decision support automations
Administration	Costs	Agency philosophy/culture
	Productivity	Priorities
	Turnover	Organizational structure
	Income	Fiscal data
	Workforce capacity	Climate data
	Safety culture	Policies and procedures
	Quality performance/benchmarks	Workflow/process data
	Effective communication	Technology capability data
	Health information exchange	Workforce positions/demand data
	Adherence to best clinical evidence	Patient population: risks and problems
		Community networks/relationships
		Educational institution relations

The aggregation and analysis of interoperable health IT data are critical to health services research, value-based payment to reward quality care, and public health functions such as real-time disease surveillance and disaster response (Office of the National Coordinator [ONC] for Health Information Technology, 2016). Data analysis is aimed at cost, safety, quality, and effectiveness outcomes. Collecting and extracting data that describe the processes and outcomes of nursing care electronically has provided evidence for the design of care protocols and delivery models (Horn & Gassaway, 2010). The formal process of using these patient data for providing evidence is termed *practice-based evidence* (PBE). PBE reflects what works in actual practice and reflects evidence of effectiveness as perceived and experienced by patients, families, or the community, thus making it more culturally sensitive (Bartgis & Bigfoot, 2010). Comparative effectiveness research is a framework to analyze a comprehensive set of patient, treatment, and outcome variables to identify treatments associated with better outcomes while controlling for patient differences (Horn & Gassaway, 2010). Although both are used to inform the delivery of practice with evidence, practice-based evidence and evidence-based practice are derived from different sources. Deriving evidence for informing practice from research is termed *evidence-based practice,* whereas informing practice from the analysis of patient data collected during the delivery of care is termed *practice-based evidence.* However, the contribution of practice-based evidence rests on structuring the input logically and providing a level of accuracy and completeness to ensure valid and reliable output. Explicit data definitions, valid linkages between datasets, and well-defined coding of input are essential in securing meaningful output that has utility. The aggregation of consistent meaningful information over time and how daily work flow affects the quality of information are especially important to uniform datasets. Using practice-based evidence requires the compilation of clinical data in a *clinical data repository.* This compilation may also be called a *data warehouse* or *data repository.* Data are stored longitudinally over multiple episodes of care. These data are accessed to provide continuity of care to the individual patient, extracted to measure care effectiveness and productivity, queried to provide evidence for care delivery, and analyzed to inform public policy.

NURSING INFORMATICS

Informatics was recognized by the American Nurses Association (ANA) as a nursing specialty in 1992 and is one of the fastest growing practice areas in health care. Nurses prepared at the master's level in nursing informatics are titled *informatics nursing specialists (INSs)* (Hannah et al., 2006). As defined by ANA (2015a), the practice of nursing informatics views the relationship of data, information, knowledge, and wisdom (DIKW) as a continuum with increasing complexity and interrelationships as nurses aggregate and apply it in decision making. *Data* are defined as discrete, objective entities, without interpretation; *information* is data that are structured, organized, or interpreted; and *knowledge* is synthesized information with identified relationships and meaning. *Wisdom* is appropriate use of knowledge in managing and solving patient problems, risks, and needs for health enhancement (e.g., nursing diagnoses). Wisdom is knowing when and how to apply evidence-based knowledge with client information to solve problems, which nurses exercise through critical thinking and clinical reasoning skills (Topaz, 2013).

The DIKW framework presents data, information, knowledge, and wisdom as building on one another to increasing levels of complexity and relationships. The concepts intersect. Data operations are naming, collecting, and organizing. Information operations are organizing and interpreting. Knowledge operations are interpreting, integrating, and understanding. Wisdom operations are understanding and applying/applying with compassion. Topaz (2013) used the nursing-specific transitions theory to investigate data related to the transition from hospital to home and DIKW to build knowledge for application/wisdom via a decision-support tool for risk of poor outcomes. Gee and colleagues (2012) used the DIKW framework to examine the HIE between clinicians and e-patients (Internet partnerships) for safety, quality, and engagement outcomes.

Nursing informatics specialists assist practitioners by providing information and evidence-based knowledge to support clinical decision making and delivery of safe patient care. Although these specialists may not be directly involved with care delivery, their effort is integrally related to reengineering work flow for clinical and administrative practice. Nursing informatics specialists participate in analysis, design, and implementation of information and communication systems; effectiveness and informatics research; education of nurses in informatics and information technology through the Technology and Informatics Guiding Education Reform (TIGER) initiative; and more recently represent nurses at the policy table in building better interoperable frameworks for care coordination and delivery through optimizing processes and technology usability (Ball et al., 2011).

The American Organization of Nurse Executives (AONE) called for the redesign of work through the use of technology to augment nursing practice in the early 2000s (Kennedy, 2003). This goal of nursing work redesign was initially to build systems and safeguards to decrease errors and enhance patient safety. In addition, AONE's (2015) competencies for nurse executives recognize the importance of information technology competence. *Keeping Patients Safe: Transforming the Work Environment of Nurses,* a report of the Institute of Medicine (IOM, now called the National Academies of Sciences, Engineering, and Medicine Health and Medicine Division [HMD]) (IOM, 2004), emphasized that risks to patient safety are embedded in many of nurses' work processes. In 2011 the IOM published *The Future of Nursing: Leading Change, Advancing Health.* It asks nurses to be partners to redesign and improve care (lead change) and find ways to improve data collection and analysis for workforce planning and policy making. This encourages the full scope of practice for nurses to not only intervene when diagnosing problems and risks but to also intervene when diagnosing needs for health promotion (advancing health).

Health Care Technology and Nursing Applications

Health Information Technology

Information management technologies are critical at every stage of health care delivery. Effective care delivery requires timely access to clinical, administrative, financial, and logistical information flows. Once acquired, these large databases need to be analyzed to identify opportunities for effective interventions to enhance the management of care and services. Deployment of information is reflected in strategies of notification, alerts, reports, and assessment of trends and the impact of interventions—all components of the latest health information technology (HIT).

According to HealthIT.gov (2015a) *meaningful use* "sets specific objectives that eligible professionals (EPs) and hospitals must achieve to qualify for Centers for Medicare & Medicaid Services (CMS) Incentive Programs":

> *Meaningful use is using certified EHR technology to improve quality, safety, efficiency, and reduce health disparities; engage patients and family; improve care coordination, and population and public health; and maintain privacy and security of patient health information. Ultimately, it is hoped that the meaningful use compliance will result in better clinical outcomes, improved population health outcomes, increased transparency and efficiency, empowered individuals, and more robust research data on health systems*
>
> **(Health IT.gov, 2015a).**

There are three stages to *meaningful use.* Meaningful use objectives evolved in three stages:

2011–2012 Stage 1
Data capture and sharing
2014 Stage 2
Advance clinical processes
2016 Stage 3
Improved outcomes (HealthIT.gov, 2015a)

Meaningful use of HIT brought with it four goals: improve quality of care and safety, engage patients and their families in care, improve care coordination, and improve population health (Calhoun et al., 2016).

Population health management is one major example of HIT. With improving population health paramount to the success of meaningful use, it is critical for organizations to define successful strategies to develop optimal programming. Table 26.2 shows 10 recommended HIT tools to achieve population health management (Shaljian & Nielsen, 2013). However, amid the rapid expansion of HIT products and adoption, there is a lag in access to and proficiency with the technology needed to implement a sophisticated population health approach (see Chapter 16). In one international survey, 50% to 90% of doctors in developed countries routinely use advanced HIT tools to manage their patients (e.g., computerized alerts, reminder systems to notify patients about preventive or follow-up care, or prompts to provide patients with test results). In the United States, only 25% had such a system, although 40% or more reported they have neither a manual nor electronic system to

TABLE 26.2   Ten Recommended Health Information Technology Tools

Tool	Elaboration
Electronic health records (EHRs)	EHRs document diagnoses, vital signs, and tests and treatments; populate registries; and create the structured data needed for advanced analytics.
Patient registries	The central database of population health management (PHM) registries are used for patient monitoring, patient outreach, point-of-care reminders, care management, health risk stratification, care gap identification, quality reporting, and performance evaluation.
Health information exchange	Enables effective coordination of care across the medical neighborhood and between care team members. Secure messaging that uses the standardized direct protocol to exchange information between providers.
Risk stratification	Analytic tools used to classify patients by their current health status and their health risk. Risk stratification and predictive modeling applications enable providers to intervene appropriately with high-risk patients and those who might become high risk.
Automated outreach	By applying analytics to registries, organizations can generate automated messaging to patients who need preventive or chronic disease care, per standardized clinical protocols.
Referral tracking	Referral management tools help practices keep track of referrals to other providers and make sure they receive the results back from those consultations.
Patient portals	Web portals attached to EHRs help providers share records with patients and engage patients in self-management. They are also important to the process of continuous care, an essential component of PHM.
Telehealth/telemedicine	Remote examination and treatment of patients using audio and video conferencing is another method of engaging and caring for patients between face-to-face visits and can also reduce the need for those encounters.
Remote patient monitoring	Whether patients are monitored at home or using mobile devices, this approach makes it possible for providers to intervene quickly when high-risk patients show signs of distress. Remote monitoring can also help patients control chronic conditions such as diabetes and hypertension.
Advanced population analytics	Applied to the data in registries and data warehouses, these analytics can be used to evaluate how different segments of patient populations are doing and to assess the clinical and financial performance of individual providers, sites of care, and the organization as a whole.

Data from Shaljian, M., & Nielsen, M. (2013). *Managing populations, maximizing technology: Population health management in the medical neighborhood.* Washington, DC: Patient-Centered Primary Care Collaborative.

complete the same activities (Shaljian & Nielsen, 2013). The ability of patient portals to send patients and their caregivers educational materials and preventive and chronic care alerts makes them invaluable. However, portals are often underused by patients if not providers (Terry, 2015).

Technological innovations in informatics have made possible the rapid analysis of large databases. The health care industry historically has generated among the largest amounts of data, much driven by record keeping, compliance and regulatory requirements, and patient care (Raghupathi & Raghupathi, 2014). In turn, statistical analyses have become more sophisticated.

Health care technology is a powerful tool for effective and efficient care delivery that needs to be harnessed for nursing's needs. System designers need to focus on how to communicate and exchange information for the automation and coordination of health care work. According to Stetson and colleagues (2001), there is no instance in which coordination of care takes place in the absence of communication, and there is no instance in which clinical information exchange occurs in the absence of clinical communication. It is now possible to integrate smartphones, handheld devices, global positioning systems, barcode scanners with medication administration systems, and

HIE networks with traditional information systems through secure wireless intranets and Internet connections for the immediate communication of information to the correct person, at the correct time, in the correct format. For example, it is now possible to link laboratory systems with nursing call systems to alert a patient's nurse when laboratory values fall outside of set limits. It is now possible to connect nursing homes and homecare nurses to a web portal with access to the HIE network to obtain client data from multiple providers. It is now possible for clients to have access to their personal health record of information and to securely send and receive direct messages from their health care providers.

Improved communication through the use of health information technology has many applications, often designed to reduce errors. Among systems and techniques that are used to prevent and reduce medical errors, computerized provider order entry (CPOE), clinical decision support systems (CDSS), electronic health records (EHR), barcode medication administration (BCMA), and radio frequency identification (RFID) are well known. Studies show that in reducing errors and improving quality of care, CPOE, CDSS, and EHR are more effective than other technologies. The integration of CPOE with CDSS also likely leads to a further reduction of medical errors. CPOE covers all three health care quality problems (low use, misuse, and overuse).

Implementing technological solutions such as provider order sets, clinical decision-support interventions, evidence-based knowledge database resources, and PHRs in health care is extremely expensive, and it has been difficult to show a return on investment (ROI) for these expenditures. Based on the size of a health system and the level of implementation with these solutions, benefits for large hospitals can range from $37 to $59 million over a 5-year period in addition to incentive payments (Bell & Thornton, 2011). The growing trend is to regard these expenditures as part of the cost of institutional infrastructure and to tie them to the cost savings gained by improving patient outcomes, provider efficiencies, and avoiding errors. Especially powerful is the drive to reduce medication errors and the associated harm. All eligible providers and health care organizations had added CPOE, CDS, and other solutions to achieve stages of meaningful use indictors by 2015, although a few EHRs failed to perform these functions (CMS, 2016b).

Other Emerging Technologies and Use of Big Data

Huston (2013) identified other emerging technologies that will change nursing practice. They are (1) genetics and genomics, (2) less invasive tools for diagnosis and treatment, (3) 3D printing, (4) robotics, and (5) biometrics. In addition to the emerging technology, Big Data are an emerging trend.

The McKinsey Global Institute defines Big Data as "data sets whose size are beyond the ability of typical database software tools to capture, store, manage, and analyze" (Manyika et al., 2011, p. 1). Although there are many general and technical definitions of Big Data, it has most frequently been described in terms of volume (amount), variety (including structured or semistructured nursing documentation, data from monitoring devices and imaging studies, scheduling and human resource data, and patient-generated data), velocity (the rate at which data accumulates), and veracity (certainty of the data, in terms of how appropriate it is for either its original purpose, perhaps at the point of use, or for secondary use in research and analytics) (SAS Institute, n.d.).

Familiar sources of Big Data that inform nursing practice include digitized clinical records from the EHR, such as encounter notes, laboratory reports, and medication data; standardized survey measures; staffing figures; public health databases; and costs and claims data. Other sources of Big Data include mobile and personal health technologies such as biosensors, sleep monitors, and patient communication portals for reporting self-care and tracking outcomes.

Analysis of these datasets can reveal patterns and correlations that can be used to predict future activity. Big Data from existing and emerging sources offer a vast modeling and analytic resource with the potential to inform nursing practice and drive innovative approaches to improve patient care outcomes. Sensmeier (2015) concluded that the use of Big Data offers tremendous opportunity to accelerate the growth and synthesis of new knowledge to make a positive impact on the health of individuals and populations. Nurses need to embrace all of these technologies and become experts in their use in order to demonstrate their ability to cope with uncertainty and also be irreplaceable.

ELECTRONIC HEALTH RECORDS

In 1965, El Camino Hospital in Mountain View, California, was one of the first to attempt to develop an electronic health record (EHR). Along with Technicon Medical

Information Systems and Lockheed Missiles and Space Company, the hospital created an information system that communicated physicians' orders, retrieved laboratory results, and supported the documentation of nursing care (Staggers et al., 2001). The development of early information systems designed to support an EHR were confined to large tertiary care centers and federal agencies such as the US Department of Veterans Affairs (VA) and the National Institutes of Health (NIH). The high cost of these systems provided little incentive for most health care institutions to change. The US Department of Health and Human Services (HHS)-funded programs stimulated EHR implementation across eligible providers in ambulatory settings and critical access hospitals through incentives from CMS, regional training curriculums, and regional extension centers staffed with HIT skilled workers (HHS, 2014). In 2014 over one-half of eligible ambulatory providers and more than 80% of hospitals were meaningfully using EHRs and exchanging standardized patient information to support safe care at home or other settings (HealthIT.gov, 2014b).

The purpose of an EHR is to document patient care in a single repository as a clinical, financial, and legal record. The electronic digital format supports the storage and exchange of the CCD from the record that is accessible and available among health care members regardless of their location. The EHR is a virtual record of retrospective, concurrent, and prospective information to support continuous, efficient, and integrated health care (Häyrinen et al., 2008). The record does not originate from one place; rather the record is a compilation of information from a variety of integrated systems and through HIE networks regionally or via state organizations.

With the use of standards and interoperability framework for data collection, patient-protected health information within an EHR can be accessed across health exchange networks, linking clinical and business processes, reducing data replication, and increasing the availability and accessibility of information. Well-designed EHRs and clinical data repositories can facilitate the collection and exchange of complete and accurate data in a form that is easily accessible to enhance clinical practice (Minthorn & Lunney, 2010; ONC for Health IT, 2016), support reuse of historical data for current care decisions, analyze patient outcomes over time (Brokel et al., 2011b), continuously improve patient safety and quality (Horn & Gassaway, 2010), or manage institutional resources.

Clinical documentation used to be collected in paper charts. The shift to EHRs generates vast amounts of electronic data about the patient, facility, population, and finances. "Expecting the right data at the correct time to the appropriate healthcare provider in the proper format can be challenging. . ." (Moerbe & Kelemen, 2014, p. 366). Moerbe and Kelemen provided an example of using Structured Query Language and nursing informatics knowledge such as workflow analysis to address pressure ulcer (PU) documentation incongruence. The 76% incidence rate of incongruent documentation of PU present on admission between nurses and doctors is a potential for lost reimbursement and patient harm that can be corrected by using the EHR in a meaningful way.

The shift from retrospective fee for service and managed care to prospective payment with financial structures such as accountable care organizations (ACO) changes how partners develop their informational, technical, financial, and professional capabilities related to capturing savings for coordinated, longitudinal, population-based care (Fisher et al., 2011). Currently patient data are of interest not only to health care providers and ACOs but also to governmental payers, who want to ensure that specific data and information are present and distributed to patients or public health entities along with incentives while they achieve meaningful use indicators (CMS, 2010). These data are also analyzed by health care providers to ensure that patient needs are transpiring in the most efficient and cost-effective manner with these required indicators. An indicator such as the quality of the patient problem list can meet the demands of the final rule, but does the list also inform the providers using a clinicians' vernacular of patient conditions, co-morbidities, or long-term risks (e.g., hyperlipidemia, diabetes type 2, risk for falls) (Ochylski et al., 2012)? In 2016, CMS delayed the objectives for meaningful use stage 3 because more than 60% of the proposed measures required interoperability, which is up from 33% in stage 2. These objectives include public health reporting measures and clinical quality measures that are part of CMS agenda.

The adoption of electronic health records has driven dramatic change in the health care industry. Increasingly, EHR systems are going mobile, which means nurses will be able to pull up records at the point of care rather than back at the nursing station. Data is also becoming increasingly important to health care facilities of all sizes, driven by the ease with which written and oral communications can be digitized

(American Nurses Association, 2015b).

But can such ease of access be potentially harmful? "On any given day, a nurse is managing information about patients, unit priorities, other nurses, and team members—all at once. The vulnerability for cognitive or information overload is real" (Sitterding & Broome, 2015, p. 11).

Here is an example of how technology may be shifting power away from experts:

> "Before the ubiquity of social media, opinions and ideas were largely left to the identified experts in the field. Now ordinary people are able to reach and influence a larger arena through the use of technology such as Facebook, Twitter, LinkedIn and various blogs and websites. This has greatly influenced effective thought and behavior of followers and has shifted the paradigm away for the leader as the all-knowing, all-powerful expert"
>
> **(Sitterding & Broome, 2015, p. 56).**

HEALTH INFORMATION EXCHANGES

Because care is complex and delivered across settings and sites, efficient and seamless linkage and access to health data are critical. The health information exchange (HIE) is the electronic movement of health-related information among organizations according to nationally recognized standards that allows health care providers to access and securely share vital medical information electronically (HealthIT.gov, 2014a). The HIE is a process within a state health information network or a regional health information organization (RHIO), often for a geographical area. All 50 states have some of the services for HIE to support patient care (HealthIT.gov, 2015b). The organizations provide oversight to authorize the locations of health information and the process for secure access and use of the information. In 2010 the Office of the National Coordinator provided direction in guiding state-based entities in operational plans to implement HIEs across the nation using Health Information Technology for Economic and Clinical Health (HITECH) Act funding (HHS, 2014). In 2014 over 50% of hospitals were able to electronically search for patient information from another health care provider. Initial services included a statewide provider directory, secure provider–provider messaging, e-prescribing for ambulatory medications, exchanging the CCD (e.g., problem lists, medications, plan of care, advance directive, patient instructions), laboratory results, immunization registry, and public health surveillance of contagious diseases (CMS, 2010). Expansion of services would include PHRs and exchanging of other vital diagnostic, outcome, and coordinated care information.

In 2004, President George W. Bush created the position of Office of the National Coordinator for Health Information Technology (ONC for Health IT) within the HHS. The coordinator's role involved leadership to develop the standards and interoperability framework and to establish the infrastructure necessary to harness the use of information technology and exchange of health information nationwide to improve patient care and reduce health care costs through support of CMS, the Agency for Healthcare Research and Quality (AHRQ), and HIT committees. The president's mandate was for each American to have an EHR by 2014. In 2009 President Barack Obama advanced this agenda with HHS and other federal agencies though funding state and regional programs to encourage adoption of EHR systems and build the infrastructure for HIEs. To facilitate the development of interoperable EHR systems across the country, standardized vocabularies such as Systematized Nomenclature of Medicine Clinical Terms (SNOMED CT) have been purchased by the federal government and made available for download through the National Library of Medicine (HHS, 2011).

SNOMED CT is a comprehensive clinical terminology, originally created and compiled by the College of American Pathologists (CAP) using multiple clinical classifications such as evidence-based nursing classifications. In April 2007, the International Health Terminology Standards Development Organisation (IHTSDO), a not-for-profit association in Denmark, took over ownership, maintenance, and license distribution. The National Library of Medicine is the US member of the IHTSDO and distributes SNOMED CT at no cost in accordance with the IHTSDO's uniform international license terms, which have been incorporated in the License for Use of the Unified Medical Language System (UMLS) Metathesaurus. This includes both English and Spanish versions as part of the UMLS Metathesaurus, where nurses can find the origins of the biomedical terminologies.

During the past 15 years, the development of EHRs has been escalated by the public's demand to be partners in decisions about their health care (HHS, 2011). This client partnership with providers is necessary to improve continuity and avoid errors among the client's different care providers. This began by avoiding errors in the medication process. Kopp and colleagues (2006) reported that lack of drug knowledge was the cause of 10% of errors and that slips and memory lapses were responsible for 40% of errors at the administration phase. Because health care work flow transpires in an interruption-driven environment, it was not surprising that medication administration errors were attributable to omissions. Integrating an EHR with pharmacy, laboratory, and documentation of clinical assessments with the implementation of computerized provider order entry (CPOE), clinical decision support (CDS), and barcode scanning and electronic medication administration records (eMAR) applications is designed to reduce errors during all phases of the medication process in health care systems.

EFFECTIVENESS

The first person to analyze patient outcomes associated with nursing care delivery was Florence Nightingale in the nineteenth century. Research on patient outcomes was not funded until health care cost and quality became social and policy issues. Health care systems continue to contain costs but need to achieve effective evidence-based care through ACOs and partnerships (CMS, 2011). Earlier measures that focused solely on reduced mortality, length of stay, and hospital costs provided little information about the quality of health care provided. Health information technology and the development of nursing classification systems have made the measurement and evaluation of nursing-sensitive outcomes feasible (Brokel et al., 2011b; Sampaio Santos et al., 2010).

Nurses spend approximately 19% of their time in patient care, 7% with assessments, 17% managing medications, 20% coordinating care, and 35% documenting patient information in EHRs (Burnes-Bolton, 2009). Fortunately, more data are documented in standardized formats that are now accessible to extract and analyze. The standardized nursing data captured within information tables and well-defined data fields allow the extraction of any standard data object into a report. Nursing informatics specialists work to organize and aggregate these data for real-time decision making in care delivery management and to a degree are involved in the analysis of patient outcomes. These activities require extracting data that can be organized in nursing outcomes databases. Without clinical outcomes databases

that reflect nursing care across the patient care providers, only data available in current coding and billing systems will provide for generic outcome evaluation. However, coding and billing databases do not yield data for many of nursing's operational needs. Nursing outcome databases are critical for two reasons: (1) nurses are able to measure and document how nurses influence patient outcomes across care providers for populations of patients, and (2) the study of nursing-sensitive outcomes allows comparisons among interventional strategies and advances the science of nursing care delivery (Furukawa et al., 2011; Minthorn & Lunney, 2010; Muller-Staub, 2009; Scherb et al., 2011).

STANDARDIZED CLINICAL TERMINOLOGY

Nurses spend a great deal of their time collecting and documenting information related to patient care delivery. Vast amounts of data are compiled, describing every holistic detail of the patient's encounter, including PHRs and messages and calls with the health care system or ambulatory care services. These data are more often encoded and recorded in a standard way that makes them amenable to analysis. For example, when documenting the description of the same surgical incision, five different nurses may use picklist or narration to capture five different entries. They may describe the size of the wound in centimeters or inches, which the HIT can convert and then display both. The wound color could be depicted as pink, slightly reddened, or slightly inflamed. When different terms are used to describe the same observable fact, it is difficult to know that everyone is referring to the same phenomenon. Defined and evidence-based descriptions associated with clinical terminologies provide nurses a method of harmonizing the documentation to foster consistency in accurately describing the wound. The access to reference-text definitions and databases to define and disclose the context of clinical concepts helps in the quality of nursing information documented.

June Clark and Norma Lang, pioneers in nursing informatics, once wrote "If we cannot name it, we cannot control it, practice it, research it, teach it, finance it, or put it into public policy" (Clark & Lang, 1992, p. 109). For nearly 40 years, nurses have been developing classification systems that itemize the diagnoses, interventions, and outcomes of the professional domain. More recently this process has been supported by different taxonomic infrastructures for classification. These variations were viewed as disruptive to the profession. However, the result has been a richer, more inclusive representation of what nurses do in different practice environments. Currently, the ANA recognizes 13 standardized terminologies. These include terminologies for nursing administration, home health care, perioperative nursing, acute care, and other nursing scopes of practice. The ANA-recognized terminologies (ANA, 2012) for nursing are:

- NANDA International Nursing Diagnoses, Definitions, and Classification
- Nursing Interventions Classification (NIC) interventions with associated activities
- Nursing Outcomes Classification (NOC) outcomes with measureable indicators
- Nursing Management Minimum Data Set (NMMDS)
- Clinical Care Classification (CCC)
- Omaha System
- PeriOperative Nursing Data Set (PNDS)
- SNOMED CT
- Nursing Minimum Data Set (NMDS)
- International Classification for Nursing Practice (ICNP)
- ABC Codes
- Logical Observation Identifier Names and Codes (LOINC)

Classification systems are non-combinatorial hierarchical languages designed to categorize objects. In health care classification systems, objects classified are generally patient diagnoses, outcomes, and care interventions. Nursing classifications, also referred to as *interface terminologies,* are generally implemented at the point of care to describe and document clinical practice (Coenen et al., 2001). Classification systems help provide the evidence-based terms used in documenting practice, and the reference terminology model provides the structure for organization with other interdisciplinary teams' documentation in the database (Bakken et al., 2001). The International Standards Organization (ISO) Technical Committee ISO/TC 215 Health Informatics, Working Group 3 Health Concept Representation (ISO/TC 215/WG 3) focused specifically on the conceptual structure required by a nursing reference terminology model (ISO, 2002). Through the use of these terminology models, diagnosis, patient outcomes, and intervention terms contained within existing clinical classification systems can be mapped for harmonization across medical and nursing terminologies.

NURSING MANAGEMENT MINIMUM DATA SET

Awareness of the need for standardized, uniformly collected, retrievable, and comparable service-related management data elements was the impetus for the original research to develop and test a Nursing Management Minimum Data Set (NMMDS) (Huber et al., 1992, 1997). Fig. 26.1 is the original NMMDS. More recent work (Garcia et al., 2015; Pruinelli et al., 2016) has been restricted to a select subset of the original NMMDS. The NMMDS was developed to meet the need for "sharable and comparable" data, especially regarding the nursing workforce and the processes of patient care (Garcia et al., 2015). Such data are crucial for nurses to have in order to compare nursing practice and evaluate costs of care.

The foundational work was the Nursing Minimum Data Set (NMDS) (Werley & Lang, 1988). Formulation of the NMDS was an effort to standardize the collection of essential nursing information for comparison of nursing data across patient populations. Three categories of data elements are included in the NMDS: nursing care, demographic, and service. Data elements related to nursing care include nursing diagnosis, intervention, outcome, and intensity of nursing care. Expanding on the use of the NMDS as a guide now helps ensure that data are collected regarding institutional structure (having the right things), process (doing things right), and outcomes (having the right things happen). Linking nursing care data to structure, process, and outcomes is necessary for the accurate evaluation of efficiency and effectiveness, following the quality framework of Donabedian (1986). The NMMDS identified the data essential for inclusion in clinical information systems necessary to support decision making in clinical and administrative nursing practice (Brokel, 2007). The challenge has been capturing nursing decisions and care without variation in documentation. Harrington and colleagues (2011) identified where HIT fails nursing usability of EHRs by violating heuristic principles. They found three of the 14 principles accounting for most of the concerns with usability. The highest concern was the mismatch between the EHR design and nursing care

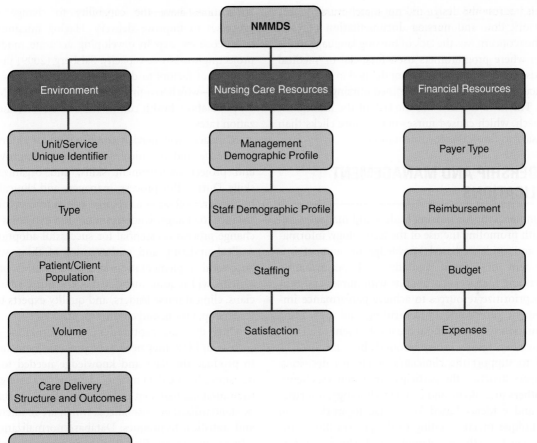
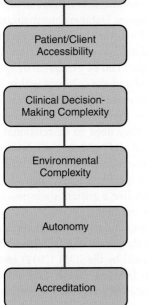

FIG. 26.1 Nursing Management Minimum Data Set (NMMDS) variables. These elements are at the unit-of-service level. (Copyright 2008 D. Huber, C. Delaney. All rights reserved.)

models because the design did not match nursing process work flow and nursing documentation of care. Another concern was the lack of nursing language in the design where programmers used financial or medical records coded terms that were not defined in the nurses' vernacular or evidence-based defined nursing classifications. The third concern was the lack of the minimalist approach, which caused nurses many more clicks than necessary to finish the documentation.

LEADERSHIP AND MANAGEMENT IMPLICATIONS

The implications for nursing leaders and managers begin with promoting the use of the technology, information, and evidence-based knowledge to support improvement of clinical and financial performance. Leaders and managers collaborate with nurses and others to prioritize resources to achieve performance improvement directions. Implementing and upgrading information systems without the involvement of all user groups often results in workarounds because the HIT failed to support the clinician's or client's decisions. Managers structure the participation of nurses, clients, and others to evaluate and enable technology, information, and evidence-based knowledge to work within each unique practice setting to design workflow processes specific to the population served. The data, information, and knowledge resources that exist need to be fully used to support wise decision making at all levels, including at the bedside, with practice councils, in the boardroom, and for policy guidance. The opportunity to advance the health of individuals and health care processes will continue to change with innovation. Leaders need to engage in understanding practical applications for patient care while avoiding undesirable consequences. Leaders have the opportunity to use the aggregated data to measure effectiveness and outcomes and make decisions with those who know the work flow and services to advance evidence-base practices.

The IOM (2011) recommended acquiring better data on the health care workforce in *The Future of Nursing: Leading Change, Advancing Health*. The data should include numbers and types of professionals available to meet future needs. Nurse leaders will need to understand the impact of bundled payments, medical homes, ACOs, health information technologies, comparative effectiveness, patient engagement with PHRs, the diversity of the population, and the level of safety. Technological applications have the capability to change system processes to improve delivery. Having nursing's data is a necessary step in developing accurate models for projecting workforce capacity. Salsberg (2009) provided a model of factors to determine health care workforce demand—which requires elements of the NMMDS—on population, health conditions and disease, and utilization rates.

Managers will need a combination of informatics knowledge and technical skills, quality improvement and project management skills, and organizational skills. During this process, managers and clinical nursing leaders will serve as change agents to overcome resistance to change. Understanding the dynamics of the change process is essential for successful adoption and cyclical updating and maintenance of these systems. Successful implementation and sustainability of these systems will require nurse managers, nurse informaticians, clinical nurse leaders, and quality experts to have leadership, vision, and commitment.

Once data are captured in an informatics system such as an EHR, they need to be processed and analyzed to produce the data and knowledge needed to make decisions. Before data mining, data preprocessing needs to occur. One first step is data normalization. Data can be standardized or normalized, which are mathematical and statistical techniques. Database normalization is a refinement process. First, the data objects that need to be in the relational database and their relationships are identified. Then a report can be generated by specifying the data tables desired and the columns within each table. Data tables are then used to track variables or items of interest. Because of the variety of databases used in health care delivery, they need to be relational so that the data can be merged and produce consolidated information. Making databases relational depends on using a *primary key*. This is a specific linkage, such as a unique identification number like a patient's admission number or social security number.

One direct leadership and management application of nursing informatics is the pursuit of learning health system (LHS) goals as presented by the IOM (2012) report *The Path to Continuously Learning Health Care in America:* managing rapidly increasing complexity, achieving greater value, and capturing opportunities from technology, industry, and policy. A continuously learning health system provides the best care at lower costs. There is an underlying information infrastructure enabling iterative cycles using actionable data/evidence to improve health and decrease costs. Nurses have a key role to play in the data analytic infrastructure, clinical decision support, and IT-supported communication/collaboration mechanisms embedded in the practice environment. To coordinate care and promote teamwork and collaboration, nurse leaders can become intimately involved in IT infrastructure development and innovation. Focal points include care transitions, continuity of care, clinical work flow, process analyses, HIE, and human factors (Cummins, 2014). Comprehensive resources on the LHS are available on the IOM website.

CURRENT ISSUES AND TRENDS

A current trend with nursing and other health care providers is to increase the use of electronic HIEs to access historical documents from many health care providers across many locations. The use of an HIE can improve the completeness of a person's health and medical records among all providers. The complete scope of a person's information accessible from a central record locator can support the providers' decisions and avoid costs from repeating tests and examinations, especially when care is provided across settings and sites. This network to exchange information now includes meaningful information within EHRs from most hospitals, laboratories, eligible ambulatory providers, pharmacies, and more and more long-term care facilities (ONC for Health IT, 2016).

One issue of concern is the lack of accessibility to a person's health record extending beyond the information stored in the confines of the health care system (ONC for Health IT, n.d.). The health records need to connect with community providers who provide health care services within schools, home, and work settings where individuals spend a majority of their time. The networks will need to expand their access to occupational health nurses, school nurses, public health and community health professionals, dentists, optometrists, hospice and homecare nurses, and therapists and social and behavioral professionals. This allows health care professionals in the community to coordinate health care with health care system providers and make informed decisions with the client, parents, and family while keeping the client active in making decisions about self-care and functional health patterns within the home and work settings.

The HIE networks will never replace provider–patient communications, but the networks will consolidate access to the person's records with current and past diagnoses, medications, and treatments through a query process using the common record locator. The access to the record locator often has been integrated within the EHR application so that providers can review it during that provider–patient visit. Most advanced HIE networks support not only this query process but also secure messaging between providers, alert messaging to providers, and collection of data for state and public health registries for cancer, immunizations, and disease surveillance. The networks are posed to advance the use of information for both patient and public health purposes with technology and clinical informatics interoperability (ONC for Health IT, 2016).

A second issue for all providers is the interoperability of the data. Clearly there is a need for standardization of language, but the type of information presented in the continuous care documents that are shared among providers also must have commonality. Any significant variation in the process for generating continuous care documents could instigate confusion between the sender and receiver of that clinical information. CCD formats that are inclusive of detailed information will provide subsequent nursing caregivers appropriate details not only for medications and a surgical plan, but also for the scheduled nursing interventions, nutrition plan, exercise/activity plan, and treatment plan when the person moves between providers and settings. Much of this information in CCD is absent or missing for the client to safely continue the treatment plan beyond the hospital setting. The efforts to improve an interoperable HIT system offer this consistent defined vocabulary, structure, and format. Interoperability is guided by leaders and managers who take action to build on the existing health IT infrastructure to increase functionality with interoperable data. One size does not fit all, so leaders need to strive for baseline data to vary the user experience to meet the user's data need based on their use of care delivery (i.e., nursing process data) with the available technology, the clinical work flow (i.e., nursing process), personal preferences, and other factors. This will support evidence-based knowledge and safe care and prevent the potential for error. Some proposals have suggested a dual model approach: meeting the needs for practicing nurses and other professionals who need the concept model for evidence-based practice according to professional processes and meeting the needs for HIM/MIS to extract and send data using the information reference model.

A third issue for nurse leaders is the role of health care professionals (nurses and nurse practitioners) who need to use the HIE networks to gain access to their patients' health and medical records and share their clinical documentation in a standard format for others to understand and use. For this reason, nursing and health care organizations continue to redesign and reengineer the existing work environment and patient-centered work flow to include the use of the HIE network in daily practice. The responsibility to complete timely documentation is important for patient access and for other providers.

A fourth consideration for nurse leaders is data analytics and meaningful use rules of engagement for the Affordable Care Act of 2010 as directed by the Office of the National Coordinator for Health Information Technology within the Centers for Medicare & Medicaid Services (CMS). CMS advocates the need for ACOs' data to measure 34 indicators of health care access, quality, costs, and outcomes (CMS, 2017). These data are helpful for leaders to improve work flow, to improve clinician and client satisfaction, client outcomes, and client access to their information, and for the affordability and sustainability of all health care organizations and services. Nursing and health care organizations are starting to store and increase trending toward using data analytics based on datasets from cooperative data warehouses, recently called Big Data. Big Data analytics makes use of the massive quantity of digitalized data that promises to support clinical decision making, disease surveillance, and population health management (Raghupathi & Raghupathi, 2014).

Short-staffing leaves nurses exhausted from running from task to task, potentially generating errors of omission with scheduled treatments, medications, or therapies. Through the ACO and health care system, incentive payments are received for quality of care health care outcomes and reduced for categories of hospital-acquired conditions. These health care outcomes are based on the appropriateness, accuracy, and frequency of specific types of interventions. Nurses enter the data, including patients' assessments and preferred outcomes, to reach a quality outcome and to complete the client's PHR for CCD with instructions at discharge. Clinical decision support strategies with reminders and alerts can message nurses after undocumented care, but the timing of the reminders needs to align with the nurses' work flow. Data analytic measures for the 14 categories of hospital-acquired conditions that affect reimbursement (such as air embolism, pressure ulcers stage III and IV, falls and trauma, poor glycemic control, surgical site infection, or catheter-associated urinary tract infection [CAUTI]) can be part of the managers' dashboard. (See Chapter 19 for more on what is a patient day and dashboards.) Monitoring dashboards display common administrative numbers for the day such as census, average length of stay of inpatients, number of RNs staffed per unit, number of patients with diagnosed infections (e.g., CAUTI, VAP), the problem list, and up-to-date plans of care.

Sharing nursing diagnoses within the problem lists and uploading scheduled and unscheduled nursing procedures and interventions to the CCD can facilitate the discharge for clients to the next level of care or other facility. The appropriate, timely sharing of client information can save nurses time when they know the preexisting nursing diagnoses from the problem lists. This allows informed decision making at the new location for point of care and allows providers to avoid readmissions when the client goes home, avoid medication errors when at home or a new facility, and decreases reassessments and duplicate testing when diagnoses are known for the client.

⁴ RESEARCH NOTE

Source

Roth, C., Payne, P.R.O, Weier, R.C., Shoben, A.B., Fletcher, E.N., Lai, A.M., et al. (2016). The geographic distribution of cardiovascular health in the stroke prevention in healthcare delivery environments (SPHERE) study. *Journal of Biomedical Informatics, 60*(1), 95–103

Purpose

Cardiovascular disease morbidity and mortality have not uniformly decreased across the population. The purpose of this study was to link community and electronic health record (EHR) data from an older female patient cohort participating in an ongoing intervention within a medical center to associate community-level data with patient-level cardiovascular health.

Discussion

Nurses collect and review many of the data for the Life's Simple 7 measures for cardiovascular health (CVH), which uses seven modifiable values found in EHRs: total cholesterol, blood pressure, fasting blood glucose, smoking status, body mass index (BMI), physical activity, and diet. CVH is evaluated as ideal, intermediate, or poor as it relates to the parameters. The community data are characteristics of the census tracks' data that include weekly per capita expenditures on various healthy food groups, socioeconomic data for income, poverty, walkability, education, and unemployment that are collected by the US census. Community data are used with patient-level data to identify geographical populations that need tailored clinical

RESEARCH NOTE—cont'd

recommendations to improve outcomes as measured by the Life's Simple 7.

Application to Practice

Nurses have a central role in assessing functional health patterns for chronic disease management and prevention. Five of the seven components of Life's Simple 7 parameters are collected in standard methods and available within the EHR, whereas standard methods to document diet and physical activity data are missing. In this study functionality within the EHR was added to enable patients to complete a short survey within the patient health record (PHR) to populate the fields of data on nutrition pattern regarding diet and activity/rest pattern. These lifestyle data available through the PHR and census track-level characteristics for geographical information provide data to tailor best practice alerts to prioritize client preventive care. The development of information architecture and automation to design best practice alerts for settings where clients are more often seen can guide practice for nurses and nurse practitioners.

CASE STUDY

Kim, Mark, and Joyce are chief nursing executives (CNEs) at three different large community hospitals in cities within 100 miles of one another. All three work with the nearby nursing schools to discuss their need for nurses with bachelor of science in nursing (BSN) degrees and nurse practitioners. All three have identified common administrative and clinical questions that must be answered to plan for workforce capacity and to support clinical experiences for students at the nursing schools. Each hospital and community uses standardized nursing classifications to support documentation requirements within the clinical information systems and shares some of the same client population. The nurse managers have access to basic reports using data warehouse repositories. The repositories include client medical diagnoses as well as problems, risks, and needs for health promotion. Nursing diagnoses are used in the diagnoses and problem list tables. All three surgery departments use the perioperative nursing dataset to record care for the operating room services. The state and local communities have promoted the use of personal health records with patient populations, and clients who are using the hospitals and ambulatory clinics have been involved at the time of admission to request a set of preferred measurable patient outcomes using a standardized nursing classification (e.g., postprocedure recovery, ambulation/walking, infection severity) and their outcome level achieved at time of departure. The nursing departments evaluate competencies using the well-defined evidence-based standardized nursing classification for interventions and have asked nurses to document these same interventions when providing care to clients using the standardized documentation terms within their respective electronic health records (EHRs).

Each of the CNEs has asked his or her unit managers and nurse informatics specialists to help identify workforce capacity and competencies by extracting data from the EHR data repositories on frequency of nursing interventions per quarter per unit, numbers of staff in each position, and hours worked by staff position per quarter per unit. The CNEs' other questions relate to types of patient populations by medical diagnoses per unit and the types and frequency of nursing diagnoses the nurses must care for per quarter per unit. The CNEs were also interested in what outcomes the clients are asking for within their respective hospitals. The CNEs asked the MIS/HIM data analysts to work with the informatics nurse specialist, two nurse managers, and two clinical nurse leaders to design various reports to extract the correct data fields from the data warehouse information tables. The EHRs were designed differently so that the clinical nurse leaders could help operationally define where the data had been documented by the RNs and other personnel on the units. The data analysts were asked to ensure there was a *primary key* (such as a unique identification number) that would link the nurse provider to not only their educational competencies from orientation, position, and nursing education level, but also linked to their frequency of documented interventions, clients, client outcomes preferred, their unit setting, their hospital setting, and the primary medical and nursing diagnoses that nurses cared for.

The data analyst, nurse informatics specialist, and CNEs were all aware that these administrative and clinical questions would require many smaller reports, initially extracted from the repository from base reports and subsequently divided up for each nurse manager or aggregated for the CNE. Once the reports were extracted, they provided multiple tables of information that the quality department staff or clinical data analyst—with the help of nurse managers—could use with data analysis tools to find frequencies, averages, ranges, and modes and then begin to show distinct similarities or differences with

Continued

comparisons between units and between hospitals on the types of staff deployed to obtained existing outcomes. Often the comparative analysis will require statistical tools to identify any significant differences. Many of the analytical tools are part of the package of tools hospitals and health systems use to answer questions.

Many of these reports that were initially generated can be programmed to run and extract the data at regular intervals such as weekly, monthly, quarterly, or annually. When the reports are basic and it is simple to extract basic data elements into a table of information, the query can run efficiently. The simpler reports with primary key variables can be aggregated in a common database for use of analytic tools that allow the linking of multiple tables of information and more robust analysis and comparison. Once the queries are well tested and of proven value, steps can be taken with MIS/HIM departments to add the extraction of data and analysis to monitoring dashboards. This can lead to real-time, effective, and efficient care delivery decision making.

CRITICAL THINKING EXERCISE

No nurse wants to make a wrong decision, mistake, or omission of care. However, the nurses on a busy and short-staffed medical–surgical floor of an acute care tertiary-level hospital know that many decisions about client diagnoses, assessments, outcomes to monitor, and the timing of interventions and administered medications need to be implemented and documented in real time. The nurse manager meets with the nurse practice council from time to time to discuss this problem of high rates of missed interventions, medication omissions, and never events (Kalisch & Xie, 2014). The council needs to improve the work flow to reduce and eliminate the opportunity to miss care that could cause the never events while maintaining staffing levels on respective units.

The nursing practice council has questions about omissions and commissions with care provided. The council needs to find information from the documented data to address these unanswered questions about errors of omission and errors of commission. The council can better support the clinical work flow when data are analyzed from the EHR repository. The council first determined the clinical work flows for both medical patients and surgical patients using the nursing process. Both clinical work flows include data needs for admission activities that include assessment documentation from nurses, nursing assistants, and other health care professionals. The second type of data is diagnosed patient problems, risks, and needs for health promotion. The interventions are more likely determined by the extent and causes on the problem list, which guides treatment plans. The third type of data is the patients' preferences for outcomes and treatment. The fourth type of data is the documentation on interventions, medications, and treatments ordered and given or omitted by all the health care professionals on the unit. The fifth type of data is the documentation on changes in the patients' assessments from the time of admission through the continued care. These data provide nurses information to evaluate care and whether the ordered care has the patient progressing, unchanged in status, or declining in status toward the patient's desired outcomes.

Each type of data is stored within a table in the EHR's data warehouse. The data analyst will join the nurses at a meeting to better understand their questions about omission of care and where these data associated with the nursing process work flow are actually documented in the EHR. The documented data are stored in tables and under classes of data.

1. What factors do the nurses and the nurse manager need to assess and analyze?
2. What data are needed to understand errors of omission and commission?
3. What time was the care treatment or medication to be provided?
4. Who was responsible for providing that intervention (medication or treatment)?
5. Where was the intervention to be completed?
6. Can the clinical decision support be designed to support nurses to prevent the omissions?
7. What nursing evidence-based knowledge exists to build clinical decision support systems for nurses in the practice setting to improve performance?
8. What can the nurse manager do to form a persuasive data management plan?
9. Who needs to be involved in developing the clinical queries?
10. Are each of the practice settings at their appropriate staffing levels? Who is and who is not?

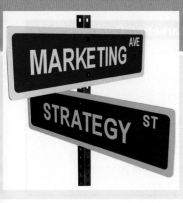

Marketing

Slimen Saliba

http://evolve.elsevier.com/Huber/leadership

You may be tempted to skip this chapter. The nurse leader's agenda is so crowded that marketing can seem a nonessential concern. After all, there are dedicated marketing personnel in most hospitals and other health care organizations. Why should nurses get involved? What does marketing have to do with the practice of nursing care? Your answer to this question depends, in part, on your definition of marketing.

One prominent textbook definition indicates that marketing is "the art and science of choosing target markets and getting, keeping, and growing customers through creating, delivering, and communicating superior customer value" (Kotler & Keller, 2016, p. 5). Much of what the average person understands about marketing focuses on the last four words of this definition: "communicating superior customer value." When many imagine the tools and methods employed to achieve this goal, what comes to mind is an unforgettable Super Bowl commercial, powerful tagline, or moving product endorsement that draws consumers to purchase a particular brand of chips or fly with a specific airline. It can be difficult, then, to think of hospitals as organizations that require marketing. When health fails, who has time to "shop" for a hospital, and who can even understand or compare the costs of the services hospitals provide? Further, busy short-staffed nurses might not recognize or value the resources that organizations spend on branding and marketing.

The focus, however, in health care marketing is not only on developing a brand and attracting customers but also also on "creating and delivering superior customer value." More simply, marketing is focused on establishing customer relationships and satisfying customer needs and wants. And it is here that nurses are crucial members of the hospital marketing team. Nurse leaders may provide input regarding the hospital's brand or communication strategy, but more importantly, nurse leaders also manage the team that most directly affects the value that a customer (the patient) receives and reports. Every interaction between a patient and a nurse creates and communicates value—the very definition of marketing. Therefore in a health care environment built and billed on patient satisfaction, this chapter is a crucial part of training for nurses and nurse leaders.

Marketing activities within hospitals and other health care organizations occur at the organizational (hospital), departmental (women's health), and unit (labor and delivery) levels. Such activities are also classified as internal or external, with each targeting a different audience or market. Target audiences can be patients and families, physicians, payers, and employees. Marketing departments within health care agencies take the lead in organizational-level activities and ensure that customer-driven marketing strategies and programs are in alignment with the organization's strategic plan. The primary product that is marketed by hospitals is their patient care, and nurses deliver most of that product. Patient satisfaction is an accepted indicator of product (care) quality, and a high level of satisfaction is imperative to viability in today's competitive marketplace (Kennedy et al., 2013). For example, as noted in part B of the Critical Thinking Exercise later in this chapter, the nurse communication section of the Hospital Consumer Assessment of Healthcare Providers and Systems (HCAHPS) survey, which is a standardized survey of patients' perspectives about hospital care, has an important impact on patients' satisfaction with hospitalization. See Chapter 15 for more on HCAHPS. Thus nurses and nurse leaders are important members of the marketing team because of their primary focus on providing patient care and managing patients' health care needs.

Not only are nurses at the center of health care delivery, but nurse leaders also are accountable for the workforce that provides this service. Marketing initiatives that focus on care delivery, customer satisfaction, and recruitment and retention of the nursing workforce are essential in hospitals. Nurse leaders who possess marketing acumen within their business skill set are invaluable to the development of more sensitive customer/patient service programs delivered by a competent, experienced nursing workforce.

Previous chapters in this text have addressed the challenges faced by top-level and frontline nurse leaders. These challenges include delivery of high-quality patient-centered care; recruitment and retention of a culturally diverse, competent workforce; promotion of a positive and inspiring image of nursing; design of a healthy work environment; and development of practices to satisfy patients and improve outcomes. Marketing initiatives can be designed and implemented to help meet these challenges.

The purpose of this chapter is to present key marketing concepts and definitions, applications of marketing to health care, and implications for nurse leaders and managers. Familiarity with marketing terminology will position a nurse leader to better understand the organization and possess the tools and techniques to respond to the challenges faced (Montoya & Kimball, 2012).

DEFINITIONS AND CORE CONCEPTS

Box 27.1 lists core marketing concepts that are the building blocks of modern marketing.

Marketing begins with understanding customer **needs** and **wants.** Needs are basic human requirements that include food, clothing, and shelter. These needs are translated to wants as a person begins to differentiate

---

BOX 27.1   **Core Marketing Concepts**
Needs and wants
Offerings and brands
Value and satisfaction
Relationships and exchange
Marketing
Company orientation
Market research
Market
Segmentation, target markets, and positioning
Competition

---

between various objects, each of which satisfies the same need. A nearly limitless list of factors influences our wants, including society, culture, family, religion, ethnicity, and location. For instance, the need for food may be translated into wanting a cheesesteak sandwich in Philadelphia or carbonara in Rome. A recent study explored the factors that influence what patients want. Researchers found, for instance, that patients want safety more than savings when differentiating between various providers for necessary health care. In fact, 97% of the time consumers will choose hospitals that are rated safer, regardless of cost (Byrnes, 2015). However, wants are not fixed. Related factors can shift and priorities change. For example, insurance mitigates the impact of cost on patient choices. If the insurance environment changes, cost may become a more important factor in the choices patients make to meet their health care needs.

Companies address customer needs by putting forth a value proposition or a way of seeing the world that satisfies those needs. What begins as an intangible value proposition is made tangible through an **offering,** which can be a combination of services, information, and experiences. For example, safety is an intangible value proposition. Patients look for tangible cues to signal adherence to this abstract value. A pristine environment and articulate, efficient nurses translate a value proposition like safety into tangible offerings for a patient. A **brand** is an offering from a known source. It is "a promise to consumers that a hospital will deliver on the kind of care needed" (Kemp et al., 2014, p. 126). In satisfying **wants,** a buyer chooses the offerings he or she perceives to deliver the most **value,** which can be understood as the sum of tangible and intangible benefits and costs. **Satisfaction** reflects a person's judgment of a product's perceived performance in relationship to expectations. Because the services provided in health care settings are highly technical and specialized, patients' expectations may be set by what health care providers tell them about a particular service (Kemp et al., 2014). The relationship between expectation and performance can result in disappointment, satisfaction, or delight (Kotler & Keller, 2016, p. 11).

Expectations and satisfaction depend significantly on the quality of the relationship between the brand and its customers. Social psychologists describe two broad categories of human relationships: **exchange relationships** in which we trade for mutual benefit and **communal relationships,** which are based on mutual caring and support (Barro, 2015). Health care is caught between these two kinds of relationships. In its strictest sense, the *business* of health care is transactional and is an exchange relationship. However, the *practice* of health care is more like a communal relationship. Health care workers are always trying to balance these two kinds of relationships. The marketing of health care is caught in this tension between an exchange relationship (the business of health care) and a communal relationship (the practice of health care).

Marketing, therefore, describes a range of relationships that facilitates transactions in which products (i.e., goods or services) are exchanged in a market. The process begins with understanding what the customer needs and wants, includes the design of offerings that fulfill these needs and wants, and ends with creating **value** for and with the customers (Kotler & Keller, 2016). Marketing ensures a focus on a company's annual, long-range, and strategic plans. Strategic, long-range plans are informed by a company's culture. Companies develop distinctive **orientations,** or **viewpoints,** that define their organizational culture. Hospital organizational cultures also have distinctive orientations. What follows is a description of four such orientations.

- **Product orientation:** An organizational culture that assumes what the customer wants is the very best quality, regardless of cost.
- **Selling orientation:** An organizational culture that assumes the customers must be persuaded to buy the firm's products.
- **Marketing orientation:** An organizational culture that assumes the customer's needs and wants should determine the quality, price, and availability of the product.
- **Holistic orientation:** An organizational culture that focuses on the customer's needs and wants, as well as the societal impact of products that meet those needs and wants. Communication and promotion of the products involve both employees and potential customers.

Institutions that are committed to sustaining a relationship with their customers strive for a culture that can be labeled as a **marketing** or **holistic orientation**. Nurses can reflect on and evaluate these four orientations (product orientation, selling orientation, marketing orientation, and holistic orientation) and describe which of these most closely resembles their current workplace (or a prior workplace). What practices can be identified as evidence of the company's orientation? How does this company orientation affect the nurses' work? How are nurses' relationships with patients and colleagues affected by the culture that this orientation describes?

Market research applies a scientific approach to ascertain insights in and information about customers and potential target markets. Steps in this approach begin with defining the problem and research objectives, proceeding to data collection and analysis, and ending with interpretation of findings relevant to a specific marketing situation or decision making (Kotler & Keller, 2016).

A **market** was once defined as the physical place where buyers and sellers assembled and exchanged goods, often via a bartering system. Today, however, a market is "a collection of buyers and sellers who transact over a particular product or product class" (Kotler & Keller, 2016, p. 7). Actual and potential customers are categorized as external markets, and employees comprise internal markets. Exchange has always been the defining concept underlying marketing (Kotler & Keller, 2016). Today, exchange can take place in person, by phone, by mail, or in a digital or virtual environment like the Internet.

Segmentation is the process of dividing a market into distinct groups of buyers "by identifying demographic, psychographic, and behavioral differences between them" (Kotler & Keller, 2016, p. 9). Segmentation has become particularly crucial as hospitals work to refine ways of predicting which patients are more or less likely to be hospitalized initially or readmitted after discharge. Identifying such segments of the population and creating relevant, effective interventions can save significant health care costs (Sanky et al., 2012). **Targeting,** then, is identifying which segment is most relevant or presents the greatest opportunity for a given business (Kotler & Keller, 2016). **Positioning** is "the act of designing a company's offering and image to occupy a distinctive place in the minds of the target market" (Kotler & Keller, 2016, p. 275). Finally, **competition** includes all the actual and potential rival offerings and substitutes a buyer might consider.

BACKGROUND

The business goal of a for-profit company is to maximize value so that shareholders will eventually benefit from their financial investment. The business goal of a non-profit or social sector organization, which includes many health care organizations, is to fulfill its mission of meeting consumer needs. Thus marketing is fundamental to creating value for customers that in turn leads to financial viability. Because of its for-profit roots, the term *marketing* often carries a negative connotation when applied to health care. Many question the appropriateness of marketing initiatives that seem focused on net income at the expense of patient care. These questions are of particular interest to nurses because nursing care composes much of the health care product.

Profitable may be the word that at first consideration seems foreign to the fabric of nursing. Nurses are educated and socialized to *give* care, not to *sell* care. Although nurses experience the impact of marketing in their daily lives as consumers, they are unlikely to be exposed to it as an essential ingredient of their professional practice. However, when basic marketing concepts and aspects of the marketing process are explored and understood, their importance to not only the health care organization at large, but also to nurses and nurse leaders, becomes clear.

Nurses are essential providers of the health care product and, as such, are engaged in marketing when delivering care. This is in part because interpersonal relationships are an important part of the therapeutic "product" of care. A health care organization dedicated to achieving excellence realizes this and works hard to inform all care providers and support staff about meeting customer needs. In excellence-driven organizations, particularly those with a holistic company orientation, marketing is more than a department; it is at the core of the organizational business framework. The American Organization of Nurse Executives (AONE) has noted the identification of marketing opportunities and the development of marketing strategies as key business skills for nurse leaders in executive practice and for those with a career goal of leadership (AONE, 2015). Nurse leaders and aspiring nurse leaders who operate within a business framework benefit from understanding marketing concepts that underlie programs and initiatives in health care organizations.

MARKETING STRATEGY

Strategic planning, a process discussed in previous chapters of this text, sets the overall direction for an organization. Defining the business, determining the mission, and developing long-term objectives form the basis of an organization's strategic plan. Marketing strategies and programs must be aligned and guided by the organization-wide strategic plan (Kotler & Keller, 2016). This cannot be done effectively without investing adequate time and resources in evaluating the organization's competitive environment.

A market research approach is used for environmental scanning and is a critical step in both the strategic and marketing planning processes. During the environmental scanning, marketing departments explore and evaluate the internal and external environments to gain an understanding of demographic and societal trends, competition, and potential customers. Also, internal business performance indicators such as profits (or losses), customer and staff satisfaction, and quality indicators are evaluated. To be most effective, compilation, review, and analysis of environmental data should involve every functional area in an organization, including the nursing department. The results of the market research need to be shared across business units, and all key stakeholders need to participate in the subsequent planning process.

Marketing strategy is based on how target markets are defined. Markets are both broad and narrow. *Mass marketing,* which is broad, offers a product to an entire external market. *Niche marketing* represents a narrower view and focuses on capturing a small but important part of the market. Consider the difference between a full-service community hospital and a children's hospital. The former serves a broad market; the latter targets very specific customers: children and their families. Understanding the application of four critical concepts of segmentation, targeting, product differentiation, and positioning is essential to becoming fluent in the language of marketing.

Segmentation and targeting are the means of making decisions about which customers will be served. *Segmentation* involves identifying pieces of the total market that contain potential customers with distinguishable characteristics such as age, gender, geographical location, or ethnicity. The essence of segmentation is to break down the mass market into submarkets of individuals with similar needs. *Targeting* takes into account the whole market that can then be considered in terms of attractive smaller market segments. Differentiation and positioning clarify how customers will be served. A product offering's *differentiation* calls for the creation of superior customer value and is typically what strengthens its position in the market against competitors. *Positioning* the product such that customers perceive it to be distinctive and desirable is the foundation of the marketing process (Kotler & Keller, 2016).

By analyzing information about the competitive market, a hospital can determine key strategies to meet the unmet needs in its service area. A small rural community hospital in a market 200 miles from any other hospital will adopt strategies for defining and serving its market that are very different from the strategies of a large suburban hospital in a market with four other hospitals within a 25-mile radius. The rural hospital would likely position itself as a full-service facility capable of meeting the most frequently occurring needs of their target audience or the local community. For example, its profile of services is likely to include women's services, emergency care, diagnostic care, and general surgery. On the other hand, the large suburban hospital in a highly competitive market might seek to differentiate itself from competitors by creating a specialty center for heart disease or cancer. However, product or service lines are not the only way to differentiate. Differentiation can be based on quality measures and other distinctions that are prevalent today. These include:

- The Joint Commission (TJC) accreditation for meeting performance standards
- Malcolm Baldrige National Quality Award for performance excellence
- Beacon Award for Excellence in critical care nursing
- Truven Health Analytics 100 Top Hospitals award
- American Nurses Credentialing Center's Magnet Recognition Program® for excellence in nursing

- Planetree Designation Program for excellence in patient- and person-centered care

Heightened patient and regulatory scrutiny, fueled by more frequent accounts in the media of medical errors, has motivated hospitals to refocus on patient care excellence and seek ways to promote this excellence to the public to gain a competitive advantage. Logos depicting the previously mentioned designations of excellence are displayed on the organization's website home page and are used to promote differentiating distinctions.

Setting marketing strategy is a shared responsibility within a health care organization. This critical activity must be guided by the strategic plan with input from every key stakeholder group, especially nursing, that is engaged in meeting customer needs during many and varied exchanges. Likewise, the organization's marketing team is engaged at the start when new services are planned. With multiple perspectives represented at the planning table, an organization will respond more effectively to the needs and challenges of its markets.

THE MARKETING PROCESS: FOCUS ON MARKETING MIX

Previous sections of this chapter have focused on marketing at the organizational level to external markets. Familiarity with the marketing terminology and concepts that have been presented are imperative to building business skills and to applying the marketing mix. There are many complex marketing models that depict steps in the marketing process. Most begin with an appraisal and understanding of the environment and potential customers, include the design and delivery of a customer-driven marketing strategy, and end with customer loyalty and equity. A more in-depth understanding of such models is required as nurses advance in their career. At this point, understanding basic aspects of the marketing process is more meaningful. The marketing mix is the set of tactical tools used in the marketing process. The marketing mix was introduced almost 50 years ago (McCarthy, 1964) but remains a useful organizing framework for successful marketing programs. Nurse leaders at all levels can apply this framework in programs and initiatives designed to meet everyday challenges.

The specific tools in the mix are custom designed to influence the buyer's decision to purchase the product or service and to be the basis for operational marketing activities. From the seller's point of view, the marketing mix emerges as a unique combination of the four Ps of (1) product, (2) price, (3) place, and (4) promotion. From the customer's point of view, a more customer-centric (patient-centric) marketing framework emphasizes the customer values of (1) acceptability, (2) affordability, (3) accessibility, and (4) awareness. This is commonly referred to as the four As (Sheth & Sisodia, 2012).

Although the four Ps framework has been in existence for more than five decades, both frameworks (the four Ps and the four As) are helpful in understanding how nurses can deliver health care effectively. Table 27.1

TABLE 27.1   Marketing Mix Elements

Seller (Hospital) Perspective	Customer (Patient) Perspective
A product is the basis of any business and is the focus of exchange between the provider and customer. It is whatever is offered to satisfy a target market's need, desire, or preference. Products generally include objects, services, and ideas. Goods and services may also be combined into a product. The primary hospital product is the care delivered by nurses.	**Acceptability** is the extent to which a firm's total product offering exceeds customer expectations. Functional aspects of design can be boosted by, for instance, enhancing the core benefit or increasing reliability of the product; psychological acceptability can be improved with changes to brand image, packing and design, and positioning.
In a narrow sense, **price** is described as the amount of money customers pay to obtain the product. Customers consider the cost in terms of reasonableness. However, in a broader sense, cost is more than the money that is exchanged. Customers place value on products and services not only according to financial issues, but also according to psychosocial and emotional concerns. For example, delayed services that result in an excessive time commitment by the customer may be a greater price than they are willing to pay. The "price" that is perceived by the customer may be very subjective.	**Affordability** is the extent to which customers in the target market are able and willing to pay the product's price. It has two dimensions: economic (ability to pay) and psychological (willingness to pay). Acceptability combined with affordability determines the product's value proposition.
The **place** refers not only to the location of the product exchange but also to activities that make the product available to the customer. Examples of obvious places for health care delivery are hospitals, which are composed of individual departments and units, practitioner offices in ambulatory settings, and outpatient surgical centers. Less obvious factors to consider are *hours of* and *access to* the service.	**Accessibility,** the extent to which customers are able to readily acquire the product, has two dimensions: availability and convenience. Questions of access continue to transform health care delivery in environments that are becoming increasingly virtual and digital. Where health care delivery once required patients to travel to a specific, brick and mortar *place* to receive care, the Internet now has the power to transform nearly any concrete location into an access point for care.
Promotion is comprised of communications with target markets about the product offered to meet needs, desires, or preferences. It is inclusive of publicity and advertising that seeks to persuade target markets that a given health care organization can deliver on their promise, meaning they provide a high-quality product. Promotion often initiates relationships with customers.	**Awareness** is the extent to which customers are informed regarding the product's characteristics, persuaded to try it, and reminded to repurchase. It has two dimensions: brand awareness and product knowledge. Sheth and Sisodia (2012) say awareness is ripest for improvement because most companies are either ineffectual or inefficient at developing it. For instance, properly done advertising can be incredibly powerful, but word-of-mouth marketing and comarketing can more effectively reach potential customers.

Data from Kotler, P., & Keller, K.L. (2016). *Marketing management* (15th ed.). New York, NY: Pearson; Sheth, J.N., & Sisodia, R. (2012). *The 4 A's of marketing: Creating value for customer, company and society.* New York, NY: Routledge.

provides brief descriptions of the four Ps and the four As as they pertain to the marketing mix.

The four Ps framework is particularly well suited to a manufacturing and industrial economy and reflects a business-centric perspective. As the US economy has become more service oriented, an alternative framework that assumes a customer-centric perspective might be more helpful in conceptualizing the ways in which a hospital's products are priced, placed, and promoted. The four As, therefore, describe a business environment in which the patient has far more influence over the marketing mix. This has been facilitated, in particular, by the development of a digital marketplace, where services can be delivered without the more traditional boundaries established by brick and mortar buildings and regular business hours. The health care market is increasingly located in digital environments like computers and smartphones. In fact, Deloitte predicted that 75 million physician visits in North America annually would occur via some form of electronic technology (Deloitte, 2014).

A recent example of such technology is the web-based application Doctor on Demand. The company offers video chats at any time of day with board-certified physicians, licensed psychologists, and lactation consultants. Applications like Doctor on Demand (which is one of many such apps) provide a current case study for understanding the customer-oriented marketing mix represented by the four As (outlined in Table 27.2).

LEADERSHIP AND MANAGEMENT IMPLICATIONS

At a glance, nurses may consider that nursing and marketing go together like oil and water. However, nurses (and nursing) are critical components to health care marketing. This is because marketing is about building relationships with customers so that needs and wants are satisfied and value is created. Marketing goals are incorporated in the organizational strategic plan. These goals focus on satisfying and creating value with respect to customers. They also may be focused on attracting new customers or increasing volume to enhance financial viability. Nursing is affected by such strategies and also can have an impact on goal achievement.

An understanding of the marketing framework as well as basic marketing concepts allows nurse leaders and managers to be knowledgeable contributors at the table where high-level goals are established and decisions about meeting goals are made. As shown in Box 27.2, there are three levels of market planning:
- Corporate strategic planning
- Strategic marketing
- Marketing management

Nursing executive leadership generally would be involved in the first two levels. Nurse leaders and managers then implement corporate strategies at the marketing management level by **promoting** the value nursing brings to the organization and managing the implementation of the marketing mix. Financial viability comes

TABLE 27.2 Customer-Oriented Marketing Mix: Telemedicine	
Marketing Mix	**Application to Telemedicine**
Acceptability	Doctor on Demand has a Net Promoter Score (NPS), a customer loyalty metric that *exceeds* the same scores for Amazon, Netflix, and other well-established digital brands *(http://npsbenchmarks.com)*.
Affordability	Although a visit with a health care provider costs more than the average copay ($40/appointment), the Doctor on Demand website points out that the visit is still less expensive than urgent care and is covered by several health plans, including United Healthcare. Additionally, downloading the app and signing up for the service is free.
Accessibility	The company's tagline is "Your personal waiting room." Video visits with providers on this app can happen at any time of day using a smartphone or computer. Additionally, the app uses the Global Positioning System (GPS) to locate nearby pharmacies and place relevant prescriptions for pickup.
Awareness	As of the writing of this chapter, the number of installations of this app on Android phones alone was approaching 1 million *(https://play.google.com)*.

BOX 27.2   The Marketing Framework

CORPORATE STRATEGIC PLANNING—Future Focus
(The art of attracting and keeping profitable customers)
Mission: Defining the corporate mission
Vision: Translating the corporate mission
Company Orientations:
- Product orientation
- Selling orientation
- Marketing orientation
- Holistic orientation

Planning Tools:
- Marketing research/market intelligence gathering
- Environmental analysis
- Value proposition analysis
- Satisfaction measurement
- SWOT (strengths, weaknesses, opportunities, and threats) analysis

Marketing Plan Development

STRATEGIC MANAGEMENT—Present/Near Future Focus
Tools: Segment
  Target
  Position

MARKETING MANAGEMENT—Present Focus
(Tactical marketing/implementation)

Marketing Mix: The Four As	Marketing Mix: The Four Ps
• Product	• Acceptability
• Price	• Affordability
• Place	• Accessibility
• Promotion	• Awareness

through the delivery of high quality care (**product**) across varied settings (**place**) and in a timely and efficient manner (**price**). Nurse leaders can challenge themselves and their colleagues to ask and answer questions such as:

1. How do I create value for my organization?
2. How do I help my organization become more patient centric?
3. How do I help my organization recognize the centrality of nursing care in affecting the organization's reputation and brand?

The nurse's interactions with patients and their families are critical to patent **satisfaction** and good clinical outcomes. Nursing relationship management is a major component of the **product/service** element of the marketing mix. All employees should focus on establishing and maintaining satisfactory customer relationships. In hospitals and other health care organizations, frontline nurses are critical in creating value for customers. There is no question that marketing is an important mindset in organizations, and "good nursing care goes hand-in-hand with good marketing efforts" (Montoya & Kimball, 2012, p. 186).

Advertising messages (promotion) about nurses and nursing care can reinforce a positive image of nursing to internal and external markets. One opportunity for promotion of nursing to all markets is to have a nursing focus on the hospital's website. Nurse leaders can ensure the promotion of nursing and nursing roles in as many venues as possible to communicate the importance of nursing, nursing practice, or nursing care to potential target markets (Ten Hoeve et al., 2014; Walker, 2014). This can be done by capturing stories of nurses who have been exemplars of compassionate and skilled care and featuring them on the hospital's intranet. These stories help define the profession and strengthen the organization's self-image as a place where branding tag lines such as "the skill to heal" and "the spirit to care" intersect with and exemplify the commitment to health and healing.

Kotler and Keller (2016) believe the future of marketing will be horizontal: consumer-to-consumer. They say that the recent economic downturn has not fostered trust in the marketplace and that customers now increasingly turn to one another for credible advice and information when selecting products (Kotler & Keller, 2016). In their book *Social Media for Nurses: Educating Practitioners and Patients in a Networked World,* Nelson and colleagues (2013, p. 2) noted that, "Over the last several decades, the role of the patient has been evolving from passive recipient of health care to informed, empowered, and engaged patient/consumer." Digital marketplaces have empowered consumers to improve their own health literacy, research providers, and write reviews of health care services (Hotopf, 2013). Nurse managers can work with their colleagues to creatively imagine how social media (promotion) can be used to leverage this technology as well as this growing cultural trend of patient-to-patient trust to build patient loyalty and brand strength. Nurse leaders and managers are responsible for promoting the merits of nursing service internally and externally.

Finally, another marketing application for nurse leaders and managers relates to workforce characteristics. Nurses who are employed make up an internal market, and the pool of nurses who are potential new hires makes up an external market. In these instances, nurses are the customers. Nurse leaders can use marketing to increase "customer" retention and attraction. When considering nurse retention and recruitment, leaders consider what **value proposition** (product) the nursing department or unit offers to nurses. Highlighting department or unit characteristics deemed important, such as shared governance and professional development opportunities, provides details about the product. Leaders can give attention to the unit (place) where nurses provide service. Consideration of the physical layout and whether the unit design is conducive to an efficient and effective workflow is important. Nurse leaders can ensure that nurses' salaries are competitive and that nurses do not feel underpaid and undervalued (Evans, 2013). Market research in collaboration with the human resources department can analyze salaries (price) in the external market and make adjustments accordingly.

One recent study also indicated that "employees who feel that they are personally cared for by their organization and managers have higher levels of commitment, are more conscious about responsibilities, have greater involvement in the organization, and are more innovative" (Moneke & Umeh, 2013, p. 201). In a health care environment where nurse–patient relationships are a key factor in patient satisfaction and willingness to recommend, similar relationships between nurse leaders and the nurses that they manage create significant value in terms of recruitment and retention of a qualified workforce.

CURRENT ISSUES AND TRENDS

A brief environmental analysis of marketing in health care reveals an emphasis on issues of cost and transparency, patient-centered care, the nursing shortage, geriatric workforce shortage, and work–life balance.

Cost and Transparency

"The lack of price transparency in healthcare threatens to erode public trust in our healthcare system" (Ellison, 2015). Access to price information is important to consumers. It is becoming more critical, particularly as accountable payment models are mandating that organizations improve performance and quality and thus customer satisfaction with the patient care experience.

An important consideration for nurses related to cost and value is that current payment models do not unbundle nursing care from room and board, thus making adjustments for nursing intensity in billing mechanisms impossible. Recommendations for incorporating a nursing intensity adjustment to existing inpatient billing could lead to determination of the economic value of that care. The marketing mix could more closely reflect the "price" of nursing care, which would contribute to the establishment of a value-based purchasing system for hospitals (Kavanagh et al., 2012).

There will be continued efforts and initiatives to address the costs of nursing care and subsequent reimbursement decisions in order to deliver and market cost-effective and efficient care. Nurses must also stay informed about, and engaged in, evolving accountable payment models in order to create care delivery systems that prevent negative outcomes for which reimbursement will be withheld. The shift away from fee-for-service models places an increasing emphasis on customer relationships and, in turn, increasing pressure on nurses to manage such relationships and build value for the customer and the system (Healthcare Financial Management Association, 2015).

Patient-Centered Care

A focus on patient-centered care began in the 1970s, but implementation remains an issue for many health care organizations. Varied patient-centered models and frameworks exist. Attributes in patient-centeredness include patient satisfaction, the patient experience of care, patient engagement, and shared decision making. Evidence supports the view that patient-centered care improves patient outcomes and is one approach to addressing racial, ethnic, and socioeconomic disparities in health care and health care outcomes (Long, 2012; Radwin et al., 2013).

Planetree is a designation that differentiates a hospital on the basis of excellence in patient- and person-centered care. The Planetree philosophy reveals a simple view of what it means to be patient-centered (Planetree, 2014). Components of the Planetree model that move an organization toward a culture of patient-centeredness can be found on their website. It is easy to determine the importance of patient-centeredness to marketing goals and ultimately to patient satisfaction, therefore models for delivery of patient-centered care will continue to evolve (Millenson & Macri, 2012).

Nursing Shortage

Though there is a debate regarding whether the nursing shortage is over, there is sufficient evidence to support the position that nurses who are baby boomers are on the cusp of retirement (Irish, 2014). The American Association of Colleges of Nursing projects a shortage of 260,000 nurses nationally by 2024 (Irish, 2014). This trend calls for internal marketing initiatives that address nurse turnover, job satisfaction, and occupational and organizational commitment. External marketing challenges will be encountered by hospitals seeking a more qualified nurse workforce (i.e., those with baccalaureate [BSN] degrees). This is supported by the American Nurses Credentialing Center's (ANCC) Magnet Recognition Program® (ANCC, 2016) as well as recent studies finding that higher percentages of registered nurses with baccalaureate degrees in hospitals are linked to lower patient mortality rates (Aiken et al., 2014; Blegen et al., 2013; Kutney-Lee et al., 2013). This calls for competitive marketing strategies to recruit successfully from the target market of BSN-prepared nurses.

Geriatric Workforce Shortage

The baby boomer population as a whole will increase the demand for health care services over the next several decades (Irish, 2014). The combination of the aging of the baby boom population, increases in life expectancy, and decreases in the number of younger persons will mean that older adults make up a much larger percentage of the US population than ever before. As a result, the scarcity of workers specializing in the care of older adults, the eldercare workforce, will be even more pronounced (Bureau of Labor Statistics, 2015).

Work–Life Balance

About two-thirds of the close to 3 million nurses who live in the United States work in hospitals. Generally

---

> **BOX 27.3   Marketing Lifestyle Management**
>
> Florida Hospital in Orlando, Florida, has developed a program of lifestyle management and is actively using it in employee self-management programs. It encourages each employee to practice eight principles of successful living in aspiring to achieve work–life balance. They are as follows:
>
> **C**hoice, **R**est, **E**nvironment, **A**ctivity, **T**rust, **I**nterpersonal relationships, **O**utlook, and **N**utrition
>
> For more information, see http://www.creationhealth.com/

speaking, hospitals are high-stress environments. In a recent study, only 23% of female participants who worked in health care indicated that they were able to balance their personal and professional lives well (Delina & Raya, 2013). Research is showing the importance of caring for oneself in order to provide outstanding patient care. Fatigue can lead to dangerous or costly mistakes, thereby affecting one's professional reputation and mental well-being (Steege & Pinekenstein, 2016). Nurse leaders need to advocate for policies that promote work–life balance in health care organizations in order to improve retention of qualified nurses and increase the value of care provided to their customers. One such initiative is described in Box 27.3.

SUMMARY

In a market in which patient needs and wants are the primary drivers of value, nurses are crucial participants in the marketing efforts of the health care organizations where they work. An understanding of the concepts and tools that are the foundation of modern marketing will enable nurses and nurse managers to advocate for their profession within health care organizations, recruit and retain high-quality peers, and build relationships with patients that facilitate meaningful exchange.

▲ RESEARCH NOTE

Source

Chen, S-Y., Wu, W-C., Chang, C-S., & Lin, C-T. (2015). Job rotation and internal marketing for increased job satisfaction and organisational commitment in hospital nursing staff. *Journal of Nursing Management, 23*, 297–306.

Purpose

The purpose of this study was to investigate how job rotation and internal marketing affect job satisfaction and organizational commitment in nurses. The concept of internal marketing emphasizes that organizations should value

RESEARCH NOTE—cont'd

and respect their employees by treating them as internal customers. Internal marketing can be essential for attracting, developing, motivating, and retaining employees such as experienced nurses. Job rotation is a planned change in the job assignment of an employee that provides employees with an opportunity to learn new skills and improves personnel management through labor utilization efficiency.

Discussion

This was a cross-sectional descriptive study of 266 (81.8% response rate) registered nurses in two hospitals in southern Taiwan. Although the study was not conducted in the United States, the authors studied job rotation and internal marketing as an innovative approach to understanding and enhancing job satisfaction and organizational commitment of nurses. The data collection survey used five-point Likert-type scaled items (1–5, strongly disagree to strongly agree) based on well-established, reliable scales. All participants were female; 42.5% had a bachelor's degree. The major findings are that job rotation and internal marketing are positively associated with job satisfaction and organizational commitment, and job satisfaction is positively associated with organizational

commitment. Although both job rotation and internal marketing enhanced job satisfaction and organizational commitment, there are fundamental differences between them. Job rotation improves efficiency in managing human resources; internal marketing is effective for attracting, selecting, training, and motivating nurses. The article contains a useful table displaying the items used to measure each of the four constructs.

Application to Practice

Job rotation enables nurses to acquire new competencies, expand their professional knowledge, and reduce job burnout. Internal marketing complements the positive effects of job rotation. Nurse leaders and managers can enhance nurses' job satisfaction and organizational commitment by using these strategies in a well-structured program that incorporates targeted education about the job rotation system and strong communication. Implementation suggestions are clarification of and advocacy for job rotation, transparency about the rotation procedure and participation in its administration, and use of job rotation as a strategic tool for training and developing staff. Combining job rotation with internal marketing can decelerate the recruitment–training–turnover cycle in nursing.

CASE STUDY

Nurses must often manage patient care circumstances that require a complex balance between respecting individual autonomy, maintaining a high standard of care, and providing excellent customer service that is the basis for marketing. Consider these two short scenarios as a way of exploring such concerns.

A. An indigenous patient is nearing the end of his life. As you discuss palliative care with the patient, who is now unable to leave his hospital bed, he makes a request. Because he subscribes to a deeply held set of religious beliefs, the patient asks that you facilitate adherence to end-of-life rituals involving ceremonies performed around an open fire.
   1. What are the priorities and guidelines that would inform your response to this request?

   2. What elements of this request would you be able to honor and in what way?
B. An elderly adult is admitted to the hospital with a list of complications. While waiting for test results, members of the family pull you aside and, citing the patient's age, request that you "do not tell Grandma" if something life-threatening is discovered. The test results reveal that the patient has late-stage cancer.
   1. What are the priorities and guidelines that would inform your response to this request?
   2. What practical steps would you take to honor both the patient and her family?

CRITICAL THINKING EXERCISE

A. Simon Sinek (2009), author of the national bestseller *Start With Why*, argues that good marketing and good leadership begin with purpose, not product.

Sinek explains this concept using what he refers to as the Golden Circle (Fig. 27.1). The circle describes the relationship between purpose and product.

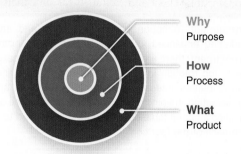

FIG. 27.1 The Golden Circle. (Based on Sinek, S. [2009]. *Start with why: How great leaders inspire everyone to take action.* New York, NY: Penguin Group.)

Successful brands and people, Sinek explains, are created and communicated from the inside of the circle out—they sell their purpose by way of their product. Sinek famously said "Good marketing offers us a view of the world. Bad marketing offers us a product to buy. . . . People don't buy *what* you do; they buy *why* you do it" (Briginshaw, 2013).

The Mayo Clinic is a primary example of a health care organization that follows these principles. Mayo's "why" has remained the same for more than a century, and the organization's ability to consistently communicate its purpose has resulted in the highest brand preference among academic medical centers. This is almost three times more than the second-leading center (Berry & Seltman, 2014). In terms of Sinek's model, the Mayo Clinic's Golden Circle might look something like Fig. 27.2.

"The needs of the patient come first" is a powerful articulation of the Mayo Clinic's purpose. This purpose informs the clinic's "how," known as the Mayo Clinic Model

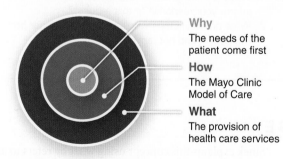

FIG. 27.2 The Golden Circle: Mayo Clinic.

of Care, which includes ideas like "an unhurried examination," "teamwork with multispecialty integration," and "professional compensation that allows a focus on quality, not quantity" (Berry & Seltman, 2014, p. 145). The "what"—the health care services that Mayo delivers—simply proves the organization's commitment to its purpose.

Interestingly, researchers have discovered a strong connection between purpose, the "why," of an individual and his or her personal health. In a study presented at the 2015 American Heart Association EPI/Lifestyle Sessions, researchers led by a team from Mount Sinai found that a sense of meaning results in better heart health and lower adverse effects from stress (Depra, 2015). Understanding and being able to articulate the "why" can help a person live longer. Perhaps one could say, then, that good marketing is good for your health.

1. What is your personal "why," "how," and "what"? Fill in a version of the Golden Circle for yourself.
2. What is the relationship between your own "why" and the "why" of the organization for which you work?
3. As a nurse manager, how can you screen for the "why" in your recruitment process?
4. How can you help those who report to you articulate and value the "why" in their work?

B. In their book *Marketing Management*, Kotler and Keller (2016, p. 558) suggested that "marketing communications allow companies to link their brands to other people, places, events, experiences, feelings, and things." Often such communications are understood in terms of advertisements or social media campaigns designed to promote a company's brand. In health care, however, the most important link between brands and experiences or feelings depends largely on communication between one patient and one nurse.

The Hospital Consumer Assessment of Healthcare Providers and Systems (HCAHPS) is one measure of such links. HCAHPS has become a national standard for collecting information on patient satisfaction. These standards are used by Medicare to determine a Total Performance Score (TPS) for each hospital, and this score determines payments for services rendered (referred to as value-based purchasing). Twenty-five percent of a hospital's TPS is determined by standards related to the patient experience of care, which are overwhelmingly tied to communication. Of these standards, a recent study published in the journal *Nursing Management* found that "the nurse communication section of the HCAHPS has the highest impact on patients' overall hospital satisfaction and likeliness to recommend the hospital to others" (Long, 2012, p. 37). The nurse's ability to explain clearly and listen carefully is the most important link between a hospital's brand and other people, experiences, and feelings. Good communication is both good care and good business.

Some hospitals have found that clear, honest communication can even create valuable connections when care has been delivered in error. An article in the *Wall Street Journal* had the following headline: "Hospitals Learn to Say 'I'm Sorry' to Patients." The article described how Stanford Hospital has developed a program to admit responsibility to patients when medical errors occur by listening attentively to patients' concerns, offering compensation, and engaging the patient in measures to ensure that the error is not repeated. It is an almost counterintuitive idea that clear communication about the *failure* of a company's service would be the hallmark of good marketing. However, over the 5 years since this program has been implemented, "the frequency of lawsuits was 50% lower, and indemnity costs in paid cases were 40% lower" than the previous 5-year period (Landro, 2016, p. D3). Empathetic communication can, retroactively, create positive links between a brand and an experience. As Mother Teresa said, "Kind words can be short and easy to speak, but their echoes are truly endless."

1. HCAHPS scores for physician communication are consistently lower than those for nurses. A recent study in the *Journal of Nursing Care Quality* indicated "An overwhelming number of patients are shown to accept the instructions of their physicians without question, despite having concerns about these instructions" (Kennedy et al., 2013, p. 333). How can you purposefully create communication links between your patients and other members of the care team, including physicians?

2. In a study titled "Compassion Practices and HCAHPS," the authors noted that "The extent to which a hospital rewards compassionate acts and compassionately supports its employees is significantly and positively associated with hospital ratings and the likelihood of recommending" (McClelland & Vogus, 2014, p. 1670). What might be the implications of this finding for you, as a nurse manager, in creating value for your floor or hospital's brand?

3. How can you most effectively communicate the value of nursing to senior management at your organization?

Chapter 1

Adams, K. L., & Iseler, J. I. (2014). The relationship of bedside nurses' emotional intelligence with quality of care. *Journal of Nursing Care Quality*, *29*(2), 174–181.

American Nurses Association (ANA). (2014). *Fast facts: The nursing workforce 2014: Growth, salaries, education, demographics & trends.* Retrieved from http://www.nursingworld.org/MainMenuCategories/ThePracticeof ProfessionalNursing/workforce/Fast-Facts-2014-Nursing-Workforce.pdf.

American Nurses Credentialing Center (ANCC). (2016a). *Magnet Recognition Program® Overview.* Retrieved from http://www.nursecredentialing.org/ Magnet/ProgramOverview.

American Nurses Credentialing Center (ANCC). (2016b). *Magnet model.* Retrieved from http://www.nursecredentialing.org/Magnet/Program Overview/New-Magnet-Model.

American Organization of Nurse Executives. (2015). *Nurse executive competencies.* Chicago, IL: Author. Retrieved from http://www.aone.org/resources/ nurse-executive-competencies.pdf.

Avolio, B. J., & Gardner, W. L. (2005). Authentic leadership development: Getting to the root of positive forms of leadership. *The Leadership Quarterly*, *16*(3), 315–338.

Bahrampour, T. (2013). *Huge shortage of caregivers looms for baby boomers, report says.* Retrieved from https://www.washingtonpost.com/national/ health-science/huge-shortage-of-caregivers-looms-for-baby-boomers- report-says/2013/08/25/665fb2aa-0ab1-11e3-b87c-476db8ac34cd_story .html.

Barker, A. M., & Young, C. E. (1994). Transformational leadership: The feminist connection in postmodern organizations. *Holistic Nursing Practice*, *9*(1), 16–25.

Bass, B., & Avolio, B. (1990). *Transformational leadership development: Manual for the Multifactor Leadership Questionnaire.* Palo Alto, CA: Consulting Psychologists Press.

Bass, B., & Riggio, R. (2006). *Transformational leadership* (2nd ed.). New York, NY: Doubleday.

Bennis, W. G. (1994). *On becoming a leader.* Reading, MA: Addison-Wesley.

Bennis, W. G. (2004). The seven ages of the leader. *Harvard Business Review*, *82*(1), 46–53.

Bennis, W. G., & Nanus, B. (1985). *Leaders: The strategies for taking charge.* New York, NY: Harper & Row.

Bennis, W. G., & Thomas, R. J. (2002). Crucibles of leadership. *Harvard Business Review*, *80*(9), 39–45.

Berry, B. (n.d.). *There is a relationship between systems thinking and W. Edwards Deming's theory of profound knowledge.* The Berrywood Group. Retrieved from http://www.berrywood.com/wp-content/uploads/2011/08/ demingpaper.pdf.

Buck, S., & Doucette, J. N. (2015). Transformational leadership practices of CNOs. *Nursing Management*, *46*(9), 42–48.

Bureau of Health Professions (BHPr), National Center for Health Workforce Analysis. (2014). *Future of the nursing workforce: National- and state-level projections, 2012–2025.* Rockville, MD: Health Resources and Services Ad- ministration (HRSA). Retrieved from http://bhpr.hrsa.gov/healthworkforce/ supplydemand/nursing/workforceprojections/index.html.

Burns, J. (1978). *Leadership.* New York, NY: Harper & Row.

BusinessDictionary.com. (2016a). *Planning.* Retrieved from http://www. businessdictionary.com/definition/planning.html.

BusinessDictionary.com. (2016b). *Organizing.* Retrieved from http://www. businessdictionary.com/definition/organizing.html.

BusinessDictionary.com. (2016c). *Directing.* Retrieved from http://www. businessdictionary.com/definition/directing.html.

BusinessDictionary.com. (2016d). *Controlling.* Retrieved from http://www. businessdictionary.com/definition/controlling.html.

Campbell, G. (2016). Growing and developing our future nurse leaders. *Voice of Nursing Leadership*, *14*(4), 4–6.

Castle, N. G., & Decker, F. H. (2011). Top management leadership style and quality of care in nursing homes. *The Gerontologist*, *51*(5), 630–642.

Chaleff, I. (2003). *The courageous follower: Standing up to and for our leaders* (2nd ed.). San Francisco, CA: Berrett-Koehler.

Chandler, J., Rycroft-Malone, J., Hawkes, C., & Noyes, J. (2015). Application of simplified complexity theory concepts for healthcare social systems to explain the implementation of evidence into practice. *Journal of Advanced Nursing*, *72*(2), 461–480.

Clay-Williams, R., Nosrati, H., Cunningham, F. C., Hillman, K., & Braithwaite, J. (2014). Do large-scale hospital- and system-wide interventions improve patient outcomes: A systematic review. *BMC Health Services Research*, *14*, 369. doi:10.1186/1472-6963-14-36.

Curtin, L. (2016). The shape of things to come. *American Nurse Today*, *11*(5), 60.

Deschamps, C., Rinfret, N., Lagace, M. C., & Prive, C. (2016). Transformational leadership and change: How leaders influence their followers' motivation through organizational justice. *Journal of Healthcare Management*, *61*(3), 194–222.

Downey, M., Parslow, S., & Smart, M. (2011). The hidden treasure in nursing leadership: Informal leaders. *Journal of Nursing Management*, *19*(4), 517–521.

Drucker, P. F. (2004). What makes an effective executive. *Harvard Business Review*, *82*(6), 58–63.

Dunham, J., & Klafehn, K. (1990). Transformational leadership and the nurse executive. *Journal of Nursing Administration*, *20*(4), 28–34.

Fayol, H. (1949). *General and industrial management.* London, UK: Pitman & Sons.

Fiedler, F., & Garcia, J. (1987). *New approaches to effective leadership: Cognitive resources and organizational performance.* New York, NY: John Wiley & Sons.

Foust, J. (1994). Creating a future for nursing through interactive planning at the bedside. *Image*, *26*(2), 129–131.

Gittell, J. H. (2009). *High performance healthcare: Using the power of relationships to achieve quality, efficiency and resilience.* New York, NY: McGraw-Hill.

Givens, R. J. (2008). Transformational leadership: The impact on organiza- tional and personal outcomes. *Emerging Leadership Journeys*, *1*(1), 4–24.

Goleman, D. (2007). *Social intelligence: The new science of social relationships.* New York, NY: Bantam Dell Publishing Group.

Görgens-Ekermans, G., & Brand, T. (2010). Emotional intelligence as a moderator of the stress-burnout relationship: A questionnaire study on nurses. *Journal of Clinical Nursing*, *21*(15–16), 2275–2285.

Gosling, J., & Mintzberg, H. (2003). The five minds of a manager. *Harvard Business Review*, *81*(11), 54–63.

Greenleaf, R. K. (2002). *Servant leadership: A journey into the nature of legitimate power and greatness* (25th anniversary ed.). Mahwah, NJ: Paulist Press.

Grossman, S. C., & Valiga, T. M. (2013). *The new leadership challenge: Creating the future of nursing* (4th ed.). Philadelphia, PA: F.A. Davis Company.

Haigh, C. A. (2008). Using simplified chaos theory to manage nursing services. *Journal of Nursing Management*, *16*, 298–304.

Hanse, J. J., Harlin, U., Jarebrant, C., Ulin, K., & Winkel, J. (2016). The impact of servant leadership dimensions on leader-member exchange among health care professionals. *Journal of Nursing Management*, *24*, 228–234.

Helgeson, S. (1995a). *The web of inclusion: A new architecture for building organizations*. New York, NY: Doubleday.

Helgeson, S. (1995b). *The female advantage: Women's ways of leadership* (2nd ed.). New York, NY: Doubleday.

Hersey, P. (2009). *The Situational Leader*. Escondido, CA: The Center for Leadership Studies.

Hersey, P. H., Blanchard, K. H., & Johnson, D. E. (2013). *Management of organizational behavior: Leading human resources* (10th ed.). Upper Saddle River, NJ: Pearson Education.

Huber, D. L., Maas, M., McCloskey, J., Scherb, C. A., Goode, C. J., & Watson, C. (2000). Evaluating nursing administration instruments. *Journal of Nursing Administration, 30*(5), 251–272.

Institute for Healthcare Improvement. (2016). *Triple aim for populations*. Retrieved from http://www.ihi.org/Topics/TripleAim/Pages/default.aspx.

Institute of Medicine (IOM). (2001). *Crossing the quality chasm: A new health system for the 21st Century*. Washington, DC: National Academies Press.

Institute of Medicine (IOM). (2004). *Keeping patients safe: Transforming the work environment of nurses*. Washington, DC: National Academies Press.

Institute of Medicine (IOM). (2011). *The future of nursing: Leading change, advancing health*. Washington, DC: National Academies Press.

Jennings, B. M., Scalzi, C. C., Rodgers, J. D., III, & Keane, A. (2007). Differentiating nursing leadership and management competencies. *Nursing Outlook, 55*, 169–175.

Joseph, M. L. (2015). Organizational culture and climate for promoting innovativeness. *Journal of Nursing Administration, 45*(3), 172–178.

Joseph, M. L., & Huber, D. L. (2015). Clinical leadership development and education for nurses: Prospects and opportunities. *Journal of Healthcare Leadership, 2015*(7), 55–64.

Joseph, M. L., Rhodes, A., & Watson, C. A. (2016). Preparing nurse leaders to innovate: Iowa's innovation seminar. *Journal of Nursing Education, 55*(2), 113–117.

Kanter, R. M. (1989). The new managerial work. *Harvard Business Review, 69*(6), 85–92.

Kellerman, B. (2008). *Followership: How followers are creating change and changing leaders*. Boston, MA: Harvard Business Press.

Kelley, R. E. (1992). *The power of followership: How to create leaders people want to follow and followers who lead themselves*. New York, NY: Doubleday.

Kleinman, C. (2004). The relationship between managerial leadership behaviors and staff nurse retention. *Hospital Topics, 82*(4), 2–9.

Knickman, J. R., & Snell, E. K. (2002). The 2030 problem: Caring for aging baby boomers. *Health Services Research, 37*(4), 849–884.

Koloroutis, M. (Ed.). (2004). *Relationship-based care: A model for transforming practice*. Minneapolis, MN: Creative Health Care Management.

Kotter, J. (2001). What leaders really do. *Harvard Business Review, 79*(11), 85–96.

Kouzes, J., & Posner, B. (1995). *The leadership challenge: How to keep getting extraordinary things done in organizations*. San Francisco, CA: Jossey-Bass.

Kouzes, J. M., & Posner, B. Z. (2012). *The leadership challenge: How to make extraordinary things happen in organizations* (5th ed.). San Francisco, CA: The Leadership Challenge/Wiley.

Lorenz, E. N. (1993). *The essence of chaos*. Seattle, WA: University of Washington Press.

Mackoff, B. L., Glassman, K., & Budin, W. (2013). Developing a leadership laboratory for nurse managers based on lived experiences: A participatory action research model for leadership development. *Journal of Nursing Administration, 43*(9), 447–454.

Malloch, K. (2002). Trusting organizations: Describing and measuring employee-to-employee relationships. *Nursing Administration Quarterly, 26*(3), 12–19.

Mannix, J., Wilkes, L., & Daly, J. (2013). Attributes of clinical leadership in contemporary nursing: An integrative review. *Contemporary Nurse, 45*(1), 10–21.

McCauley, G. (2005). *Leadership in a quantum age*. Ottawa, Ontario, Canada: WEL-Systems Institute. Retrieved from http://www.wel-systems.com/articles/Leadership.htm.

McClure, M. (1991). Introduction. In I. Goertzen (Ed.), *Differentiating nursing practice: Into the twenty-first century* (pp. 1–11). Kansas City, MO: American Academy of Nursing.

Mintzberg, H. (1973). *The nature of managerial work*. New York, NY: Harper & Row.

Mintzberg, H. (1975). The manager's job: Folklore and fact. In M. Matteson & J. Ivancevich (Eds.), *Management classics* (3rd ed., pp. 63–85). Plano, TX: Business Publications.

Mintzberg, H. (1994). Managing as blended care. *Journal of Nursing Administration, 24*(9), 29–36.

Mintzberg, H. (1998). Covert leadership: Notes on managing professionals. *Harvard Business Review, 76*(6), 140–147.

Mortier, A. V., Vlerick, P., & Clays, E. (2016). Authentic leadership and thriving among nurses: The mediating role of empathy. *Journal of Nursing Management, 24*, 357–365.

O'Neil, E., Morjikian, R. L., Cherner, D., Hirschkorn, C., & West, T. (2008). Developing nursing leaders: An overview of trends and programs. *Journal of Nursing Administration, 38*(4), 178–183.

Patrick, A., Laschinger, H. K. S., Wong, C., & Finegan, J. (2011). Developing and testing a new measure of staff nurse clinical leadership: The clinical leadership survey. *Journal of Nursing Management, 19*, 499–460.

Peake, S., & McDowall, A. (2012). Chaotic careers: A narrative analysis of career transition themes and outcomes using chaos theory as a guiding metaphor. *British Journal of Guidance & Counseling, 40*(4), 395–410.

Pediani, R. (1996). Chaos and evolution in nursing research. *Journal of Advanced Nursing, 23*(4), 645–646.

Pipe, T. B. (2008). Illuminating the inner leadership journey by engaging intention and mindfulness as guided by caring theory. *Nursing Administration Quarterly, 32*(2), 117–125.

Quoidbach, J., & Hansenne, M. (2009). The impact of trait emotional intelligence on nursing team performance and cohesiveness. *Journal of Professional Nursing, 25*(1), 23–29.

Read, E. A., & Laschinger, H. K. S. (2015). The influence of authentic leadership and empowerment on nurses' relational social capital, mental health and job satisfaction over the first year of practice. *Journal of Advanced Nursing, 71*(7), 1611–1623.

Reynolds, K. (2011). Servant-leadership as gender-integrative leadership: Paving a path for more gender-integrative organizations through leadership education. *Journal of Leadership Education, 10*(2), 155–171.

Rosenhead, J. (1998). *Complexity theory and management practice*. Operational Research working papers, LSEOR 98.25. London, UK: Department of Operational Research, London School of Economics and Political Science.

Shirey, M. R. (2006). Building authentic leadership and enhancing entrepreneurial performance. *Clinical Nurse Specialist, 20*(6), 280–282.

Spano-Szekely, L., Quinn Griffin, M. T., Clavelle, J., & Fitzpatrick, J. J. (2016). Emotional intelligence and transformational leadership in nurse managers. *Journal of Nursing Administration, 46*(2), 101–108.

Steaban, R. L. (2016). Health care reform, care coordination, and transformational leadership. *Nursing Administration Quarterly, 40*(2), 153–163.

Stetler, C. B., Ritchie, J. A., Rycroft-Malone, J., & Charns, M. P. (2014). Leadership for evidence-based practice: Strategic and functional behaviors for institutionalizing EBP. *Worldviews on Evidence-Based Nursing, 11*(4), 219–226. doi:10.1111/wvn.12044.

Tannenbaum, R., & Schmidt, W. H. (1973). How to choose a leadership pattern. *Harvard Business Review, 51*(3), 162–180.

Thomson, N. B., Rawson, J. V., Slade, C. P., & Bledsoe, M. (2016). Transformation and transformational leadership: A review of the current and relevant literature for academic radiologists. *Academic Radiology, 23*(5), 592–599.

Upenieks, V. (2003a). Nurse leaders' perceptions of what compromises successful leadership in today's acute inpatient environment. *Nursing Administration Quarterly, 27*(2), 140–152.

Upenieks, V. (2003b). What constitutes effective leadership? *Journal of Nursing Administration, 33*(9), 456–467.

US Census Bureau. (2014). *The baby boom cohort in the United States: 2012 to 2060: Population estimates and projections*. Retrieved from https://www.census.gov/prod/2014pubs/p25-1141.pdf.

W. Edwards Deming Institute. (2016). *The system of profound knowledge*. Retrieved from https://deming.org/theman/theories/profoundknowledge.

Weberg, D. (2010). Transformational leadership and staff retention: An evidence review with implications for healthcare systems. *Nursing Administration Quarterly, 34*(3), 246–258.

Weberg, D. (2012). Complexity leadership: A healthcare imperative. *Nursing Forum, 47*(4), 268–277.

Wheatley, M. J. (2006). *Leadership and the new science: Discovering order in a chaotic world* (3rd ed.). San Francisco, CA: Berrett-Koehler.

Wong, C. A., & Laschinger, H. K. S. (2013). Authentic leadership, performance, and job satisfaction: The mediating role of empowerment. *Journal of Advanced Nursing, 69*(4), 947–959.

Chapter 2

Agency for Healthcare Research and Quality (AHRQ). (n.d.). *AHRQ health care innovations exchange*. Retrieved from https://innovations.ahrq.gov/.

American Organization of Nurse Executives (AONE). (2015). AONE nurse executive competencies. *Nurse Leader, 3*(1), 15–21.

Anderson, L. A., & Anderson, D. (2009). *Awake at the wheel: Moving beyond change management to conscious change leadership*. Retrieved from http://www.beingfirst.com/.

Appelbaum, S. H., Habashy, S., Malo, J., & Shafiq, H. (2012). Back to the future: revisiting Kotter's 1996 change model. *Journal of Management Development, 31*(8), 764–782. http://dx.doi.org/10.1108/02621711211253231.

Axelrod, R. H., Axelrod, E., Jacobs, R. W., & Beedon, J. (2006). Beat the odds and succeed in organizational change. *Consulting Management-C2M, 17*(2), 6–9.

Balfour, M., & Clarke, C. (2001). Searching for sustainable change. *Journal of Clinical Nursing, 10*, 44–50.

Balogun, J. (2006). Managing change: Steering a course between intended strategies and unanticipated outcomes. *Long Range Planning, 39*, 29–49.

Bartunek, J. M., Rousseau, D. M., Rudolph, J., & DePalma, J. A. (2006). On the receiving end: Sensemaking, emotion, and assessments of an organizational change initiated by others. *Journal of Applied Behavioral Science, 42*, 182–206.

Bennis, W. G., Benne, K. D., & Chin, R. (Eds.). (1961). *The planning of change: Readings in the applied behavioral sciences*. New York, NY: Holt, Rinehart & Winston.

Burns, J. (1978). *Leadership*. New York, NY: Harper & Row.

Burnes, B. (2004). Kurt Lewin and complexity theories: Back to the future? *Journal of Change Management, 4*(4), 309–325.

Cambridge Dictionary. (2016). *Cambridge dictionary*. Retrieved from http://dictionary.cambridge.org/us/.

Center for Creative Leadership (CCL). (2014). *Innovation leadership: How to use innovation to lead effectively, work collaboratively, and drive results*. Greensboro, NC: Author.

Centers for Medicare & Medicaid Services (CMS). (n.d.). *CMS Innovation Center*. Retrieved from https://innovation.cms.gov/.

Christensen, C. M., Bohmer, R., & Kenagy, J. (2000). Will disruptive innovations cure health care? *Harvard Business Review, 78*(5), 102–112.

Clarke, C. S. (2013). Resistance to change in the nursing profession: Creative transdisciplinary solutions. *Creative Nursing, 19*, 70–76. http://dx.doi.org/10.1891/1078-4535.19.2.70.

Copnell, B., & Bruni, N. (2006). Breaking the silence: Nurses' understandings of change in clinical practice. *Journal of Advanced Nursing, 55*(3), 301–309. http://dx.doi.org/10.1111/j.1365-2648.2006.03911.x.

Cullen, L. (2015). Evidence into practice: Awakening the innovator in every nurse. *Journal of PeriAnesthesia Nursing, 30*, 430–435.

Drucker, P. F. (1992). *Managing for the future: The 1990s and beyond*. New York, NY: Dutton.

Estrada, N. (2009). Exploring perceptions of a learning organization by RNs and relationship to EBP beliefs and implementation in the acute care setting. *Worldviews on Evidence-Based Nursing, 6*(4), 200–209.

Falk-Rafael, A. R. (2000). Nurses' orientations to change: Debunking the "resistant to change" myth. *Journal of Professional Nursing, 16*(6), 336–344.

Hallencreutz, J., & Turner, D. (2011). Exploring organizational change best practice: Are there any clear-cut models and definitions? *International Journal of Quality and Service Sciences, 3*, 60–68. http://dx.doi.org/10.1108/17566691111115081.

Hernandez, S. E., Conrad, D. A., Marcus-Smith, M. S., Reed, P., & Watts, C. (2013). Patient-centered innovation in health care organizations: A conceptual framework and case study application. *Health Care Management Review, 38*(2), 166–175. doi:10.1097/HMR.0b013e31825e718a.

Hersey, P., Blanchard, K. H., & Johnson, D. E. (2013). *Management of organizational behavior: Leading human resources* (10th ed.). Upper Saddle River, NJ: Pearson Education.

Hughes, F. (2006). Nurses at the forefront of innovation. *International Nursing Review, 53*, 94–101.

Institute of Medicine (IOM). (2011). *The future of nursing: Leading change, advancing health*. Washington, DC: National Academies Press.

Issel, L. M., & Anderson, R. A. (1996). Take charge: Managing six transformations in healthcare delivery. *Nursing Economic$, 14*(2), 78–85.

Jansson, N. (2013). Organizational change as practice: A critical analysis. *Journal of Organizational Change Management, 26*, 1003–1019. http://dx.doi.org/10.1108/JOCM-09-2012-0152.

Joseph, M. L. (2015). Organizational culture and climate for promoting innovativeness. *Journal of Nursing Administration, 45*, 172–178. doi:10.1097/NNA.0000000000000178.

Kapoor, K. K., Dwivedi, Y. K., & Williams, M. D. (2014). Rogers' innovation adoption attributes: A systematic review and synthesis of existing research. *Information Systems Management, 31*, 74–91. doi:10.1080/10580530.2014.854103.

Kerfoot, K. (1998). Leading change is leading creativity. *Nursing Economic$, 16*(2), 98–99.

Kotter, J. P. (2012). *Leading change*. Boston, MA: Harvard Business Review Press.

Leeman, J., Baernholdt, M., & Sandelowski, M. (2007). Developing a theory-based taxonomy of methods for implementing change in practice. *Journal of Advanced Nursing, 58*(2), 191–200. http://dx.doi.org/10.1111/j.1365-2648.2006.04207.x.

Lewin, K. (1947). Frontiers in group dynamics: Concept, method, and reality in social science; social equilibrium and social change. *Human Relations, 1*(1), 5–41.

Lewin, K. (1951). *Field theory in social science: Selected theoretical papers*. New York, NY: Harper & Row.

Lippitt, G. (1973). *Visualizing change: Model building and the change process*. La Jolla, CA: University Associates.

Longenecker, C. O., & Longenecker, P. D. (2014). Why hospital improvement efforts fail: A view from the front line. *Journal of Healthcare Management, 59*, 147–157.

Mills, J. H., Dye, K., & Mills, A. J. (2009). *Understanding organizational change*. New York, NY: Routledge.

Packard, T., & Shih, A. (2014). Organizational change tactics: The evidence base in the literature. *Journal of Evidence-Based Social Work, 11*, 498–510. http://dx.doi.org/10.1080/15433714.2013.831006.

Porter-O'Grady, T., & Malloch, K. (2015). *Quantum leadership: Building better partnerships for sustainable health* (4th ed.). Sudbury, MA: Jones and Bartlett.

Prochaska, J. O., & DiClemente, C. C. (1983). Stages and processes of self-change of smoking: Toward an integrative model of change. *Journal of Consulting and Clinical Psychology, 51*(3), 390–395.

Robbins, B., & Davidhizar, R. (2007). Transformational leadership in health-care today. *The Health Care Manager, 26*, 234–239.

Robert Wood Johnson Foundation (RWJF). (2015). *The transforming care at the bedside (TCAB) toolkit.* Princeton, NJ: Robert Wood Johnson Foundation. Retrieved from http://www.rwjf.org/en/library/research/2008/06/the-transforming-care-at-the-bedside-tcab-toolkit.html.

Rogers, E. M. (2003). *Diffusion of innovations* (5th ed.). New York, NY: Free Press.

Romano, C. (1990). Diffusion of technology innovation. *Advances in Nursing Science, 13*(2), 11–21.

Rost, J. C. (1994). Leadership: A new conception. *Holistic Nursing Practice, 9*(2), 1–8.

Senge, P., Kleiner, A., Roberts, C., Ross, R., & Smith, B. (1994). *The fifth discipline fieldbook.* New York, NY: Doubleday.

Shanley, C. (2007). Management of change for nurses: Lessons from the discipline of organizational studies. *Journal of Nursing Management, 15,* 538–546.

Thomas, R., & Hardy, C. (2011). Reframing resistance to organizational change. *Scandinavian Journal of Management, 27,* 322–331.

Tonges, M., Ray, J. D., Overman, A. S., & Willis, B. (2015). Creating a culture of rapid change adoption: Implementing an innovations unit. *Journal of Nursing Administration, 45*(7/8), 384–390.

Valente, S. (2011). Rapid cycle change projects improve quality of care. *Journal of Nursing Care Quality, 26*(1), 54–60.

Van Woerkum, C., Aarts, N., & Van Herzele, A. (2011). Changed planning for planned and unplanned change. *Planning Theory, 10,* 144–161. http://dx.doi.org/10.1177/1473095210389651.

Vestal, K. (2013). Change fatigue: A constant leadership challenge. *Nurse Leader, 11*(5), 10–11. http://dx.doi.org/10.1016/j.mnl.2013.07.005.

Weimer, B. J., Amick, H., & Lee, S. D. (2008). Conceptualization and measurement of organizational readiness for change: A review of the literature in health services research and other fields. *Medical Care Research and Review, 65*(4), 379–436.

Wheatley, M. J. (2007). *Finding our way: Leadership for an uncertain time.* San Francisco, CA: Berrett-Koehler.

Workman, R., & Kenney, M. (1988). The change experience. In S. Pinkerton & P. Schroeder (Eds.), *Commitment to excellence: Developing a professional nursing staff* (pp. 17–25). Rockville, MD: Aspen.

Chapter 3

Afendulis, C. C., Caudry, D. J., O'Malley, A. J., Kemper, P., & Grabowski, D. C. for the THRIVE Research Collaborative. (2016). Green house adoption and nursing home quality. *Health Services Research, 51*(1 Pt 2), 454–474.

Aiken, L. H., Lake, E. T., Sochalski, J., & Sloane, D. M. (1997). Design of an outcomes study of the organization of hospital AIDS care. *Research in the Sociology of Health Care, 14,* 3–26.

Aiken, L. H., Smith, H. L., & Lake, E. T. (1994). Lower Medicare mortality among a set of hospitals known for good nursing care. *Medical Care, 32,* 771–785.

Al-Hamdan, Z., Nussera, H., & Masa'deh, R. (2015). Conflict management style of Jordanian nurse managers and its relationship to staff nurses' intent to stay. *Journal of Nursing Management, 24*(2), E137–E145.

American Nurses Association. (2010). *Position statement: Just culture.* Retrieved from http://nursingworld.org/psjustculture.

American Nurses Association. (2016). *Healthy work environment.* Retrieved from http://nursingworld.org/MainMenuCategories/WorkplaceSafety/Healthy-Work-Environment.

American Nurses Credentialing Center (ANCC). (2016). *ANCC Magnet Recognition Program®.* Retrieved from http://www.nursecredentialing.org/Magnet.

Barnes, H., Rearden, J., & McHugh, M. D. (2016). Magnet® hospital recognition linked to lower central line-associated bloodstream infection rates. *Research in Nursing & Health, 39*(2), 96–104.

Bellot, J. (2011). Defining and assessing organizational culture. *Nursing Forum, 46*(1), 29–37.

Bellot, J. (2012). Nursing home culture change: What does it mean to nurses? *Research in Gerontological Nursing, 5*(4), 264–273.

Blegen, M. A., Pepper, G. A., & Rosse, J. (2005). *Safety climate on hospital units: A new measure.* Retrieved from http://www.ncbi.nlm.nih.gov/books/NBK20592/.

Carthon, J. M. B., Lasater, K. B., Sloane, D. M., & Kutney-Lee, A. (2015). The quality of hospital work environments and missed nursing care is linked to heart failure readmissions: A cross-sectional study of US hospitals. *BMJ Quality & Safety, 24*(4), 255–263.

D'ambra, A. M., & Andrews, D. R. (2014). Incivility, retention and new graduate nurses: An integrated review of the literature. *Journal of Nursing Management, 22*(6), 735–742.

DeJoy, D. M., Schaffer, B. S., Wilson, M. G., Vandenbert, R. J., & Butts, M. M. (2004). Creating safer workplaces: Assessing the determinants and role of safety climate. *Journal of Safety Research, 35,* 81–90.

Feather, R. A., Ebright, P., & Bakas, T. (2015). Nurse manager behaviors that RNs perceive to affect their job satisfaction. *Nursing Forum, 50*(2), 125–136.

Gershon, R. R. M., Stone, P. W., Baaken, S., & Larson, E. (2004). Measurement of organizational culture and climate in healthcare. *Journal of Nursing Administration, 34*(1), 33–40.

Grabowski, D. C., Afendulis, C. C., Caudry, D. J., O'Malley, A. J., Kemper, P. for the THRIVE Research Collaborative. (2016). The impact of green house adoption on Medicare spending and utilization. *Health Services Research, 51*(1 Pt 2), 433–453.

Hatch, M. J., & Cunliffe, A. L. (2013). *Organization theory: Modern, symbolic and postmodern perspectives.* New York: Oxford University Press.

Higgins, E. A. (2015). The influence of nurse manager transformational leadership on nurse and patient outcomes: Mediating effects of supportive practice environments, organizational citizenship behaviours, patient safety culture and nurse job satisfaction. *Electronic Thesis and Dissertation Repository.* Paper 3184. Retrieved from http://ir.lib.uwo.ca/cgi/viewcontent.cgi?article=4453&context=etd.

Institute of Medicine (IOM). (2001). *Crossing the quality chasm.* Washington, DC: National Academies Press.

Institute of Medicine (IOM). (2011). *The future of nursing: Leading change, advancing health.* Washington, DC: National Academies Press.

Jackson, G. L., Powers, B. J., Chatterjee, R., Bettger, J. P., Kemper, A. R., Hasselblad, V., et al. (2013). The patient-centered medical home: A systematic review. *Annals of Internal Medicine, 158*(3), 169–178.

Kutney-Lee, A., Stimpfel, A. W., Sloane, D. M., Cimiotti, J. P., Quinn, L. W., & Aiken, L. H. (2015). Changes in patient and nurse outcomes associated with Magnet hospital recognition. *Medical Care, 53*(6), 550–557.

Litwin, G., & Stringer, R. (1968). *Motivation and organizational climate.* Boston, MA: Division of Research, Graduate School of Business Administration, Harvard University.

Ma, C., & Park, S. H. (2015). Hospital Magnet status, unit work environment, and pressure ulcers. *Journal of Nursing Scholarship, 47*(6), 565–573.

Mark, B. A. (1996). Organizational culture. In J. J. Fitzpatrick & J. Norbeck (Eds.), *Annual Review of Nursing Research, 14,* 145–163.

McHugh, M. D., & Ma, C. (2013). Hospital nursing and 30-day readmissions among Medicare patients with heart failure, acute myocardial infarction, and pneumonia. *Medical care, 51*(1), 52.

McHugh, M. D., Rochman, M. F., Sloane, D. M., Berg, R. A., Mancini, M. E., Nadkarni, V. M., et al. (2016). Better nurse staffing and nurse work environments associated with increased survival of in-hospital cardiac arrest patients. *Medical Care, 54*(1), 74–80.

Parry, J. S., Calarco, M. M., & Hensinger, B. (2014). Unit-based interventions: De-stressing the distressed. *Nursing Management, 45*(8), 38–44.

Peters, T., & Waterman, R. H. (1982). *In search of excellence.* New York, NY: Warner Communications.

Quality and Safety Education for Nurses (QSEN). (2014). *QSEN Institute.* Retrieved from http://qsen.org/.

Reason, J. (1997). *Managing the risks of organisational accidents*. London, UK: Ashgate Publishing.

Reeves, S., Perrier, L., Goldman, J., Freeth, D., & Zwarenstein, M. (2013). Interprofessional education: Effects on professional practice and healthcare outcomes (update). *Cochrane Database Syst Rev, 3*(3).

Schein, E. H. (1996). Culture: The missing concept in organization studies. *Administrative Science Quarterly, 41*(2), 229–240.

Sleutel, M. R. (2000). Climate, culture, context, or work environment? Organizational factors that influence nursing practice. *Journal of Nursing Administration, 30*, 53–58.

Snow, J. (2002). Enhancing work climate to improve performance and retain valued employees. *Journal of Nursing Administration, 33*(2), 111–117.

Stokowski, L. A. (2014). The risky business of nursing. *Medscape*, January 14, 2014. Retrieved from http://www.medscape.com/viewarticle/818437.

Stone, P. W., Harrison, M. I., Feldman, P., Linzer, M., Peng, T., Roblin, D., et al. (2005). *Organizational climate of staff working conditions and safety: An integrative model*. Retrieved from http://www.ncbi.nlm.nih.gov/books/NBK20497/.

Tourangeau, A. E., Thomson, H., Cummings, G., & Cranley, L. A. (2013). Generation-specific incentives and disincentives for nurses to remain employed in acute care hospitals. *Journal of Nursing Management, 21*(3), 473–482.

US Department of Health and Human Services: Health Resources and Services Administration. (2010). *The registered nurse population: Findings from the 2008 National Sample Survey of Registered Nurses*. Retrieved from https://bhw.hrsa.gov/sites/default/files/bhw/nchwa/rnsurveyfinal.pdf.

Uttal, B. (1983). The corporate culture vultures. *Fortune Magazine, 108*(8), 66.

Van Bogaert, P., Timmermans, O., Weeks, S. M., van Heusden, D., Wouters, K., & Franck, E. (2014). Nursing unit teams matter: Impact of unit-level nurse practice environment, nurse work characteristics, and burnout on nurse reported job outcomes, and quality of care, and patient adverse events—A cross-sectional survey. *International Journal of Nursing Studies, 51*(8), 1123–1134.

Wooten, L. P., & Crane, P. (2003). Nurses as implementers of organizational culture. *Nursing Economic$, 21*, 275–279.

Zimmerman, S., Bowers, B. J., Cohen, L. W., Grabowski, D. C., Horn, S. D., & Kemper, P. (2016). New evidence on the green house model of nursing home care: Synthesis of findings and implications for policy, practice, and research. *Health Services Research, 51*(Suppl.), 475–496.

Chapter 4

Altman, S. H., Butler, A. S., & Shern, L. (2015). *Assessing progress on the Institute of Medicine report The Future of Nursing*. Retrieved from http://www.nap.edu/catalog/21838/assessing-progress-on-the-institute-of-medicine-report-the-future-of-nursing.

American Nurses Association. (n.d.). *ANA CAUTI prevention tool*. Retrieved from http://nursingworld.org/ANA-CAUTI-Prevention-Tool.

American Nurses Association. (2016). *Nursing administration: Scope and standards of practice* (2nd ed.). Silver Spring, MD: Author.

American Nurses Credentialing Center. (2016). *Magnet model*. Retrieved from http://www.nursecredentialing.org/Magnet/ProgramOverview/New-Magnet-Model.

American Organization of Nurse Executives. (2015). *Nurse executive competencies*. Chicago, IL: Author. Retrieved from http://www.aone.org/resources/nurse-executive-competencies.pdf.

American Society for Quality. (n.d.). *What is Six Sigma?* Retrieved from http://asq.org/learn-about-quality/six-sigma/overview/overview.html.

Baghbanian, A., Hughes, I., Kebriaei, A., & Khavarpour, F. A. (2012). Adaptive decision-making: How Australian healthcare managers decide. *Australian Health Review, 36*, 49–56. doi:http//dx.doi.or/10.1071/AH10971.

Benner, P. (1984). *From novice to expert: Excellence and power in clinical practice*. Menlo Park, CA: Addison-Wesley.

Benner, P., Sutphen, M., Leonard, V., & Day, L. (2010). *Educating nurses: A call for radical transformation*. San Francisco, CA: Jossey-Bass.

Braaten, J. S. (2015). Hospital system barriers to rapid response team activation: A cognitive work analysis. *American Journal of Nursing, 115*(2), 22–32. doi:10.1097/01.NAJ.0000460673.82070.af.

Cappelletti, A., Engel, J. K., & Prentice, D. (2014). Systematic review of clinical judgment and reasoning in nursing. *Journal of Nursing Education, 53*(4), 453–458. doi:10.3928/01484834-20104724-01.

Centers for Medicare and Medicaid Services (CMS). (2015). *Accountable care organizations (ACO)*. Retrieved from https://www.cms.gov/Medicare/Medicare-Fee-for-Service-Payment/ACO/index.html?redirect=/ACO/.

Centers for Medicare and Medicaid Services (CMS). (2016). *Payment adjustments and hardship information*. Retrieved from https://www.cms.gov/Regulations-and-Guidance/Legislation/EHRIncentivePrograms/PaymentAdj_Hardship.html.

Craig, K. (2010). Patient acuity. In D. L. Huber (Ed.), *Leadership and nursing care management* (4th ed., pp. 503–521). Maryland Heights, MO: Elsevier.

Dickson, G. L., & Flynn, L. (2012). Nurses' clinical reasoning: Processes and practices of medication safety. *Qualitative Health Research, 22*, 3–16. doi:10.1177/10499732311440448.

Doughtery, L., Sque, M., & Crouch, R. (2012). Decision-making processes used by nurses during intravenous drug preparation and administration. *Journal of Advanced Nursing, 68*(6), 1302–1311.

Dunham-Taylor, J., & Pinczuk, J. Z. (2015). *Financial management for nurse managers: Merging the heart with the dollar* (3rd ed.). Burlington, MA: Jones & Bartlett.

Effken, J. A., Brewer, B. B., Logue, M. D. Gephart, S. M., & Verran, J. (2011). Using cognitive work analysis to fit decision support tools to nurse managers' work flow. *International Journal of Medical Informatics, 80*, 698–707. doi:10.1016/j.ijmedinf.2011.07.003.

Ek, B., & Svedlund, M. (2015). Registered nurses' experiences of their decision-making at an Emergency Medical Dispatch Centre. *Journal of Clinical Nursing, 24*(7/8), 1122–1131. doi:10.1111/jocn.12701.

Endacott, R., Scholes, J., Cooper, S., McConnell-Henry, T., Porter, J., Missen, K., et al. (2012). Identifying patient deterioration: Using simulation and reflective interviewing to examine decision making skills in a rural hospital. *International Journal of Nursing Studies, 49*, 710–717. doi:10.1016/j.ijnurstu.2011.11.018.

Frith, K. H., & Anderson, E. F. (2012). Improve care delivery with integrated decision support. *Nursing Management, 43*, 52–54.

Ganz, F. D., Wagner, N., & Toren, O. (2015). Nurse middle manager ethical dilemmas and moral distress. *Nursing Ethics, 22*, 43–51. doi:10.1177/0969733013515490.

Gifford, W., Lefebre, N., & Davies, B. (2014). An organizational intervention to influence evidence-informed decision making in home health nursing. *Journal of Nursing Administration, 44*, 395–402. doi:10.1097/NNA.0000000000000089.

Goudreau, J., Pepin, J., Larue, C., Dubois, S., Descôteaux, R., Lavoie, P., et al. (2015). A competency-based approach to nurses' continuing education for clinical reasoning and leadership through reflective practice in a care situation. *Nurse Education in Practice, 15*(6), 572–578. doi:http://dx.doi.org/1016/j.npr.2015.10.013.

Graham-Dickerson, P., Houser, J., Thomas, E., & Casper, C. (2013). The value of staff nurse involvement in decision making. *Journal of Nursing Administration, 43*, 286–292. doi:10.1097/NNA.0b013e31828eec15.

Guo, K. L. (2008). DECIDE: A decision-making model for more effective decision making by healthcare managers. *The Health Care Manager, 27*, 118–127.

Haenke, R., & Stichler, J. F. (2015). Applying Lean Six Sigma for innovative change to the post-anesthesia care unit. *Journal of Nursing Administration, 45*, 185–187. doi:10.1097/NNA.0000000000000181.

Hart, M. A. (2012). Accountable care organizations: The future of care delivery? *American Journal of Nursing, 112*(2), 23–26.

Institute of Medicine (IOM). (1999). *To err is human: Building a safer health system*. Washington, DC: National Academies Press.

Institute of Medicine (IOM). (2011). *The future of nursing: Leading change, advancing health*. Washington, DC: National Academies Press.

Interprofessional Education Collaborative. (2011). *Core competencies for interprofessional collaborative practice*. Retrieved from https://ipecollaborative.org/uploads/IPEC-Core-Competencies.pdf.

Jansson, I., & Forsberg, A. (2016). How do nurses and ward managers perceive that evidence-based sources are obtained to inform relevant nursing interventions?: An exploratory study. *Journal of Clinical Nursing, 25*, 769–776. doi:10.1111/jocn.13095.

Johansen, M. L., & O'Brien, J. L. (2015). Decision making in nursing practice: A concept analysis. *Nursing Forum, 51*, 40–48. doi:10.1111/nuf.12119.

Jones, T. L. (2015). A descriptive analysis of implicit rationing of nursing care: Frequency and patterns in Texas. *Nursing Economic$, 33*, 144–154.

Kagan, I., & Barnoy, S. (2013). Organizational safety culture and medical error reporting by Israeli nurses. *Journal of Nursing Scholarship, 45*, 273–280. doi:10.1111/jnu.12026.

Kerr, N. (2013). 'Creating a protective picture': A grounded theory of RN decision making when using a charting-by-exception documentation system. *MEDSURG Nursing, 22*(2), 110–116.

Koharchik, L., Caputi, L., Robb, M., & Culleiton, A. L. (2015). Fostering clinical reasoning in nursing students: How can instructors in practice settings impart this essential skill? *American Journal of Nursing, 115*(1), 58–61. doi:10.1097/01.NAJ.0000459638.68657.9b.

Kontio, E., Lundgren-Laine, H., Kontio, J., Korvenranta, H., & Salanterä, S. (2013). Information utilization in tactical decision making of middle management health managers. *Computers, Informatics, Nursing, 31*, 9–16. doi:10.1097/NXN.0b013e318261f192.

Kramer, M., Maguire, P., Halfer, D., Budin, W. C., Hall, D. S., Goodloe, L., et al. (2012). The organizational transformative power of nurse residency programs. *Nursing Administration Quarterly, 36*, 155–168. doi:10.1097/naq.0b013e318249fdaa.

Lancaster, R. J., Westphal, J., & Jambunathan, J. (2015). Using SBAR to promote clinical judgment in undergraduate nursing students. *Journal of Nursing Education, 54*(Suppl.), S31–S34. doi:10.3928/01484834-20150218-08.

Lankarani, K. B., Alinejad, Z. M., Mooghali, A., Joulaei, H., Akbari, M., & Hashmati, B. (2015). An analytical study of health system managers' decision-making models. *Shiraz E-Medical Journal, 16*, e31330, 1–5. doi:10.17795/semj31330.

Lasater, K., Nielsen, A. E., Stock, M., & Ostrogorsky, T. L. (2015). Evaluating the clinical judgment of newly hired staff nurses. *Journal of Nursing Education, 46*, 563–571. doi:10.3928/00220124-20151112-09.

Levett-Jones, T., Hoffman, K., Dempsey, J., Yeun-Sim Jeong, S., Noble, D., Norton, C. A., et al. (2010). The 'five rights' of clinical reasoning: An educational model to enhance nursing students' ability to identify and manage clinically 'at risk' patients. *Nurse Education Today, 30*, 510–520. doi:10.1016/jnedt.2009.10.020.

Linderman, A., Pesut, D., & Disch, J. (2015). Sense making and knowledge transfer: Capturing the knowledge and wisdom of nurse leaders. *Journal of Professional Nursing, 31*, 290–297. doi:http://dx.doi.org/10.1016/j.profnurs2015.02.004.

Makary, M. A., & Daniel, M. (2016). Medical error-the third leading cause of death in the US. *BMJ, 353*. doi:10:1136/bmj.i2139. Retrieved from http://www.bmj.com/content/353/bmj.i2139.

Melnyk, B. M., Gallagher-Ford, L., Thomas, B. K., Troseth, M., Wyngarden, K., & Szalacha, L. (2016). A study of chief nurse executives indicates low prioritization of evidence-based practice and shortcomings I hospital performance metrics across the United States. *Worldviews on Evidenced-Based Nursing, 13*, 6–14. doi:10.1111/wvn.12133.

Merrill, K. C. (2015). Leadership style and patient safety. *Journal of Nursing Administration, 45*, 319–324. doi:10.1097/NNA.0000000000000207.

Molpus, J. (2013). Redesigning ED throughput. *HealthLeaders Magazine, 16*(6), 67–70.

Murphy, L. S., Wilson, M. L., & Newhouse, R. P. (2013). Data analytics: Making the most of input with strategic output. *Journal of Nursing Administration, 43*, 367–370. doi:10.1097/NNA.0b013e31829d60c7.

Nickitas, D. M., & Mensik, J. (2015). Exploring nurse staffing through excellence: A data-driven model. *Nurse Leader, 13*, 40–47. doi:10.1016/j.mnl.2014.11.005.

Patient Protection and Affordable Care Act 42 U.S.C. 300gg–11. (2010). Retrieved from http://www.hhs.gov/healthcare/about-the-law/read-the-law/.

Porter-O'Grady, T. (2015). Through the looking glass: Predictive and adaptive capacity in a time of great change. *Nursing Management, 46*(6), 22–29. doi:10.1097/01.NUMA.0000465397.67041.bc.

Quality and Safety Education for Nurses (QSEN). (2014). *Competencies*. Retrieved from http://qsen.org/competencies/.

Rambur, B., Vallett, C., Cohen, J. A., & Tarule, J. M. (2013). Metric-driven harm: An exploration of unintended consequences of performance measurement. *Applied Nursing Research, 26*, 269–272. doi:http://dx.doi.org/10.1016/j.apnr.2013.09.001.

Renz, S. M., Boltz, M. P., Wagner, L. M., Capezuti, E. A., & Lawrence, T. (2013). Examining the feasibility and utility of an SBAR protocol in long-term care. *Geriatric Nursing, 34*, 295–301. doi:http://dx.doi.org/10.1016/j.gerinurse.2013.04.010.

Sadler-Smith, E., & Burke-Smalley, L. A. (2015). What do we really understand about how managers make important decisions? *Organizational Dynamics, 44*, 9–16. doi:http://dx.doi.org/10.1016/j.orgdyn.2014.11.002.

Satyadi, C. (2013). Lean Six Sigma applications in healthcare. *Clinical Leadership and Management Review, 27*(3), 21–24.

Sedgwick, M. G., Grigg, L., & Dersch, S. (2014). Deepening the quality of clinical reasoning and decision-making in rural hospital nursing practice. *Rural and Remote Health, 14*(3), 1–12.

Shirey, M. R., Ebright, P. R., & McDaniel, A. M. (2013). Nurse manager cognitive decision-making amidst stress and work complexity. *Journal of Nursing Management, 21*, 17–30. doi:10.1111/j.1365-2834.2012.01380.x.

Sitterding, M. C., Broome, M. E., Everett, L. Q., & Ebright, P. (2012). Understanding situation awareness in nursing work: A hybrid concept analysis. *Advances in Nursing Science, 35*(1), 77–92.

Stec, M. W. (2016). Health as expanding consciousness: Clinical reasoning in baccalaureate nursing students. *Nursing Science Quarterly, 29*, 54–61. doi:10.1177/0894318415614901.

Stiegler, M. P., & Ruskin, K. J. (2012). Decision-making and safety in anesthesiology. *Current Opinion in Anesthesiology, 25*, 724–729. doi:10.1097/ACO.0b013e328359307a.

Sveinsdóttir, H., Ragnarsdóttir, E. D., & Blöndal, K. (2016). Praise matters: The influence of nurse unit managers' praise on nurses' practice, work environment and job satisfaction: A questionnaire study. *Journal of Advanced Nursing, 72*, 558–568. doi:10.1111/jan.12849.

Tanner, C. A. (2006). Thinking like a nurse: A research-based model of clinical judgment in nursing. *Journal of Nursing Education, 45*, 204–211.

Tower, M., Chaboyer, W., Green, Q., Dyer, K., & Wallis, M. (2012). Registered nurses' decision-making regarding documentation in patients' progress notes. *Journal of Clinical Nursing, 21*, 2917–2929. doi:10.1111/j.1365-2702.2012.04135.x.

Van Bogaert, P., Kowalski, C., Weeks, S. M., Van Heusden, D., & Clarke, S. P. (2013). The relationship between nurse practice environment, nurse work characteristics, burnout and job outcome and quality of nursing care: A cross-sectional study. *International Journal of Nursing Studies, 50*, 1667–1677. doi:10.1016/j.ijnurstu.2013.05.010.

Van Oostveen, C. J., Braaksma, A., & Vermeulen, H. (2014). Developing and testing a computerized decision support system for nurse-to-patient assignment. *Computers, Informatics, Nursing, 32*, 276–285. Doi:10.1097/CIN.0000000000000056.

Vestal, K. (2015). A double-edged sword: Don't bring me problems, bring me solutions. *Nurse Leader, 13*(2), 10–11. doi:10.1016/j.mnl.2015.01.010.

Weidema, F. C., Molewijk, A. C., Kamsteeg, F., & Widdershoven, G. A. M. (2015). Managers' views on and experiences with moral case deliberation in nursing teams. *Journal of Nursing Management, 23*(8), 1067–1075.

Westra, B. I., Clancy, T. R., Sensmeier, J., Warren, J. J., Weaver, C., & Delaney, C. W. (2015). Nursing knowledge: Big data science-implications for nurse leaders. *Nursing Administration Quarterly, 39*, 304–310. doi:10.1097/NAQ.0000000000000130.

Wheatley, M. (1999). *Leadership and the new science.* San Francisco, CA: Bennett-Koehler Publishers.

Zydziunaite, V., Lepaite, D., & Suominen, T. (2013). Leadership styles in ethical dilemmas when head nurses make decisions. *International Nursing Review, 60*, 228–235. doi:10.1111/inr.12018.

Chapter 5

Aiken, L. H., Clarke, S. P., Sloane, D. M., Lake, E. T., & Cheney, T. (2008). Effects of hospital care environment on patient mortality and nurse outcomes. *Journal of Nursing Administration, 38*(5), 223–229. doi:10.1097/01.NNA.0000312773.42352.d7.

Aiken, L. H., Clarke, S. P., Sloane, D. M., Sochalski, J., & Silber, J. H. (2002). Hospital nurse staffing and patient mortality, nurse burnout, and job dissatisfaction. *The Journal of the American Medical Association (JAMA), 288*(16), 1987–1993. doi:10.1001/jama.288.16.1987.

American Association of Critical-Care Nurses (AACN). (2005). *AACN standards for establishing and sustaining healthy work environments: A journey to excellence.* Aliso Viejo, CA: AACN.

American Institute of Stress (AIS). (n.d.). *Workplace stress.* Retrieved from http://www.stress.org/workplace-stress/.

American Nurse Credentialing Center (ANCC). (2016a). *ANCC Magnet Recognition Program®.* Retrieved from http://www.nursecredentialing.org/Magnet.

American Nurse Credentialing Center (ANCC). (2016b). *ANCC Pathway to Excellence®.* Retrieved from http://www.nursecredentialing.org/Pathway.

American Psychological Association (APA). (2013). *By the numbers: A psychologically healthy workplace fact sheet.* Retrieved from https://www.apaexcellence.org/assets/uploads/2013-phw-fact-sheet.pdf.

Barnes, R. (2015, June 25). *Affordable Care Act survives Supreme Court challenge.* Washington Post. Retrieved from https://www.washingtonpost.com/politics/courts_law/obamacare-survives-supreme-court-challenge/2015/06/25/af87608e-188a-11e5-93b7-5eddc056ad8a_story.html.

Centers for Medicare & Medicaid Services (CMS). (2014). *HCAHPS: Patients' perspectives of care survey.* Retrieved from https://www.cms.gov/Medicare/Quality-Initiatives-Patient-Assessment-instruments/HospitalQualityInits/HospitalHCAHPS.html.

Claessens, B. J. C., van Eerde, W., Rutte, C. G., & Roe, R. A. (2007). A review of the time management literature. *Personal Review, 36*(2), 255–276. doi:10.1108/00483480710726136.

Creation. (n.d.). *Merriam-Webster's online dictionary.* Retrieved from http://www.merriam-webster.com/dictionary/creation.

de Berker, A. O., Rutledge, R. B., Mathys, C., Marshall, L., Cross, G. F., Dolan, R. J., et al. (2016). Computations of uncertainty mediate acute stress responses in humans. *Communications, 7*, 10996. doi:10.1038/ncomms10996.

Ditkoff, M. (2010). Intention: The root of creativity. *Innovation Excellence.* Retrieved from http://www.innovationexcellence.com/blog/2010/07/12/intention-the-root-of-creativity/.

Federal Antitrust Policy in the Health Care Marketplace: Hearing before the Committee on Judiciary, Senate, 105th Congress. 84. (1997). (Prepared statement of John C. McMeekin on behalf of the American Hospital Association). Retrieved from https://books.google.com/books.

Fetter, R. B., Shin, Y., Freeman, J. L., Averill, R. F., & Thompson, J. D. (1980). Case mix definition by diagnosis related groups. *Medical Care, 18*(2), 1–53.

Fischer, J., & Keenan, N. (2010). *Prioritizing self-care: The key to stress management.* Retrieved from http://ezinearticles.com/?Prioritizing-Self-Care:-The-Key-to-Stress-Management&id=5499316.

Gilbert, D. (2007). *Stumbling on happiness.* New York, NY: Vintage Books.

Gionta, D. (2009). Setting boundaries at work: Steps to making them a reality. *Psychology Today.* Retrieved www.psychologytoday.com/blog/occupational-hazards/200901/setting-boundaries-work-steps-making-them-reality.

Johansen, M. L., & Cadmus, E. (2016). Conflict management style, supportive work environments and the experience of work stress in emergency nurses. *Journal of Nursing Management, 24*(2), 211–218.

Kanter, R. M. (1977). *Work and family in the United States: A critical review and agenda for research and policy.* New York, NY: Russell Sage Foundation.

Kath, L. M., Stichler, J. F., & Ehrhart, M. G. (2012). Moderators of the negative outcomes of nurse manager stress. *Journal of Nursing Management, 42*(4), 215–221. doi:10.1097/NNA.0b013e31824ccd25.

Krichbaum, K., Diemert, C., Jacox, L., Jones, A., Koenig, P., Mueller, C., et al. (2007). Complexity compression: Nurses under fire. *Nursing Forum, 42*(2), 86–94.

Lacey, S. R., Goodyear-Bruch, C., Olney, A., Hanson, M. D., Altman, M., Brinker, D., et al. (2016). Driving nurse leader development and organizational change from the bedside: The AACN Clinical Scene Investigator Academy. *Critical Care Nurse.* (In review).

Lacey, S. R., Olney, A., & Cox, K. (2012). The Clinical Scene Investigator Academy: The power of staff nurses improving patient and organizational outcomes. *Journal of Nursing Care Quality, 27*(1), 56–62.

Lundberg, U., & Cooper, C. L. (2011). *The science of occupational health: Stress, psychobiology and the new world of work.* Chichester, West Sussex, UK: Wiley-Blackwell.

Marshall, D. (2013, April 11). There's a critical difference between creativity and innovation. *Business Insider Australia.* Retrieved from http://www.businessinsider.com.au/difference-between-creativity-and-innovation-2013-4.

McCarthy, J., & Deady, R. (2008). Moral distress reconsidered. *Nursing Ethics, 15*(2), 254–262. doi:10.1177/0969733007086023.

McCarthy, J., & Gastmans, C. (2015). Moral distress: A review of the argument-based nursing ethics literature. *Nursing Ethics, 22*(1), 131–152.

McCowen, K. C., Malhotra, A., & Bistrian, B. R. (2001). Stress-induced hyperglycemia. *Critical Care Clinics, 17*(1), 107–124.

McMillan, K., & Perron, A. (2013). Nurses amidst change: The concept of change fatigue offers an alternative perspective on organizational change. *Policy, Politics, & Nursing Practice, 14*(1), 26–32.

Moreland, J. J., & Apker, J. (2016). Conflict and stress in hospital nursing: Improving communicative responses to enduring professional challenges. *Health Communication, 31*(7), 815–823.

Nelson, D. L., & Simmons, B. L. (2004). Eustress: An elusive construct, an engaging pursuit. In P. L. Perrewé & D. C. Ganster (Eds.), *Research in occupational stress and well-being* (Vol. 3., 265–322). Oxford, UK: Elsevier.

Nowrouzi, B., Lightfoot, N., Lariviere, M., Carter, L., Rukholm, E., Schinke, R., et al. (2015). Occupational stress management and burnout interventions in nursing and their implications for healthy work environments. *Workplace Health & Safety, 63*(7), 308–315.

Öhman, A. (2000). Fear and anxiety: Evolutionary, cognitive, and clinical perspectives. In M. Lewis & J. M. Haviland-Jones (Eds.), *Workplace health & safety, handbook of emotions* (pp. 573–593). New York, NY: The Guilford Press.

Peckham, C. (2015). Nurses tell all! Salaries, benefits, and whether they'd do it again. *Medscape.* Retrieved from http://www.medscape.com/viewarticle/854372.

Pines, E. W., Rauschhuber, M. L., Norgan, G. H., Cook, J. D., Canchola, L., Richardson, C., et al. (2012). Stress resiliency, psychological empowerment and conflict management styles among baccalaureate nursing students. *Journal of Advanced Nursing, 68*(7), 1482–1493. doi:10.1111/j.1365-2648.2011.05875.x.

Prediction. (n.d.). *Merriam-Webster's online dictionary.* Retrieved from http://www.merriam-webster.com/dictionary/prediction.

Ratanasiripong, P., Park, J. F., Ratanasiripong, N., & Kathalae, D. (2015). Stress and anxiety management in nursing students: Biofeedback and mindfulness mediation. *Journal of Nursing education, 54*(9), 520–524.

Richmond, P. A., Book, K., Hicks, M., Pimpinella, A., & Jenner, P. A. (2009). C.O.M.E. be a nurse manager. *Nursing Management, 40*(2), 52–54. doi:10.1097/01.NUMA.0000345875.99318.82.

Rosch, P. J. (2001). The quandary of job stress compensation. *Health and Stress, 3*, 1–4.

Rosenfeld, P., & Glassman, K. (2016). The long-term effect of a nurse residency program, 2005–2012: Analysis of former nurse residents. *Journal of Nursing Administration, 46*(6), 336–344.

Rosenthal, M. S. (2002). *50 ways to prevent and manage stress.* New York, NY: The McGraw-Hill Companies, Inc.

Rush, K. L., Adamack, M., Gordon, J., Lilly, M., & Janke, R. (2013). Best practices of formal new graduate nurse transition programs: An integrative review. *International Journal of Nursing Studies, 50*(3), 345–356. doi:http://dx.doi.org/10.1016/j.ijnurstu.2012.06.009.

Rushton, C. H. (2006). Defining and addressing moral distress: Tools for critical care nursing leaders. *AACN Advanced Critical Care, 17*(2), 161–168.

Sasso, L., Bagnasco, A., Bianchi, M., & Bressan, V. (2016). Moral distress in undergraduate nursing students: A systematic review. *Nursing Ethics, 23*(5), 523–534.

Saunders, E. G. (2013). *The 3 secrets to effective time investment: Achieve more success with less stress.* New York, NY: McGraw-Hill.

Scott, D. L. (2003). *Wall Street words: An A to Z guide to investment terms for today's investor.* Boston, MA: Houghton Mifflin Company.

Seaward, B. L. (2013). *Essentials of managing stress* (3rd ed.). Burlington, MA: Jones & Bartlett Learning.

Seyle, H. (1950). Stress and general adaption syndrome. *British Medical Journal, 1*(4667), 1383–1392.

Shirey, M. R., McDaniel, A. M., Ebright, P. R., Fisher, M. L., & Doebbeling, B. N. (2010). Understanding nurse manager stress and work complexity. *Journal of Nursing Administration, 40*(2), 82–91. doi:10.1097/NNA.0b013e3181cb9f88.

Ullrich, P. M., & Lutgendorf, S. K. (2002). Journaling about stressful events: Effects of cognitive processing and emotional expression. *Annals of Behavioral Medicine, 24*(3), 244–250.

US Department of Health and Human Services. (2014). *Key features of the Affordable Care Act.* Retrieved from http://www.hhs.gov/healthcare/facts-and-features/key-features-of-aca/index.html.

White, G. B. (2015, February 12). The alarming, long-term consequences of workplace stress. *The Atlantic.* Retrieved from http://www.theatlantic.com/business/archive/2015/02/the-alarming-long-term-consequences-of-work-place-stress/385397/.

Woods, E. (2005). *Employee development at the workplace: Achieving empowerment in a continuous learning environment* (2nd ed.). Dubuque, IA: Kendall Hunt.

World Wide Web Foundation. (2015). *Sir Tim Berners-Lee.* Retrieved from http://webfoundation.org/about/sir-tim-berners-lee.

Chapter 6

Agency for Healthcare Research and Quality (AHRQ). (2007). *Nurse staffing and quality of patient care.* Evidence report/Technology assessment Number 151. Retrieved from http://archive.ahrq.gov/downloads/pub/evidence/pdf/nursestaff/nursestaff.pdf.

American Hospital Association (AHA). (2002). *In our hands: How hospital leaders can build a thriving workforce.* Chicago, IL: Author.

American Nurses Association (ANA). (2010). *Nursing's social policy statement: The essence of the profession.* Silver Spring, MD: Author.

American Nurses Association (ANA). (2015a, December 21). *News release: Nurses rank as most honest, ethical profession for 14th straight year.*

Retrieved from http://www.nursingworld.org/2015-NursesRanked MostHonestEthicalProfession.

American Nurses Association (ANA). (2015b). *Code of ethics for nurses with interpretive statements.* Silver Spring, MD: Author. Retrieved from http://www.nursingworld.org/codeofethics.

American Nurses Association (ANA). (2016). *The nursing process.* Retrieved from http://www.nursingworld.org/EspeciallyForYou/StudentNurses/Thenursingprocess.aspx.

APRN Joint Dialogue Group Report. (2008, July 7). *Consensus model for APRN regulation: Licensure, accreditation, certification & education.* Retrieved from http://www.nursingworld.org/ConsensusModelforAPRN.

Buerhaus, P. I., Donelan, K., Ulrich, B. T., DesRoches, C., & Dittus, R. (2007). Trends in the experiences of hospital employed registered nurses: Results from three national surveys. *Nursing Economic$, 25*(2), 69–80.

Carroll, J. (2007). *Americans: 2.5 children is "ideal" family size.* Retrieved from http://www.gallup.com/poll/27973/americans-25-children-ideal-family-size.aspx.

Cooper, R. W. (2014). Legal and ethical issues. In D. L. Huber (Ed.), *Leadership and nursing care management* (5th ed., pp. 94–110). St. Louis, MO: Elsevier.

Family. (n.d.). In *Cambridge Dictionaries Online.* Retrieved from http://dictionary.cambridge.org/us/dictionary/english/family.

Hassmiller, S. B., & Cozine, M. (2006). Addressing the nurse shortage to improve the quality of patient care. *Health Affairs, 25*(1), 268–274.

Hewitt, T. A., & Chreim, S. (2015). Fix and forget or fix and report: A qualitative study of tensions at the front line of incident reporting. *BMJ Quality & Safety, 24*, 303–310.

Hill, G., & Hill, K. (2016). *Cross examination.* Retrieved from http://dictionary.law.com/Default.aspx?selected=408.

Institute of Medicine (IOM). (2011). *The future of nursing: Leading change, advancing health.* Washington, DC: National Academies Press.

Legal Information Institute. (2015). *Federal rules of evidence.* Retrieved from https://www.law.cornell.edu/rules/fre.

Milken Institute School of Public Health. (2012). *Individual access to medical records: 50 state comparison.* Retrieved from http://www.healthinfolaw.org/comparative-analysis/individual-access-medical-records-50-state-comparison.

Muller, L. S. (2007). Legal issues in case management practice. In S. Powell & H. Tahan (Eds.), *CMSA core curriculum for case management.* Philadelphia, PA: Wolters Kluwer.

Muller, L. S. (2008). Power of attorney and guardianship: What we think we know. *Professional Case Management, 13*(3), 169–172.

Muller, L. S. (2011). The case manager as expert witness. *Professional Case Management, 16*(5), 261–265.

Muller, L. S., & Fink-Samnick, E. (2015). Mandatory reporting: Let's clear up the confusion. *Professional Case Management, 20*(4), 199–203.

National Council of State Boards of Nursing (NCSBN). (2011). *Uniform licensure requirements.* Retrieved from https://www.ncsbn.org/3884.htm.

National Council of State Boards of Nursing (NCSBN). (2016a). *Boards and regulation.* Retrieved from https://www.ncsbn.org/boards.htm.

National Council of State Boards of Nursing (NCSBN). (2016b). *Nurse licensure compact.* Retrieved from https://www.ncsbn.org/nurse-licensure-compact.htm.

NCLEX. (2016). *NCLEX & other exams.* Retrieved from https://www.ncsbn.org/nclex.htm.

National Conference of State Legislatures (NCSL). (2015, September 28). *Mental health professionals' duty to warn.* Retrieved from http://www.ncsl.org/research/health/mental-health-professionals-duty-to-warn.aspx.

Needleman, J., Buerhaus, P., Pankratz, S., Leibson, C. L., Stevens, S. R., & Harris, M. (2011). Nurse staffing and inpatient mortality. *New England Journal of Medicine, 364*(11), 1037–1045.

NursingLicensure.org. (2013). *LPN/LVN and registered nurse license requirements by state.* Retrieved from http://www.nursinglicensure.org/.

Obama, B. H. (2016, January 6). *New executive actions to reduce gun violence and make our communities safer.* Retrieved from https://www.whitehouse.gov/the-press-office/2016/01/04/fact-sheet-new-executive-actions-reduce-gun-violence-and-make-our.

Obergefell v. Hodges, 576 U.S. 11. (The Supreme Court of the United States June 26, 2015).

Popa, I. E., Tudor, A. T., Span, G. A., & Fulop, M. T. (2011). Essential characteristics of a correct professional judgment process. *International Journal of Business Research, 11*(1). Retrieved from http://www.freepatentsonline.com/article/International-Journal-Business-Research/272511058.html.

PricewaterhouseCoopers (PwC). (2007). *What works: Healing the healthcare staffing shortage.* New York, NY: Author. Retrieved from https://council.brandeis.edu/pdfs/2007/PwC Shortage Report.pdf.

Profession. (n.d.). In *Cambridge Dictionaries Online.* Retrieved from http://dictionary.cambridge.org/us/dictionary/english/profession.

Skehan, J., & Muller, L. (2016a). Case management matter: Reducing disparities in the LGBT community. *Professional Case Management, 21*(3), 156–160.

Skehan, J., & Muller, L. (2016b). Reducing disparities in the LGBT community. *Professional Case Management Journal, 21*(3), 156–160.

Stavropoulou, C., Doherty, C., & Tosey, P. (2015). How effective are incident-reporting systems for improving patient safety? A systematic literature review. *Milbank Quarterly, 93*(4), 826–866.

Tarasoff v. Regents of the University of California, 17 Cal.3d 425, 131 Cal. Rptr. 14. (California Supreme Court 1976).

US Department of Health and Human Services (HHS). (2016). *Personal representatives.* Retrieved from http://www.hhs.gov/hipaa/for-professionals/privacy/guidance/personal-representatives/.

Vrbnjak, D., Denieffe, S., O'Gorman, C., & Pajnkihar, M. (2016). Barriers to reporting medication errors and near misses among nurses: A systematic review. *International Journal of Nursing Studies, 63*, 162–178.

Chapter 7

Agency for Healthcare Research and Quality (AHRQ). (2016). *TeamSTEPPS: Strategies and tools to enhance performance and patient safety.* Rockville, MD: Author. Retrieved from http://www.ahrq.gov/professionals/education/curriculum-tools/teamstepps/index.html.

Anderson, J., Malone, L., & Manning, J. (2014). Nursing bedside clinical handover—an integrated review of issues. *Journal of Clinical Nursing, 24*, 662–671.

Battey, B. (2012). Perspectives of spiritual care for nurse managers. *Journal of Nursing Management, 20*(8), 1012–1020.

Burkhart, L., Schmidt, L., & Hogan, N. (2011). Development and psychometric testing of the Spiritual Care Inventory instrument. *Journal of Advanced Nursing, 67*(11), 2463–2472. doi:10.1111/j.1365-2648.2011.05654.

Compton, J., Copeland, K., Flanders, S., Cassity, C., Spetman, M., Xiao, Y., et al. (2012). Implementing SBAR across a large multihospital health system. *Joint Commission Journal on Quality & Patient Safety, 38*(6), 261–268.

Cornell, P., Gervis, M. T., Yates, L., & Vardaman, J. M. (2014). Impact of SBAR on nurse shift reports and staff rounding. *MEDSURG Nursing, 23*(5), 334–342.

Fackler, C., Chambers, A., & Bourbonniere, M. (2015). Hospital nurses' lived experience of power. *Journal of Nursing Scholarship, 47*(3), 267–274.

Foronda, C. L., Alhusen, J., Budhathoki, C., Lamb, M., Tinsley, K., MacWilliams, B., et al. (2015). A mixed-methods, international, multisite study to develop and validate a measure of nurse-to-physician communication in simulation. *Nursing Education Perspectives, 36*(6), 383–388.

Glymph, D. C., Olenick, M., Barbera, S., Brown, E. L., Prestianni, L., & Miller, C. (2015). Healthcare utilizing deliberate discussion linking events (HUDDLE): A systematic review. *AANA Journal, 83*(3), 183–188.

Green, A., Albanese, B., Cafri, G., & Aarons, G. (2014). Leadership, organizational climate, and working alliance in a children's mental health service system. *Community Mental Health Journal, 50*(7), 771–777.

Hawkes, D., Hingley, D., Wood, S., & Blackhall, A. (2015). Evaluating the VERA framework for communication. *Nursing Standard, 30*(3), 44–48.

Hersey, P., Blanchard, K., & Johnson, D. (2013). *Management of organizational behavior: Leading human resources* (10th ed.). Upper Saddle River, NJ: Pearson Education.

Hettema, J. E., Ernst, D., Williams, J. R., & Miller, K. J. (2014). Parallel processes: Using motivational interviewing as an implementation coaching strategy. *Journal of Behavioral Health Services & Research, 42*(3), 324–336.

Institute of Medicine (IOM). (2011). *The future of nursing: Leading change, advancing health.* Washington, DC: National Academies Press.

Joyce, J., & Herbison, G. (2015). Reiki for depression and anxiety. *Cochrane Database of Systematic Reviews,* (4), CD006833. doi:10.1002/14651858.CD006833.pub2.

Kear, T., & Ulrich, B. (2015). Patient safety and patient safety culture in nephrology nurse practice settings: Issues, solutions and best practices. *Nephrology Nursing Journal, 42*(2), 113–122.

Kleiner, C., Link, T., Maynard, M., & Carpenter, K. (2014). Coaching to improve the quality of communication during briefings and debriefings. *AORN Journal, 100*(4), 358–368.

Kotter, J. (1996). *Leading change.* Boston, MA: Harvard Business School Press.

Krieger, D. (1979) *Therapeutic touch: How to use your hands to help or heal.* Englewood Cliffs, NJ: Prentice Hall.

Matzke, B., Houston, S., Fischer, U., & Bradshaw, M. J. (2014). Using a team-centered approach to evaluate effectiveness of nurse-physician communications. *JOGNN: Journal of Obstetric, Gynecologic & Neonatal Nursing, 43*(6), 684–694. doi:10.1111/1552-6909.12486.

Maxfield, D., Grenny, J., Lavandero, R., & Groah, L. (n.d.). *The silent treatment: Why safety tools and checklists aren't enough to save lives.* Retrieved from http://www.silenttreatmentstudy.com/silencekills/.

Nicotera, A., Mahon, M., & Wright, K. (2014). Communication that builds teams: Assessing a nursing conflict intervention. *Nursing Administration Quarterly, 38*(3), 248–260.

Patterson, K., Grenny, J., McMillan, R., & Switzler, A. (2011). *Crucial conversations: Tools for talking when stakes are high* (2nd ed.). New York, NY: McGraw-Hill Education.

Plonien, C., & Williams, M. (2015). Stepping up teamwork via TeamSTEPPS. *AORN Journal, 101*(4), 465–470.

Pryse, Y., McDaniel, A., & Schafer, J. (2014). Psychometric analysis of two new scales: The Evidence-Based Practice Nursing Leadership and Work Environment Scales. *Worldviews on Evidence-Based Nursing, 11*(4), 240–247.

Rand, W. (n.d.). *Reiki in hospitals.* Retrieved from http://www.reiki.org/healing/reiki_in_hospitalsold.html.

Rosenberg, M. B. (2004). *We can work it out: Resolving conflicts peacefully and powerfully.* Encinitas, CA: Puddledancer Press.

Sears, M. (2010). *Humanizing health care: Creating cultures of compassion with nonviolent communication.* Encinitas, CA: Puddledancer Press.

The Joint Commission (TJC). (2008). *Comprehensive accreditation manual for hospitals.* Oakbrook Terrace, IL: Author.

Tuckman, B. (1965). Developmental sequence in small groups. *Psychological Bulletin, 63*(6), 384–399. Retrieved from http://dx.doi.org/10.1037/h0022100.

US Department of Labor, Bureau of Labor Statistics. (2012). *Occupational outlook handbook: Registered nurses.* Retrieved from http://www.bls.gov/ooh/healthcare/registered-nurses.htm.

Vertino, K. A. (2014a, September 30). Effective interpersonal communication: A practical guide to improve your life. *OJIN: The Online Journal of Issues in Nursing, 19*(3), 1.

Vertino, K. A. (2014b). Evaluation of a TeamSTEPPS initiative on staff attitudes toward teamwork. *Journal of Nursing Administration, 44*(2), 97–102.

Warrell, M. (2012, August 27). Hiding behind email? Four times you should never use email. *Forbes.* Retrieved from http://www.forbes.com/sites/margiewarrell/2012/08/27/do-you-hide-behind-email/#dc8f0e97bf00.

Workplace Bullying Institute (WBI). (2016). *WBI—the Workplace Bullying Institute.* Retrieved from http://www.workplacebullying.org/.

Wu, L., Koo, M., Tseng, H, Liao, Y., & Chen, Y. (2015). Concordance between nurses' perception of their ability to provide spiritual care and the identified spiritual needs of hospitalized patients: A cross-sectional observational study. *Nursing & Health Sciences, 17*(4), 426–433.

Chapter 8

Adams, A., & Bond, S. (2000). Hospital nurses' job satisfaction, individual and organizational characteristics. *Journal of Advanced Nursing, 32*(3), 536–543.

Agency for Healthcare Research and Quality (AHRQ). (2016). *TeamSTEPPS strategies and tools to enhance performance and patient safety.* Retrieved from http://www.ahrq.gov/professionals/education/curriculum-tools/teamstepps/index.html.

American Association of Critical-Care Nurses (AACN). (2005). *AACN standards for establishing and sustaining healthy work environments: A journey to excellence.* Retrieved from http://www.aacn.org/wd/hwe/docs/hwestandards.pdf.

Book, C., & Galvin, K. (1975). *Instruction in and about small group discussion.* Falls Church, VA: Speech Communication Association.

Budin, W. C., Brewer, C. S., Chao, Y. Y., & Kovner, C. (2013). Verbal abuse from nurse colleagues and work environment of early registered nurses. *Journal of Nursing Scholarship, 45*(3), 308–316.

Cherniss, C., & Goleman, D. (2001). *The emotionally intelligent workplace: How to select for, measure, and improve emotional intelligence in individuals, groups, and organizations.* San Francisco, CA: Jossey-Bass.

Debono, D. S., Greenfield, D., Travaglia, J. F., Long, J. C., Black, D., Johnson, J., et al. (2013). Nurses' workarounds in acute healthcare settings: A scoping review. *BMC Health Services Research, 13*(1), 175–175. Retrieved from http://bmchealthservres.biomedcentral.com/articles/10.1186/1472-6963-13-175.

DiMeglio, K., Padula, C., Piatek, C., Korber, S., Barrett, A., Ducharme, M., et al. (2005). Group cohesion and nurse satisfaction: Examination of a team-building approach. *Journal of Nursing Administration, 35*(3), 110–120.

Farley, M., & Stoner, M. (1989). The nurse executive and interdisciplinary team building. *Nursing Administration Quarterly, 13*(2), 24–30.

Fewster-Thuente, L., & Velsor-Friedrich, B. (2008). Interdisciplinary collaboration for healthcare professionals. *Nursing Administration Quarterly, 32*(1), 40–48.

Goldratt, E. M., & Cox, J. (2016). *The goal: A process of ongoing improvement* (3rd ed.). Milton Park, Abingdon, Oxon, UK: Routledge.

Grenier, A. C., & Knebel, E. (Eds.). (2003). *Health professions education: A bridge to quality. Executive summary.* Washington, DC: National Academies Press. http://www.ncbi.nlm.nih.gov/books/NBK221525/?report=reader.

Harter, J. K., Schmidt, F. L., Asplund, J. W., Killham, E. A., & Agrawal, S. (2010). Causal impact of employee work perceptions on the bottom line of organizations. *Perspectives on Psychological Science, 5*(4), 378–389.

Hersey, P., Blanchard, K. H., & Johnson, D. E. (2013). *Management of organizational behavior: Leading human resources* (10th ed.). Upper Saddle River, NJ: Pearson Education.

Houser, J., Erken Brack, L., Handberry, L., Ricker, F., & Stroup, L. (2012). Involving nurses in decisions: Improving both nurse and patient outcomes. *Journal of Nursing Administration, 42*(7/8), 375–382.

Institute for Healthcare Improvement (IHI). (2016). *Triple aim initiative.* Retrieved from http://www.ihi.org/engage/initiatives/tripleaim/pages/default.aspx.

Institute of Medicine (IOM). (1999). *To err is human: Building a safer health system.* Washington, DC: National Academies Press.

Institute of Medicine (IOM). (2001). *Crossing the quality chasm: A new health system for the 21st Century.* Washington, DC: National Academies Press.

Jacobs, B., & Rosenthal, T. (1984). Managing effective meetings. *Nursing Economic$, 2*(2), 137–141.

Jay, A. (1982). How to run a meeting. *Journal of Nursing Administration, 12*(1), 22–28.

Kalisch, B., & Begeny, S. (2005). Improving nursing unit teamwork. *Journal of Nursing Administration, 35*(12), 550–556.

Kalisch, B., & Lee, K. H. (2010). The impact of teamwork on missed nursing care. *Nursing Outlook, 58*(5), 233–241.

Katzenbach, J. R., & Smith, D. K. (1993). *The wisdom of teams: Creating the high-performance organization.* New York, NY: HarperCollins.

Katzenbach, J. R., & Smith, D. K. (2015). *The wisdom of teams: Creating the high-performance organization* (reprint ed.). Boston, MA: Harvard Business Review Press.

Lancaster, J. (1981). Making the most of meetings. *Journal of Nursing Administration, 11*(10), 15–19.

Lancaster, G., Kolakowsky-Hayner, S., Kovacich, J., & Greer-Williams, N. (2015). Interdisciplinary communication and collaboration among physicians, nurses, and unlicensed assistive personnel. *Journal of Nursing Scholarship, 47*(3), 275–284.

Laramee, A. (1999). The building blocks of successful relationships. *The Journal of Care Management, 5*(4), 40, 42, 44–45.

Lencioni, P. (2002). *The five dysfunctions of a team.* San Francisco, CA: Jossey-Bass.

Lencioni, P. (2004). *Death by meeting.* San Francisco, CA: Jossey-Bass.

Lencioni, P. (2006). *Silos, politics and turf wars.* San Francisco, CA: Jossey-Bass.

Lu, H., Barriball, K. L., Zhang, X., & While, A. E. (2012). Job satisfaction among hospital nurses revisited: A systematic review. *International Journal of Nursing Studies, 49*(8), 1017–1038.

Manion, J. (2004). Strengthening organizational commitment: Understanding the concept as a basis for creating effective workforce retention strategies. *The Health Care Manager, 23*(2), 167–176.

Manion, J. (2009). *The engaged workforce: Proven strategies to build a positive healthcare workplace.* Chicago, IL: AHA Press.

Manion, J. (2011). *From management to leadership: Strategies for transforming health care.* San Francisco, CA: Jossey-Bass.

Manion, J., Lorimer, W., & Leander, W. J. (1996). *Team based healthcare organizations: Blueprint for success.* Gaithersburg, MD: Aspen.

Read, E., & Laschinger, H. K. (2013). Correlates of new graduate nurses' experiences of workplace mistreatment. *Journal of Nursing Administration, 43*(4), 221–228.

Riley, W., Davis, S. E., Miller, K. K., & McCullough, M. (2010). A model for developing high-reliability teams. *Journal of Nursing Management, 18,* 556–563.

Ronco, W. (2005). *Partnering solutions.* Franklin Lakes, NJ: Career Press.

Roth, C., Wieck, K. L., Fountain, R., & Haas, B. K. (2015). Hospital nurses' perceptions of human factors contributing to nursing errors. *Journal of Nursing Administration, 45*(5), 263–269.

Salas, E., & Rosen, M. A. (2013). Building high reliability teams: Progress and some reflections on teamwork training. *BMJ Quality & Safety, 22*(5), 369–373.

Veninga, R. (1982). *The human side of health administration: A guide for hospital, nursing, and public health administrators.* Englewood Cliffs, NJ: Prentice-Hall.

Wellins, R., Byham, W., & Wilson, J. (1991). *Empowered teams.* San Francisco, CA: Jossey-Bass.

Wong, C. A., Cummings, G. G., & Ducharme, L. (2013). The relationship between nursing leadership and patient outcomes: A systematic review update. *Journal of Nursing Management, 21*(5), 709–724.

Wynia, M. K., Von Kohorn, I., & Mitchell, P. H. (2012). Challenges at the intersection of team based and patient-centered health care: Insights from the IOM working group. *Journal of the American Medical Association, 308*(13), 1327–1328.

Chapter 9

Agency for Healthcare Research and Quality [AHRQ]. (2013). *TeamSTEPPS® 2.0: Team strategies & tools to enhance performance and patient safety.* (AHRQ Publication No. 14-0001-2). Retrieved from http://www.ahrq.gov/

sites/default/files/wysiwyg/professionals/education/curriculum-tools/ teamstepps/instructor/essentials/pocketguide.pdf.

Airth-Kindree, N. M. M., & Kirkhorn, L. E. C. (2016). Ethical grand rounds: Teaching ethics at the point of care. *Journal of Nursing Education Perspectives, 37*(1), 48–50. doi:10.5480/13-1128.

Altschuler, J., Margolius, D., Bodenheimer, T., & Grumbach, K. (2012). Estimating a reasonable patient panel size for primary care physicians with team-based task delegation. *Annals of Family Medicine, 10*(5), 396–400. doi:10.1370/afm.1400.

Amer, K. S. (2013). *Quality and safety for transformational nursing: Core competencies.* Boston, MA: Pearson.

American Association of Colleges of Nursing. (2008). *The essentials of bacca-laureate education for professional nursing practice.* Retrieved from http:// www.aacn.nche.edu/education-resources/BaccEssentials08.pdf.

American Association of Critical-Care Nurses (AACN). (2004). *AACN delegation handbook* (2nd ed.). Aliso Viejo, CA: Author.

American Nurses Association (ANA). (2009). *Patient safety: Rights of registered nurses when considering a patient assignment.* Retrieved from http:// nursingworld.org/rnrightsps.

American Nurses Association (ANA) and the National Council of State Boards of Nursing (NCSBN). (2005). *Joint statement on delegation.* Retrieved from https://www.ncsbn.org/Delegation_joint_statement_NCSBN-ANA.pdf.

Bowles, D. J. (2015). *Gerontology nursing case studies* (2nd ed.). New York, NY: Springer Publishing Company.

Brady, A., Fealy, G., Casey, M., Hegarty, J., Kennedy, C., McNamara, M., et al. (2015). Am I covered? An analysis of a national enquiry database on scope of practice. *Journal of Advanced Nursing, 71*(10), 2402–2412. doi:10:1111/ jan.12711.

Bryant, E. (2015). Delegation in practice. *Practice Nurse, 45*(8), 22–25.

Catalano, J. T. (2015). *Nursing now! Today's issues and tomorrow's trends* (7th ed.). Philadelphia, PA: F.A. Davis.

College of Registered Nurses of British Columbia. (2013). *Assigning and delegating to unregulated care providers.* Vancouver, BC, Canada: Author. Retrieved from https://www.crnbc.ca/Standards/Lists/StandardResources/ 98AssigningDelegatingUCPs.pdf.

Craftman, A. G., von Strauss, E., Rudberg, S. L., & Westerbotn, M. (2012). *Journal of Clinical Nursing, 22*, 569–578, doi:10.1111/j.1365-2702.2012/04262/x.

Day, L., Turner, K., Anderson, R. A., Mueller, C., McConnell, E. S., & Corazzini, K. N. (2014). Teaching delegation to RN students. *Journal of Nursing Regulation, 5*(2), 10–14. doi:10.1016/S2155-8256(15)30083-1.

Finkelman, A., & Kenner, C. (2013) *Professional nursing concepts: Competencies for quality leadership* (2nd ed.). Burlington, MA: Jones & Bartlett.

Graham, L., West, C., & Bauer, D. (2014). Faculty development focused on team-based collaborative care. *Education for Primary Care, 25*(4), 227–229.

Hand, T. (2016). The developing role of the HCA in general practice. *Practice Nurse, 42*(19), 14–17.

Hansten, R. (2014). Coach as chief correlator of tasks to results through delegation skill and teamwork development. *Nurse Leader, 12*(4), 69–73. doi:10.1016/j.mnl.2013.10.007.

Hasson, F., McKenna, H. P., & Keeney, S. (2013). Delegating and supervising unregistered professionals: The student nurse experience. *Nurse Education Today, 33*(3), 229–235. doi:10.1016/j.nedt.2012.02.008.

Haughton, B., & Stang, J. (2012). Population risk factors and trends in health care and public policy. *Journal of the Academy of Nutrition and Dietetics, 112*(3), 535–546. doi:10.1016/j.jand.2011.12.011.

Heath, H. (2012). How to optimize the registered nurse contribution in care homes. *Nursing Older People, 2*(24), 23–28.

Henderwood, M. (2015). ICU nurses' role in ventilation. *Kai Tiaki Nursing New Zealand, 21*(7), 14–15.

Idaho Health Care Association. (2016). *Nurse delegation tool kit.* Retrieved from http://www.idhca.org/nurse-delegation-toolkit/.

Johnson, M., Magnusson, C., Allan, H., Evans, K., Ball, E., Horton, K., et al. (2015). 'Doing the writing' and 'working in parallel': How 'distal nursing' affects delegation and supervision in the emerging role of the newly

qualified nurse. *Nurse Education Today, 35*, e29–e33. doi:10.1016/j. nedt.2014.11.020.

Josephsen, J., & Butt, A. (2014). Virtual multipatient simulation: A case study. *Clinical Simulation in Nursing, 10*, e235–e240. doi:10.1016/j.ecns.2013. 12.004.

Kaernested, B., & Bragadottier, H. (2012). Delegation of registered nurses revisited: Attitudes towards delegation and preparedness to delegate effectively. *Nordic Journal of Nursing Research & Clinical Studies, 103*(32), 10–15.

Keogh, K. (2014). Lecturer says delegation should be a part of pre-registration courses. *Nursing Standard, 29*(1), 9. doi:10.7748/ns.29.1.9.s7.

Kovner, A. R., & Knickman, J. R. (Eds.). (2011). *Jonas & Kovner's health care delivery in the United States* (10th ed.). New York, NY: Springer Publishing.

Lake, S., Moss, C., & Duke, J. (2009). Nursing prioritization of the patient need for care: A tacit knowledge embedded in the clinical decision-making literature. *International Journal of Nursing Practice, 15*, 376–388.

Lamb, G. (2013). *Care coordination: The game changer—how nursing is revolu-tionizing quality care.* Silver Spring, MD: American Nurses Association.

Lanfranchi, J. A. (2013). Instituting code blue drills in the OR. *Association of periOperative Registered Nurses Journal, 97*(4), 428–434. doi:10.1016/j. aorn.2013.01.017.

Lee, C., Beanland, C., Goeman, D., Johnson, A., Thorn, J., Koch, S., et al. (2015). Evaluation of a support worker role, within a nurse delegation and supervision model, for provision of medicines support for older people living at home: The Workforce Innovation for Safe and Effective (WISE) Medicines care study. *BMC Health Services Research, 15*(460), 1–11. doi:10.1186/s12913-015-1120-9.

Lichtenstein, B. J., Reuben, D. B., Karlamangla, A. S., Han, W., Roth, C. P., & Wenger, N. S. (2015). Effect of physician delegation to other healthcare providers on the quality of care for geriatric conditions. *Journal of American Geriatrics Society, 63*, 2164–2170. doi:10.1111/jgs.13654.

Magnusson, C. (2013). Tool designed to improve delegation skills will be trialed at three trusts. *Nursing Standard, 27*(52), 6. doi:10.7748/ns2013.08.27. 52.6.s4.

McDonald, K. M., Schultz, E., Albin, L., Pineda, N., Lonhart, J., Sundaram, V., et al. (2010). *Care coordination atlas version 3* (Prepared by Stanford University under subcontract to Battelle on Contract No. 290-04-0020. AHRQ publication No. 11-0023-EF.) Rockville, MD: Agency for Health Care Research and Quality. Retrieved from http://archive.ahrq.gov/ professionals/systems/long-term-care/resources/coordination/atlas/ care-coordination-measures-atlas.pdf.

National Council of State Boards of Nursing (NCSBN). (2005a). *Working with others: A position paper.* Retrieved from https://www.ncsbn.org/Working_ with_Others.pdf.

National Council of State Boards of Nursing (NCSBN). (2005b). *Joint statement on delegation.* Retrieved from https://www.ncsbn.org/Delegation_joint_ statement_NCSBN-ANA.pdf.

National Council of State Boards of Nursing (NCSBN). (2016). National guidelines for nursing delegation. *Journal of Nursing Regulation, 7*(1), 5–14.

Nelson, J. L. (2010). Helping new nurses set priorities. *American Nurse Today, 5*(5). Retrieved from https://www.americannursetoday.com/helping-new-nurses-set-priorities/.

O'Keefe, C. (2014). The authority for certain clinical tasks performed by unlicensed patient care technicians and LPNs/LVNs in the hemodialysis setting: A review. *Nephrology Nursing Journal, 41*(3), 247–255.

O'Malley, A. S., Gourevitch, R., Draper, K., Bond, A., & Tirodkar, M. A. (2014). Overcoming challenges to teamwork in patient-centered medical homes: A qualitative study. *Journal of General Internal Medicine, 30*(2), 183–192. doi:10.1007/s11606-014-3065-9.

Owsley, T. (2013). The paradox of nursing regulation: Politics or patient safety? *Journal of Legal Medicine, 34*, 483–503. doi:10.1080/01947648.2013.859974.

Papastavrou, E., Andreou, P., & Efstathiou, G. (2014). Rationing of nursing care and nurse–patient outcomes: A systematic review of quantitative studies. *International Journal of Health Planning Management, 29*, 3–25. doi:10.1002/hpm.2160.

Patterson, E. S., Ebright, P. R., & Saleem, J. J. (2011). Investigating stacking: How do registered nurses prioritize their activities in real-time? *International Journal of Industrial Ergonomics, 41*, 389–393.

Patton, D., Fealy, G., McNamara, M., Casey, M., O Connor, T., Doyle, L., et al. (2013). Individual-level outcomes from a national clinical leadership development programme. *Contemporary Nurse, 45*(1), 56–63.

Pittman, P., & Forrest, E. (2015). The changing roles of registered nurses in Pioneer Accountable Care Organizations. *Nursing Outlook, 63*, 554–565. doi:10.1016/j.outlook.2015.05.008.

Saccomano, S. J., & Pinto-Zipp, G. (2014). Integrating delegation into the undergraduate curriculum. *Creative Nursing, 20*(2), 106–115. doi:10.1891/1078-4535.20.2.106.

Trossman, S. (2012). OK to delegate? *The American Nurse, 44*(6), 1, 6.

True, G., Stewart, G. L., Lampman, M., Pelak, M., & Solimo, S. L. (2014). Teamwork and delegation in medical homes: Primary care staff perspectives in the Veterans Health Administration. *Journal of General Internal Medicine, 29*(Suppl. 2), S632–S639. doi:10.1007/s11606-013-2666-z.

Wilkinson, K. (2016). Sharing supervision and liability as a nurse manager. *Nursing Management, 47*(4), 11–13. doi:10.1097/01.

Wilt, L., & Foley, M. (2016). Delegation of Glucagon® in the school setting: A comparison of state legislation. *The Journal of School Nursing, 27*(3), 185–196. doi:10.1177/1059840511398240.

Chapter 10

Aiken, L. H., Sloane, D. M., Bruyneel, L., Van den Heede, K., Griffiths, P., Busse, R., et al. (2014). Nurse staffing and education and hospital mortality in nine European countries: A retrospective observational study. *Lancet, 383*(9931), 1824–1830.

Aiken, L. H., Sloane, D. M., Griffiths, P., Rafferty, A. M., Bruyneel, L., McHugh, M., et al. (2016). Nursing skill mix in European hospitals: Cross-sectional study of the association with mortality, patient ratings, and quality of care. *BMJ Quality & Safety, 0*, 1–10. Retrieved from http://qualitysafety.bmj.com/content/early/2016/11/03/bmjqs-2016-005567.full.pdf+html.

Amason, A. (1996). Distinguishing effects of functional and dysfunctional conflict on strategic decision making: Resolving a paradox for top management teams. *Academy of Management Journal, 39*(1), 123–148.

Amason, A., & Sapienza, H. (1997). The effects of top management team size and interaction norms on cognitive and affective conflict. *Journal of Management, 23*(4), 495–516.

Arms, D., & Stalter, A. M. (2016). Serving on organizational boards: What nurses need to know. *Online Journal of Issues in Nursing, 21*(2).

Augsburger, D. (1973). *Caring enough to confront.* Glendale, CA: Regal Books.

Barki, H., & Hartwick, J. (2001). Interpersonal conflict and its management in information system development. *MIS Quarterly, 25*(2), 195–228.

Barki, H., & Hartwick, J. (2004). Conceptualizing the construct of interpersonal conflict. *International Journal of Conflict Management, 15*(3), 216–244.

Bender, M., & Feldman, M. S. (2015). A practice theory approach to understanding the interdependency of nursing practice and the environment: Implications for nurse-led care delivery models. *Advances in Nursing Science, 38*(2), 96–109.

Bennis, W., & Nanus, B. (1985). *Leaders: The strategies for taking charge.* New York, NY: Harper & Row.

Blake, R., & Mouton, J. S. (1964). *The managerial grid.* Houston, TX: Gulf Publishing.

Boynton, B. (2012). *Disruptive behavior, bullying, & incivility: A glossary of violence in healthcare workplaces.* Retrieved from http://www.confidentvoices.com/2012/04/04/disruptive-behavior-bullying-incivility-workplace-abuse-a-glossary-of-violence/.

Briles, J. (2007). Snakes at the nursing station. *American Nurse Today, 2*(8), 52–53.

Brown, L. D. (1983). *Managing conflict at organizational interfaces.* Reading, MA: Addison-Wesley.

Brubaker, D., Noble, C., Fincher, R., & Kee-Young Park, S. (2014). Conflict resolution in the workplace: What will the future bring? *Conflict Resolution Quarterly, 31*(4), 357–386. doi:10.1002/crq.21104.

Bureau of Health Professions (BHPr), National Center for Health Workforce Analysis. (2014). *Future of the nursing workforce: National- and state-level projections, 2012–2025.* Rockville, MD: Health Resources and Services Administration (HRSA). Retrieved from http://bhpr.hrsa.gov/healthworkforce/supplydemand/nursing/workforceprojections/index.html.

Charmaz, K. (1990). 'Discovering' chronic illness: Using grounded theory. *Social Science and Medicine, 30*, 1161–1172.

Chavez, V. (2016). *Presenteeism could be more expensive than absenteeism.* Visionarity. Retrieved from http://visionarity.com/presenteeism-expensive-absenteeism/.

Conrad, C. (1990). *Strategic organizational communication: An integrated perspective* (2nd ed.). Fort Worth, TX: Holt, Rinehart & Winston.

Cox, K. B. (2014). The new Intragroup Conflict Scale: Testing and psychometric properties. *Journal of Nursing Measurement, 22*(1), 59–76.

Cziraki, K., & Laschinger, H. (2015). Leader empowering behaviours and work engagement: The mediating role of structural empowerment. *Nursing Leadership, 28*(3), 10–22.

Daft, R. L. (2013). *Organization theory and design* (11th ed.). Mason, OH: South-Western Cengage Learning.

Dahl, R. A. (1957). The concept of power. *Systems Research and Behavioral Science, 2*(3), 202–210.

DeDreu, C. K. W., & Weingart, L. R. (2003). Task versus relationship conflict, team performance, and team member satisfaction: A meta-analysis. *Journal of Applied Psychology, 88*(4), 741–750.

De La Roche, A. S. R. (2015, May 15). *Managing the cost of conflict.* Retrieved from http://www.mediate.com/articles/SgubiniA6.cfm.

Deutsch, M. (1973). *The resolution of conflict: Constructive and destructive processes.* New Haven, CT: Yale University Press.

Ehteshami, A., Rezaei1, P., Tavakoli, N., & Kasaei, M. (2013). The role of health information technology in reducing preventable medical errors and improving patient safety. *International Journal of Health System and Disaster Management, 1*(4), 195–199.

Emerson, R. M. (1957). Power-dependence relations. *American Sociological Review, 27*(1), 31–40.

Filley, A. C. (1975). *Interpersonal conflict resolution.* Glenview, IL: Scott Foresman.

Filley, A., House, R., & Kerr, S. (1976). *Managerial process and organizational behavior.* Glenview, IL: Scott Foresman.

Fisher, R., Ury, W., & Patton, B. (1992). *Getting to yes: Negotiating agreement without giving in* (2nd ed.). New York, NY: Penguin Books.

French, J., & Raven, B. (1959). The bases of social power. In D. Cartwright (Ed.), *Studies in social power* (pp. 150–167). Ann Arbor, MI: University of Michigan, Institute for Social Research.

Gardner, D. L. (1992). Conflict and retention of new graduate nurses. *Western Journal of Nursing Research, 14*(1), 76–85.

Glaser, B. G. (1978). *Theoretical sensitivity: Advances in the methodology of grounded theory.* Mill Valley, CA: The Sociology Press.

Glaser, B. G., & Strauss, A. L. (1967). *The discovery of grounded theory: Strategies for qualitative research.* Chicago, IL: Aldine Transaction.

Hart, C. (2015). The elephant in the room: Nursing and nursing power on an interprofessional team. *The Journal of Continuing Education in Nursing, 46*(8), 349–355.

Health Quality Council of Alberta (HQCA). (2013, March). *Managing disruptive behavior in the healthcare workplace-Provincial framework.* Calgary, AB, Canada. Retrieved from http://hqca.ca/health-care-provider-resources/frameworks/managing-disruptive-behavior-in-the-healthcare-workplace-provincial-framework/.

Hersey, P. H., Blanchard, K. H., & Johnson, D. E. (2013). *Management of organizational behavior: Leading human resources* (10th ed.). Upper Saddle River, NJ: Pearson Education.

Hersey, P., Blanchard, K. H., & Natemeyer, W. E. (1979). Situational leadership, perception, and the impact of power. *Group and Organization Studies, 4*(4), 418–428.

Hickson, D. J., Hinings, C. R., Lee, C. A., Schneck, R. E., & Pennings, J. M. (1971). A strategic contingencies theory of intraorganizational power. *Administrative Science Quarterly*, 16(2), 216–229.

Huston, C. J. (2008). Eleven strategies for building a personal power base. *Nursing Management*, 39(4), 58–61.

Institute of Medicine (IOM). (1999). *To err is human: Building a safer health system*. Washington, DC: National Academies Press.

Institute of Medicine (IOM). (2010). *The future of nursing: Leading change, advancing health*. Washington, DC: National Academies Press.

James, J. T. (2013). A new, evidence-based estimate of patient harms associated with hospital care. *Journal of Patient Safety*, 9(3), 122–128.

Jehn, K. A. (1997). A qualitative analysis of conflict types and dimensions in organizational groups. *Administrative Science Quarterly*, 42(3), 530–557.

Jehn, K. A., Northcraft, G., & Neale, M. (1999). Why differences make a difference: A field study of diversity, conflict, and performance in workgroups. *Administrative Science Quarterly*, 44(4), 741–763.

Johansen, M. L. (2012). Keeping the peace: Conflict management strategies for nurse managers. *Nursing Management*, 43(2), 50–54.

Kane, R. L., Shamliyan, T., Mueller, C., Duvai, S., & Wilt, T. (2007). *Nursing staffing and quality of patient care. Evidence report/technology Assessment No. 151*(prepared by the Minnesota Evidence-based Practice Center under Contract No. 290-0009) . AHRQ Publication No. 07-E005. Rockville, MD: Agency for Healthcare Research and Quality.

Kanter, R. M. (1993). *Men and women of the corporation* (2nd ed.). New York, NY: Basic Books.

King, I. M. (1981). *A theory for nursing: Systems, concepts, process*. New York, NY: Wiley & Sons.

Kipnis, D., Schmidt, S. M., Swaffin-Smith, C., & Wilkinson, I. (1984). Patterns of managerial influence: Shotgun managers, tacticians, and bystanders. *Organizational Dynamics*, 12(3), 58–67.

Kipnis, D., Schmidt, S. M., & Wilkinson, I. (1980). Intraorganizational influence tactics: Explorations in getting one's way. *Journal of Applied Psychology*, 65(4), 440–452.

Kirschbaum, K. (2012). Physician communication in the operating room: Expanding application of face-negotiation theory to the health communication context. *Health Communication*, 27(3), 292–301.

Knickle, K., McNaughton, N., & Downar, J. (2012). Beyond winning: Mediation, conflict resolution, and non-rational sources of conflict in the ICU. *Critical Care*, 16, 308. doi:10.1186/cc11141.

Kotter, J. P. (1979). *Power in management: How to understand, acquire, and use it*. New York, NY: AMACOM.

Kouzes, J., & Posner, B. (2012). *The leadership challenge: How to make extraordinary things happen in organizations* (5th ed.). San Francisco, CA: Wiley.

Kovner, C. T., Brewer, C. S., Fatehi, F., & Jun, J. (2014). What does nurse turnover rate mean and what is the rate? *Policy, Politics, & Nursing Practice*, 15(3/4), 64–71.

Kuperschmidt, B. R. (2008). Conflicts at work: Try carefronting. *Journal of Christian Nursing*, 25(1), 10–17.

Liberatore, P., Brown-Williams, R., Brucker, J., Dukes, N., Kimmey, L., McCarthy, K., et al. (1989). A group approach to problem-solving. *Nursing Management*, 20(9), 68–72.

Lyon, A. (2012, March 18). *Unresolved conflict develops into unpredictable consequences*. Western Pennsylvania Healthcare News. Retrieved from http://www.wphealthcarenews.com/unresolved-conflict-develops-into-unpredictable-consequences/.

Makary, M. A., & Daniel, M. (2016). Medical error—the third leading cause of death in the US. *British Medical Journal*, 353, i2139. doi:http://dx.doi.org/10.1136/bmj.i2139. Retrieved from http://www.bmj.com/content/353/bmj.i2139.

Mannix, J., Wilkes, L., & Daly, J. (2013). Attributes of clinical leadership in contemporary nursing: An integrative review. *Contemporary Nurse*, 45(1), 10–21.

Manojlovich, M. (2007). Power and empowerment in nursing: Looking back to inform the future. *The Online Journal of Issues in Nursing*, 12(1). Retrieved from http://www.nursingworld.org/MainMenuCategories/ANAMarketplace/ANAPeriodicals/OJIN/TableofContents/Volume122007/No1Jan07/LookingBackwardtoInformtheFuture.htmlWhile.

NSI Nursing Solutions, Inc. (2016). *2016 national healthcare retention & RN staffing report*. East Petersburg, PA: NSI Nursing Solutions, Inc. Retrieved from http://www.nsinursingsolutions.com/Files/assets/library/retention-institute/NationalHealthcareRNRetentionReport2016.pdf.

Oetzel, J. G., & Ting-Toomey, S. (2003). Face concerns in interpersonal conflict: A cross-cultural empirical test of the face negotiation theory. *Communication Research*, 30(6), 599–624.

Oetzel, J. G., Ting-Toomey, S., Masumoto, T., Yokochi, Y., Pan, X., Takai, J., et al. (2001). Face and facework in conflict: A cross-cultural comparison of China, Germany, Japan, and the United States. *Communication Monographs*, 68, 235–258.

Patton, C. M. (2014). Conflict in health care: A literature review. *The Internet Journal of Healthcare Administration*, 9(1), 1–11.

Pfeffer, J. (1981). *Power in organizations*. Boston, MA: Pitman Books.

Pondy, L. R. (1967). Organizational conflict: Concepts and models. *Administrative Science Quarterly*, 12(2), 296–320.

Putnam, L. L., & Poole, M. S. (1987). Conflict and negotiation. In F. M. Jablin, L. L. Putnam, K. Roberts, & L. W. Porter (Eds.), *Handbook of organizational communication* (pp. 549–599). Newbury Park, CA: Sage.

Rahim, M. A. (1983a). A measure of styles of handling interpersonal conflict. *Academy of Management Journal*, 26(2), 368–376.

Rahim, M. A. (1983b). Measurement of organizational conflict. *Journal of General Psychology*, 109(2), 189–199.

Rahim, M. A. (1983c). *Rahim organizational conflict inventories: Experimental edition: Professional manual*. Palo Alto, CA: Consulting Psychologists Press.

Rahim, M. A. (2010). *Managing conflict in organizations* (4th ed.). Piscataway, NJ: Transaction Publishers.

Rahim, M. A., & Bonoma, T. V. (1979). Managing organizational conflict: A model for diagnosis and intervention. *Psychological Reports*, 44(3), 1323–1344.

Rao, A. (2012). The contemporary construction of nurse empowerment. *Journal of Nursing Scholarship*, 44(4), 396–402.

Raven, B., & Kruglanski, W. (1975). Conflict and power. In P. Swingle (Ed.), *The structure of conflict* (pp. 177–219). New York, NY: Academic Press.

Richards, D. (2016, February 23). What is the average cost of absenteeism? *rMagazine*. Retrieved from http://www.wellworksforyou.com/faq/what-is-the-average-cost-of-absenteeism/.

Robbins, S. P., & Judge, T. A. (2016). *Organizational behavior* (17th ed.). Upper Saddle River, NJ: Prentice Hall Publishing.

Robert Wood Johnson Foundation (RWJF). (2015). *Nurses and nursing. Future of nursing: Campaign for action*. Retrieved from http://www.rwjf.org/en/our-topics/topics/nurses-and-nursing.html.

Shargh, F. S., Soufi, M., & Dadashi, M. A. (2013). Conflict management and negotiation. *Journal of Applied Basic Science*, 5(5), 538–543.

Sieloff, C. L. (2003). Measuring nursing power within organizations. *Journal of Nursing Scholarship*, 35(2), 183–187.

Skehan, J. (2015). Nurse leader, nursing leaders: Strategies for eradicating bullying in the Workplace. *Nurse Leader*, 13(2), 60–62. http://dx.doi.org/10.1016/j.mnl.2014.07.015.

Small, C. R., Porterfield, S., & Gordon, G. (2015). Disruptive behavior within the workplace. *Applied Nursing Research*, 28(2), 57–71.

Sportsman, S., & Hamilton, P. (2007). Conflict management styles in the health professions. *Journal of Professional Nursing*, 23(3), 157–166.

Thew, J. (2016). *4 strategies for nurses who want to enter the boardroom*. HealthLeadersMedia. Retrieved from http://www.healthleadersmedia.com/nurse-leaders/4-strategies-nurses-who-want-enter-boardroom.

Thomas, K. W. (1976). Conflict and conflict management. In M. D. Dunnette (Ed.), *The handbook of industrial and organizational psychology* (pp. 889–935). Chicago, IL: Rand McNally.

Thomas, K. W. (1977). Toward multi-dimensional values in teaching: The example of conflict behaviors. *Academy of Management Review*, 2(3), 484–490.

Thomas, K. W. (1992). Conflict and negotiation processes in organizations. In M. D. Dunnette, & L. M. Hough (Eds.), *The handbook of industrial and organizational psychology* (2nd ed., Vol. 3., pp. 651–717). Palo Alto, CA: Consulting Psychologists Press.

Thomas, K. W., & Kilmann, R. H. (1974). *Thomas-Kilmann conflict mode instrument.* Tuxedo, NY: Xicom.

Ting-Toomey, S. (1988). Intercultural conflict styles: A face negotiation theory. In Y. Y. Kim & W. Gudykunst (Eds.), *Theories in intercultural communication* (pp. 213–235). Newbury Park, CA: Sage.

Ting-Toomey, S., & Kurogi, A. (1998). Facework competence in intercultural conflict: An updated face-negotiation theory. *International Journal of Intercultural Relations, 22,* 187–225.

Tomajan, K. (2012). Advocating for nurses and nursing. *OJIN: The Online Journal of Issues in Nursing, 17*(1), 4.

Wall, J. A., & Callister, R. R. (1995). Conflict and its management. *Journal of Management, 21*(3), 515–558.

Walton, R. E. (1966). Theory of conflict in lateral organizational relationships. In J. R. Lawrence (Ed.), *Operational research and the social sciences* (pp. 409–426). London: Tavistock Publications.

Weber, M. (1947). *The theory of social and economic organization* (A.M. Henderson & T. Parsons, Trans.). New York, NY: Oxford University Press (Original work published 1923).

Yukl, G., & Falbe, C. M. (1991). Importance of different power sources in downward and lateral relations. *Journal of Applied Psychology, 76*(3), 416–423.

Yukl, G., Falbe, C., & Joo, Y. Y. (1993). Patterns of influence behavior for managers. *Group and Organization Management, 18*(1), 5–28.

Yukl, G., Lepsinger, R., & Lucia, T. (1992). Preliminary report on development and validation of the Influence Behavior Questionnaire. In K. E. Clar, M. B. Cla, & D. P. Campbell (Eds.), *The impact of leadership* (pp. 417–427). Greensboro, NC: Center for Creative Leadership.

Yukl, G., Seifert, C. F., & Chavez, C. (2008). Validation of the extended Influence Behavior Questionnaire. *The Leadership Quarterly, 19*(5), 609–621.

Chapter 11

Agency for Healthcare Research and Quality (AHRQ). (2014). *The SHARE approach—Taking steps toward cultural competence: A fact sheet.* Rockville, MD: Author. Retrieved from http://www.ahrq.gov/professionals/education/curriculum-tools/shareddecisionmaking/tools/tool-7/index.html.

Agency for Healthcare Research and Quality (AHRQ). (2015). *2014 National healthcare quality and disparities report.* Retrieved from http://www.ahrq.gov/research/findings/nhqrdr/nhqdr14/index.html.

Alegria, M., Lin, J., Chen, C. N., Duan, N., Cook, B., & Meng, X. L. (2012). The impact of insurance coverage in diminishing racial and ethnic disparities in behavioral health services. *Health Services Resources Journal, 47*(3pt2), 1322–1344.

Ayanian, J. Z. (2015, October 15). The costs of racial disparities in health care. *Harvard Business Review.* Retrieved from https://hbr.org/2015/10/the-costs-of-racial-disparities-in-health-care.

Boekhorst, J. A. (2015). The role of authentic leadership in fostering workplace inclusion: A social information processing perspective. *Human Resource Management, 54*(2), 241–264.

Clearly Cultural. (2004–2016a). *Power distance index.* Retrieved from http://www.clearlycultural.com/geert-hofstede-cultural-dimensions/power-distance-index/.

Clearly Cultural. (2004–2016b). *Individualism.* Retrieved from http://www.clearlycultural.com/geert-hofstede-cultural-dimensions/individualism/.

Cultural diversity. (2016). *Oxford Dictionaries.* Retrieved from http://www.oxforddictionaries.com/us/definition/american_english/cultural-diversity.

Culture. (n.d.). *Merriam-Webster.* Retrieved from http://www.merriam-webster.com/dictionary/culture.

Diversity. (n.d.). *Merriam-Webster.* Retrieved from http://www.merriam-webster.com/dictionary/diversity.

Frey, W. H. (2014). *New projections point to a majority minority nation in 2044.* Washington, DC: Brookings. Retrieved from http://www.brookings.edu/blogs/the-avenue/posts/2014/12/12-majority-minority-nation-2044-frey.

Goode, T. D., Dunne, M. C., & Bronheim, S. M. (2006). *The evidence base for cultural and linguistic competency in health care.* New York, NY: The Commonwealth Fund. Retrieved from http://www.commonwealthfund.org/usr_doc/Goode_evidencebasecultlinguisticcomp_962.pdf.

Health Research & Educational Trust. (2013). *Becoming a culturally competent health care organization.* Chicago, IL: Health Research & Educational Trust. Retrieved from http://www.diversityconnection.org/diversityconnection/membership/Resource%20Center%20Docs/Equity%20of%20Care%20Report%20FINAL.pdf.

Hendricks, J. M., & Cope, V. C. (2013). Generational diversity: What nurse managers need to know. *Journal of Advanced Nursing, 69*(3), 717–725.

Kaiser Family Foundation. (2015). *Key facts about the uninsured population.* Retrieved from http://kff.org/uninsured/fact-sheet/key-facts-about-the-uninsured-population/.

Lewis, B. (2017). *Negotiation tactics: How to haggle like your life depends on it.* Retrieved from https://www.fluentin3months.com/negotiation-tactics/.

Malik, S. (2015). *How to overcome the major challenges in cross cultural communication.* Retrieved from https://www.linkedin.com/pulse/how-overcome-major-challenges-cross-cultural-iim-shillong-pgpex.

McKirnan, D. J., DuBois, S. N., Alvy, L. M., & Jones, K. (2013). Health care access and health behaviors among men who have sex with men: The cost of health disparities. *Health Education & Behavior, 40*(1), 32–41.

MinorityNurse.com. (2015). *Nursing statistics.* Retrieved from http://minoritynurse.com/nursing-statistics/.

National Center for Cultural Competence. (n.d.a). *The compelling need for cultural and linguistic competence.* Retrieved from http://nccc.georgetown.edu/foundations/need.html.

National Center for Cultural Competence. (n.d.b). *Self-assessment checklist for personnel providing primary health care services.* Retrieved from http://nccc.georgetown.edu/documents/checklist_PHC.html.

Nelson, L. R., Signorella, M. L., & Botti, K. G. (2016). Accent, gender, and perceived competence. *Hispanic Journal of Behavioral Sciences, 38*(2), 166–185.

Office of Minority Health (OMH). (n.d.). *Think cultural health.* Retrieved from https://www.thinkculturalhealth.hhs.gov/.

Office of Minority Health (OMH). (2013). *National standards for culturally and linguistically appropriate services in health and health care: A blueprint for advancing and sustaining CLAS policy and practice.* Retrieved from https://www.thinkculturalhealth.hhs.gov/pdfs/EnhancedCLASStandardsBlueprint.pdf.

Refugee Health Technical Assistance Center. (2011). *Best practices for communicating through an interpreter.* Retrieved from http://refugeehealthta.org/access-to-care/language-access/best-practices-communicating-through-an-interpreter/.

Smith, J. C., & Medalia, C. (2014, September). *Health insurance coverage in the United States: 2013.* United States Census Bureau. http://www.census.gov/content/dam/Census/library/publications/2014/demo/p60-250.pdf.

The California Endowment. (2003). Improving access to health care for limited English proficient health care consumers. *Health . . . In brief, 2*(1). Retrieved from http://www.hablamosjuntos.org/resources/pdf/2003TCE_%20improving_access_to_healthcare.pdf.

ToughNickel. (2016). *High-context vs. low-context communication.* Retrieved from https://toughnickel.com/business/High-Context-vs-Low-Context-Communication.

US Census Bureau. (n.d.). *State and county quick facts.* Retrieved from https://www.census.gov/quickfacts/table/PST045216/00.

US Census Bureau. (2012). *Most children younger than age 1 are minorities, Census Bureau reports.* Retrieved from http://www.census.gov/newsroom/releases/archives/population/cb12-90.html.

US Census Bureau. (2014). *2014 National population projections.* Retrieved from http://www.census.gov/population/projections/data/national/2014.html.

US Equal Employment Opportunity Commission. (2002). *Americans with Disabilities Act: Questions and answers.* Retrieved from https://www.ada.gov/q&aeng02.htm.

Virginia.gov. (2016). *What is health inequity?* Retrieved from http://www.vdh.virginia.gov/health-equity/unnatural-causes-is-inequality-making-us-sick/what-is-health-inequity/.

Ward, A., Ravlin, E. C., Klass, B. S., Ployhart, R. E., & Buchan, N. R. (2016). When do high-context communicators speak up? Exploring contextual communication orientation and employee voice. *Journal of Applied Psychology, 101*(10), 1498–1511.

Williams, D. A., Berger, J. B., & McClendon, S. A. (2005). *Toward a model of inclusive excellence and change in postsecondary institutions.* Association of American Colleges and Universities (AAC&U). Retrieved from https://www.aacu.org/sites/default/files/files/mei/williams_et_al.pdf.

World Health Organization (WHO). (2016). *Health systems.* Retrieved from http://www.who.int/healthsystems/topics/equity/en/.

Chapter 12

Alidina, S., & Funke-Furber, J. (1988). First line nurse managers: Optimizing the span of control. *Journal of Nursing Administration, 18*(5), 34–39.

Altaffer, A. (1998). First-line managers: Measuring their span of control. *Nursing Management, 29*(7), 36–39.

ASQ (American Society for Quality). (n.d.). *Malcolm Baldrige National Quality Award (MBNQA).* Retrieved from http://asq.org/learn-about-quality/malcolm-baldrige-award/overview/overview.html.

Bradley, C. (2014). Leading nursing through influence and structure: The system nurse executive role. *Journal of Nursing Administration, 44*(12), 619–621.

Carayon, P., Xie, A., & Kianfar, S. (2014). Human factors and ergonomics as a patient safety practice. *BMJ Quality & Safety, 23*(3), 196–205.

Charnes, M., & Tewksbury, L. (1993). The continuum of organization structures. In *Collaborative management in health care: Implementing the integrative organization* (pp. 20–43). San Francisco, CA: Jossey-Bass.

Choi, S., Jang, I., Park, S., & Lee, H. (2014). Effects of organizational culture, self-leadership and empowerment on job satisfaction and turnover intention in general hospital nurses. *Journal of Korean Academy of Nursing Administration, 20*(2), 206–214.

Cicolini, G., Comparcini, D., & Simonetti, V. (2014). Workplace empowerment and nurses' job satisfaction: A systematic literature review. *Journal of Nursing Management, 22*(7), 855–871.

Clegg, S. R. (1990). *Modern organizations: Organization studies in the postmodern world.* London, UK: Sage Publications.

Dale Carnegie Training. (2016). *Organizational assessments.* Retrieved from http://www.dalecarnegie.com/organizational-assessment/.

Dartmouth Institute for Health Policy & Clinical Practice. (2010). *Microsystems at a glance.* Retrieved from http://clinicalmicrosystem.org/wp-content/uploads/2014/07/glance_booklet.pdf.

DiCuccio, M. H. (2015). The relationship between patient safety culture and patient outcomes: A systematic review. *Journal of Patient Safety, 11*(3), 135–142.

Donabedian, A. (1980). *Explorations in quality assessment and monitoring: The definition of quality and approaches to its assessment* (Vol. 1). Ann Arbor, MI: Health Administration Press.

Doran, D., McCutcheon, A. S., Evans, M. G., MacMillan, K., McGillis Hall, L., Pringle, D., et al. (2004). *Impact of the manager's span of control on leadership and performance.* Ottawa, ON, Canada: Canadian Health Services Research Foundation.

Edgren, L., & Barnard, K. (2012). Complex adaptive systems for management of integrated care. *Leadership in Health Services, 25*(1), 39–51.

Eisenstein, H. (1995). The Australian femocratic experiment: A feminist case for bureaucracy. In M. M. Ferree & P. Y. Martin (Eds.), *Feminist organizations: Harvest of the new women's movement* (pp. 69–83). Philadelphia, PA: Temple University Press.

Farmer, D. J. (1997). The postmodern turn and the Socratic gadfly. In H. T. Miller & C. J. Fox (Eds.), *Postmodernism "reality" and public administration* (pp. 105–117). Burke, VA: Chatelaine Press.

Filerman, G. (2003). Closing the management competence gap. *Human Resources for Health, 1*(7), 1–3.

Gantz, N. R., Sherman, R., Jasper, M., Choo, C. G., Herrin-Griffith, D., & Harris, K. (2012). Global nurse leader perspectives on health systems and workforce challenges. *Journal of Nursing Management, 20*(4), 433–443.

Gittell, J. H. (2002). Coordinating mechanisms in care provider groups: Relational coordination as a mediator and input uncertainty as a moderator of performance effects. *Management Science, 48*(11), 1408–1426.

Gittell, J. H. (2004). Achieving focus in hospital care: The role of relational coordination. In R. E. Herzlinger (Ed.), *Consumer-driven health care: Implications for providers, payers, and policymakers* (pp. 683–695). San Francisco, CA: Jossey-Bass.

Hatch, M. J., & Cunliffe, A. L. (2013). *Organization theory: Modern, symbolic, and postmodern perspectives* (3rd ed.). Oxford, UK: Oxford University Press.

Institute for Healthcare Improvement (IHI). (2016). *Clinical Microsystem Assessment Tool.* Retrieved from http://www.ihi.org/resources/pages/tools/clinicalmicrosystemassessmenttool.aspx and http://clinicalmicrosystem.org/wp-content/uploads/2014/07/microsystem_assessment.pdf.

Jaques, E. (1990). In praise of hierarchy. *Harvard Business Review, 68*(1), 127–133.

Kanter, R. M. (1977). *Men and women of the corporation.* New York, NY: Basic Books.

Kerfoot, K. M., & Luquire, R. (2012). Alignment of the system's chief nursing officer: Staff or direct line structure? *Nursing Administration Quarterly, 36*(4), 325–331.

Laschinger, H. K. S. (1996). A theoretical approach to studying work empowerment in nursing: A review of studies testing Kanter's theory of structural power in organizations. *Nursing Administration Quarterly, 20*(2), 25–41.

Laschinger, H. K. S., & Fida, R. (2014). A time-lagged analysis of the effect of authentic leadership on workplace bullying, burnout, and occupational turnover intentions. *European Journal of Work and Organizational Psychology, 23*(5), 739–753.

Laschinger, H. K., Wong, C. A., Cummings, G. G., & Grau, A. (2014). Resonant leadership and workplace empowerment: The value of positive organizational cultures in reducing workplace incivility. *Nursing Economics, 32*(1), 5–15, 44.

Laschinger, H. K., Wong, C. A., & Grau, A. (2013). Authentic leadership, empowerment and burnout: A comparison in new graduates and experienced nurses. *Journal of Nursing Management, 21*(3), 541–552.

Laschinger, H. K., Wong, C. A., Grau, A. L., Read, E. A., & Pineau Stam, L. M. (2012). The influence of leadership practices and empowerment on Canadian nurse manager outcomes. *Journal of Nursing Management, 20*(7), 877–888.

Leatt, P., Lemieux-Charles, L., & Aird, C. (1994). Program management: Introduction and overview. In L. Lemieux-Charles, P. Leatt, & C. Aird (Eds.), *Program management and beyond: Management innovations in Ontario hospitals* (pp. 1–10). Ottawa, ON, Canada: Canadian College of Health Service Executives.

Lorenz, H. L. (2008). Service line leadership. *Nurse Leader, 6*(1), 42–43.

Mahon, A., & Young, R. (2006). Health care managers as a critical component of the health care workforce. In C. Dubois, M. McKee, & E. Nolte (Eds.), *Human resources for health in Europe* (pp. 116–139). Berkshire, United Kingdom: Open University Press.

Mark, B. A., Sayler, J., & Smith, C. S. (1996). A theoretical model for nursing systems outcomes research. *Nursing Administration Quarterly, 20*(4), 12–27.

Matthews, S., Laschinger, H. K. S., & Johnstone, L. (2006). Staff nurse empowerment in line and staff organizational structures for chief nurse executives. *Journal of Nursing Administration, 6*(11), 526–533.

McCutcheon, A. S. (2004). *Relationships between leadership style, span of control and outcomes.* Unpublished doctoral dissertation, Toronto, ON, Canada: University of Toronto.

McDaniel, R. R., Driebe, D., & Lanham, H. J. (2013). Health care organizations as complex systems: New perspectives on design and management. *Advances in Health Care Management*, 15, 3–26.

McIntosh, N., Meterko, M., Burgess, J. F., Jr., Restuccia, J. D., Kartha, A., Kaboli, P., et al. (2014). Organizational predictors of coordination in inpatient medicine. *Health Care Management Review*, 39(4), 279–292.

Meier, K. J., & Bohte, J. (2003). Span of control and public organizations: Implementing Luther Gulick's research design. *Public Administration Review*, 63(1), 61–70.

Meyer, R. M. (2008). Span of management: Concept analysis. *Journal of Advanced Nursing*, 63(1), 104–112.

Meyer, R. M., & O'Brien-Pallas, L. (2010). Nursing Services Delivery Theory: An open system approach. *Journal of Advanced Nursing*, 66(12), 2828–2838.

Morash, R., Brintnell, J., & Rodger, G. L. (2005). A span of control tool for clinical managers. *Canadian Journal of Nursing Leadership*, 18(3), 83–93.

O'Connor, E. S. (1999). The politics of management thought: A case study of the Harvard Business School and the Human Relations School. *Academy of Management Review*, 24(1), 117–131.

Pabst, M. K. (1993). Span of control on nursing inpatient units. *Nursing Economic$*, 11(2), 87–90.

Porter-O'Grady, T. (2015). Confluence and convergence: Team effectiveness in complex systems. *Nursing Administration Quarterly*, 39(1), 78–83.

Porter-O'Grady, T., & Malloch, K. (2014). *Quantum leadership: Building better partnerships for sustainable health* (4th ed.). Burlington, MA: Jones & Bartlett Learning.

Prins, G. (2000). *Testing theories on structure and strategy: An assessment of organizational knowledge*. Delft, The Netherlands: Eburon.

Read, E. A. (2014). Workplace social capital in nursing: An evolutionary concept analysis. *Journal of Advanced Nursing*, 70(5), 997–1007.

Redman, R. W., & Jones, K. R. (1998). Effects of implementing patient centered care models on nurse and non-nurse managers. *Journal of Nursing Administration*, 28(11), 46–53.

Reed, M. I. (1992). *The sociology of organizations: Themes, perspectives and prospects*. New York, NY: Harvester Wheatsheaf.

Rouse, W. B. (2008). Health care as a complex adaptive system: Implications for design and management. *Bridge-Washington-National Academy of Engineering*, 38(1), 17.

Scott, W. R. (1992). *Organizations: Rational, natural, and open systems* (3rd ed.). Englewood Cliffs, NJ: Prentice-Hall.

Shirey, M. R., & White-Williams, C. (2015). Boundary spanning leadership practices for population health. *Journal of Nursing Administration*, 45(9), 411–415.

Smith, L., Andrusyszyn, M. A., & Spence Laschinger, H. K. (2010). Effects of workplace incivility and empowerment on newly-graduated nurses' organizational commitment. *Journal of Nursing Management*, 18(8), 1004–1015.

Tichy, N. M., Tushman, M. L., & Fombrun, C. (1979). Social network analysis for organizations. *Academy of Management Review*, 4(4), 507–519.

Weber, M. (1978). *Economy and society: An outline of interpretive sociology* (E. Fischoff, H. Gerth, A. M. Henderson, F. Kolegar, C. W. Mills, T. Parsons, M. Rheinstein, G. Roth, E. Shils, & C. Wittich, Trans., Vol. 2). Berkeley, CA: University of California Press.

Wenger, E. (2008). *Communities of practice: A brief introduction*. Retrieved from https://scholarsbank.uoregon.edu/xmlui/bitstream/handle/1794/11736/A%20brief%20introduction%20to%20CoP.pdf.

West, E., & Barron, D. N. (2005). Social and geographical boundaries around senior nurse and physician leaders: An application of social network analysis. *Canadian Journal of Nursing Research*, 37(3), 132–148.

Willem, A., Buelens, M., & De Jonghe, I. (2007). Impact of organizational structure on nurses' job satisfaction: A questionnaire survey. *International Journal of Nursing Studies*, 44, 1011–1020.

Wong, C. A., & Laschinger, H. K. (2013). Authentic leadership, performance and job satisfaction: The mediating role of empowerment. *Journal of Advanced Nursing*, 69(4), 947–959.

Wong, C. A., Elliot-Miller, P., Laschinger, H. K., Cuddihy, M., Meyer, R., Keatings, M., et al. (2015). Examining the relationships between span of control and manager and unit work outcomes in Ontario academic hospitals. *Journal of Nursing Management*, 23(2), 156–168.

Yang, J., Liu, Y., Huang, C., & Zhu, L. (2013). Impact of empowerment on professional practice environments and organizational commitment among nurses: A structural equation approach. *International Journal of Nursing Practice*, 19(S1), 44–55.

Young, G. J., Charnes, M. P., & Heeren, T. C. (2004). Product line management in professional organizations: An empirical test of competing theoretical perspectives. *Academy of Management Journal*, 47(5), 723–734.

Chapter 13

American Hospital Association. (2016). *2016 American Hospital Association Environmental scan*. Retrieved from http://www.hhnmag.com/articles/3199-american-hospital-association-environmental-scan.

American Nurses Association. (2015). *4 health care trends that will affect American nurses*. Retrieved from http://nursingworld.org/MainMenuCategories/CareerCenter/Resources/4-Health-Care-Trends-That-Will-Affect-American-Nurses.html.

American Nurses Credentialing Center. (2016). *Find a Magnet hospital*. Retrieved from http://www.nursecredentialing.org/Magnet/FindaMagnetFacility.

Aston, G. (2015). Telehealth promises to reshape health care: Hospitals embrace powerful new tools to continuously connect to patients. *H&HN Hospitals & Health Networks*. Retrieved from http://www.hhnmag.com/articles/3648-telehealth-promises-to-reshape-health-care.

Brull, S. (2015). Successful shared governance through education. *Nursing Economic$*, 33(6), 314–319.

Centralization. In *BusinessDictionary.com*. (2016). Retrieved from http://www.businessdictionary.com/definition/centralization.html.

Clavelle, J. T., Porter-O'Grady, T., & Drenkard, K. (2013). Structural empowerment and the nursing practice environment in Magnet organizations. *Journal of Nursing Administration*, 43(11), 566–573.

Davidson, S., Weberg, D., Porter-O'Grady, T., & Malloch, K. (Eds.). (2016). *Leadership for evidence-based innovation in nursing and health professions*. Sudbury, MA: Jones & Bartlett.

Decentralization. *BusinessDictionary.com*. (2016). Retrieved from http://www.businessdictionary.com/definition/decentralization.html.

Elsevier. (2014). *Is Magnet status worth the cost?* Retrieved from http://confidenceconnected.com/blog/2014/10/30/is-magnet-status-worth-the-cost/.

Finkelman, A., & Kenner, C. (2016). *Professional nursing concepts*. Burlington, MA: Jones & Bartlett Learning.

French-Bravo, M., & Crow, G. (2015). Shared governance: The role of buy-in in bringing about change. *Online Journal of Issues in Nursing*, 20(2), 8.

Gallup Inc. (2014). *State of the American workplace*. Retrieved from http://www.gallup.com/poll/181289/majority-employees-not-engaged-despite-gains-2014.aspx.

Gray, B. B. (2013). *Taking control through shared governance*. Retrieved from https://www.nurse.com/blog/2013/02/18/taking-control-through-shared-governance-2/.

Hoying, C., & Allen, S. (2011). Enhancing shared governance for interdisciplinary practice. *Nursing Administration Quarterly*, 35(3), 252–259.

Hoying, C., Lecher, W. T., Mosko, D. D., Roberto, N., Mason, C., Murphy, S. W., et al. (2014). On the scene: Cincinnati. *Nursing Administration Quarterly*, 38(1), 28–29.

Institute of Healthcare Improvement (IHI). (2016). *The IHI triple aim*. Retrieved from http://www.ihi.org/engage/initiatives/tripleaim/pages/default.aspx.

Jordan, B. A. (2016). Designing a unit practice council structure. *Nursing Management*, 47(1), 15, 16, 18.

Kastelle, T. (2013). Hierarchy is overrated. *Harvard Business Review*. Retrieved from https://hbr.org/2013/11/hierarchy-is-overrated/.

Kneflin, N., O'Quinn, L., Geigle, G., Mott, B., Nebrig, D., & Munafo, J. (2016). Direct care nurses on the shared governance journey towards positive patient outcomes. *Journal of Clinical Nursing, 25*(5/6), 875–882.

Kurian, G. T. (2013). *AMA dictionary of business and management.* New York, NY: AMACOM.

Legare, F., & Witterman, H. (2013). Shared decision making: Examining key elements and barriers to adoption into routine clinical practice. *Health Affairs, 32*(2), 276–284.

Mathias, J. M. (2015). Shared governance teaches staff to take ownership of decision making. *OR Manager.* Retrieved from http://web.a.ebscohost.com/ehost/detail/detail?vid=2&sid=41bf6ac2-89fb-4d2c-aab1-24b58624ccba%40sessionmgr4003&hid=4112&bdata=JnNpdGU9ZWhvc3QtbGl2ZSZzY29wZT1zaXRl#AN=103794440&db=rzh.

McHugh, M. D., Kelly, L. A., Smith, H. L., Wu, E. S., Vanak, J. M., & Aiken, L. H. (2013). Lower mortality in Magnet hospitals. *Medical Care, 51*(5), 382–388.

Mitchell, P., Wynia, M., Golden, R., McNellis, B., Okun, S., Webb, C. E., et al. (2012). *Core principles & values of effective team-based health care.* Discussion paper. Washington, DC: Institute of Medicine. Retrieved from https://www.nationalahec.org/pdfs/vsrt-team-based-care-principles-values.pdf.

Porter-O'Grady, T., & Malloch, K. (2015). *Quantum leadership: Advancing innovation, transforming health care* (4th ed.). Burlington, MA: Jones & Bartlett.

Swihart, D., & Hess, R. (2014). *Shared governance: A practical approach to transforming interprofessional healthcare* (3rd ed.). Danvers, MA: HCPro.

Wilson, J., Speroni, K. G., Jones, R. A., & Daniel, M. G. (2014). Exploring how nurses and managers perceive shared governance. *Nursing, 44*(7), 19–22.

Chapter 14

American Nurses Association. (2013). *ANA Leadership Institute™ competency model.* Retrieved from https://learn.ana-nursingknowledge.org/template/ana/publications_pdf/leadershipInstitute_competency_model_brochure.pdf.

American Nurses Credentialing Center. (2013). *2014 Magnet® application manual.* Silver Spring, MD: Author. http://www.nursecredentialing.org/MagnetApplicationManual.

American Organization of Nurse Executives (AONE). (2015). *Nurse executive competencies.* Retrieved from http://www.aone.org/resources/nec.pdf.

Centers for Disease Control and Prevention. (2015). *Public Health Information Network Communities of Practice: Do a SWOT analysis.* Retrieved from http://www.cdc.gov/phcommunities/resourcekit/evaluate/swot_analysis.html.

Institute for Healthcare Improvement (IHI). (2016). *IHI Triple Aim initiative.* Retrieved from http://www.ihi.org/engage/initiatives/tripleaim/pages/default.aspx.

Institute of Medicine (IOM). (2011). *The future of nursing: Leading change, advancing health.* Washington, DC: National Academies Press.

Jasper, M., & Crossan, F. (2012). What is strategic management? *Journal of Nursing Management, 20*(7), 838–846. doi:10.1111/jonm.12001.

Jones, B. (2015). Mission versus purpose: What's the difference? Talking Point: *The Disney Institute* blog. Retrieved from https://disneyinstitute.com/blog/2015/04/mission-versus-purpose-whats-the-difference/346/.

Kotter, J. P. (2014). *Accelerate: Building strategic agility for a faster-moving world.* Boston, MA: Harvard Business Review Press.

Management Study Guide. (n.d.). *Strategic management—meaning and important concepts.* Retrieved from http://www.managementstudyguide.com/strategic-management.htm.

Nag, R., Hambrick, D. C., & Chen, M.-J. (2007). What is strategic management, really? Inductive derivation of a consensus definition of the field. *Strategic Management Journal, 28*(9), 935–955.

National Academies of Sciences, Engineering, and Medicine (NAM). (2015). *Assessing progress on the Institute of Medicine Report The Future of Nursing.* Washington, DC: National Academies Press. Retrieved from http://www.nap.edu/catalog/21838/assessing-progress-on-the-institute-of-medicine-report-the-future-of-nursing.

Oermann, M. H. (2002). Developing a professional portfolio in nursing. *Orthopaedic Nursing, 21*(2), 73–78.

Pearce, J. A., & Robinson, R. (2012). *Strategic management* (13th ed.). New York, NY: McGraw-Hill/Irwin.

Rand Health. (n.d.). *The Affordable Care Act in depth.* Retrieved from http://www.rand.org/health/key-topics/aca/in-depth.html.

Shirey, M. R. (2015). Strategic agility for nursing leadership. *Journal of Nursing Administration, 45*(6), 305–308. doi:10.1097/NNA.0000000000000204.

Society for Human Resource Management (SHRM). (2012). *Mission and vision statements: What is the difference between mission, vision and value statements?* Retrieved from http://www.shrm.org/templatestools/hrqa/pages/isthereadifferencebetweenacompany'smission,visionandvaluestatements.aspx.

Stakeholder. (n.d.). In *BusinessDictionary.com.* Retrieved from http://www.businessdictionary.com/definition/stakeholder.html.

The Joint Commission. (2016). *Certification Comprehensive Stroke Center.* Retrieved from http://www.jointcommission.org/certification/advanced_certification_comprehensive_stroke_centers.aspx.

Titzer, J., Phillips, T., Tooley, S., Hall, N., & Shirey, M. (2013). Nurse manager succession planning: Synthesis of the evidence. *Journal of Nursing Management, 21*, 971–979.

Wadsworth, B., Felton, F., & Linus, R. (2016). SOARing into strategic planning: Engaging nurses to achieve significant outcomes. *Nursing Administration Quarterly, 40*(4), 299–306.

Whittington, J. W., Nolan, K., Lewis, N., & Torres, T. (2015). Pursuing the Triple Aim: The first 7 years. *Milbank Quarterly, 93*(2), 263–300. Retrieved from http://www.milbank.org/uploads/documents/featured-articles/pdf/Milbank_Quarterly_Vol-93_No-_2_Pursuing_the_Triple_Aim_The_First_7_Years.pdf.

Chapter 15

Adams, D. (2004). *The pillars of planning: Mission values, vision.* Washington, DC: National Endowment for the Arts. Retrieved from https://4good.org/morrie-warshawski-consultant/the-pillars-of-planning-mission-vision-values-by-don-adams.

Aiken, L., Cimiotti, J., Sloane, D., Smith, H., Lynn, L., & Neff, D. (2011). Effects of nurse staffing and nurse education on patient deaths in hospitals with different nurse work environments. *Medical Care, 49*(12), 1047–1053.

Aiken, L., Sloane, D., Bruyneel, L., Van den Heede, K., Sermeus, W., & RN4CAST Consortium. (2013). Nurses' reports of working conditions and hospital quality of care in 12 countries in Europe. *International Journal of Nursing Studies, 50*(2), 143–153.

Aiken, L. H., Sloane, D. M., Griffiths, P., Rafferty, A. M., Bruyneel, L., McHugh., et al. (2016). Nursing skill mix in European hospitals: Cross-sectional study of the association with mortality, patient ratings, and quality of care. *BMJ Quality & Safety,* 1–10. Retrieved from http://qualitysafety.bmj.com/content/early/2016/11/03/bmjqs-2016-005567.full.pdf+html.

American Association of Critical-Care Nurses (AACN). (n.d.). *Synergy Model: Basic information about the AACN Synergy Model for Patient Care.* Retrieved from https://www.aacn.org/nursing-excellence/aacn-standards/synergy-model.

American Nurses Association. (2015). *The Registered Nurse Safe Staffing Act.* Retrieved from http://www.nursingworld.org/MainMenuCategories/Policy-Advocacy/State/Legislative-Agenda-Reports/State-StaffingPlansRatios.

American Organization of Nurse Executives (AONE). (2012). *AONE guiding principles for the role of the nurse in future care delivery toolkit.* Washington, DC: Author.

Brookes, J. (2011). Engaging staff in the change process. *Nursing Management, 18*(5), 16–19.

Burman, M., Robinson, B., & Hart, A. M. (2013). Linking evidence-based nursing practice and patient-centered care through patient preferences. *Nursing Administration Quarterly, 37*(3), 231–241.

Canadian Institute for Health Information. (2017). *Hospital reportsSeries*. Retrieved from https://secure.cihi.ca/estore/productSeries.htm?pc= PCC219.

Case Management Society of America (CMSA). (2016). *What is a case manager?* Little Rock, AR: Author. Retrieved from http://www.cmsa.org/Home/CMSA/WhatisaCaseManager/tabid/224/Default.aspx.

Chow, S. K. Y., & Wong, F. K. Y. (2010). Health-related quality of life in patients undergoing peritoneal dialysis: Effects of a nurse-led case management programme. *Journal of Advanced Nursing, 66*(8), 1780–1792.

Cole, L., & Houston, S. (1999). Structured care methodologies: Evolution and use in patient care delivery. *Outcomes Management for Nursing Practice, 3*(2), 53–59.

Donabedian, A. (1988). The quality of care: how can it be assessed? *Journal of the American Medical Association, 260*, 1743–1748.

Dubois, C-A., D'Amour, D., Tchouaket, E., Clarke, S., Rivard, M., & Blais, R. (2013). Association of patient safety outcomes with models of nursing care organization at unit level in hospitals. *Journal for Quality in Health Care, 25*(2), 110–117.

Engelke, M. K., Guttu, M., Warren, M. B., & Swanson, M. (2008). School nurse case management for children with chronic illness: Health, academic, and quality of life outcomes. *The Journal of School Nursing, 24*(4), 205–214.

Epstein, R. M., & Street, R. L. (2011). The values and value of patient-centered care. *The Annals of Family Medicine, 9*(2), 100–103.

Erickson, J. I., & Ditomassi, M. (2011). Professional practice model: Strategies for translating models into practice. *Nursing Clinics of North America, 46*, 35–44.

Fernandez, R., Johnson, M., Tran, D. T., & Miranda, C. (2012). Models of care in nursing: A systematic review. *International Journal of Evidence-Based Healthcare, 10*(4), 324–337.

Gaudine, A., & Thorne, L. (2012). Nurses' ethical conflict with hospitals: A longitudinal study of outcomes. *Nursing Ethics, 19*(6), 727–737.

Grabowski, D., Elliot, A., Leitzell, B., Coehn, L., & Zimmerman, S. (2014). Who are the innovators? Nursing homes implementing cultural change. *The Gerontologist, 54*(S1), S65–S75.

Hajewski, C., & Shirey, M. (2014). Care coordination: A model for the acute care hospital setting. *Journal of Nursing Administration, 44*(11), 577–585.

Hardcastle, L. E., Record, K. L., Jacobson, P. D., & Gostin, L. O. (2011). Improving the population's health: The Affordable Care Act and the importance of integration. *The Journal of Law, Medicine & Ethics, 39*(3), 317–327.

Hayes, L., O'Brien-Pallas, L., Duffield, C., Shamian, J., Buchan, J., Hughes, F., et al. (2012). Nurse turnover: a literature review–an update. *International Journal of Nursing Studies, 49*(7), 887–905.

Houston, S., Leveille, M., Luquire, R., Fike, A., Ogola, G. O., & Chando, S. (2012). Decisional involvement in Magnet®, Magnet-aspiring, and non-Magnet hospitals. *Journal of Nursing Administration, 42*(12), 586–591.

Huber, D. L. (2013). Professional practice models. In D. L. Huber (Ed.), *Leadership and nursing care management* (5th ed., pp. 256–273). St. Louis, MO: Elsevier.

Institute of Medicine (IOM). (2001). *Crossing the quality chasm: A new health system for the 21st century*. Washington, DC: National Academies Press.

Jackson, G. L., Powers, B. J., Chatterjee, R., Bettger, J. P., Kemper, A. R., Hasselblad, V., et al. (2013). The patient-centered medical home: A systematic review. *Annals of Internal Medicine, 158*(3), 169–178.

Jost, S. G., & Rich, V. L. (2010). Transformation of a nursing cuture through actualization of a nursing professional practice model. *Nursing Administration Quarterly, 34*(1), 30–40.

Kalisch, B., & Lee, K. H. (2011). Nurse staffing levels and teamwork: A cross-sectional study of patient care units in acute care hospitals. *Journal of Nursing Scholarship, 43*(1), 82–88.

Katon, W. J., Lin, E. H. B., Von Korff, M., Ciechanowski, P., Ludman, E. J., Young, B., Peterson, D., Rutter, C. M., McGregor, M., & McCulloch, D. (2010). Collaborative care for patients with depression and chronic illnesses. *New England Journal of Medicine, 363*(27), 2611–2620.

Katz, R. E., & Frank, R. G. (2010). A vision for the future: New care delivery models can play a vital role in building tomorrow's eldercare workforce. *Generations: Journal of the American Society on Aging, 34*(4), 82–88.

Kimball, B., Joynt, J., Cherner, D., & O'Neil, E. (2007). The quest for new innovative care delivery models. *Journal of Nursing Administration, 37*(9), 392–398.

Kramer, M., Schmalenberg, C., & Maguire, P. (2010). Nine structures and leadership practices essential to a magnetic (healthy) work environment. *Nursing Administration Quarterly, 34*(1), 4–17.

Landman, N., Aannestad, L., Smoldt, R., & Cortese, D. (2014). Teamwork in health care. *Nursing Administration Quarterly, 38*(3), 198–205.

Légaré, F., & Witteman, H. O. (2013). Shared decision making: Examining key elements and barriers to adoption into routine clinical practice. *Health Affairs, 32*(2), 276–284.

Luzinski, C. (2012). Exemplary professional practice: The core of a Magnet® organization. *The Journal of Nursing Administration, 42*(2), 72–73.

MacPhee, M. (2007). Strategies and tools for managing change. *Journal of Nursing Administration, 37*(9), 405–413.

MacPhee, M. (2014). *Valuing patient safety: Responsible workforce design*. Ottawa, ON, Canada: Canadian Federation of Nurses' Unions. Retrieved from https://nursesunions.ca/sites/default/files/valuing_patient_safety_web_may_2014.pdf.

Mattila, E., Pitkanen, A., Alanen, S., Leino, K., Luojus, K., Rantanen, A., & Aalto, P. (2014). The effects of the primary nursing care model: A systematic review. *Journal of Nursing & Care, 3*(205). doi:10.4172/2167-1168.1000205.

McHugh, M., Kelly, L., Smith, H., Wu, E., Vanak, J., & Aiken, L. H. (2013). Lower mortality in magnet hospitals. *Medical Care, 51*(5), 382.

Minnick, A. F., Mion, L. C., Johnson, M. E., & Catrambone, C. (2007). How unit level nursing responsibilities are structured in U.S. hospitals. *Journal of Nursing Administration, 37*(10), 452–458.

Murphy, M., Hinch, B., Llewellyn, J., Dillon, P., & Carlson, E. (2011). Promoting professional nursing practice: Linking a professional practice model to performance expectations. *Nursing Clinics of North America, 46*, 67–79.

Naylor, M. (2012). Advancing high value transitional care: The central role of nursing and its leadership. *Nursing Administration Quarterly, 36*(2), 115–126.

Porter, M. (2010). What is value in health care? *New England Journal of Medicine, 363*(26), 2477–2481.

Rathert, C., Wyrwich, M. D., & Austin, S. (2013). Patient-centered care and outcomes: A systematic review of the literature. *Medical Care Research and Review, 70*(4), 351–379.

Reverby, S. (1987). *Ordered to care: The dilemma of American nursing, 1850–1945*. Cambridge, MA: Cambridge University Press.

Shirey, M. R. (2008). Nursing practice models for acute and critical care: Overview of care delivery models. *Critical Care Nursing Clinics of North America, 20*, 365–373.

Stiggelbout, A. M., Van der Weijden, T., De Wit, M. P. T., Frosch, D., Légaré, F., Montori, V. M., Trevena, L., & Elwyn, G. (2012). Shared decision making: Really putting patients at the centre of healthcare. *British Medical Journal, 344*(7842), 28–31.

Stimpfel, A., Rosen, J., & McHugh, M. (2014). Understanding the role of the professional practice environment on quality of care in Magnet® and non-magnet hospitals. *Journal of Nursing Administration, 44*(1), 10–16.

Tran, D., Johnson, M., Fernandez, R., & Jones, S. (2010). A shared care model vs. a patient allocation model of nursing care delivery: Comparing nursing staff satisfaction and stress outcomes. *International Journal of Nursing Practice, 16*, 148–158.

Vanhaecht, K., Panella, M., Van Zelm, R., & Sermeus, W. (2010). An overview on the history and concept of care pathways as complex interventions. *International Journal of Care Pathways, 14*(3), 117–123.

Watts, T. (2012). End-of-life care pathways as tools to promote and support a good death: A critical commentary. *European Journal of Cancer Care, 21*(1), 20–30.

White, H., & Glazier, R. (2011). Do hospitalist physicians improve the quality of inpatient care delivery? A systematic review of process, efficiency and outcome measures. *BMC Medicine, 9*(58), 1–22.

Chapter 16

Advancing Integrated Mental Health Solutions (AIMS) Center. (2016). *Our projects*. University of Washington, Psychiatry and Behavioral Sciences Division of Integrated Care and Public Health. Retrieved from http://aims.uw.edu/projects.

Ahmed, O. I. (2016). Disease management, case management, care management, and care coordination: A framework and brief manual for care programs and staff. *Professional Case Management, 21*(3), 137–146.

American Case Management Association (ACMA). (2013). *Standards of practice & scope of services for health care delivery system case management and transitions of care (TOC) professionals*. Little Rock, AR: Author.

American Nurses Association (ANA). (2016). *Title "nurse" protection: Summary of language by state, policy and advocacy, title protection*. Retrieved from http://www.nursingworld.org/MainMenuCategories/Policy-Advocacy/State/Legislative-Agenda-Reports/State-TitleNurse/Title-Nurse-Summary-Language.html.

American Organization of Nurse Executives (AONE). (2015). *Nurse executive competencies: Population health*. Washington, DC: Author.

Ashford, J. B., & LeCroy, C. W. (2013). *Human behavior in the social environment: A multi-dimensional perspective* (5th ed.). Belmont, CA: Cengage Learning.

Berger, C. S. (2009). Social work case management in medical settings. In A. R. Roberts (Ed.), *Social workers' desk reference* (2nd ed., pp. 790–796). New York, NY: Oxford University Press.

Berwick, D. M., Nolan, T. W., & Whittington, J. (2008). The Triple Aim: Care, health, and cost. *Health Affairs, 27*(3), 759–769.

Braden, C. J. (2002). *State of the science paper #2: Involvement/participation, empowerment and knowledge outcome indicators of case management*. Little Rock, AR: Case Management Society of America.

Brown, R. S., Peikes, D., Peterson, G., Schore, J., & Razafindrakoto, C. M. (2012). Six features of Medicare coordinated care demonstration programs that cut hospital admissions of high-risk patients. *Health Affairs, 31*(6), 1156–1166.

Butler, M., Kane, R. L., McAlpine, D., Kathol, R. G., Fu, S. S., Hagedorn, H., et al. (2008). *Integration of mental health/substance abuse and primary care*. Evidence reports/technology assessments No. 173 (Prepared by the Minnesota Evidence-based Practice Center under Contract No. 290-02-0009.) AHRQ Publication No. 09-E003. Rockville, MD: Agency for Healthcare Research and Quality.

Calhoun, C., Hall, L. K., & Kemper, D. (2016). Patient engagement: Engaging patients in the care process by leveraging meaningful use goals. In D. B. Nash, R. J. Fabius, A. Skoufalos, J. L. Clarke, & M. R. Horowitz (Eds.), *Population health: Creating a culture of wellness* (2nd ed., Chapter 7). Burlington, MA: Jones and Bartlett Learning.

Canadian Interprofessional Health Collaborative (CIHC). (2010). *A national interprofessional competency framework*. College of Health Disciplines, University of British Columbia. Vancouver, Canada: Author.

Care Continuum Alliance (CCA). (2012a). *Implementation and evaluation: A population health guide for primary care models*. Retrieved from http://www.populationhealthalliance.org/publications/population-health-guide-for-primary-care-models.html.

Care Continuum Alliance (CCA). (2012b). *Participant engagement and the use of incentives considerations*. Retrieved from http://www.populationhealthalliance.org/publications.html.

Carr, D. (2009). Building collaborative partnerships in critical care: The RN case manager/social work dyad in critical care. *Professional Case Management, 14*(3), 121–132.

Case Management Society of America (CMSA). (2016a). *Standards of practice for case management*. Little Rock, AR: Author.

Case Management Society of America (CMSA). (2016b). *e4: Engage, empower, enhance, enable*. Little Rock, AR: Author. Retrieved from http://solutions.cmsa.org/acton/fs/blocks/showLandingPage/a/10442/p/p-0015/t/page/fm/0/r/-/s/?sid=jz4BYiipa.

Case Management Society of America (CMSA). (2017). *CMSA core curriculum for case management*. Little Rock, AR: Author.

Centers for Disease Control and Prevention (CDC). (2012). *Chronic disease prevention and health promotion*. Atlanta, GA: Author.

Centers for Medicare & Medicaid Services (CMS). (2003). Medicare program; Demonstration: Capitated disease management for beneficiaries with chronic illnesses. *Federal Register, 68*(40), 9673–9680.

Chen, A., Brown, R., Archibald, N., Aliotta, S., & Fox, P. D. (2000). *Best practices in coordinated care*. MPR 8534-004. Mathematica Policy Research, Inc. Retrieved from https://innovation.cms.gov/files/x/cc-executive-summary.pdf.

Clark, K. A. (1996). Alternate case management models. In D. L. Flarey & S. S. Blancett (Eds.), *Handbook of nursing case management* (pp. 295–304). Gaithersburg, MD: Aspen.

Cline, B. G. (1990). Case management: Organizational models and administrative methods. *Caring: National Association for Home Care Magazine, 9*(7), 14–18.

Coleman, J. R. (1999). Integrated case management: The 21st century challenge for HMO case managers, Part 1. *The Case Manager, 10*(5), 28–34.

Commission for Case Manager Certification (CCMC). (2015). *Code of professional conduct for case managers with standards, rules, procedures, and penalties*. Mount Laurel, NJ: Author.

Commission for Case Manager Certification (CCMC). (2016). *Case management body of knowledge (CMBOK)*. Mount Laurel, NJ: Author.

Daniels, S. (2015). Hospital case management: A new view from the C-Suite. *Professional Case Management, 20*(3), 156–158. doi:10.1097/NCM.0000000000000095.

Disease management. (n.d.). *PHM glossary*. Retrieved from http://www.populationhealthalliance.org/research/phm-glossary/d.html.

Edington, D. W., Schultz, A. B., & Pitts, J. S. (2016). The future of population health at the workplace: Trends, technology, and the role of mind-body and behavioral science. In D. B. Nash, R. J. Fabius, A. Skoufalos, J. L. Clarke, & M. R. Horowitz (Eds.), *Population health: Creating a culture of wellness* (2nd ed., Chapter 20). Burlington, MA: Jones and Bartlett Learning.

Eghaneyan, B. H., Sanchez, K., & Mitschke, D. B. (2014). Implementation of a collaborative care model for the treatment of depression and anxiety in a community health center: Results from a qualitative case study. *Journal of Multidisciplinary Healthcare, 7*, 503–513. dx.doi.org/10.2147/JMDH.S69821.

Ellsworth, J. (2015). Case managers: A key to reducing admissions. *Professional Case Management, 20*(3), 147–149.

Epstein Becker Green. (2015, October 12). *Population health challenges and rewards of integrating behavioral health into primary care*. Webinar. Retrieved from http://www.ebglaw.com/announcements/complimentary-webinar-addresses-challenges-and-rewards-of-integrating-behavioral-health-into-primary-care/.

Fink-Samnick, E., & Muller, L. (2015). Case management practice: Is technology helping or hindering practice in legal and regulatory issues. *Professional Case Management, 20*(2), 98–102.

Fleisher, P., & Henrickson, M. (2002). *Toward a typology of case management. White paper*. Washington DC: National Institutes of Health.

Forbes, M. A. (1999). The practice of professional nurse case management. *Nursing Case Management, 4*(1), 28–33.

Fortney, J., Sladek, R., Unützer, J., Alfred, L., Carneal, G., Emmet, B., et al. (2015). *Fixing behavioral health care in America: A national call for integrating and coordinating specialty behavioral health care with the medical system*. Issue Brief. The Kennedy Forum in Partnership with Advancing Integrated Mental Health Solutions (AIMS) Center, The Kennedy Center for Mental Health Policy and Research, Satcher Health Leadership Institute, Morehouse School of Medicine. Retrieved from http://www.thekennedyforum.com.

Gartner, Inc. (2016). *Predictive modeling*. Retrieved from http://www.gartner.com/it-glossary/predictive-modeling/.

Gillespie, L. (2016, May 21). *Hospitals push Medicare to soften readmission penalties in light of socioeconomic risks*. Modern Healthcare. Retrieved from http://www.modernhealthcare.com/article/20160521/MAGAZINE/305219914.

Goodman, R. A., Bunnell, R., & Posner, S. F. (2014). What is "community health"? Examining the meaning of an evolving field in public health. *Preventive Medicine, 67*(Supp. 1), S58–S61. dx.doi.org/10.1016/j.ypmed.2014.07.028.

Graf, T., Erskine, A., & Steele, G. D. (2014). Leveraging data to systematically improve care coronary artery disease management at Geisinger. *Journal of Ambulatory Care Management, 37*(3), 199–205.

Gupta, A. (2015). *Tech is driving collaboration in behavioral health*. TechCrunch. Retrieved from http://techcrunch.com/2015/09/19/tech-is-driving-collaboration-in-behavioral-health/.

Hawkins, J. W., Veeder, N. W., & Pearce, C. W. (1998). *Nurse–social worker collaboration in managed care*. New York, NY: Springer.

Hawkins, K., Wells, T. S., Hommer, C. E., Ozminkowski, R. J., Richards, D. M., & Yeh, C. S. (2014). Factors driving engagement decisions in care coordination programs. *Professional Case Management, 19*(5), 216–223.

Health Enhancement Research Organization (HERO) and Population Health Alliance (PHA). (2015). *Program measurement & evaluation guide: Core metrics for employee health management*. Retrieved from http://population-healthalliance.org/publications/program-measurement-evaluation-guide-core-metrics-for-employee-health-management.html.

Health Sciences Institute. (2016). *Chronic care professional (CCP) certification*. Retrieved from http://healthsciences.org/Chronic-Care-Professional-Certification.

Herman, C. (2013). *The evolving context of social work case management: NASW releases revised standards of practice, practice perspective*. Washington, DC: National Association of Social Workers.

Hickam, D. H., Weiss, J. W., Guise, J-M., Buckley, D., Motu'apuaka, M., Graham, E., et al. (2013). *Outpatient case management for adults with medical illness and complex care needs*. Comparative Effectiveness Review No. 99. (Prepared by the Oregon Evidence based Practice Center under Contract No. 290-2007-10057-I.) AHRQ Publication No.13-EHC031-EF. Rockville, MD: Agency for Healthcare Research and Quality. Retrieved from http://effectivehealthcare.ahrq.gov/index.cfm/search-for-guides-reviews-and-reports/?pageaction=displayproduct&productid=1369.

Hu, J., Gonsahn, M. D., & Nerenz, D. R. (2014). Socioeconomic status and readmissions: Evidence from an urban teaching hospital. *Health Affairs, 33*(5), 778–785. doi:10.1377/hlthaff.2013.0816.

Huber, D. L. (2002). The diversity of case management models. *Lippincott's Case Management, 7*(6), 212–220.

Huber, D. L. (2005). The diversity of service delivery models. In D. Huber (Ed.), *Disease management: A guide for case managers* (pp. 55–67). Philadelphia, PA: Saunders.

Improving Chronic Illness Care. (2006–2016). *The chronic care model*. Retrieved from http://www.improvingchroniccare.org/index.php?p=The_Chronic_CareModel&s=2.

Institute for Healthcare Improvement (IHI). (2017). *Triple aim for populations*. Retrieved from http://www.ihi.org/Topics/TripleAim/Pages/default.aspx.

Institute of Medicine (IOM). (2001). *Crossing the quality chasm: A new health system for the 21st century*. Washington, DC: National Academies Press.

Interprofessional Education Collaborative (IPEC). (2011). *Core competencies for interprofessional collaborative practice: Report of an expert panel*. Washington, DC: Author.

Katon, W. J., Lin, E. H., Von Korff, M., Ciechanowski, P., Ludman, E. J., Young, B., et al. (2010). Collaborative care for patients with depression and chronic illnesses. *New England Journal of Medicine, 363*(27), 2611–2620.

Kindig, D. A. (2007). Understanding population health terminology. *Milbank Quarterly, 85*(1), 139–161. doi:10.1111/j.1468-0009.2007.00479.x.

Kolbasovsky, A., Zeitlin, J., & Gillespie, W. (2012). Impact of point-of-care case management on readmissions and costs. *The American Journal of Managed Care, 18*(8), 300–306.

Kongstvedt, P. R. (2013). *Essentials of managed health care* (6th ed.). Sudbury, MA: Jones and Bartlett.

Lee, J. (2016). Behavioral economics: How BE influences and changes health. In D. B. Nash, R. J. Fabius, A. Skoufalos, J. L. Clarke, & M. R. Horowitz (Eds.), *Population health: Creating a culture of wellness* (2nd ed., Chapter 8). Burlington, MA: Jones and Bartlett Learning.

Lipold, A. G. (2002, June 19). Disease management comes of age, not a moment too soon. *Business & Health, 7*. Retrieved from http://managedhealthcareexecutive.modernmedicine.com/managed-healthcare-executive/content/disease-management-comes-age-not-moment-too-soon.

Lyles, C. A. (2016). The political landscape in relation to the health and wealth of nations. In D. B. Nash, R. J. Fabius, A. Skoufalos, J. L. Clarke, & M. R. Horowitz (Eds.), *Population health: Creating a culture of wellness* (2nd ed., Chapter 5). Burlington, MA: Jones and Bartlett Learning.

Milliman, Inc. (2014). *Economic impact of integrated medical-behavioral healthcare: Implications for psychiatry*. Milliman American Psychiatric Association Report. Denver, CO: Author.

Momany, E. T., Flach, S. D., Nelson, F. D., & Damiano, P. C. (2006). A cost analysis of the Iowa Medicaid primary care case management program. *Health Services Research, 41*(4 Pt. 1), 1357–1371.

Nagasako, E., Waterman, B., & Dunagan, W. C. (2014). Adding socioeconomic data to hospital readmissions calculations may produce more useful results. *Health Affairs, 33*(5), 786–791. doi:10.1377/hlthaff.2013.1148.

Nash, D., Fabius, R. J., Skoufalos, A., Clarke, J. L., & Horowitz, M. R. (2016). *Preface. Population health: Creating a culture of wellness* (2nd ed.). Burlington, MA: Jones and Bartlett Learning.

National Association of Social Workers (NASW). (2013). *Standards of practice for social work case management*. Washington, DC: Author.

National Association of Chronic Disease Directors (NACDD). (2016). *About NACDD*. Retrieved from http://www.chronicdisease.org/?page=AboutUs.

National Council of State Boards of Nursing (NCSBN). (2016). *Nurse licensure compact*. Retrieved from https://www.ncsbn.org/nurse-licensure-compact.htm.

Nobel, J. J., & Norman, G. K. (2003). Emerging information management technologies and the future of disease management. *Disease Management, 6*(4), 219–231.

Older Americans Act. (1965). *42 U.S.C. 3056*. Retrieved from http://www.gpo.gov/fdsys/pkg/STATUTE-79/pdf/STATUTE-79-Pg218.pdf.

Plocher, D. W. (2013). Fundamentals and core competencies of disease management. In P. R. Kongstvedt (Ed.), *Essentials of managed health care* (6th ed., Chapter 8). Sudbury, MA: Jones and Bartlett.

Population Health Alliance (PHA). (2015). *2015 Population health alliance outcomes guidelines report*. Washington, DC: Author.

Population health management. (n.d.). *PHM glossary*. Retrieved from http://www.populationhealthalliance.org/research/phm-glossary/p.html.

Prochaska, J. O., & Prochaska, J. M. (2016). *Behavior change, population health: Creating a culture of wellness* (2nd ed.). Burlington, MA: Jones and Bartlett Learning.

Raiff, N. R., & Shore, B. K. (1993). *Advanced case management: New strategies for the nineties*. Newbury Park, CA: Sage.

Rheaume, A., Frisch, S., Smith, A., & Kennedy, C. (1994). Case management and nursing practice. *Journal of Nursing Administration, 24*(3), 30–36.

Rice, S. (2016, January 12). Adjusting for social determinants in value-based payments still fuzzy. *Modern Healthcare*. Retrieved from http://www.modernhealthcare.com/article/20160112/NEWS/160119972.

Ridgely, M. S., & Willenbring, M. C. (1992). Application of case management to drug abuse treatment: Overview of models and research issues. *NIDA Monograph, 127*, 12–33.

Robbins, C., & Birmingham, J. (2005). The social worker and nurse roles in case management applying the three Rs. *Lippincott's Case Management, 10*(3), 120–127.

Robert Wood Johnson Foundation. (2011). *Mental disorders and medical co-morbidity, research synthesis*. Report 21. Princeton, NJ: Author.

Rushton, S. (2015). The population care coordination process. *Professional Case Management, 20*(5), 230–238.

SAS. (2016). *What is Big Data?* Retrieved from http://www.sas.com/en_us/insights/big-data.html.

Schore, J. L., Brown, R. S., & Cheh, V. A. (1999). Case management for high-cost Medicare beneficiaries. *Health Care Financing Review, 20*(4), 87–101.

Shaljian, M., & Nielsen, M. (2013). *Managing populations, maximizing technology: Population health management in the medical neighborhood*. Washington, DC: Patient-Centered Primary Care Collaborative.

Shortell, S. M., Anderson, D. A., Gilles, R. R., Mitchell, J. B., & Morgan, K. L. (1993). The holographic organization. *Healthcare Forum Journal, 36*(2), 20–26.

Sidorov, J., & Romney, M. (2016). The spectrum of care. In D. B. Nash, R. J. Fabius, A. Skoufalos, J. L. Clarke, & M. R. Horowitz (Eds.), *Population health: Creating a culture of wellness* (2nd ed., Chapter 2). Burlington, MA: Jones and Bartlett Learning.

Social Security Act of 1935. (2013). *Legislative history*. Retrieved from http://www.ssa.gov/history/35act.html.

Stellefson, M., Dipnarine, K., & Stopka, C. (2013). The chronic care model and diabetes management in US primary care settings: A systematic review. *Preventing Chronic Disease, 10*, 1–21. doi:http://dx.doi.org/10.5888/pcd10.120180.

Summers, N. (2016). *Fundamentals of case management practice: Skills for the human services* (5th ed.). Boston, MA: Cengage Learning.

Tahan, H. A. (2017). The case management process. In H. A. Tahan & T. M. Treiger (Eds.), *CMSA core curriculum for case management* (3rd ed.). Philadelphia, PA: Wolters Kluwer.

Takeda, A., Taylor, S. J. C., Taylor, R. S., Kahn, F., Krum, H., & Underwood, M. (2012). *Clinical service organisation for heart failure. Cochrane Database of Systematic Reviews*, (9), CD002752. doi:10.1002/14651858.CD002752.pub3.

The Joint Commission (TJC). (2015). *Facts about disease-specific care certification*. Retrieved from https://www.jointcommission.org/facts_about_disease-specific_care_certification/.

The Joint Commission (TJC). (2016). *What is certification?* Retrieved from https://www.jointcommission.org/certification/certification_main.aspx.

Treadwell, J., & Bean, G. (2009). Supporting disease management through inventions in the medical home. *Professional Case Management, 14*(4), 192–197.

Treiger, T. M. (2011). Case management: Prospects in definition, education, and settings of practice. *The Remington Report, 19*(1), 46–48.

Treiger, T. M. (2012). Helping clients bridge gaps to self-advocacy, self-management. *Healthcare Intelligence Network*. [interview] Retrieved from http://hin.com/blog/2012/09/14/meet-healthcare-case-management-manager-teresa-treiger-helping-clients-bridge-gaps-to-self-advocacy-self-management.

Treiger, T. M., & Fink-Samnick, E. (2013). COLLABORATE: A universal competency based paradigm for professional case management, part I: Introduction, historical validation, and competency presentation. *Professional Case Management, 18*(3), 122–135.

Treiger, T. M., & Fink-Samnick, E. (2016). *COLLABORATE for professional case management: A universal competency-based paradigm*. Philadelphia, PA: Wolters Kluwer.

Unützer, J., Harbin, H., Schoenbaum, M., & Druss, B. (2013). *The collaborative care model: An approach to integrating physical and mental health care in Medicaid health homes*. Center for Health Care Strategies and Mathematica Policy Research. Centers for Medicare and Medicaid Services. Washington, DC: CMS.

Walters, B. H., Adams, S. A., Nieboer, A. P., & Bal, R. (2012). Disease management projects and the Chronic Care Model in action: Baseline qualitative research. *BMC Health Services Research, 12*(1), 114. doi:10.1186/1472-6963-12-114.

Ward, B. W., Schiller, J. S., & Goodman, R. A. (2013). Multiple chronic conditions among US adults: A 2012 update. *Preventing Chronic Disease, 11*, E62.

Watson, A. (2016). Evaluating and measuring quality and outcomes: A new "essential activity" of case management practice. *Professional Case Management, 21*(1), 51–52.

Weil, M., & Karls, J. M. (1985). *Case management in human service practice: A systematic approach to mobilizing resources for clients*. San Francisco, CA: Jossey-Bass.

World Health Organization (WHO). (2010). *Framework for action on inter-professional education and collaborative practice*. Geneva, Switzerland: Author.

World Health Organization (WHO). (2016). *What are social determinants of health?* Retrieved from http://www.who.int/social_determinants/sdh_definition/en/.

Young, B., Clark, C., Kansky, J., & Pupo, E. (2014). *Health information exchange committee ambulatory toolkit*. Chicago, IL: Health Information Management and Systems Society (HIMSS).

Young, T. K. (2004). *Population health: Concepts and methods* (2nd ed.). New York, NY: Oxford University Press.

Young, S. (2009). Professional relationships and power dynamics between urban community-based nurses and social work case managers: Advocacy in action. *Professional Case Management, 14*(6), 312–320.

Zander, K. (2002). Nursing case management in the 21st century: Intervening where margin meets mission. *Nursing Administration Quarterly, 26*(5), 58–67.

Zimmerman, J., & Dabelko, H. I. (2007). Collaborative models of patient care. *Social Work in Health Care, 44*(4), 33–47. doi:10.1300/j010v44n04_03.

Chapter 17

AACN Practice Alert. (2011). *Family presence: Visitation in the adult ICU*. Retrieved from http://www.aacn.org/wd/practice/docs/practicealerts/family-visitation-in-the-adult-icu-pa-2015.pdf.

Aarons, G. A. (2006). Transformational and transactional leadership: Association with attitudes toward evidence-based practice. *Psychiatric Services, 57*(8), 1162–1169. doi:10.1176/appi.ps.57.8.1162.

Aarons, G. A., Ehrhart, M. G., & Farahnak, L. R. (2014). The Implementation Leadership Scale (ILS): Development of a brief measure of unit level implementation leadership. *Implementation Science, 9*(1), 45. doi:10.1186/1748-5908-9-45.

Aarons, G. A., Ehrhart, M. G., Farahnak, L. R., & Hurlburt, M. S. (2015). Leadership and organizational change for implementation (LOCI): A randomized mixed method pilot study of a leadership and organization development intervention for evidence-based practice implementation. *Implementation Science, 10*(1), 11. doi:10.1186/s13012-014-0192-y.

Aarons, G. A., Ehrhart, M. G., Farahnak, L. R., & Sklar, M. (2014). Aligning leadership across systems and organizations to develop a strategic climate for evidence-based practice implementation. *Annual Review of Public Health, 35*, 255–274. doi:10.1146/annurev-publhealth-032013-182447.

Abdullah, G., Rossy, D., Ploeg, J., Davies, B., Higuchi, K., Sikora, L., et al. (2014). Measuring the effectiveness of mentoring as a knowledge translation intervention for implementing empirical evidence: A systematic review. *Worldviews on Evidence-Based Nursing, 11*(5), 284–300. doi:10.1111/wvn.12060.

Adams, S., Farrington, M., & Cullen, L. (2012). Evidence into practice: Publishing an evidence-based practice project. *Journal of PeriAnesthesia Nursing, 27*(3), 193–202. doi:10.1016/j.jopan.2012.03.004.

Advisory Board. (2015). *Motivational interviewing 101*. Retrieved from https://www.advisory.com/-/media/Advisory-com/Research/NEC/Research-Study/2015/Motivational-Interviewing-101/30618-NEC-Motivational-Interviewing-Toolkit-WEB.pdf.

Agency for Healthcare Research and Quality (AHRQ). (2014). *Toolkit for using the AHRQ quality indicators*. Rockville, MD: Agency for Healthcare

Research and Quality. Retrieved from http://www.ahrq.gov/professionals/systems/hospital/qitoolkit/index.html.

Ament, S. M., de Groot, J. J., Maessen, J. M., Dirksen, C. D., van der Weijden, T., & Kleijnen, J. (2015). Sustainability of professionals' adherence to clinical practice guidelines in medical care: A systematic review. *BMJ Open, 5*(12), e008073. doi:10.1136/bmjopen-2015-008073.

American Association of Colleges of Nursing. (2015). *The doctor of nursing practice. Current issues and clarifying recommendations.* Retrieved from http://www.aacn.nche.edu/aacn-publications/white-papers/DNP-Implementation-TF-Report-8-15.pdf.

American Nurses Credentialing Center. (2016). *ANCC Magnet Recognition Program*®. Retrieved from http://www.nursecredentialing.org/Magnet.aspx.

Atamna, Z., Chazan, B., Nitzan, O., Colodner, R., Kfir, H., Strauss, M., et al. (2016). Seasonal influenza vaccination effectiveness and compliance among hospital health care workers. *Israel Medical Association Journal, 18*(1), 5–9.

Avorn, J., & Soumerai, S. B. (1983). Improving drug-therapy decisions through educational outreach. A randomized controlled trial of academically based "detailing." *New England Journal of Medicine, 308*(24), 1457–1463. doi:10.1056/NEJM198306163082406.

Baggett, M., Batcheller, J., Blouin, A. S., Behrens, E., Bradley, C., Brown, M. J., et al. (2014). Excellence and evidence in staffing: A data-driven model for excellence in staffing (2nd ed.). *Nursing Economic$, 32*(Suppl. 3), 3–35.

Balakas, K., Sparks, L., Steurer, L., & Bryant, T. (2013). An outcome of evidence-based practice education: Sustained clinical decision-making among bedside nurses. *Journal of Pediatric Nursing, 28*(5), 479–485. doi:10.1016/j.pedn.2012.08.007.

Balik, B., Conway, J., Zipperer, L., & Watson, J. (2011). *Achieving an exceptional patient and family experience of inpatient hospital care. IHI Innovation Services white paper.* Cambridge, MA: Institute for Healthcare Improvement. Retrieved from http://www.ihi.org/resources/pages/ihiwhitepapers/achievingexceptionalpatientfamilyexperienceinpatienthospitalcarewhitepaper.aspx.

Ball, J. E., Griffiths, P., Rafferty, A. M., Lindqvist, R., Murrells, T., & Tishelman, C. (2016). A cross-sectional study of 'care left undone' on nursing shifts in hospitals. *Journal of Advanced Nursing, 72*(9), 2086–2097. doi:10.1111/jan.12976.

Bassett, R. D., Vollman, K. M., Brandwene, L., & Murray, T. (2012). Integrating a multidisciplinary mobility programme into intensive care practice (IMMPTP): A multicentre collaborative. *Intensive and Critical Care Nursing, 28*(2), 88–97. doi:10.1016/j.iccn.2011.12.001.

Bates, D. W., Saria, S., Ohno-Machado, L., Shah, A., & Escobar, G. (2014). Big data in health care: Using analytics to identify and manage high-risk and high-cost patients. *Health Affairs, 33*(7), 1123–1131. doi:10.1377/hlthaff.2014.0041.

Berenholtz, S. M., Pham, J. C., Thompson, D. A., Needham, D. M., Lubomski, L. H., Hyzy, R. C., et al. (2011). Collaborative cohort study of an intervention to reduce ventilator-associated pneumonia in the intensive care unit. *Infection Control & Hospital Epidemiology, 32*(4), 305–314. doi:10.1086/658938.

Bick, D., & Graham, I. D. (2010). *Evaluating the impact of implementing evidence-based practice.* United Kingdom: Wiley-Blackwell.

Bisognano, M., & Schummers, D. (2015). Governing for improved health. Hospital trustees play an important role in community health. *Healthcare Executive, 30*(3), 80–82.

Block, J., Lilienthal, M., Cullen, L., & White, A. (2012). Evidence-based thermoregulation for adult trauma patients. *Critical Care Nursing Quarterly, 35*(1), 50–63. doi:10.1097/CNQ.0b013e31823d3e9b.

Borenstein, J. E., Aronow, H. U., Bolton, L. B., Dimalanta, M. I., Chan, E., Palmer, K., et al. (2016). Identification and team-based interprofessional management of hospitalized vulnerable older adults. *Nursing Outlook, 64*(2), 137–145. doi:10.1016/j.outlook.2015.11.014.

Breimaier, H. E., Halfens, R. J., Wilborn, D., Meesterberends, E., Haase Nielsen, G., & Lohrmann, C. (2013). Implementation interventions used in nursing homes and hospitals: A descriptive, comparative study between Austria, Germany, and The Netherlands. *ISRN Nursing, 2013*, 706054. doi:10.1155/2013/706054.

Cahill, N. E., Murch, L., Cook, D., Heyland, D. K., & Canadian Critical Care Trials Group. (2014). Implementing a multifaceted tailored intervention to improve nutrition adequacy in critically ill patients: Results of a multi-center feasibility study. *Critical Care, 18*(3), R96. doi:10.1186/cc13867.

Centers for Medicare & Medicaid Services. (2011). *HCAHPS: Patients' perspective of care survey.* Retrieved from https://www.cms.gov/Medicare/Quality-Initiatives-Patient-Assessment-instruments/HospitalQualityInits/HospitalHCAHPS.html.

Centers for Medicare & Medicaid Services. (2015a). *Overview: Hospital-based purchasing.* Retrieved from https://www.cms.gov/Medicare/Quality-Initiatives-Patient-Assessment-Instruments/hospital-value-based-purchasing/index.html?redirect=/Hospital-Value-Based-Purchasing/.

Centers for Medicare & Medicaid Services. (2015b). *Medicare shared savings program: Accountable care organizations.* Retrieved from https://www.federalregister.gov/articles/2015/06/09/2015-14005/medicare-program-medicare-shared-savings-program-accountable-care-organizations.

Centers for Medicare & Medicaid Services. (2015c). *Electronic health record incentive program—Stage 3 and modifications to meaningful use in 20015 through 2017.* Retrieved from https://www.federalregister.gov/articles/2015/10/16/2015-25595/medicare-and-medicaid-programs-electronic-health-record-incentive-program-stage-3-and-modifications.

Chun, G. J., Sautter, J. M., Patterson, B. J., & McGhan, W. F. (2016). Diffusion of pharmacy-based influenza vaccination over time in the United States. *American Journal of Public Health, 106*(6), 1099–1100. doi:10.2105/AJPH.2016.303142.

Clay-Williams, R., Nosrati, H., Cunningham, F. C., Hillman, K., & Braithwaite, J. (2014). Do large-scale hospital- and system-wide interventions improve patient outcomes: A systematic review. *BMC Health Services Research, 14*, 369. doi:10.1186/1472-6963-14-369.

Crabtree, E., Brennan, E., Davis, A., & Coyle, A. (2016). Improving patient care through nursing engagement in evidence-based practice. *Worldviews on Evidence-Based Nursing, 13*(2), 172–175. doi:10.1111/wvn.12126.

Crowe, S., Fenton, M., Hall, M., Cowan, K., & Chalmers, I. (2015). Patients', clinicians' and the research communities' priorities for treatment research: There is an important mismatch. *Research Involvement and Engagement, 1*(1), 1–10. doi:10.1186/s40900-015-0003-x.

Cullen, L. (2015). Evidence into practice: Awakening the innovator in every nurse. *Journal of PeriAnesthesia Nursing, 30*(5), 430–435. doi:10.1016/j.jopan.2015.08.003.

Cullen, L., & Adams, S. L. (2012). Planning for implementation of evidence-based practice. *Journal of Nursing Administration, 42*(4), 222–230. doi:10.1097/NNA.0b013e31824ccd0a.

Cullen, L., Dawson, C. J., Hanrahan, K., & Dole, N. (2014). Evidence-based practice: Strategies for nursing leaders. In D. L. Huber (Ed.), *Leadership and nursing care management* (5th ed., pp. 274–290). St. Louis, MO: Elsevier.

Cullen, L., Hanrahan, K., Tucker, S., Rempel, G., & Jordan, K. (2012). *Evidence-based practice building blocks: Comprehensive strategies, tools and tips.* Iowa City, IA: Office of Nursing Research and Evidence-Based Practice, Department of Nursing Services and Patient Care, University of Iowa Hospitals and Clinics. Available from: https://uihc.org/evidence-based-practice-building-blocks-comprehensive-strategies-tools-and-tips.

Cullen, L., Titler, M. G., & Rempel, G. (2010). An advanced educational program promoting evidence-based practice. *Western Journal of Nursing Research, 33*(3), 345–364. doi:10.1177/0193945910379218.

Dang, D., Melnyk, B. M., Fineout-Overholt, E., Ciliska, D., DiCenso, A., Cullen, L., et al. (2011). Models to guide implementation and sustainability of evidence based practice. In B. M. Melnyk & E. Fineout-Overholt (Eds.), *Evidence-based practice in nursing and healthcare: A guide to best practice* (3rd ed., pp. 274–315). Philadephia, PA: Wolters Kluwer Health.

Davies, B., Edwards, N., Ploeg, J., Virani, T., Skelly, J., & Dobbins, M. (2006). *Determinants of the sustained use of research evidence in nursing.* Canadian Foundation for Healthcare Improvement. Retrieved from http://www.cfhi-fcass.ca/SearchResultsNews/06-12-01/2740e0cb-33b1-45be-aee8-860d09c48f8d.aspx.

Davies, B., Tremblay, D., & Edwards, N. (2010). Sustaining evidence-based practice systems and measuring the impacts. In D. Bick & I. D. Graham (Eds.), *Evaluating the impact of implementing evidence-based practice* (pp. 165–188). Oxford, United Kingdom: STTI/Wiley-Blackwell.

Davison, C. M., Ndumbe-Eyoh, S., & Clement, C. (2015). Critical examination of knowledge to action models and implications for promoting health equity. *International Journal for Equity in Health, 14,* 49. doi:10.1186/s12939-015-0178-7.

Debourgh, G. A. (2012). Synergy for patient safety and quality: Academic and service partnerships to promote effective nurse education and clinical practice. *Journal of Professional Nursing, 28*(1), 48–61.

DECIDE. (2015). *Key DECIDE tools.* Retrieved from http://www.decide-collaboration.eu/.

Dee, C. R., & Reynolds, P. (2013). Lifelong learning for nurses-building a strong future. *Medical Reference Services Quarterly, 32*(4), 451–458. doi:10.1080/02763869.2013.837741.

Dembe, A. E., Lynch, M. S., Gugiu, P. C., & Jackson, R. D. (2014). The translational research impact scale: Development, construct validity, and reliability testing. *Evaluation & the Health Professions, 37*(1), 50–70. doi:10.1177/0163278713506112.

Department of Health and Human Services. (2009). Breach notification for unsecured protected health information. *Federal Registry, 74*(162), 42740.

Dogherty, E. J., Harrison, M. B., Baker, C., & Graham, I. D. (2012). Following a natural experiment of guideline adaptation and early implementation: A mixed-methods study of facilitation. *Implementation Science, 7,* 9. doi:10.1186/1748-5908-7-9.

Doyle, C., Howe, C., Woodcock, T., Myron, R., Phekoo, K., McNicholas, C., et al. (2013). Making change last: Applying the NHS Institute for Innovation and Improvement Sustainability model to healthcare improvement. *Implementation Science, 8,* 127. doi:10.1186/1748-5908-8-127.

Duffy, J. R., Culp, S., Sand-Jecklin, K., Stroupe, L., & Lucke-Wold, N. (2016). Nurses' research capacity, use of evidence, and research productivity in acute care: Year 1 findings from a partnership study. *Journal of Nursing Administration, 46*(1), 12–17. doi:10.1097/NNA.0000000000000287.

Ellen, M. E., Leon, G., Bouchard, G., Lavis, J. N., Ouimet, M., & Grimshaw, J. M. (2013). What supports do health system organizations have in place to facilitate evidence-informed decision-making? A qualitative study. *Implementation Science, 8,* 84. doi:10.1186/1748-5908-8-84.

Everett, L. Q., & Sitterding, M. C. (2011). Transformational leadership required to design and sustain evidence-based practice: A system exemplar. *Western Journal of Nursing Research, 33*(3), 398–426. doi:10.1177/0193945910383056.

Farrington, M., Hanson, A., Laffoon, T., & Cullen, L. (2015). Low-dose ketamine infusions for postoperative pain in opioid-tolerant orthopaedic spine patients. *Journal of PeriAnesthesia Nursing, 30*(4), 338–345. doi:10.1016/j.jopan.2015.03.005.

Fleuren, M., Wiefferink, K., & Paulussen, T. (2004). Determinants of innovation within health care organizations: Literature review and Delphi study. *International Journal for Quality in Healthcare, 16*(2), 107–123. doi:10.1093/intqhc/mzh030.

Flodgren, G., Parmelli, E., Doumit, G., Gattellari, M., O'Brien, M. A., Grimshaw, J., & Eccles, M. P. (2011). Local opinion leaders: Effects on professional practice and health care outcomes. *Cochrane Database of Systematic Reviews,* (8), CD000125. doi:10.1002/14651858.CD000125.pub4.

Foote, J. M., Conley, V., Williams, J. K., McCarthy, A. M., & Countryman, M. (2015). Academic and institutional review board collaboration to ensure ethical conduct of doctor of nursing practice projects. *Journal of Nursing Education, 54*(7), 372–377. doi:10.3928/01484834-20150617-03.

Forberg, U., Wallin, L., Johansson, E., Ygge, B. M., Backheden, M., & Ehrenberg, A. (2014). Relationship between work context and adherence to a clinical practice guideline for peripheral venous catheters among registered nurses in pediatric care. *Worldviews on Evidence-Based Nursing, 11*(4), 227–239. doi:10.1111/wvn.12046.

Gagliardi, A. R., Webster, F., Perrier, L., Bell, M., & Straus, S. (2014). Exploring mentorship as a strategy to build capacity for knowledge translation research and practice: A scoping systematic review. *Implementation Science, 9,* 122. doi:10.1186/s13012-014-0122-z.

Garcia, A., Caspers, B., Westra, B., Pruinelli, L., & Delaney, C. (2015). Sharable and comparable data for nursing management. *Nursing Administration Quarterly, 39*(4), 297–303. doi:10.1097/NAQ.0000000000000120.

Gawlinski, A., & Becker, E. (2012). Infusing research into practice: A staff nurse evidence-based practice fellowship program. *Journal for Nurses in Staff Development, 28*(2), 69–73. doi:10.1097/NND.0b013e31824b418c.

Gerrish, K., Nolan, M., McDonnell, A., Tod, A., Kirshbaum, M., & Guillaume, L. (2012). Factors influencing advanced practice nurses' ability to promote evidence-based practice among frontline nurses. *Worldviews on Evidence-Based Nursing, 9*(1), 30–39. doi:10.1111/j.1741-6787.2011.00230.x.

Gifford, W. A., Davies, B. L., Graham, I. D., Tourangeau, A., Woodend, A. K., & Lefebre, N. (2013). Developing leadership capacity for guideline use: A pilot cluster randomized control trial. *Worldviews on Evidence-Based Nursing, 10*(1), 51–65. doi:10.1111/j.1741-6787.2012.00254.x.

GRADE. (2012). *GRADE working group.* Retrieved from http://www.gradeworkinggroup.org/.

Granger, B. B., Prvu-Bettger, J., Aucoin, J., Fuchs, M. A., Mitchell, P. H., Holditch-Davis, D., et al. (2012). An academic-health service partnership in nursing: Lessons from the field. *Journal of Nursing Scholarship, 44*(1), 71–79. doi:10.1111/j.1547-5069.2011.01432.x.

Greenhalgh, T., Robert, G., Bate, P., Macfarlane, F., & Kyriakidou, O. (2005). *Diffusion of innovations in health service organizations.* Malden, MA: Blackwell Publishing Ltd.

Grimshaw, J. M., Eccles, M. P., Lavis, J. N., Hill, S. J., & Squires, J. E. (2012). Knowledge translation of research findings. *Implementation Science, 7,* 50. doi:10.1186/1748-5908-7-50.

Hakko, E., Guvenc, S., Karaman, I., Cakmak, A., Erdem, T., & Cakmakci, M. (2015). Long-term sustainability of zero central-line associated bloodstream infections is possible with high compliance with care bundle elements. *Eastern Mediterranean Health Journal, 21*(4), 293–298.

Hanrahan, K., Wagner, M., Matthews, G., Stewart, S., Dawson, C., Greiner, J., et al. (2015). Sacred cow gone to pasture: A systematic evaluation and integration of evidence-based practice. *Worldviews on Evidence-Based Nursing, 12*(1), 3–11. doi:10.1111/wvn.12072.

Harrison, M. B., Graham, I. D., van den Hoek, J., Dogherty, E. J., Carley, M. E., & Angus, V. (2013). Guideline adaptation and implementation planning: A prospective observational study. *Implementation Science, 8,* 49. doi:10.1186/1748-5908-8-49.

Harvey, G., & Kitson, A. (2016). PARIHS revisited: From heuristic to integrated framework for the successful implementation of knowledge into practice. *Implementation Science, 11,* 33. doi:10.1186/s13012-016-0398-2.

Hauck, S., Winsett, R. P., & Kuric, J. (2013). Leadership facilitation strategies to establish evidence-based practice in an acute care hospital. *Journal of Advanced Nursing, 69*(3), 664–674. doi:10.1111/j.1365-2648.2012.06053.x.

Herzer, K. R., Niessen, L., Constenla, D. O., Ward, W. J., Jr., & Pronovost, P. J. (2014). Cost-effectiveness of a quality improvement programme to reduce central line-associated bloodstream infections in intensive care units in the USA. *BMJ Open, 4*(9), e006065. doi:10.1136/bmjopen-2014-006065.

Hoke, L. M., & Guarracino, D. (2016). Beyond socks, signs, and alarms: A reflective accountability model for fall prevention. *American Journal of Nursing, 116*(1), 42–47. doi:10.1097/01.NAJ.0000476167.43671.00.

Hosking, J., Knox, K., Forman, J., Montgomery, L. A., Valde, J. G., & Cullen, L. (In press). Evidence into practice: Leading new graduate nurses to evidence-based practice through a nurse residency program. *Journal of PeriAnesthesia Nursing.*

Huis, A., Holleman, G., van Achterberg, T., Grol, R., Schoonhoven, L., & Hulscher, M. (2013). Explaining the effects of two different strategies for promoting hand hygiene in hospital nurses: A process evaluation alongside a cluster randomised controlled trial. *Implementation Science*, 8, 41. doi:10.1186/1748-5908-8-41.

Hulscher, M. E., Schouten, L. M., Grol, R. P., & Buchan, H. (2013). Determinants of success of quality improvement collaboratives: What does the literature show? *BMJ Quality & Safety*, 22(1), 19–31. doi:10.1136/bmjqs-2011-000651.

Institute for Healthcare Improvement. (2015a). *The science improvement on a whiteboard!* Retrieved from http://www.ihi.org/education/IHIOpenSchool/resources/Pages/BobLloydWhiteboard.aspx.

Institute for Healthcare Improvement. (2015b). *Family of measures.* Retrieved from http://www.ihi.org/education/IHIOpenSchool/resources/Pages/AudioandVideo/Whiteboard15.aspx.

Institute for Healthcare Improvement. (2016). *Governance leadership of safety and improvement.* Retrieved from http://www.ihi.org/topics/governance-leadership/pages/default.aspx.

Institute of Medicine. (2011a). *Clinical guidelines we can trust.* Washington, DC: National Academies Press.

Institute of Medicine. (2011b). *Finding what works in health care: Standards for systematic reviews.* Washington, DC: National Academies Press.

Institute of Medicine. (2012). *Communicating with patients on health care evidence.* Washington, DC: National Academies Press.

Institute of Medicine. (2015a). *Integrating research and practice: Health system leaders working toward high-value care: Workshop summary.* Washington, DC: National Academies Press. Available at: http://www.nap.edu/catalog/18945/integrating-research-and-practice-health-system-leaders-working-toward-high.

Institute of Medicine. (2015b). *Assessing progress on the Institute of Medicine report The Future of Nursing.* Washington, DC: National Academies Press. Retrieved from http://www.nationalacademies.org/hmd/Reports/2015/Assessing-Progress-on-the-IOM-Report-The-Future-of-Nursing.aspx.

Ivanovska, V., Hek, K., Mantel Teeuwisse, A. K., Leufkens, H. G., Nielen, M. M., & van Dijk, L. (2016). Antibiotic prescribing for children in primary care and adherence to treatment guidelines. *Journal of Antimicrobial Chemotherapy*, 71(6), 1707–1714. doi:10.1093/jac/dkw030.

Ivers, N., Jamtvedt, G., Flottorp, S., Young, J. M., Odgaard-Jensen, J., French, S. D., et al. (2012). Audit and feedback: Effects on professional practice and healthcare outcomes. *Cochrane Database of Systematic Reviews*, (6), CD000259. doi:10.1002/14651858.CD000259.pub3.

Jackson, N. (2016). Incorporating evidence-based practice learning into a nurse residency program: Are new graduates ready to apply evidence at the bedside? *Journal of Nursing Administration*, 46(5), 278–283. doi:10.1097/NNA.0000000000000343.

Jacobs, S. R., Weiner, B. J., & Bunger, A. C. (2014). Context matters: Measuring implementation climate among individuals and groups. *Implementation Science*, 9, 46. doi:10.1186/1748-5908-9-46.

Johnson, L., Grueber, S., Schlotzhauer, C., Phillips, E., Bullock, P., Basnett, J., & Hahn-Cover, K. (2014). A multifactorial action plan improves hand hygiene adherence and significantly reduces central line-associated bloodstream infections. *American Journal of Infection Control*, 42(11), 1146–1151. doi:10.1016/j.ajic.2014.07.003.

Khan, S., Timmings, C., Moore, J. E., Marquez, C., Pyka, K., Gheihman, G., & Straus, S. E. (2014). The development of an online decision support tool for organizational readiness for change. *Implementation Science*, 9, 56. doi:10.1186/1748-5908-9-56.

Kissoon, N. (2015). Sepsis guidelines: Suggestions to improve adherence. *Journal of Infection*, 71(Suppl. 1), S36–S41. doi:10.1016/j.jinf.2015.04.017.

Klompas, M., Branson, R., Eichenwald, E. C., Greene, L. R., Howell, M. D., Lee, G., et al. (2014). Strategies to prevent ventilator-associated pneumonia in acute care hospitals: 2014 update. *Infection Control & Hospital Epidemiology*, 35(8), 915–936. doi:10.1086/677144.

Kouzes, J. M., & Posner, B. Z. (2012). *The leadership challenge: How to make extraordinary things happen in organizations.* San Francisco, CA: Jossey-Bass.

Kramer, M., Maguire, P., Halfer, D., Budin, W. C., Hall, D. S., Goodloe, L., et al. (2012). The organizational transformative power of nurse residency programs. *Nursing Administration Quarterly*, 36(2), 155–168. doi:10.1097/NAQ.0b013e318249fdaa.

Kruk, M. E., Yamey, G., Angell, S. Y., Beith, A., Cotlear, D., Guanais, F., et al. (2016). Transforming global health by improving the science of scale-up. *PLoS Biology*, 14(3), e1002360. doi:10.1371/journal.pbio.1002360.

Letzkus, L., Hengartner, M., Yeago, D., & Crist, P. (2013). The immobile pediatric population: Can progressive mobility hasten recovery? *Journal of Pediatric Nursing*, 28(3), 296–299. doi:10.1016/j.pedn.2013.02.029.

Levin, R. F. (2014). Developing the infrastructure to support EBP: It takes partnerships. *Research and Theory for Nursing Practice*, 28(3), 199–203.

Lewis, L. C. (2014). Charting a new course: Advancing the next generation of nursing-sensitive indicators. *Journal of Nursing Administration*, 44(5), 247–249. doi:10.1097/NNA.0000000000000061.

Liira, H., Saarelma, O., Callaghan, M., Harbour, R., Jousimaa, J., Kunnamo, I., et al. (2015). Patients, health information, and guidelines: A focus-group study. *Scandinavian Journal of Primary Health Care*, 33(3), 212–219. doi:10.3109/02813432.2015.1067517.

Lord, R. K., Mayhew, C. R., Korupolu, R., Mantheiy, E. C., Friedman, M. A., Palmer, J. B., & Needham, D. M. (2013). ICU early physical rehabilitation programs: Financial modeling of cost savings. *Critical Care Medicine*, 41(3), 717–724. doi:10.1097/CCM.0b013e3182711de2.

Luke, D. A., Calhoun, A., Robichaux, C. B., Elliott, M. B., & Moreland-Russell, S. (2014). The Program Sustainability Assessment Tool: A new instrument for public health programs. *Preventing Chronic Disease*, 11, 130184. doi:10.5888/pcd11.130184.

Maher, L., Gustafson, D., & Evans, A. (2010). *Sustainability odel and guide. NHS Institute for Innovation and Improvement.* Retrieved from http://www.qihub.scot.nhs.uk/media/162236/sustainability_model.pdf.

Makic, M. B., & Rauen, C. (2016). Maintaining your momentum: Moving evidence into practice. *Critical Care Medicine*, 36(2), 13–18. doi:10.4037/ccn2016568.

Malkoc, M., Karadibak, D., & Yildirim, Y. (2009). The effect of physiotherapy on ventilatory dependency and the length of stay in an intensive care unit. *International Journal of Rehabilitation Research*, 32(1), 85–88. doi:10.1097/MRR.0b013e3282fc0fce.

Mark, D. D., Latimer, R. W., White, J. P., Bransford, D., Johnson, K. G., & Song, V. L. (2014). Hawaii's statewide evidence-based practice program. *Nursing Clinics of North America*, 49(3), 275–290. doi:10.1016/j.cnur.2014.05.002.

Mason, D. J., Keepnews, D., Holmberg, J., & Murray, E. (2013). The representation of health professionals on governing boards of health care organizations in New York City. *Journal of Urban Health: Bulletin of the New York Academy of Medicine*, 90(5), 888–901. doi:10.1007/s11524-012-9772-9.

Matthew-Maich, N., Ploeg, J., Dobbins, M., & Jack, S. (2013). Supporting the uptake of nursing guidelines: What you really need to know to move nursing guidelines into practice. *Worldviews on Evidence-Based Nursing*, 10(2), 104–115. doi:10.1111/j.1741-6787.2012.00259.x.

McMullan, C., Propper, G., Schuhmacher, C., Sokoloff, L., Harris, D., Murphy, P., & Greene, W. H. (2013). A multidisciplinary approach to reduce central line-associated bloodstream infections. *Joint Commission Journal on Quality and Patient Safety*, 39(2), 61–69.

Melnyk, B. M., Gallagher-Ford, L., Thomas, B. K., Troseth, M., Wyngarden, K., & Szalacha, L. (2016). A study of chief nurse executives indicates low prioritization of evidence-based practice and shortcomings in hospital performance metrics across the United States. *Worldviews on Evidence-Based Nursing*, 13(1), 6–14. doi:10.1111/wvn.12133.

Mick, J. (2014). Nurse interns' experience with participation in the evidence-based practice project requirement of a nursing internship program. *Nurse Educator*, 39(2), 54–55. doi:10.1097/NNE.0000000000000017.

Milat, A. J., Bauman, A., & Redman, S. (2015). Narrative review of models and success factors for scaling up public health interventions. *Implementation Science*, 10, 113. doi:10.1186/s13012-015-0301-6.

Milat, A. J., King, L., Newson, R., Wolfenden, L., Rissel, C., Bauman, A., & Redman, S. (2014). Increasing the scale and adoption of population health interventions: Experiences and perspectives of policy makers, practitioners, and researchers. *Health Research Policy and Systems, 12*, 18. doi:10.1186/1478-4505-12–18.

Milic, M. M., Puntillo, K., Turner, K., Joseph, D., Peters, N., Ryan, R., et al. (2015). Communicating with patients' families and physicians about prognosis and goals of care. *American Journal of Critical Care, 24*(4), e56–e64. doi:10.4037/ajcc2015855.

Missal, B., Schafer, B., Halm, M., & Schaffer, M. (2010). A university and health care organization partnership to prepare nurses for evidence-based practice. *Journal of Nursing Education, 49*(8), 456–461. doi:10.3928/01484834-20100430-06.

Montini, T., & Graham, I. D. (2015). "Entrenched practices and other biases": Unpacking the historical, economic, professional, and social resistance to de-implementation. *Implementation Science, 10*, 24. doi:10.1186/s13012-015-0211-7.

Morgan, L. A. (2012). A mentoring model for evidence-based practice in a community hospital. *Journal for Nurses in Staff Development, 28*(5), 233–237. doi:10.1097/NND.0b013e318269fe0f.

Morris, P. E., Goad, A., Thompson, C., Taylor, K., Harry, B., Passmore, L., et al. (2008). Early intensive care unit mobility therapy in the treatment of acute respiratory failure. *Critical Care Medicine, 36*(8), 2238–2243. doi:10.1097/CCM.0b013e318180b90e.

Mwaniki, P., Ayieko, P., Todd, J., & English, M. (2014). Assessment of paediatric inpatient care during a multifaceted quality improvement intervention in Kenyan district hospitals—use of prospectively collected case record data. *BMC Health Services Research, 14*, 312. doi:10.1186/1472-6963-14-312.

NIH Fogarty International Center. (2016). *Implementation science information and resources.* Retrieved from http://www.fic.nih.gov/researchtopics/pages/implementationscience.aspx.

Niven, D. J., Mrklas, K. J., Holodinsky, J. K., Straus, S. E., Hemmelgarn, B. R., Jeffs, L. P., & Stelfox, H. T. (2015). Towards understanding the de-adoption of low-value clinical practices: A scoping review. *BMC Medicine, 13*, 255. doi:10.1186/s12916-015-0488-z.

O'Brien, M. A., Rogers, S., Jamtvedt, G., Oxman, A. D., Odgaard-Jensen, J., Kristoffersen, D. T., et al. (2007). Educational outreach visits: Effects on professional practice and health care outcomes. *Cochrane Database of Systematic Reviews,* (4), CD000409. doi:10.1002/14651858.CD000409.pub2.

O'Connor, B. (2012). New American Association of Colleges of Nursing data show enrollment surge in baccalaureate and graduate programs amid calls for more highly educated nurses. *Journal of Professional Nursing, 28*(3), 137–138.

Office for Human Research Protections (OHRP). (2016). *Quality improvement activities FAQs.* Retrieved from https://www.hhs.gov/ohrp/regulations-and-policy/guidance/faq/quality-improvement-activities/.

Ogden, T., Bjornebekk, G., Kjobli, J., Patras, J., Christiansen, T., Taraldsen, K., & Tollefsen, N. (2012). Measurement of implementation components ten years after a nationwide introduction of empirically supported programs—a pilot study. *Implementation Science, 7*, 49. doi:10.1186/1748-5908-7-49.

Ogrinc, G., Nelson, W. A., Adams, S. M., & O'Hara, A. E. (2013). An instrument to differentiate between clinical research and quality improvement. *IRB, 35*(5), 1–8.

Oster, C. A. (2011). *Guiding principles for evidence-based practice.* Sudbury, MA: Jones & Bartlett Learning.

Paparone, P. (2015). Supporting influenza vaccination intent among nurses: Effects of leadership and attitudes toward adoption of evidence-based practice. *Journal of Nursing Administration, 45*(3), 133–138. doi:10.1097/NNA.0000000000000172.

Parkosewich, J. A. (2013). An infrastructure to advance the scholarly work of staff nurses. *Yale Journal of Biology and Medicine, 86*(1), 63–77.

Parry, G. J., Carson-Stevens, A., Luff, D. F., McPherson, M. E., & Goldmann, D. A. (2013). Recommendations for evaluation of health care improvement initiatives. *Academic Pediatrics, 13*(Suppl. 6), S23–S30. doi:10.1016/j.acap.2013.04.007.

Perme, C., & Chandrashekar, R. (2009). Early mobility and walking program for patients in intensive care units: Creating a standard of care. *American Journal of Critical Care, 18*(3), 212–221. doi:10.4037/ajcc2009598.

Piscotty, R., & Kalisch, B. (2014). Nurses' use of clinical decision support: A literature review. *Computers, Informatics, Nursing, 32*(12), 562–568. doi:10.1097/CIN.0000000000000110.

Piscotty, R. J., Jr., Kalisch, B., & Gracey-Thomas, A. (2015). Impact of healthcare information technology on nursing practice. *Journal of Nursing Scholarship, 47*(4), 287–293. doi:10.1111/jnu.12138.

Platt, R., Grossmann, C., & Selker, H. P. (2013). Evaluation as part of operations: Reconciling the common rule and continuous improvement. Commentary. *Hastings Center Report, Spec No,* S37–S39. doi:10.1002/hast.139.

Pohlman, M. C., Schweickert, W. D., Pohlman, A. S., Nigos, C., Pawlik, A. J., Esbrook, C. L., et al. (2010). Feasibility of physical and occupational therapy beginning from initiation of mechanical ventilation. *Critical Care Medicine, 38*(11), 2089–2094. doi:10.1097/CCM.0b013e3181f270c3.

Prochaska, J. J., & Sanders-Jackson, A. (2016). Patient decision aids for discouraging low-value health care procedures: Null findings and lessons learned. *JAMA Internal Medicine, 176*(1), 41–42. doi:10.1001/jamainternmed.2015.7347.

Proctor, E., Luke, D., Calhoun, A., McMillen, C., Brownson, R., McCrary, S., & Padek, M. (2015). Sustainability of evidence-based healthcare: Research agenda, methodological advances, and infrastructure support. *Implementation Science, 10*, 88. doi:10.1186/s13012-015-0274-5.

Pronovost, P. J., Demski, R., Callender, T., Winner, L., Miller, M. R., Austin, J. M., et al. (2013). Demonstrating high reliability on accountability measures at the Johns Hopkins Hospital. *Joint Commission Journal on Quality and Patient Safety, 39*(12), 531–544.

Pryse, Y., McDaniel, A., & Schafer, J. (2014). Psychometric analysis of two new scales: The evidence-based practice nursing leadership and work environment scales. *Worldviews on Evidence-Based Nursing, 11*(4), 240–247. doi:10.1111/wvn.12045.

QSEN Institute. (2012). *Competencies.* Retrieved from http://www.qsen.org/competencies.

Rangachari, P., Rissing, P., & Rethemeyer, K. (2013). Awareness of evidence-based practices alone does not translate to implementation: Insights from implementation research. *Quality Management in Health Care, 22*(2), 117–125. doi:10.1097/QMH.0b013e31828bc21d.

Rauen, C. A., Chulay, M., Bridges, E., Vollman, K. M., & Arbour, R. (2008). Seven evidence-based practice habits: Putting some sacred cows out to pasture. *Critical Care Nurse, 28*(2), 98–124.

Registered Nurses' Association of Ontario (RNAO). (2013). *Developing and sustaining nursing leadership* (2nd ed.). Toronto, ON, Canada: Author.

Rockafellow, E., Comried, L., Cullen, L., Bombei, C., & Greiner, J. (2014). Some like it HOT! (Abstract). *Critical Care Nurse, 34*(2), e36.

Rogers, E. M. (2003). *Diffusion of innovations* (5th ed.). New York, NY: Free Press.

Ronnebaum, J. A., Weir, J. P., & Hilsabeck, T. A. (2012). Earlier mobilization decreases the length of stay in the intensive care unit. *Journal of Acute Care Physical Therapy, 3*(2), 204–210.

Roski, J., Bo-Linn, G. W., & Andrews, T. A. (2014). Creating value in health care through Big Data Opportunities and policy implications. *Health Affairs, 33*(7), 1115–1122. doi:10.1377/hlthaff.2014.0147.

RWJ Aligning Forces for Quality. (2013). *Engaging patients in improving ambulatory care: A compendium of tools from Maine, Oregon, and Humboldt County, California.* Princeton, NJ: Robert Wood Johnson Foundation. Retrieved from http://www.rwjf.org/en/library/research/2013/03/engaging-patients-in-improving-ambulatory-care.html.

Ryan, R., Santesso, N., Lowe, D., Hill, S., Grimshaw, J., Prictor, M., et al. (2014). Interventions to improve safe and effective medicines use by consumers: An overview of systematic reviews. *Cochrane Database of Systematic Reviews,* (4), CD007768. doi:10.1002/14651858.CD007768.pub3.

Rycroft-Malone, J., & Bucknall, T. (2010). Using theory and frameworks to facilitate the implementation of evidence into practice. *Worldviews on Evidence-Based Nursing, 7*(2), 57–58. doi:10.1111/j.1741-6787.2010.00194.x.

Sackett, D. L., Straus, S. E., Richardson, W. S., Rosenberg, W., & Haynes, R. B. (2000). *Evidence-based medicine: How to practice and teach EBM* (2nd ed.). Edinburgh, Scotland: Churchill Livingstone.

Sadler, B. L., Joseph, A., Keller, A., & Rostenberg, B. (2009). *Using evidence-based environmental design to enhance safety and quality.* IHI Innovation Series white paper. Cambridge, MA: Institute for Healthcare Improvement. Available at http://www.ihi.org/resources/pages/ihiwhitepapers/usingevidencebasedenvironmentaldesignwhitepaper.aspx.

Sandstrom, B., Willman, A., Svensson, B., & Borglin, G. (2015). Perceptions of national guidelines and their (non) implementation in mental healthcare: A deductive and inductive content analysis. *Implementation Science, 10*, 43. doi:10.1186/s13012-015-0234-0.

Schaffer, M. A., Sandau, K. E., & Diedrick, L. (2013). Evidence-based practice models for organizational change: Overview and practical applications. *Journal of Advanced Nursing, 69*(5), 1197–1209. doi:10.1111/j.1365-2648.2012.06122.x.

Schall, M. C., Cullen, L., Pennathur, P., Chen, H., Burrell, K., & Matthews, G. (In review). *Usability evaluation and implementation of a health information technology dashboard of evidence-based quality indicators.*

Schell, S. F., Luke, D. A., Schooley, M. W., Elliott, M. B., Herbers, S. H., Mueller, N. B., & Bunger, A. C. (2013). Public health program capacity for sustainability: A new framework. *Implementation Science, 8*, 15. doi:10.1186/1748-5908-8-15.

Schweickert, W. D., & Kress, J. P. (2011). Implementing early mobilization interventions in mechanically ventilated patients in the ICU. *Chest, 140*(6), 1612–1617. doi:10.1378/chest.10-2829.

Sigma Theta Tau International Research and Scholarship Advisory Committee. (2008). Sigma Theta Tau International position statement on evidence-based practice February 2007 summary. *Worldviews on Evidence-Based Nursing, 5*(2), 57–59. doi:10.1111/j.1741-6787.2008.00118.x.

Spyridonidis, D., & Calnan, M. (2011). Opening the black box: A study of the process of NICE guidelines implementation. *Health Policy, 102*(2–3), 117–125.

Stacey, D., Legare, F., Col, N. F., Bennett, C. L., Barry, M. J., Eden, K. B., et al. (2014). Decision aids for people facing health treatment or screening decisions. *Cochrane Database of Systematic Reviews*, (1), CD001431. doi:10.1002/14651858.CD001431.pub4.

Standards for Quality Improvement Reporting Excellence (SQUIRE). (2015). *Revised standards for quality improvement reporting excellence (SQUIRE 2.0).* Retrieved from http://www.squire-statement.org/index.cfm?fuseaction=page.viewPage&pageID=471&nodeID=1.

Stenberg, M., & Wann-Hansson, C. (2011). Health care professionals' attitudes and compliance to clinical practice guidelines to prevent falls and fall injuries. *Worldviews on Evidence-Based Nursing, 8*(2), 87–95. doi:10.1111/j.1741-6787.2010.00196.x.

Stetler, C. B., Ritchie, J. A., Rycroft-Malone, J., & Charns, M. P. (2014). Leadership for evidence-based practice: Strategic and functional behaviors for institutionalizing EBP. *Worldviews on Evidence-Based Nursing, 11*(4), 219–226. doi:10.1111/wvn.12044.

Stevens, K. R. (2013). The impact of evidence-based practice in nursing and the next big ideas. *Online Journal of Issues in Nursing, 18*(2), 4.

Stillwell, S. B., Fineout-Overholt, E., Melnyk, B. M., & Williamson, K. M. (2010). Searching for the evidence: Strategies to help you conduct a successful search. *American Journal of Nursing, 110*(5), 41–47.

Straus, S. E., Tetroe, J. M., & Graham, I. D. (2011). Knowledge translation is the use of knowledge in health care decision making. *Journal of Clinical Epidemiology, 64*(1), 6–10. doi:10.1016/j.jclinepi.2009.08.016.

Taylor, N., Clay-Williams, R., Hogden, E., Braithwaite, J., & Groene, O. (2015). High performing hospitals: A qualitative systematic review of associated factors and practical strategies for improvement. *BMC Health Services Research, 15*, 244. doi:10.1186/s12913-015-0879-z.

The Iowa Model Collaborative. (In review). *The Iowa Model Revised: Development and Validation.* Worldviews on Evidence-Based Nursing.

The Joint Commission. (2017). *National patient safety goals.* Retrieved from https://www.jointcommission.org/standards_information/npsgs.aspx.

Titler, M. (2004). Methods in translation science. *Worldviews on Evidence-Based Nursing, 1*(1), 38–48.

Titler, M., & Everett, L. Q. (2001). Translating research into practice. Considerations for critical care investigators. *Critical Care Nursing Clinics of North America, 13*(4), 587–604.

Titler, M. G. (2010). Translation science and context. *Research and Theory for Nursing Practice, 24*(1), 35–55.

Titler, M. G. (2014). Overview of evidence-based practice and translation science. *Nursing Clinics of North America, 49*(3), 269–274. doi:10.1016/j.cnur.2014.05.001.

Titler, M. G., Kleiber, C., Steelman, V. J., Rakel, B. A., Budreau, G., Everett, L. Q., et al. (2001). The Iowa Model of Evidence-Based Practice to Promote Quality Care. *Critical Care Nursing Clinics of North America, 13*(4), 497–509.

Titsworth, W. L., Hester, J., Correia, T., Reed, R., Guin, P., Archibald, L., et al. (2012). The effect of increased mobility on morbidity in the neurointensive care unit. *Journal of Neurosurgery, 116*(6), 1379–1388. doi:10.3171/2012.2.JNS111881.

Tonges, M., Ray, J. D., Overman, A. S., & Willis, B. (2015). Creating a culture of rapid change adoption: Implementing an innovations unit. *Journal of Nursing Administration, 45*(7–8), 384–390. doi:10.1097/NNA.0000000000000219.

Torrey, W. C., Bond, G. R., McHugo, G. J., & Swain, K. (2012). Evidence-based practice implementation in community mental health settings: The relative importance of key domains of implementation activity. *Administration and Policy in Mental Health, 39*(5), 353–364. doi:10.1007/s10488-011-0357-9.

Tucker, S. (2014). Determining the return on investment for evidence-based practice: An essential skill for all clinicians. *Worldviews on Evidence-Based Nursing, 11*(5), 271–273. doi:10.1111/wvn.12055.

Ubbink, D. T., Guyatt, G. H., & Vermeulen, H. (2013). Framework of policy recommendations for implementation of evidence-based practice: A systematic scoping review. *BMJ Open, 3*(1). doi:10.1136/bmjopen-2012-001881.

US Preventive Services Task Force (USPSTF). (2012). *Grade definitions.* Retrieved from http://www.uspreventiveservicestaskforce.org/Page/Name/grade-definitions.

VanDeusen Lukas, C., Engle, R. L., Holmes, S. K., Parker, V. A., Petzel, R. A., Nealon Seibert, M., et al. (2010). Strengthening organizations to implement evidence-based clinical practices. *Health Care Management Review, 35*(3), 235–245. doi:10.1097/HMR.0b013e3181dde6a5.

Van Hoof, T. J., Harrison, L. G., Miller, N. E., Pappas, M. S., & Fischer, M. A. (2015). Characteristics of academic detailing: Results of a literature review. *American Health & Drug Benefits, 8*(8), 414–422.

van Klei, W. A., Hoff, R. B., van Aarnhem, E. E., Simmermacher, R. K., Regli, L. P., Kappen, T. H., et al. (2012). Effects of the introduction of the WHO "Surgical Safety Checklist" on in-hospital mortality: A cohort study. *Annals of Surgery, 255*(1), 44–49.

Vaughn, T. E., McCoy, K. D., BootsMiller, B. J., Woolson, R. F., Sorofman, B., Tripp-Reimer, T., et al. (2002). Organizational predictors of adherence to ambulatory care screening guidelines. *Medical Care, 40*(12), 1172–1185.

Von Korff, M., Turner, J. A., Shortreed, S. M., Saunders, K., Rosenberg, D., Thielke, S., & LeResche, L. (2015). Timeliness of care planning upon initiation of chronic opioid therapy for chronic pain. *Pain Medicine, 17*(3), 511–520. doi:10.1093/pm/pnv054.

Walter, M. R., Aucoin, J., Brown, R., Thompson, J. A., & Sullivan, D. T. (2014). A multimodal approach to EBP. *Nursing Management, 45*(1), 14–17. doi:10.1097/01.NUMA.0000440638.48766.a7.

Weeks, S., Moore, P., & Allender, M. (2011). A regional evidence-based practice fellowship: Collaborating competitors. *Journal of Nursing Administration, 41*(1), 10–14. doi:10.1097/NNA.0b013e318200282c.

Weiss, C. H., Moazed, F., McEvoy, C. A., Singer, B. D., Szleifer, I., Amaral, L. A., et al. (2011). Prompting physicians to address a daily checklist and process of care and clinical outcomes: A single-site study. *American Journal of Respiratory and Critical Care Medicine, 184*(6), 680–686.

Wieczorkiewicz, S., & Zatarski, R. (2015). Adherence to and outcomes associated with a clostridium difficile guideline at a large teaching institution. *Hospital Pharmacy, 50*(1), 42–50. doi:10.1310/hjp5001-042.

Wiltsey Stirman, S., Kimberly, J., Cook, N., Calloway, A., Castro, F., & Charns, M. (2012). The sustainability of new programs and innovations: A review of the empirical literature and recommendations for future research. *Implementation Science, 7,* 17. doi:10.1186/1748-5908-7-17.

World Health Organization. (2007). *Practical guidance for scaling up health service innovations.* Switzerland: Author.

Yeh, J. S., Van Hoof, T. J., & Fischer, M. A. (2016). Key features of academic detailing: Development of an expert consensus using the Delphi method. *American Health & Drug Benefits, 9*(1), 42–50.

Zomorodi, M., Topley, D., & McAnaw, M. (2012). Developing a mobility protocol for early mobilization of patients in a surgical/trauma ICU. *Critical Care Research and Practice, 2012,* 964547. doi:10.1155/2012/964547.

Chapter 18

AbuAlRub, R. F., Al-Akour, N. A., & Alatari, N. H. (2015). Perceptions of reporting practices and barriers to reporting incidents among registered nurses and physicians in accredited and nonaccredited Jordanian hospitals. *Journal of Clinical Nursing, 24*(19–20), 2973–2982.

Agency for Healthcare Research and Quality (AHRQ). (n.d.). *TeamSTEPPS: National implementation.* Retrieved from http://teamstepps.ahrq.gov/.

Agency for Healthcare Research and Quality. (2013a). *Practice facilitation handbook: Module 7. Measuring and benchmarking clinical performance.* Rockville, MD: Author. Retrieved from http://www.ahrq.gov/professionals/prevention-chronic-care/improve/system/pfhandbook/mod7.html.

Agency for Healthcare Research and Quality. (2013b). *Strategy 3: Nurse bedside shift report implementation handbook.* Rockville, MD: Author. Retrieved from http://www.ahrq.gov/professionals/systems/hospital/engagingfamilies/strategy3/index.html.

Agency for Healthcare Research and Quality (AHRQ). (2013c). *Guide to patient and family engagement in hospital quality and safety.* Rockville, MD: Author. Retrieved from http://www.ahrq.gov/professionals/systems/hospital/engagingfamilies/index.html.

Agency for Healthcare Research and Quality (AHRQ). (2014). *Patient safety primer: Voluntary patients safety event reporting (incident reporting).* Retrieved from https://psnet.ahrq.gov/primers/primer/13/voluntary-patient-safety-event-reporting-incident-reporting.

Agency for Healthcare Research and Quality (AHRQ). (2015). *Inpatient quality indicators overview.* Retrieved from http://www.qualityindicators.ahrq.gov/Modules/iqi_resources.aspx.

Ahmed, S., Manaf, N. H., & Islam, R. (2013). Effects of Lean Six Sigma application in healthcare services: A literature review. *Reviews in Environmental Health, 28*(4), 189–194.

American Nurses Association (ANA). (2010). *Position statement: Just culture.* Retrieved from http://nursingworld.org/psjustculture.

American Nurses Association (ANA). (2015). *Code of ethics for nurses with interpretive statements.* Silver Spring, MD: Author.

American Nurses Credentialing Center (ANCC). (2016). *ANCC Magnet Recognition Program®.* Retrieved from http://www.nursecredentialing.org/Magnet.

American Society for Quality (ASQ). (n.d.a). *Quality glossary—C.* Retrieved from https://asq.org/quality-resources/quality-glossary/c.

American Society for Quality (ASQ). (n.d.b). *Quality Glossary—L.* Retrieved from https://asq.org/quality-resources/quality-glossary/l.

American Society for Quality (ASQ). (n.d.c). *Quality glossary—T.* Retrieved from https://asq.org/quality-resources/quality-glossary/t.

Berwick, D. M., Godfrey, A. B., & Roessner, J. (1990). *Curing health care: New strategies for quality improvement.* San Francisco, CA: Jossey-Bass.

Berwick, D. M., & Hackbarth, A. D. (2012). Eliminating waste in US health care. *Journal of the American Medical Association, 307*(14), 1513–1516.

Berwick, D. M., Nolan, T. W., & Whittington, J. (2008). The triple aim: Care, health and cost. *Health Affairs, 27*(3), 759–769.

California Patient Safety Action Coalition (CAPSAC). (2016). *CAPSAC: Fair and just culture.* Retrieved from http://www.capsac.org/our-approach-to-safety/fair-and-just-culture/.

Caplan, W., Davis, S., Kraft, S., Berkson, S., Gaines, M. E., Schwab, W., & Pandhi, N. (2014). Engaging patients at the front lines of primary care redesign: Operational lessons for an effective program. *The Joint Commission Journal on Quality and Patient Safety, 40*(12), 533–540.

Carroll, R. (2014). *Enterprise risk management: A framework for success.* Chicago, IL: American Society for Health Risk Management.

Center for Advancing Health. (2010). *A new definition of patient engagement: What is engagement and why is it important?* Washington, DC: Author.

Centers for Medicare & Medicaid Services. (2015). *Hospital value-based purchasing: Overview.* Retrieved from https://www.cms.gov/Medicare/Quality-initiatives-patient-assessment-instruments/hospital-value-based-purchasing/index.html.

Centers for Medicare & Medicaid Services. (2016). *Hospital Compare: Compare hospitals.* Retrieved from https://www.medicare.gov/hospitalcompare/search.html.

Chassin, M. R. (1997). Assessing strategies for quality improvement. *Health Affairs, 16*(3), 151–161.

Chassin, M. R., & Loeb, J. M. (2013). High-reliability health care: Getting there from here. *The Milbank Quarterly, 91*(3), 459–490.

Committee on Enhancing Federal Healthcare Quality Programs (CEFHQP). (2002). In J. M. Corrigan, J. Eden, & B. M. Smith (Eds.), *Leadership by example: Coordinating government roles in improving health care quality.* Washington, DC: National Academies Press.

Corrigan, J. M., Eden, J., & Smith, B. M. (Eds.). (2002). *Leadership by example: Coordinating government roles in improving health care quality.* Washington, DC: National Academies Press.

Deming, W. E. (2000a). *The new economics for industry, government, education.* Cambridge, MA: MIT Center for Advanced Engineering Studies.

Deming, W. E. (2000b). *Out of the crisis.* Cambridge, MA: MIT Center for Advanced Engineering Studies.

Donabedian, A. (1980). *Explorations in quality assessment and monitoring: The definition of quality and approaches to its assessment* (Vol. 1). Ann Arbor, MI: Health Administration Press.

Erickson, I., Ditomassi, M., & Jones, D. A. (2015). *Fostering a research-intensive organization: An interdisciplinary approach for nurses from Massachusetts General Hospital.* Indianapolis, IN: Sigma Theta Tau International.

Harmon, F. G. (1997). Future present. In F. Hesselbein, M. Goldsmith, & R. Beckhard (Eds.), *The organization of the future* (pp. 239–247). San Francisco, CA: Jossey-Bass.

Harry, M., & Schroeder, R. (2000). *Six Sigma: The breakthrough strategy revolutionizing the world's top corporations.* New York, NY: Currency/Doubleday.

Hegge, M. (2015). *Faculty pak: Guide to the code of ethics for nurses with interpretive statements: Development, interpretation and application.* Silver Spring, MD: American Nurses Association. Retrieved from http://www.nursingworld.org/MainMenuCategories/EthicsStandards/CodeofEthicsforNurses/Faculty-Pak.

Hibbard, J. H., Stockard, J., Mahoney, E. R., & Tusler, M. (2004). Development of the Patient Activation Measure (PAM): Conceptualizing and measuring activation in patients and consumers. *HSR: Health Services Research, 39*(4), 1005–1026.

His Holiness the Dalai Lama, & Cutler, H. C. (1998). *The art of happiness.* New York, NY: Riverhead Books.

Hughes, R. G. (Ed.). (2008). *Patient safety and quality: An evidence-based handbook for nurses.* (AHRQ Publication No. 08-0043). Retrieved from http://archive.ahrq.gov/clinicians-providers/resources/nursing/resources/nurseshdbk/nurseshdbk.pdf.

Institute for Healthcare Improvement (IHI). (2004). *About IHI.* Retrieved from http://www.ihi.org/about/Pages/default.aspx.

Institute for Healthcare Improvement (IHI). (2005). *Going lean in health care.* Cambridge, MA: Author.

Institute for Healthcare Improvement (IHI). (2016a). *Plan-Do-Study-Act (PDSA) worksheet.* Retrieved from http://www.ihi.org/resources/pages/tools/plandostudyactworksheet.aspx.

Institute for Healthcare Improvement (IHI). (2016b). IHI Open School: *Overview.* Retrieved from http://www.ihi.org/education/ihiopenschool/overview/Pages/default.aspx.

Institute of Medicine (IOM), Committee on Enhancing Federal Health Care Quality Programs. (2002). *Enhancing federal health care quality programs.* Retrieved from http://nationalacademies.org/hmd/activities/quality/fedhcquality.aspx.

Institute of Medicine (IOM), Committee on Quality of Health Care in America (CQHCA). (2001). *Crossing the quality chasm: A new health system for the 21st century.* Washington, DC: National Academies Press.

Institute of Medicine (IOM), Committee on the National Quality Report on Health Care Delivery. (2001). *Envisioning the national health care quality report.* Washington, DC: National Academies Press.

Institute of Medicine (IOM), Committee on the Robert Wood Johnson Foundation Initiative on the Future of Nursing. (2011). *The future of nursing: Leading change, advancing health.* Washington, DC: National Academies Press.

Jones, D., & Womack, J. (2003). *Lean thinking: Banish waste and create wealth in your corporation, revised and updated.* New York, NY: Free Press.

Juran, J. M. (1989). *Juran on leadership for quality: An executive handbook.* New York, NY: The Free Press.

Juran Institute. (2009). *Product store.* Retrieved from https://www.juran.com/resources.

Kohn, L. T., Corrigan, J. M., & Donaldson, M. S. (Eds.). (2000). *To err is human: Building a safer health care system.* Washington, DC: National Academies Press.

Lake, E. T., Staiger, D., Horbar, J., Cheung, R., Kenny, M. J., Patrick, T., & Rogowski, J. A. (2012). Association between hospital recognition for nursing excellence and outcomes for low-birth-weight infants. *Journal of the American Medical Association, 307*(16), 1709–1716.

Lin, C. (2013). *Three ways to get physicians on board with clinical standards.* Retrieved from https://www.advisory.com/research/financial-leadership-council/at-the-margins/2013/05/three-strategies-for-ensuring-clinical-standardization.

Lohr, K. (Ed.). (1990). *Medicare: A strategy for quality assurance* (Vol. 2). Washington, DC: National Academies Press.

Maurer, M., Dardess, P., Carman, K., & Smeeding, I. (2014). *Guide to patient and family engagement: Environmental scan report.* Rockville, MD: Agency for Healthcare Research and Quality. Retrieved from http://www.ahrq.gov/research/findings/final-reports/ptfamilyscan/.

McHugh, M. D., Kelly, L. A., Smith, H. L., Wu, E. S., Vanak, J. M., & Aiken, L. H. (2013). Lower mortality in Magnet hospitals. *Medical Care, 51*(5), 382–388.

National Institute of Standards and Technology. (2007). *Presidential award for excellence honors five U.S. organizations: Two nonprofits recognized in first year of category.* Retrieved from www.nist.gov/public_affairs/releases/2007baldrigerecipients.cfm.

National Patient Safety Foundation. (2016). *RCA2 Improving root cause analyses and actions to prevent harm* (Vol. 2). Boston, MA: Author.

National Quality Forum (NQF). (2004). *National voluntary consensus standards for nursing-sensitive care: An initial performance measure set.* Washington, DC: Author.

National Quality Forum (NQF). (2009). *NQF patient safety terms and definitions.* Washington, DC: Author. Retrieved from https://www.qualityforum.org/Topics/Safety_Definitions.aspx.

National Quality Forum (NQF). (2011). *Measure evaluation criteria.* Retrieved from http://www.qualityforum.org/.

National Quality Forum (NQF). (2012). *Nursing-sensitive care: Initial measures.* Retrieved from http://www.qualityforum.org/Projects/n-r/Nursing-Sensitive_Care_Initial_Measures/Nursing_Sensitive_Care__Initial_Measures.aspx.

Nursing Alliance for Quality Care (NAQC). (2016). *About NAQC.* Retrieved from http://www.naqc.org/Functional/About-NAQC.

Omenn, G. (2002). *Public briefing: Opening statement—Leadership by example: Coordinating government roles in improving health care quality.* Washington, DC: Institute of Medicine.

O'Neil, E. H., The Pew Health Professions Commission (PHPC). (1998). *Recreating health professional practice for a new century: The fourth report of the Pew Health Professions Commission.* San Francisco, CA: PHPC.

Palmer, S., & Torgerson, D. J. (1999). Definition of efficiency. *British Medical Journal, 318*, 1136.

Pelletier, L. R. (1998). Guest editorial: Standardization. *Journal of Nursing Care Quality, 13*(1), vii.

Pelletier, L. R. (2000). On error-free health care: Mission possible! [Editorial]. *Journal for Healthcare Quality, 22*(3), 2, 9.

Pelletier, L. R., & Hoffman, J. A. (2002). A framework for selecting performance measures for opioid treatment programs. *Journal for Healthcare Quality, 24*(3), 24–35.

Pelletier, L. R., & Stichler, J. F. (2013). Action brief: Patient engagement and activation: A health reform imperative and improvement opportunity for nursing. *Nursing Outlook, 61*(1), 51–54.

Pelletier, L. R., & Stichler, J. F. (2014a). Ensuring patient and family engagement: A professional nurse's toolkit. *Journal of Nursing Care Quality, 29*(2), 110–114.

Pelletier, L. R., & Stichler, J. F. (2014b). Patient-centered care and engagement: Nurse leaders' imperative for health reform. *The Journal of Nursing Administration, 44*(9), 473–480.

Pelletier, L. R. (2015). Commentary on "Engagement as an Element of Safe Inpatient Psychiatric Environments." *Journal of the American Psychiatric Nurses Association, 21*(3), 191–194.

Planetree. (2014). *Reputation: Welcome to Planetree.* Retrieved from http://planetree.org/reputation/.

Plsek, P., & Omnias, A. (1989). *Juran Institute quality improvement tools: Problem solving/glossary.* Wilton, CT: Juran Institute.

Polacek, M. J., Allen, D. E., Damin-Moss, R. S., Schwartz, A. J., & Sharp, D., et al. (2015). Engagement as an element of safe inpatient psychiatric environments. *Journal of the American Psychiatric Nurses Association, 21*(3), 181–190.

Press Ganey. (2015). *Nursing Quality (NDNQI).* Retrieved from http://www.pressganey.com/solutions/clinical-quality/nursing-quality.

QSEN Institute. (2014). *Pre-licensure KSAs.* Retrieved from http://qsen.org/competencies/pre-licensure-ksas/.

Quality Interagency Coordination (QuIC). Task Force. (2000). *Doing what counts for patient safety: Federal actions to reduce medical errors and their impact.* Retrieved from http://archive.ahrq.gov/quic/report/mederr2.htm.

Robert Wood Johnson Foundation. (2014). *Aligning Forces for Quality: Patient engagement toolkit.* Retrieved from http://forces4quality.org/node/6319.html.

Roeder, A. (2014). *Reducing wasteful health care spending begs the question, what is waste?* Retrieved from http://www.hsph.harvard.edu/news/features/reducing-wasteful-health-care-spending/.

Sackett, D. L., Rosenberg, W. M. C., Gray, J. A. M., Haynes, R. B., & Richardson, W. S. (1996). Evidence-based medicine: What it is and what it isn't. *British Medical Journal, 312*(7023), 71.

Sharp HealthCare. (2016). *Mission, vision and values.* Retrieved from http://www.sharp.com/about/our-story/mission-vision-values.cfm.

The Joint Commission (TJC). (2016a). *Specification manual for Joint Commission National Quality Measures.* Retrieved from https://manual.jointcommission.org/releases/TJC2016A/AppendixDTJC.html.

The Joint Commission (TJC). (2016b). *Facts about ORYX vendors performance measurement systems.* Retrieved from http://www.jointcommission.org/facts_about_oryx_performance_measurement_systems/.

The Joint Commission (TJC). (2016c). *Sentinel events (SE): Hospital.* Retrieved from http://www.jointcommission.org/assets/1/6/CAMH_24_SE_all_CURRENT.pdf.

The Joint Commission (TJC). (2016d). *Core measure sets*. Retrieved from http://www.jointcommission.org/core_measure_sets.aspx.

The Joint Commission (TJC). (2016e). *Comprehensive accreditation manual for hospitals: Patient safety systems (Update 2)*. Retrieved from http://www.jointcommission.org/assets/1/18/PSC_for_Web.pdf.

The Joint Commission (TJC). (2016f). *Specifications manual for national hospital inpatient quality measures*. Retrieved from https://www.jointcommission.org/specifications_manual_for_national_hospital_inpatient_quality_measures.aspx.

The Joint Commission (TJC). (2016g). *Sentinel event alert/topics library updates*. Retrieved from http://www.jointcommission.org/daily_update/joint_commission_daily_update.aspx?k=721&b=&t=4.

The Joint Commission (TJC). (2016h). *National patient safety goals*. Retrieved from http://www.jointcommission.org/standards_information/npsgs.aspx.

US Department of Veterans Affairs. (2015a). *VA National Center for Patient Safety*. Retrieved from http://www.patientsafety.va.gov/index.asp.

US Department of Veterans Affairs. (2015b). *Root cause analysis tools*. Retrieved from http://www.patientsafety.va.gov/docs/joe/rca_tools_2_15.pdf.

US Department of Veterans Affairs. (2015c). *Healthcare failure mode and effect analysis (HFMEA)*. Retrieved from http://www.patientsafety.va.gov/professionals/onthejob/hfmea.asp.

Visiting Nursing Service of New York (VNSNY). (2016). *Vision and mission*. Retrieved from https://www.vnsny.org/who-we-are/about-us/mission-vision/.

Waddill-Goad, S. M., & Langster, H. J. (2016). Planning intentional quality and safety. In S. Waddill-Goad & H. J. Langster (Eds.), *Nurse burnout: Overcoming stress in nursing* (pp. 167–196). Indianapolis, IN: Nursing Knowledge International.

Weick, K. E., & Sutcliffe, K. M. (2007). *Managing the unexpected* (2nd ed.). San Francisco, CA: Jossey-Bass.

Wise, D. (2014). *Getting to know just culture*. Retrieved from https://www.outcome-eng.com/getting-to-know-just-culture/.

Yakusheva, O., Lindrooth, R., & Weiss, M. (2014). Nurse value-added and patient outcomes in acute care. *Health Services Research, 49*(6), 1767–1786.

Zou, X-J., & Zhang, Y-P. (2016). Rates of nursing errors and handoffs-related errors in a medical unit following implementation of a standardized nursing handoff form. *Journal of Nursing Care Quality, 31*(1), 61–67.

Chapter 19

Agency for Healthcare Research and Quality (AHRQ). (2000). *Outcomes research fact sheet*. Retrieved from http://archive.ahrq.gov/research/findings/factsheets/outcomes/outfact/outcomes-and-research.html.

Agency for Healthcare Research and Quality (AHRQ). (2016). *Desirable attributes of a quality measure*. Retrieved from https://www.qualitymeasures.ahrq.gov/tutorial/attributes.aspx.

Aiken, L. H., Sloane, D. M., Bruyneel, L., Van den Heede, K., Griffiths, P., Busse, R., et al. (2014). Nurse staffing and education and hospital mortality in nine European countries: A retrospective observational study. *Lancet, 383*(9931), 1824–1830.

Baker, J. D. (2015). Language of improvement: Metrics, key performance indicators, benchmarks, analytics, scorecards, and dashboards. *AORN Journal, 102*(3), 223–227.

Berkowitz, R. E., Fang, Z., Helfand, B. K., Jones, R. N., Schreiber, R., & Paasche-Orlow, M. K. (2013). Project ReEngineered Discharge (RED) lowers hospital readmissions of patients discharged from a skilled nursing facility. *Journal of the American Medical Directors Association, 14*(10), 736–740.

Black, N. (2013). Patient reported outcome measures could help transform healthcare. *British Medical Journal, 346*, f167. doi:10.1136/bmj.f167.

Brennan, P. F., & Bakken, S. (2015). Nursing needs big data and big data needs nursing. *Journal of Nursing Scholarship, 47*(5), 477–484.

Centers for Medicare & Medicaid Services (CMS). (2015, December 18). *CMS quality measure development plan: Supporting the transition to the merit-based incentive payment system (MIPS) and alternative payment models (APMs)*. Retrieved from https://www.cms.gov/Medicare/Quality-Initiatives-Patient-Assessment-Instruments/Value-Based-Programs/MACRA-MIPS-and-APMs/Draft-CMS-Quality-Measure-Development-Plan-MDP.pdf.

Cohen, M. Z., Thompson, C. B., Yates, B., Zimmerman, L., & Pullen, C. H. (2015). Implementing common data elements across studies to advance research. *Nursing Outlook, 63*(2), 181–188.

Corwin, E. J., Berg, J. A., Armstrong, T. S., DeVito Dabbs, A., Lee, K. A., Meek, P., & Redeker, N. (2014). Envisioning the future in symptom science. *Nursing Outlook, 62*(5), 346–351.

Coulter, A., Locock, L., Ziebland, S., & Calabrese, J. (2014). Collecting data on patient experience is not enough: They must be used to improve care. *British Medical Journal, 348*, g2225. doi:10.1136/bmj.g2225.

Donabedian, A. (1985). *The methods and findings of quality assessment and monitoring: An illustrated analysis* (Vol. 3). Ann Arbor, MI: Health Administration Press.

Donabedian, A. (2005). Evaluating the quality of medical care. 1966. *Milbank Quarterly, 83*(4), 691–729.

Doran, D., Mildon, B., & Clarke, S. (2011). Towards a national report card in nursing: A knowledge synthesis. *Nursing Leadership, 24*(2), 38–57.

Dusek, B., Pearce, N., Harripaul, A., & Lloyd, M. (2014). Care transitions: A systematic review of best practices. *Journal of Nursing Care Quality, 30*(3), 233–239.

Ellwood, P. M. (1988). Shattuck lecture—Outcomes management: A technology of patient experience. *New England Journal of Medicine, 318*(23), 1549–1556.

Frith, K. H., Anderson, F., & Sewell, J. P. (2010). Assessing and selecting data for a nursing services dashboard. *Journal of Nursing Administration, 40*(1), 10–16.

Gallagher, R. M., & Rowell, P. A. (2003). Claiming the future of nursing through nursing-sensitive quality indicators. *Nursing Administration Quarterly, 27*(4), 273–284.

Garcia, A., Caspers, B., Westra, B., Pruinelli, L., & Delaney, C. (2015). Sharable and comparable data for nursing management. *Nursing Administration Quarterly, 39*(4), 297–303.

Griffiths, P., Ball, J., Drennan, J., Dall'Ora, C., Jones, J., Maruotti, A., et al. (2016). Nurse staffing and patient outcomes: Strengths and limitations of the evidence to inform policy and practice. *International Journal of Nursing Studies, 63*, 213–225.

Healthcare Information and Management Systems Society (HIMSS). (2015). *HIMSS CNO-CNIO vendor roundtable guiding principles for Big Data in nursing: Using Big Data to improve the quality of care and outcomes*. Retrieved from http://www.himss.org/sites/himssorg/files/FileDownloads/HIMSS_Nursing_Big_Data_Group_Principles.pdf.

Huber, D., & Oermann, M. (1998). The evolution of outcomes management. In D. L. Flarey & S. S. Blancett (Eds.), *Cardiovascular outcomes: Collaborative, path-based approaches* (pp. 3–12). Gaithersburg, MD: Aspen.

Iezzoni, L. I. (Ed.). (2013). *Risk adjustment for measuring health care outcomes* (4th ed.). Chicago, IL: Health Administration Press.

Institute for Healthcare Improvement (IHI). (2016). *Triple Aim for populations*. Retrieved from http://www.ihi.org/Topics/TripleAim/Pages/default.aspx.

International Consortium for Health Outcomes Measurement (ICHOM). (2016). *ICHOM's mission*. Retrieved from http://www.ichom.org/why-we-do-it/.

Jeffs, L., Beswick, S., Lo, J., Lai, Y., Chhun, A., & Campbell, H. (2014). Insights from staff nurses and managers on unit-specific nursing performance dashboards. *BMJ Quality & Safety, 23*(12), 1001–1006.

Jeffs, L., MacMillan, K., McKey, C., & Ferris, E. (2009). Nursing leaders' accountability to narrow the safety chasm: Insights and implications from the collective evidence base on health care safety. *Canadian Journal of Nursing Leadership, 22*(1), 73–85.

Jeffs, L., Merkley, J., McAllister, M., Richardson, S., & Eli, J. (2011). Using a nursing balanced scorecard approach to measure and optimize nursing performance. *Nursing Leadership, 24*(1), 47–58.

Jeffs, L., Doran, D., Hayes, L., Mainville, C., VanDeVelde-Coke, S., Lamont, L., & Boal, A. S. (2015a). Implementation of the National Nursing Quality Report initiative in Canada: Insights from pilot participants. *Journal of Nursing Care Quality*, 30(4), E9–E16.

Jeffs, L., Nincic, V., White, P., Hayes, L., & Lo, J. (2015b). Leveraging data to transform nursing care: Insights from nurse leaders. *Journal of Nursing Care Quality*, 30(3), 269–274.

Jennings, B. M., Staggers, N., & Brosch, L. R. (1999). A classification scheme for outcome indicators. *Image—The Journal of Nursing Scholarship*, 31(4), 381–388.

Jha, A. K., Joynt, K. E., Orav, E. J., & Epstein, A. M. (2012). The long-term effect of premier pay for performance on patient outcomes. *New England Journal of Medicine*, 366(17), 1601–1615.

Kane, R. L. (2006). Introduction: An outcomes approach. In R. L. Kane (Ed.), *Understanding health care outcomes research* (2nd ed., pp. 3–22). Boston, MA: Jones & Bartlett.

Kerfoot, K. (2015). Intelligently managed data: Achieving excellence in nursing care. *Nursing Economic$*, 33(6), 342–343.

Kohlbrenner, J., Whitelaw, G., & Cannaday, D. (2011). Nurses critical to quality, safety, and now financial performance. *Journal of Nursing Administration*, 41(3), 122–128.

Latif, A., Rawat, N., Pustavoitau, A., Pronovost, P. J., & Pham, J. C. (2013). National study on the distribution, causes, and consequences of voluntarily reported medication errors between the ICU and non-ICU settings. *Critical Care Medicine*, 41(2), 389–398.

Lin, J., Jiao, T., Biskupiak, J. E., & McAdam-Marx, C. (2013). Application of electronic medical record data for health outcomes research: A review of recent literature. *Expert Review of Pharmacoeconomics and Outcomes Research*, 13(2), 191–200.

Loan, L. A., Patrician, P. A., & McCarthy, M. (2011). Participation in a national nursing outcomes database: Monitoring outcomes over time. *Nursing Administration Quarterly*, 35(1), 72–81.

Markovitz, A. A., & Ryan, A. M. (2016). Pay-for-performance: Disappointing results or masked heterogeneity? *Medical Care Research and Review*, 1–76. pii:1077558715619282.

Morris, R., Matthews, A., & Scott, A. P. (2014). Validity, reliability and utility of the Irish Nursing Minimum Data Set for General Nursing in investigating the effectiveness of nursing interventions in a general nursing setting: A repeated measures design. *International Journal of Nursing Studies*, 51(4), 562–571. doi:10.1016/j.ijnurstu.2013.07.011.

Mukamel, D. B., Ye, Z., Glance, L. G., & Li, Y. (2015). Does mandating nursing home participation in quality reporting make a difference? Evidence from Massachusetts. *Medical Care*, 53(8), 713–719.

Murphy, L. S., Wilson, M. L., & Newhouse, R. P. (2013). Data analytics: Making the most of input with strategic output. *Journal of Nursing Administration*, 43(7–8), 367–370.

Naci, H., & Soumerai, S. B. (2016). History bias, study design, and the unfulfilled promise of pay-for-performance policies in health care. *Preventing Chronic Disease*, 13. doi:10.5888/pcd13.160133.

National Institutes of Health (NIH). (2016). *Common data element (CDE) resource portal*. Retrieved from https://www.nlm.nih.gov/cde/.

National Quality Forum (NQF). (2004). *National voluntary consensus standards for nursing-sensitive care: An initial performance measure set—A consensus report*. Washington, DC: Author. Retrieved from http://www.qualityforum.org/Publications/2004/10/National_Voluntary_Consensus_Standards_for_Nursing-Sensitive_Care__An_Initial_Performance_Measure_Set.aspx.

National Quality Forum (NQF). (2015). *Data needed for systematically improving healthcare*. Retrieved from http://www.qualityforum.org/Publications/2015/07/Data_for_Systematic_Improvement_Final_White_Paper.aspx.

Naylor, M. D. (2007). Advancing the science in the measurement of health care quality influenced by nurses. *Medical Care Research & Review*, 64(Suppl. 2), S144–S169.

Naylor, M. D., Aiken, L. H., Kurtzman, E. T., Olds, D. M., & Hirschman, K. B. (2011). The importance of transitional care in achieving health reform. *Health Affairs*, 30(4), 746–754.

Naylor, M. D. (2012). Advancing high value transitional care. The central role of nursing and its leadership. *Nursing Administration Quarterly*, 36(2), 115–126.

Nilsson, E., Orwelius, L., & Kristenson, M. (2016). Patient-reported outcomes in the Swedish National Quality Registers. *Journal of Internal Medicine*, 279(2), 141–153.

Pelletier, L. R., & Stichler, J. F. (2013). American Academy of Nursing on Policy Action brief: Patient engagement and activation: A health reform imperative and improvement opportunity for nursing. *Nursing Outlook*, 61(1), 51–54.

Porter, M. E. (2010). What is value in health care? *New England Journal of Medicine*, 363(26), 2477–2481.

Porter, M. E., Larsson, S., & Lee, T. H. (2016). Standardizing patient outcomes measurement. *New England Journal of Medicine*, 374(6), 504–506.

Redeker, N. S., Anderson, R., Bakken, S., Corwin, E., Docherty, S., Dorsey, S. G., et al. (2015). Advancing symptom science through use of common data elements. *Journal of Nursing Scholarship*, 47(5), 379–388.

Reichert, J., & Furlong, G. (2014). Five key pillars of an analytics center of excellence, which are required to manage populations and transform organizations into the next era of health care. *Nursing Administration Quarterly*, 38(2), 159–165.

Serratt, T. (2013a). California's nurse-to-patient ratios, Part 2: 8 years later, what do we know about hospital level outcomes? *Journal of Nursing Administration*, 43(10), 549–553.

Serratt, T. (2013b). California's nurse-to-patient ratios, Part 3: Eight years later, what do we know about patient level outcomes? *Journal of Nursing Administration*, 43(11), 581–585.

Trinkoff, A. M., Lerner, N. B., Storr, C. L., Han, K., Johantgen, M. E., & Gartrell, K. (2015). Leadership education, certification and resident outcomes in US nursing homes: Cross-sectional secondary data analysis. *International Journal of Nursing Studies*, 52(1), 334–344.

Velentgas, P., Dreyer, N. A., Nourjah, P., Smith, S. R., & Torchia, M. M. (Eds.). (2013). *Developing a protocol for observational comparative effectiveness research: A user's guide*. AHRQ Publication No. 12(13)-EHC099. Rockville, MD: Agency for Healthcare Research and Quality.

Westra, B., Clancy, T., Sensmeier, J, Warren, J. J., Weaver, C., & Delaney, C. W. (2015). Nursing knowledge: Big data science—implications for nurse leaders. *Nursing Administration Quarterly*, 39(4), 304–310.

Zrelak, P. A., Utter, G. H., Sadeghi, B., Cuny, J., Baron, R., & Romano, P. S. (2012). Using the agency for healthcare research and quality patient safety indicators for targeting nursing quality improvement. *Journal of Nursing Care Quality*, 27(2), 99–108.

Chapter 20

Ametz, J. E., Hamblin, L., Essenmacher, L., Upfal, M. J., Ager, J., & Luborsky, M. (2015). Understanding patient-to-worker violence in hospitals: A qualitative analysis of documented incident reports. *Journal of Advanced Nursing*, 71(2), 338–348.

ASIS International and the Society for Human Resource Management (ASIS/SHRM). (2011). *Workplace violence prevention and intervention*. Retrieved from https://www.asisonline.org/Standards-Guidelines/Standards/published/Pages/Workplace-Violence-Prevention-and-Intervention-Standard-(Download).aspx.

Aytaç, S., & Dursun, S. (2012). The effect on employees of violence climate in the workplace. *Work*, 41, 3026–3031.

Bible, J. D. (2012). The jerk at work: Workplace bullying and the law's inability to combat it. *Employee Relations Law Journal*, 38(1), 32–51.

Branch, S., Ramsay, S., & Barker, M. (2013). Workplace bullying, mobbing, and general harassment: A review. *International Journal of Management Reviews*, 15, 280–299.

Busch, N. E., & Givens, A. D. (2012). Public-private partnerships in Homeland Security: Opportunities and challenges. *Homeland Security Affairs, 8*(18), 1–24.

Campana, K. L., & Hammond, S. (2015). Incivility from patients and their families: Can organisational justice protect nurses from burnout? *Journal of Nursing Management, 23*(6), 716–725.

Chang, C., Eatough, E. M., Spector, P. E., & Kessler, S. R. (2012). Violence-prevention climate, exposure to violence and aggression, and prevention behavior. *Journal of Organizational Behavior, 33,* 657–677.

Christie, W. (2015). Perceptions of managerial support after workplace violence. *Nursing Management, 22*(7), 32–36.

Cowin, L., Davies, R., Estall, G., Berlin, T., Fitzgerald, M., & Hoot, S. (2003). De-escalating aggression and violence in the mental health setting. *International Journal of Mental Health Nursing, 12,* 64–73.

Farkas, G. M., & Tsukayama, J. K. (2012). An integrative approach to threat assessment and management: Security and mental health response to a threatening client. *Work, 42,* 9–14.

Foley, M., & Rauser, E. (2012). Evaluating progress in reducing workplace violence: Trends in Washington State workers' compensation claim rates, 1997–2007. *Work, 42,* 67–81.

Frederickson, E. D., & McCorkle, S. (2013). Explaining organizational responses to workplace aggression. *Public Personnel Management, 42,* 223–238.

Hamblin, L. E., Essenmacher, L., Upfal, M., Russell, J., Luborsky, M. Ager, J., & Ametz, J. E. (2015). Catalysts of worker-to-worker violence and incivility in hospitals. *Journal of Clinical Nursing, 24,* 2458–2467.

Healthcare & Public Health Sector Coordinating Council. (2017). *Active shooter planning and response in a healthcare setting* 3rd edition. Retrieved from https://www.fbi.gov/file-repository/active_shooter_planning_and_response_in_a_healthcare_setting.pdf/view.

Healthy Workplace Bill. (2016). *State of the union.* Retrieved from http://healthyworkplacebill.org/states/.

Jenkins, E. L., Fisher, B. S., & Hartley, D. (2012). Safe and secure at work?: Findings from the 2002 workplace risk supplement. *Work, 42,* 57–66.

Lanctot, N., & Guay, S. (2014). The aftermath of workplace violence among healthcare workers: A systematic literature review of the consequences. *Aggression and Violent Behavior, 19*(5), 492–501.

Magnavita, N. (2014). Workplace violence and occupational stress in healthcare workers: A chicken-and-egg situation—Results of a 6-year follow-up study. *Journal of Nursing Scholarship, 46*(5), 366–376.

Mao, F. Z. (2013). Is litigation your final answer? Why the Healthy Workplace Bill should include an ADR provision. *Brooklyn Journal of Law and Policy, 21*(2), 679–723.

Mayo v. PCC Structurals, Inc., 795 F. 3d 941. (9th Cir. 2015).

National Institute for Occupational Safety and Health (NIOSH) Centers for Disease Control and Prevention, U.S. Department of Health and Human Services. (2012). *How to prevent violence on the job.* DHHS, NIOSH Publication No. 2012-118. Retrieved from http://www.cdc.gov/niosh/docs/2012-118/pdfs/2012-118.pdf.

National Institute for Occupational Safety and Health (NIOSH) Centers for Disease Control and Prevention, US Department of Health and Human Services. (2013). *Workplace violence prevention for nurses.* DHHS, NIOSH Publication No. 2013-155. Retrieved from http://www.cdc.gov/niosh/topics/violence/training_nurses.html.

National Institute for Occupational Safety and Health (NIOSH) Centers for Disease Control and Prevention, US Department of Health and Human Services. (2015). *Notable milestones in NIOSH history.* Retrieved from http://www.cdc.gov/niosh/timeline.html.

Nielsen, M. B., & Einarson, S. (2012). Outcomes of exposure to workplace bullying. *Work and Stress, 26*(4), 309–332.

Occupational Safety and Health Administration (OSHA) US Department of Labor. (2015a). *Workplace violence in healthcare: Understanding the challenge.* Retrieved from https://www.osha.gov/Publications/OSHA3826.pdf.

Occupational Safety and Health Administration (OSHA) US Department of Labor. (2015b). *Guidelines for preventing workplace violence for healthcare and social service workers.* OSHA publication 3148-04R 2015. Retrieved from https://www.osha.gov/Publications/osha3148.pdf.

Paccione, M. (n.d.). *De-escalating conflict in the healthcare setting.* Retrieved from http://www.health.ri.gov/materialbyothers/DeEscalatingConflictInTheHealthcareSetting.pdf.

Richmond, J. S., Berlin, J. S., Fishkind, A. B., Holloman, G. H., Jr., Zeller, S. L., Wilson, M. P., et al. (2012). Verbal de-escalation of the agitated patient: Consensus statement of the American Association for Emergency Psychiatry Project BETA de-escalation workgroup. *Western Journal of Emergency Medicine, 13*(1), 17–25.

Sanders, D. E., Pattison, P., & Bible, J. D. (2012). Legislating "nice": Analysis and assessment of proposed workplace bullying prohibitions. *Southern Law Journal, 2*(1), 1–36.

Secretary of Labor v. Integra Health Management, Inc., OSHRC No. 13-1124. (June 22, 2015).

Spector, P. E., Yang, L., & Zhou, Z. E. (2015). A longitudinal investigation of the role of violence prevention climate in exposure to workplace physical violence and verbal abuse. *Work and Stress, 29*(4), 325–340.

Speroni, K. G, Fitch, L., Duggan, T., Dawson, E., & Atherton, M. (2014). Incidence and cost of nurse workplace violence perpetrated by hospital patients or patient visitors. *Journal of Emergency Nursing, 40*(3), 218–228.

Stagg, S. J., Sheridan, D. J., Jones, R. A., & Speroni, K. G. (2013). Workplace bullying: The effectiveness of a workplace program. *Workplace Health and Safety, 61*(8), 333–338.

The Joint Commission (TJC). (2017). *Preventing violence in the health care setting. Sentinel Event Alert #45.* Retrieved from http://www.jointcommission.org/assets/1/18/sea_45.pdf.

Yamada, D. C. (2010). Workplace bullying and American employment law: A ten-year progress report and assessment. *Comparative Labor Law and Policy Journal, 32,* 251–284.

Chapter 21

Acree, C. M. (2006). The relationship between nurse leadership practices and hospital nursing retention. *Newborn and Infant Nursing Reviews, 6*(1), 34–40.

Aiken, L. H. (2008). Economics of nursing. *Policy, Politics, & Nursing Practice, 9*(2), 73–79.

Aiken, L. H., Clarke, S. P., Sloane, D. M., Sochalski, J., & Silber, J. H. (2002). Hospital nurse staffing and patient mortality, nurse burnout, and job dissatisfaction. *Journal of the American Medical Association, 288*(16), 1987–1993.

American Association of Colleges of Nursing (AACN). (2008). *AACN applauds Representatives Latham and Baldwin for introducing the Nurses' Higher Education and Loan Repayment Act of 2008.* Washington, DC: Author. Retrieved from http://www.aacn.nche.edu/news/articles/2008/higher-education-act.

American Association of Colleges of Nursing (AACN). (2011). *2011 Survey overview: Percentage change in enrollments in entry-level baccalaureate nursing programs: 1994–2011.* Washington, DC: Author. Retrieved from http://www.aacn.nche.edu/Media-Relations/EnrollChanges.pdf.

American Association of Colleges of Nursing (AACN). (2011–2012). *Enrollment and graduations in baccalaureate and graduate programs in nursing.* Washington, DC: Author.

American Association of Colleges of Nursing (AACN). (2012a). *New AACN data show an enrollment surge in baccalaureate and graduate programs amid calls for more highly educated nurses.* Washington, DC: Author. Retrieved from http://www.aacn.nche.edu/news/articles/2012/enrollment-data.

American Association of Colleges of Nursing (AACN). (2012b). *AACN report on 2010–2011 salaries of instructional and administrative nursing faculty in baccalaureate and graduate programs in nursing.* Washington, DC: Author. Retrieved from http://www.aacn.nche.edu/media-relations/fact-sheets/nursing-faculty-shortage.

American Association of Colleges of Nursing (AACN). (2012–2013). *Enrollment and graduations in baccalaureate and graduate programs in nursing.* Washington, DC: Author.

American Association of Colleges of Nursing (AACN). (2013–2014). *2013–2014 salaries of instructional and administrative nursing faculty in baccalaureate and graduate programs in nursing.* Washington, DC: Author.

American Association of Colleges of Nursing (AACN). (2014). *2013 Survey overview: Percentage change in enrollments in entry-level baccalaureate nursing programs: 1994–2013.* Washington, DC: Author. Retrieved from http://www.aacn.nche.edu/Media-Relations/EnrollChanges.pdf.

American Association of Colleges of Nursing (AACN). (2015a). *New AACN data confirm enrollment surge in schools of nursing.* Washington, DC: Author. Retrieved from http://www.aacn.nche.edu/faculty/news/2015/enrollment.

American Association of Colleges of Nursing (AACN). (2015b). *Fact sheet: Enhancing diversity in the nursing workforce.* Washington, DC: Author.

American Association of Colleges of Nursing (AACN). (2016). *Special survey on vacant faculty positions for academic year 2015–2016.* Washington, DC: Author.

American Association of Critical-Care Nurses. (2016). *AACN Standards for establishing and sustaining healthy work environments* (2nd ed.). Aliso Viejo, CA: Author. Retrieved from http://www.aacn.org/wd/hwe/docs/hwestandards.pdf.

American Hospital Association (AHA), Commission on Workforce for Hospitals and Health Systems. (2002). *In our hands: How hospital leaders can build a thriving workforce.* (AHA Product No. 210101). Chicago, IL: Author.

American Hospital Association (AHA). (2010). *Workforce 2015: Strategy trumps shortage.* Chicago, IL: Author.

American Hospital Association (AHA) Career Center. (2015). *2015 health care talent acquisition environmental scan.* Chicago, IL. Retrieved from http://www.healthcareercenter.com/.

American Nurses Association (ANA). (2002). *Nursing's agenda for the future: A call to the nation.* Silver Spring, MD: Author.

American Nurses Association (ANA). (2012). *ANA's Principles for nurse staffing* (2nd ed.). Silver Spring, MD: Author.

American Nurses Association (ANA). (2014). *Fast facts: The nursing workforce 2014: Growth, salaries, education, demographics & trends.* Silver Spring, MD: Author.

American Nurses Credentialing Center (ANCC). (2016). *Magnet Recognition Program® overview.* Retrieved from http://www.nursecredentialing.org/Magnet/ProgramOverview.

American Organization of Nurse Executives. (2016). *AONE's guiding principles for the newly licensed nurse's transition into practice.* Retrieved from http://www.aone.org/resources/newly-licensed-nurses-transition-practice.

Atencio, B. L., Cohen, J., & Gorenberg, B. (2003). Nurse retention: Is it worth it? *Nursing Economic$, 21*(6), 262–268, 299.

Auerbach, D. I., Buerhaus, P. I., & Staiger, D. O. (2011). Registered nurse supply grows faster than projected amid surge in new entrants ages 23–26. *Health Affairs, 30*(12), 2286–2292.

Auerbach, D. I., Staiger, D. O., Muench, U., & Buerhaus, P. I. (2013). The nursing workforce in an era of health care reform. *New England Journal of Medicine, 386*(16), 1470–1472.

Buerhaus, P. I., Auerbach, D. I., & Staiger, D. O. (2009a). The recent surge in nurse employment: Causes and implications. *Health Affairs, 28*(4), w657–w668.

Buerhaus, P. I., Auerbach, D. I., & Staiger, D. O. (2016). Recent changes in the number of nurses graduating from undergraduate and graduate programs. *Nursing Economic$, 34*(1), 46–48.

Buerhaus, P. I., DesRoches, C., Donelan, K., & Hess, R. (2009b). Still making progress to improve the hospital workplace environment? Results from the 2008 national survey of registered nurses. *Nursing Economic$, 27*(5), 289–301.

Buerhaus, P. I., Donelan, K., Ulrich, B. T., Norman, L., & Dittus, R. (2005). Is the shortage of hospital registered nurses getting better or worse? Findings from two recent national surveys of RNs. *Nursing Economic$, 2*(2), 61–71, 96.

Buerhaus, P. I., Staiger, D., & Auerbach, D. (2000). Implications of an aging registered nurse workforce. *Journal of the American Medical Association, 283*(22), 2948–2954.

Buerhaus, P. I., Staiger, D. O., & Auerbach, D. L. (2008). *The future of the nursing workforce in the United States: Data, trends, and implications.* Boston: Jones and Bartlett.

Buerhaus, P. I., Staiger, D., & Auerbach, D. (2009c). *The future of the nursing workforce in the United States: Data, trends and implications.* Burlington, MA: Jones & Bartlett Learning.

Bureau of Health Professions (BHPr). (2002). *Projected supply, demand, and shortages of Registered Nurses: 2000–2020.* Rockville, MD: US Department of Health and Human Services, Bureau of Health Professions, Health Resources and Services Administration, National Center for Health Workforce Analysis.

Bureau of Health Professions (BHPr). (2004). *What is behind HRSA's projected supply, demand, and shortage of registered nurses?* Rockville, MD: US Department of Health and Human Services, Bureau of Health Professions, Health Resources and Services Administration.

Bureau of Health Professions (BHPr). (2006). *The registered nurse population: Findings from the March 2004 national sample survey of registered nurses.* Rockville, MD: US Department of Health and Human Services, Bureau of Health Professions, Health Resources and Services Administration.

Bureau of Health Professions (BHPr). (2010). *The registered nurse population: Findings from the 2008 National Sample Survey of Registered Nurses.* Rockville, MD: US Department of Health and Human Services, Bureau of Health Professions, Health Resources and Services Administration.

Bureau of Health Professions (BHPr). (2013). *The U.S. nursing workforce: Trends in supply and education.* Rockville, MD: Department of Health and Human Services, Health Resources and Services Administration, Bureau of Health Professions, National Center for Health Workforce Analysis.

Bureau of Health Workforce. (2014). *The future of the nursing workforce: National- and state-level projections, 2012–2025.* Rockville, MD: US Department of Health and Human Services, Health Resources and Services Administration (HRSA), National Center for Health Workforce Analysis. Retrieved from http://bhw.hrsa.gov/healthworkforce/index.html.

Bureau of Labor Statistics (BLS). (2007). Employment outlook: 2006–16. Occupational employment projections into 2016. In *Monthly Labor Review.* Washington, DC: US Bureau of Labor Statistics.

Bureau of Labor Statistics (BLS). (2014). *Occupational outlook handbook: Registered nurses.* Washington, DC: US Bureau of Labor Statistics. Retrieved from http://www.bls.gov/ooh/healthcare/registered-nurses.htm#tab-1.

Carlson, S. M., Cowart, M. E., & Speaker, D. L. (1992). Perspectives of nursing personnel in the 1980s. In M. E. Cowart & W. J. Serow (Eds.), *Nurses in the workplace* (pp. 1–27). Newbury Park, CA: Sage.

Colby, S. L., & Ortman, J. M. (2015). *Projections of the size and composition of the U.S. population: 2014–2060.* Washington, DC: US Census Bureau.

Curran, C. R. (2003). Nurse recruitment: A waste of postage, paper, and people. *Nursing Economic$, 21*(1), 5–32.

Daniel, P., Chamberlain, A., & Gordon, F. (2000). Expectations and experiences of newly recruited Filipino nurses. *British Journal of Nursing, 10*(4), 256–265.

Davidhizar, R. (2005). Joining the ranks: Nurses as role models. *Caring: National Association for Home Care Magazine, 24*(1), 50–51.

Donelan, K., Buerhaus, P. I., DesRoches, C., & Burke, S. P. (2010). Health policy thought leaders' views of the health workforce in an era of health reform. *Nursing Outlook, 58*(4), 175–180. http://dx.doi.org/10.1016/j.outlook.2010.06.003.

Duchscher, J. B. (2009). Transition shock: The initial stage of role adaptation for newly graduated registered nurses. *Journal of Advanced Nursing, 65,* 1103–1113.

Duffield, C. M., Roche, M. A., Homer, C., Buchan, J., & Dimitrelis, S. (2014). A comparative review of nurse turnover rates and costs across countries. *Journal of Advanced Nursing, 70*(12), 2703–2712.

Duffield, C. M., Roche, M. A., O'Brien-Pallas, L., Diers, D., Aisbett, C., King, M., et al. (2007). *Glueing it together: Nurses, their work environment and patient safety.* Australia: University of Technology Sydney, Centre for Health Services Management.

Erickson, J. I., Holm, L. J., & Chelminiak, L. (2004). Keeping the nursing shortage from becoming a nursing crisis. *Journal of Nursing Administration, 34*(2), 83–87.

Estabrooks, C. A., Floyd, J. A., Scott-Findlay, S., O'Leary, K. A., & Gushta, M. (2003). Individual determinants of research utilization: A systematic review. *Journal of Advanced Nursing, 43*(5), 506–520.

Gagnon, S., Ritchis, J., Lynch, A., Drouin, S., Cass, V., Rinfret, N., et al. (2006). *Job satisfaction and retention of nursing staff: The impact of nurse management and leadership.* Ottawa, Ontario, Canada: Canadian Health Services Research Foundation. Retrieved from http://www.cfhi-fcass.ca/Home.aspx.

Gordon, S. (2005). *Nursing against the odds: How health care cost cutting, media stereotypes, and medical hubris undermine nurses and patient care.* Ithaca, NY: Cornell University Press.

Grando, V. T. (1998). Making do with fewer nurses in the United States, 1945–1965. *Image, 30*(2), 147–149.

Grant, R. (2016, February 3). The U.S. is running out of nurses. *The Atlantic,* 1–10. Retrieved from https://www.theatlantic.com/health/archive/2016/02/nursing-shortage/459741/.

Hairr, D., Salisbury, H., Johannsson, M., & Redfern-Vance, N. (2014). Nurse staffing and the relationship to job satisfaction and retention. *Nursing Economic$, 32*(3), 142–147.

Halfer, D. (2007). A magnetic strategy for new graduate nurses. *Nursing Economic$, 25*(1), 6–11.

Hall, L. M., Lalonde, M., Dales, L., Peterson, J., & Cripps, L. (2011). Strategies for retaining midcareer nurses. *Journal of Nursing Administration, 41*(12), 531–537.

Hart, S. M. (2006). Generational diversity: Impact on recruitment and retention of registered nurses. *Journal of Nursing Administration, 36*(1), 10–12.

Hayes, T., & Godsey, J. (2016). Nursing's identity crisis: A study describing nurses' perceptions of their brand image compared with perceptions help by the American public. *Association for Marketing and Health Care Research* (conference proceedings [abstract]). Crested Butte, CO: Association for Marketing and Health Care Research.

Hayhurst, A., Saylor, C., & Stuenkel, D. (2005). Work environmental factors and retention of nurses. *Journal of Nursing Care Quality, 20*(3), 283–288.

Henriksen, C., Page, N. E., Williams, R. I. I., & Worral, P. S. (2003). Responding to nursing's agenda for the future: Where do we stand on recruitment and retention? *Nursing Leadership Forum, 8*(2), 78–84.

Hunt, S. T. (2009). *Nursing turnover: Costs, causes, & solutions.* Woodinville, WA: SuccessFactors, Inc. Retrieved from https://www.nmlegis.gov/lcs/handouts/LHHS%20081312%20NursingTurnover.pdf.

Institute of Medicine (IOM). (2001). *Crossing the quality chasm: A new health care system for the 21st century.* Washington, DC: National Academies Press.

Institute of Medicine (IOM). (2011). *The future of nursing: Leading change, advancing health.* Washington, DC: National Academies Press.

Institute of Medicine (IOM). (2016). *Assessing progress on the Institute of Medicine Report: The future of nursing.* Washington, DC: National Academies Press.

International Council of Nurses (ICN). (2007). *Nurse retention and migration.* Geneva, Switzerland: Author. Retrieved from http://www.icn.ch/images/stories/documents/publications/position_statements/C06_Nurse_Retention_Migration.pdf.

Johnson & Johnson (J&J). (2016). *The campaign for nursing's future.* Retrieved from https://www.discovernursing.com/.

Jones, C. B. (2004a). The costs of nurse turnover. Part 1. An economic perspective. *Journal of Nursing Administration, 34*(12), 562–570.

Jones, C. B. (2004b). The costs of nurse turnover. Part 2. Application of the nursing turnover cost calculation methodology. *Journal of Nursing Administration, 35*(1), 41–49.

Juraschek, S. P., Zhang, X., Ranganathan, V., & Lin, V. W. (2012). United States registered nurse workforce report card and shortage forecast. *American Journal of Medical Quality, 27*(3), 241–249.

Kalish, B., & Lee, K. H. (2014). Staffing and job satisfaction: Nurses and nursing assistants. *Journal of Nursing Management, 22,* 465–471.

Kalish, B. J., & Xie, B. (2014). Errors of omission: Missed nursing care. *Western Journal of Nursing Research, 36*(7), 875–890.

Kane, R., Shamliyan, T., Mueller, C., Duval, S., & Wilt, T. (2007). *Nurse staffing and quality of patient care.* Rockville, MD: Report No. 151 prepared for US Department of Health and Human Services, Agency for Healthcare Research and Quality. Retrieved from https://www.ncbi.nlm.nih.gov/books/NBK38315/.

Kenny, P., Reeve, R., & Hall, J. (2016). Satisfaction with nursing education, job satisfaction, and work intentions of new graduate nurses. *Nurse Education Today, 36,* 230–235.

King, M. G. (1989). Nursing shortage, circa 1915. *Image, 21*(3), 124–127.

Kleinman, C. S. (2004). Leadership: A key strategy in staff nurse retention. *The Journal of Continuing Education in Nursing, 35*(3), 128–132.

Ko, Y. K., & Yu, S. (2014). Clinical ladder program implementation. *Journal of Nursing Administration, 44*(11), 612–616.

Kovner, C. T., Brewer, C., Fairchild, S., Poornima, S., Kim, H., & Djukic, M. (2007). Newly licensed RNs' characteristics, work attitudes, and intentions to work. *American Journal of Nursing, 10*(9), 58–70.

Kovner, C. T., Brewer, C. S., & Fatehi, F. (2014). What does nurse turnover rate mean and what is the rate? *Policy Political Nurse Practice, 15*(3–4), 64–71. Retrieved from http://www.rnworkproject.org/.

Kramer, M., & Hafner, L. (1989). Shared values: Impact on staff nurse job satisfaction and perceived productivity. *Nursing Research, 38*(3), 172–177.

Kramer, M., Halfer, D., Maguire, P., & Schmalenberg, C. (2012). Impact of healthy work environments and multistage nurse residence programs on retention of newly licensed RNs. *The Journal of Nursing Administration, 42*(3), 148–159.

Kuhar, P. A., Miller, D., Spear, B. T., Ulreich, S. M., & Mion, L. C. (2004). The meaningful retention strategy inventory: A targeted approach to implementing retention strategies. *Journal of Nursing Administration, 34*(1), 10–18.

Lartey, S., Cummings, G., & Profetto-McGrath, J. (2014). Interventions that promote retention of experienced registered nurses in health care settings: A systematic review. *Journal of Nursing Management, 22,* 1027–1041. http://dx.doi:10.1111/jonm.12105.

Laschinger, H. K., Leiter, M., Day, A., & Gilin, D. (2009). Workplace empowerment, incivility, and burnout: Impact on staff nurse recruitment and retention outcomes. *Journal of Nursing Management, 17,* 302–311. http://dx.doi:10.1111/j.1365-2834.2009.00999.x.

Lee, D. (2008). *Successful onboarding: How to get your new employees started off right.* Retrieved from http://docplayer.net/7594470-Successful-onboarding-how-to-get-your-new-employees-started-off-right-introduction.html.

Leiter, M. P., Price, S. L., & Laschinger, H. K. (2010). Generational differences in distress, attitudes and incivility among nurses. *Journal of Nursing Management, 18*(8), 970–980. http://dx.doi:10.111/j.1365-2834.2010.01168.x.

Lipsey, J. (2004). *Targeted selection.* Omaha, NE: Leadership Solutions.

Mackoff, B., & Triolo, P. (2008a). Why do nurse managers stay? Building a model of engagement. Part 1, dimensions of engagement. *Journal of Nursing Administration, 38*(3), 118–124.

Mackoff, B., & Triolo, P. (2008b). Why do nurse managers stay? Building a model of engagement. Part 2, cultures of engagement. *Journal of Nursing Administration, 38*(4), 166–171.

MacWilliams, B. R., Schmidt, B., & Bleich, M. R. (2013). Men in nursing. *American Journal of Nursing, 113*(1), 38–44.

Manion, J., & Bartholomew, K. (2004). Community in the workplace: A proven retention strategy. *Journal of Nursing Administration, 34*(1), 46–53.

May, J. H., Bazzoli, G. J., & Gerland, A. M. (2006). Hospitals' responses to nurse staffing strategies. *Health Affairs, 25*(4), 316–323.

McClure, M. L., Poulin, M. A., Sovie, M. D., & Wandelt, M. A. (1983). *Magnet hospitals: Attraction and retention of professional nurses.* Kansas City, MO: American Nurses Association.

McHugh, M. D., Aiken, L. H., Cooper, R. A., & Miller, P. (2008). The U.S. presidential election and health care workforce policy. *Policy, Politics, & Nursing Practice, 9*(1), 6–14.

Meraviglia, M., Grobe, S. J., Tabone, S. Wainwright, M., Shelton, S., Yu, L., & Jordan, C. (2008). Nurse friendly hospital project: Enhancing nurse retention and quality of care. *Journal of Nursing Care Quality, 23*(4), 305–315.

Mills, J., & Mullins, A. (2008). The California nurse mentor project: Every nurse deserves a mentor. *Nursing Economic$, 26*(5), 310–315.

Mion, L. C., Hazel, C., & Ca, M. (2006). Retaining and recruiting mature experienced nurses: A multicomponent organizational strategy. *Journal of Nursing Administration, 36*(3), 148–154.

Morris-Thompson, T., Shepherd, J., Plata, R., & Marks-Maran, D. (2011). Diversity, fulfilment and privilege: The image of nursing. *Journal of Nursing Management, 19*, 683–692.

Muench, U., Sindelar, J., Busch, S. H., & Buerhaus, P. I. (2015). Salary differences between make and female registered nurses in the United States. *Journal of the American Medical Association, 313*(12), 1265–1267.

Muslin, I., Willis, W. K., McInerney, M., & Deslich, S. (2015). Global worker migration: Crisis and opportunity in the nursing profession. *Journal of Health Management, 17*(1), 1–10.

Nall, R. (2012). *Targeted selection interview tips.* Retrieved from http://www.ehow.com/way_5347581_targeted-selection-interview-tips.html.

National Council of State Boards of Nursing (NCSBN). (2016). *Transition to Practice: Outline of NCSBN's Transition to Practice (TTP) modules.* Chicago, IL: NCSBN. Retrieved from https://www.ncsbn.org/transition-to-practice.htm.

NSI Nursing Solutions, Inc. (2016). *2016 national healthcare retention & RN staffing report.* East Petersburg, PA: Author. Retrieved from http://ww.nsinursing-solutions.com/Files/assets/library/retention-institute/NationalHealthcare RNRetentionReport2016.pdf.

Palumbo, M. V., McIntosh, B., Rambur, B., & Naud, S. (2009). Retaining an aging nurse workforce: Perceptions of human resource practices. *Nursing Economic$, 27*(4), 221–232.

Park, M., & Jones, C. (2010). A retention strategy for newly graduated nurses. An integrative review of orientation programs. *Journal for Nurses in Staff Development, 26*(4), 142–149. http://dx.doi:10.1097/NND.0b013e31819aa130.

Pierson, M. A., Liggett, C., & Moore, K. S. (2010). Twenty years of experience with a clinical ladder: A tool for professional growth, evidence-based practice, recruitment, and retention. *The Journal of Continuing Education in Nursing, 41*(1), 33–40.

Pine, R., & Tart, K. (2007). Return on investment: Benefits and challenges of a baccalaureate nurse residency program. *Nursing Economic$, 25*(1), 13–18, 39.

Pittman, P., Bass, E., Hargraves, J., Herrera, C., & Thompson, P. (2015). The future of nursing: Monitoring the progress of recommended change in hospitals, nurse-led clinics, and home health, and hospice agencies. *Journal of Nursing Administration, 45*(2), 93–99.

Press Ganey. (2016). *Nursing quality (NDNQI).* Retrieved from http://www.pressganey.com/solutions/clinical-quality/nursing-quality.

PricewaterhouseCoopers. (2007). *What works: Healing the healthcare staffing shortage.* New York, NY: PricewaterhouseCoopers Health Research Institute. Retrieved from https://council.brandeis.edu/pdfs/2007/PwC%20Shortage%20Report.pdf.

Sanders, C. L., Krugman, M., & Schloffman, D. H. (2013). Leading change to create a healthy and satisfying work environment. *Nursing Administration Quarterly, 37*(4), 346–355.

Staiger, D. O., Auerbach, D. I., & Buerhaus, P. I. (2012). Registered nurse labor supply and the recession—Are we in a bubble? *New England Journal of Medicine, 366*(16), 1463–1465.

Stam, L. M. P., Laschinger, H. K. S., Regan, S., & Wong, C. A. (2013). The influence of personal and workplace resources on new graduate nurses' job satisfaction. *Journal of Nursing Management, 23*, 190–199.

Stanley, D. (2012). Celluloid devils: A research study of male nurses in feature films. *Journal of Advanced Nursing, 68*(11), 2526–2537.

Summers, A. (1997). Sairey Gamp: Generating fact from fiction. *Nursing Inquiry, 4*(1). doi:10.111/j.1440-1800.1997.tb00132.x.

Tri-Council for Nursing. (2004). *Joint statement from the Tri-Council for Nursing on recent registered nurse supply and demand projections.* Retrieved from http://www.aacn.nche.edu/news/articles/2010/tricouncil.

Ulrich, B. T., Lavandero, R., Woods, D., & Early, S. (2014). Critical care nurse work environments 2013. A status report. *Critical Care Nurse, 34*(4), 64–79.

US Department of Health & Human Services. (2013). *The U.S. health workforce chartbook part I: Clinicians.* Rockville, MD: US Department of Health & Human Services, Health Resources Services Administration, National Center for Health Workforce Analysis.

US Department of Health & Human Services. (2015). *Sex, race, and ethnic diversity of U.S. health occupations (2010–2012).* Rockville, MD: US Department of Health & Human Services, Health Resources Services Administration, Bureau of Health Workforce, National Center for Health Workforce Analysis.

VanWyngeeren, K., & Stuart, T. (n.d.). *Increasing new graduate nurse retention from a student nurse perspective.* Retrieved from http://rn-journal.com/journal-of-nursing/increasing-new-graduate-nurse-retention-from-a-student-nurse-perspective.

Weberg, D. (2010). Transformational leadership and staff retention: An evidence review with implications for healthcare systems. *Nursing Administration Quarterly, 34*(3), 246–258.

Zastock, D., & Holly, C. (2010). Retaining nurse managers. *American Nurse Today, 5*(12), 3p-3p.

Chapter 22

Aiken, L. H., Clarke, S. P., Cheung, R. B., Sloane, D. M., & Silber, J. H. (2003). Educational levels of hospital nurses and surgical patient mortality. *Journal of the American Medical Association, 290*(12), 1617–1623.

Aiken, L. H., Clarke, S. P., Sloane, D. M., Sochalski, J., & Silber, J. H. (2002). Hospital nurse staffing and patient mortality, nurse burnout, and job dissatisfaction. *Journal of the American Medical Association, 288*(16), 1987–1993.

Aiken, L. H., Sloane, D. M., Bruyneel, L., Van den Heede, K., Griffiths, P., Busse, R., et al. (2014). Nurse staffing and education and hospital mortality in nine European countries: A retrospective observational study. *Lancet, 383*(9931), 1824–1830.

Aiken, L. H., Sloane, D. M., Griffiths, P., Rafferty, A. M., Bruyneel, L., McHugh, M., et al. (2016). Nursing skill mix in European hospitals: Cross-sectional study of the association with mortality, patient ratings, and quality of care. *BMJ Quality & Safety,* Published online first: November 15, 2016, 1–10. Retrieved from http://qualitysafety.bmj.com/content/early/2016/11/03/bmjqs-2016-005567.full.pdf+html.

Aiken, L. H., Xue, Y., Clarke, S. P., & Sloane, D. M. (2007). Supplemental nurse staffing in hospitals and quality of care. *Journal of Nursing Administration, 37*(7–8), 335–342.

American Academy of Ambulatory Care Nursing (AAACN). (2005). *Ambulatory care nurse staffing: An annotated bibliography.* Pitman, NJ: Author.

American Academy of Pediatrics (AAP) and the American College of Obstetricians and Gynecologists (ACOG). (2012). *Guidelines for perinatal care* (7th ed.). Washington, DC: March of Dimes.

American Association of Colleges of Nursing (AACN). (2007). *White paper on the education and role of the clinical nurse leader.* Washington, DC: Author.

American Association of Critical-Care Nurses. (2016). *AACN synergy model for patient care.* Retrieved from http://www.aacn.org/wd/certifications/content/synmodel.pcms?menu=certification.

American Nurses Association (ANA). (n.d.). *Safe staffing: The registered nurse safe staffing act HR 876/S.58.* Retrieved from http://www.nursingworld.org/SafeStaffingFactsheet.aspx.

American Nurses Association (ANA). (2010). *Nursing's social policy statement: The essence of the profession* (3rd ed.). Silver Spring, MD: Author.

American Nurses Association (ANA). (2012). *ANA's principles for nurse staffing* (2nd ed.). Silver Spring, MD: Author.

American Nurses Association (ANA). (2015a). *Code of ethics for nurses with interpretive statements.* Silver Spring, MD: Author.

American Nurses Association (ANA). (2015b). *The registered nurse safe staffing act HR2083/S.1132.* Retrieved from http://www.rnaction.org/site/DocServer/RN_Safe_Staffing_Act.pdf/2027989535?docID=2442&verID=1.

American Nurses Association (ANA). (2016a). *Nurse staffing.* Retrieved from http://www.nursingworld.org/nursestaffing.

American Nurses Association (ANA). (2016b). *Nurse staffing.* Retrieved from http://www.nursingworld.org/MainMenuCategories/Policy-Advocacy/State/Legislative-Agenda-Reports/State-StaffingPlansRatios.

American Organization of Nurse Executives (AONE). (2000). *Staffing management and methods: Tools and techniques for nurse leaders.* Chicago, IL: Author.

Association of periOperative Registered Nurses (AORN). (2014). *AORN position statement on perioperative safe staffing and on-call practices.* Denver, CO: Author. Retrieved from https://www.aorn.org/guidelines/clinical-resources/position-statements.

Association of Women's Health, Obstetric and Neonatal Nurses (AWHONN). (2010). *Guidelines for professional registered nurse staffing for perinatal units.* Washington, DC: Author.

Aydelotte, M. K. (1973). *Nurse staffing methodology: A review and critique of selected literature.* US Department of Health, Education and Welfare, Division of Nursing. Publication No. (NIH) 73-433. Washington, DC: Government Printing Office.

Blegen, M. A, Goode, C. J., & Reed, L. (1998). Nurse staffing and patient outcomes. *Nursing Research, 47*(1), 43-50.

Bogue, R. (2012, May 29). Nurses: Key to making or breaking your future margin. *Hospitals and Health Networks.* Retrieved from http://www.hhnmag.com/articles/5500-nurses-key-to-making-or-breaking-your-future-margin.

Brennan, C. W., & Daly, B. J. (2008). Patient acuity: a concept analysis. *Journal of Advanced Nursing, 65*(5), 1114-1126.

Case Management Society of America (CMSA). (2016). *What is a case manager?* Little Rock, AR: Author. Retrieved from http://www.cmsa.org/Home/CMSA/WhatisaCaseManager/tabid/224/Default.aspx.

Cipriano, P., & Cutruzzula, J. (2007). Over-recruiting: Breaking the short staffing and turnover cycle. *Nurse Leader, 5*(6), 28-32.

Clarke, S. P. (2005). The policy implications of staffing-outcomes research. *Journal of Nursing Administration, 35*(1), 17-19.

Dalton, K. (2007). *A study of charge compression in calculating DRG relative weights.* Centers for Medicaid & Medicare Services (CMS): Contract no. 500-00-0024-TO18. Baltimore, MD: CMS.

Dent, R. L., & Bradshaw, P. (2012). Building the business case for acuity-based staffing. *Nurse Leader, 10*(2), 26-28.

Donabedian, A. (1966). Evaluating the quality of medical care. *Milbank Memorial Fund Quarterly, 44*(3), 166-206.

Eck Birmingham, S. (2010). Evidenced-based staffing: The next step. *Nurse Leader, 8*(3), 24-26, 35.

Eck Birmingham, S., Nell, K., & Abe, N. (2011). Determining staffing needs based on patient outcomes vs. patient interventions. In P. Cowan & S. Moorhead (Eds.), *Current issues in nursing* (8th ed., pp. 391-404). St. Louis, MO: Mosby Elsevier.

Edwardson, S. (2007). Conceptual frameworks used in funded nursing health services research projects. *Nursing Economic$, 25*(4), 222-227.

Emergency Nurses Association (ENA). (2015). *Staffing and productivity in the emergency care setting.* Retrieved from https://www.ena.org/SiteCollection Documents/Position%20Statements/StaffingandProductivityEmergency Department.pdf.

Finkler, S. A., Jones, C. B., & Kovner, C. T. (2013). *Financial management for nurse managers and executives* (4th ed.). Philadelphia, PA: Saunders.

Fitzpatrick, T. (2015, June 24). *Clinical labor optimization: Managing supply and demand in a dynamic environment.* International webinar innovations for advancing nursing administration [Webinar].

Fitzpatrick, T. A., & Brooks, B. A. (2010). The nurse leader as a logistician: Optimizing human capital. *Journal of Nursing Administration, 40*(2), 69-74.

Flanders, K., & Carr, D. (2016). Staffing by acuity: Building a bridge to support nursing effectiveness. *Voice of Nursing Leadership, 14*(5), 12-14.

Frith, K., Anderson, F., Caspers, B., Tseng, F., Sanford, K., Hoyt, N., et al. (2010). Effects of nurse staffing on hospital-acquired conditions and length of stay in community hospitals. *Quality Management in Health Care, 19*(2), 147-155.

Gavigan, M., Fitzpatrick, T. A., & Miserendino, C. (2016). Effective staffing takes a village: Creating the staffing ecosystem. *Nursing Economic$, 34*(2), 58-65.

Guanci, G., & Felgen, J. (2016). How relationship-based care supports the Magnet journey. *Nursing Management, 47*(1), 9-12.

Haas, S. A., Vlasses, F., & Havey, J. (2016). Developing staffing models to support population health management and quality outcomes in ambulatory care settings. *Nursing Economic$, 34*(3), 126-133.

Habasevich, B. (2012, July 26). *Re: Defining acuity* [Online forum blog]. Retrieved from https://www.mediware.com/rehabilitation/blog/defining-acuity/.

Joseph, M. L., & Fowler, D. (2016). Innovating traditional nursing administration challenges. *Journal of Nursing Administration, 46*(3), 120-121.

Kane, R., Shamliyan, T., Mueller, C., Duval, S., & Wilt, T. (2007a). *Nurse staffing and quality of patient care.* US Department of Health and Human Services. AHRQ Publication No. 07-E005. Washington, DC: Author.

Kane, R., Shamliyan, T., Mueller, C., Duval, S., & Wilt, T. (2007b). The association of registered nurse staffing levels and patient outcomes. *Medical Care, 45*(12), 1195-1204.

Kelly, L. A., McHugh, M. D., & Aiken, L. H. (2011). Nurse outcomes in Magnet and non-Magnet hospitals. *Journal of Nursing Administration, 41*(10), 428-433.

Koloroutis, M. (Ed.). (2004). *Relationship-based care: A model for transforming practice.* Minneapolis, MN: Creative Health Care Management.

Koning, C. (2014). Does self-scheduling increase nurses' job satisfaction? An integrative literature review. *Nursing Management, 21*(6), 24-28.

Kullberg, A., Bergenmar, M., & Sharp, L. (2016). Changed nursing scheduling for improved safety culture and working conditions-patients' and nurses' perspectives. *Journal of Nursing Management, 24*(4), 524-532.

Lauw, C., & Gares, D. (2005). Resource management: What's right for you? *Nursing Management, 36*(12), 46-49.

Lawson, L. D., Miles, K. S., Vallish, R. O., & Jenkins, S. A. (2011). Recognizing nursing professional growth and development in a collective bargaining environment. *Journal of Nursing Administration, 41*(5), 197-200.

Liang, B., & Turkcan, A. (2016). Acuity-based nurse assignment and patient scheduling in oncology clinics. *Health Care Management Science, 19*(3), 207-226.

Litvak, E., Buerhaus, P., Davidoff, F., Long, M., McManus, M., & Berwick, D. (2005). Managing unnecessary variability in patient demand to reduce nursing stress and improve patient safety. *Journal on Quality and Patient Safety, 31*(6), 330-338.

MacPhee, M., & Borra, L. S. (2012). *Flexible work practices in nursing.* Geneva, Switzerland: International Council of Nurses.

Malloch, K. (2015). Measurement of nursing's complex health care work: Evolution of the science for determining the required staffing for safe and effective patient care. *Nursing Economic$, 33*(1), 20-25.

Maloney, S., Fencl, J. L., & Hardin, S. R. (2015). Is nursing care missed? A comparative study of three North Carolina hospitals. *MEDSURG Nursing, 24*(4), 229-235.

Mark, B. A., Harless, D. W., & Berman, W. F. (2007). Nurse staffing and adverse events in hospitalized children. *Policy, Politics, and Nursing Practice, 8*(2), 83-92.

McDonough, K. S. (2013). Development of the McDonough Optimum Staffing Method: Evidence-driven recommendations based on patient demand. *Virginia Nurses Today*, 21(2), 8–11.

McHugh, M. D., Rochman, M. F., Sloane, D. M., Berg, R. A., Mancini, M. E., Nadkarni, V. M., et al. (2016). Better nurse staffing and nurse work environments associated with increased survival of in-hospital cardiac arrest patients. *Medical Care*, 54(1), 74–80.

McKinley, J., & Cavouras, C. (2000). Evolving staffing measures. In American Organization of Nurse Executives (AONE), *Staffing management and methods: Tools and techniques for nurse leaders* (pp. 1–33). San Francisco, CA: Jossey-Bass.

Mensik, J. (2014). What every nurse should know about staffing. *American Nurse Today*, 9(2), 1–11.

Mitchell, P. (2008). *Nurse staffing–A summary of current research, opinion and policy* (pp. 1–37). Pullman, WA: The William D. Ruckelshaus Center.

Morris, R., MacNeela, P., Scott, A., Treacy, P., & Hyde, A. (2007). Reconsidering the conceptualization of nursing workload: Literature review. *Journal of Advanced Nursing*, 57(5), 463–471.

National Association of Neonatal Nurses (NANN). (2014). *RN staffing in the neonatal intensive care unit.* NANN Position Statement No. 3061. Chicago, IL: Author.

National Council of State Boards of Nursing (NCSBN). (2016). A changing environment: 2016 NCSBN environmental scan national council. *Journal of Nursing Regulation*, 6(4), 4–37.

National Labor Relations Board (NLRB). (2016). *National Labor Relations Act.* Washington, DC: Author. Retrieved from https://www.nlrb.gov/resources/national-labor-relations-act.

Needleman, J., Buerhaus, P., Mattke, S., Stewart, M., & Zelevinski, K. (2002). Nurse-staffing levels and the quality of care in hospitals. *New England Journal of Medicine*, 346(22), 1715–1722.

Needleman, J., Buerhaus, P., Pankratz, S., Leibson, C., Stevens, S., & Harris, M. (2011). Nurse staffing and inpatient hospital mortality. *New England Journal of Medicine*, 364(11), 1037–1045.

Needleman, J., Buerhaus, P. I., Stewart, M., Zelevinsky, K., & Mattke, S. (2006). Nurse staffing in hospitals: Is there a business case for quality? *Health Affairs*, 25(1), 204–211.

Norrish, B. R., & Rundall, T. G. (2001). Hospital restructuring and the work of registered nurses. *Milbank Quarterly*, 79(1), 55–79.

Pappas, S., Davidson, N., Woodard, J., Davis, J., & Welton, J. (2015). Risk-adjusted staffing to improve patient value. *Nursing Economic$*, 33(2), 72–87.

Person, C. (2004). Patient care delivery. In M. Koloroutis (Ed.), *Relationship-based care: A model for transforming practice* (pp. 159–182). Minneapolis, MN: Creative Health Care Management.

Pickard, B., & Warner, M. (2007). Demand management: A methodology for outcomes-driven staffing and patient flow management. *Nurse Leader*, 4(2), 30–34.

Porter, C. (2010). A nursing labor management partnership model. *Journal of Nursing Administration*, 40(6), 272–276.

Pruinelli, L., Delaney, C., Garcia, A., Caspers, B., & Westra, B. L. (2016). Nursing management minimum dataset: Cost effective tool to demonstrate the value of nurse staffing in the Big Data science era. *Nursing Economic$*, 34(2), 66–89.

Robertson, R., & Samuelson, C. (1996). Should nurse patient ratios be legislated? Pros and cons. *Georgia Nursing*, 56(5), 2.

Seago, J. A., Spetz, J., Coffman, J., Rosenoff, E., & O'Neil, E. (2003). Minimum staffing ratios: The California workforce initiative survey. *Nursing Economic$*, 21(2), 65–70.

Simpson, R. (2012). Technology enables value-base nursing care. *Nursing Administration Quarterly*, 36(1), 85–87.

The Joint Commission (TJC). (2016). *Joint Commission FAQ page.* Oakbrook Terrace, IL: Author. Retrieved from https://www.jointcommission.org/about/jointcommissionfaqs.aspx.

Thompson, J. D., & Diers, D. (1985). DRGs and nursing intensity. *Nursing & Health Care*, 6(8), 434–439.

Unruh, L. (2008). Nurse staffing: Patient, nurse, financial outcomes. *American Journal of Nursing*, 108(1), 62–71.

Unruh, L., & Fottler, M. D. (2004, June). *Patient turnover and nursing staff adequacy.* Paper presented at Academy Health Annual Research Meeting, San Diego, CA.

Welton, J. M. (2010). Value-based nursing care. *Journal of Nursing Administration*, 40(10), 399–401.

Welton, J. M., & Dismuke, C. E. (2008). Testing an inpatient nursing intensity billing model. *Policy, Politics, & Nursing Practice*, 9(2), 103–111.

Welton, J. M., & Harris, K. (2007). Hospital billing and reimbursement: Charging for inpatient nursing care. *Journal of Nursing Administration*, 30(6), 309–315.

Welton, J. M., Zone-Smith, L., & Fischer, M. H. (2006). Adjustment of inpatient care reimbursement for nursing intensity. *Policy, Politics, & Nursing Practice*, 7(4), 270–280.

Chapter 23

Abass, I., Helton, J., Mhatre, S., & Sansgiry, S. (2012). Impact of electronic health records on nurses' productivity. *CIN: Computers, Informatics, Nursing*, 30(5), 237–241.

Aiken, L. H., Sloane, D., Bruyneel, L., Van den Heede, K., Griffiths, P., Busse, R., et al. (2014). Nurse staffing and education and hospital mortality in nine European countries: A retrospective observational study. *Lancet*, 383(9931), 1824–1830.

Bureau of Labor Statistics. (2015). *Occupational outlook handbook: Registered nurses.* Retrieved from http://www.bls.gov/ooh/healthcare/registered-nurses.htm.

Centers for Medicare & Medicaid Services. (2015). *National healthcare expenditures (NHE) fact sheet 2015.* Retrieved from https://www.cms.gov/research-statistics-data-and-systems/statistics-trends-and-reports/nationalhealthexpenddata/nhe-fact-sheet.html.

Finkler, S. A., Jones, C. B., & Kovner, C. T. (2013). *Financial management for nurse managers and nurse executives* (4th ed.). St. Louis, MO: Elsevier Health Sciences.

Jenkins, P., & Welton, J. (2014). Measuring direct patient cost per patient in the acute care setting. *Journal of Nursing Administration*, 44(5), 257–262.

Keehan, S. P., Sisko, A. M., Truffer, C. J., Poisal, J. A., Cuckler, G. A., Madison, A. J., et al. (2011). National health spending projections through 2020: Economic recovery and reform drive faster spending growth. *Health Affairs*, 30(8), 1594–1605.

Kovner, C. T., Brewer, C. S., Fatehi, F., & Jun, J. (2014). What does nurse turnover rate mean and what is the rate? *Policy, Politics & Nursing Practice*, 15(3/4), 64–71.

Lucero, R. J., Lake, E. T., & Aiken, L. H. (2009). Variations in nursing care quality across hospitals. *Journal of Advanced Nursing*, 65(11), 2299–2310.

Murray, M. E. (2012). Economics of the health care delivery system. In J. Zerwekh & A. Z. Garneau (Eds.), *Nursing Today* (7th ed., pp. 331–350). St. Louis, MO: Elsevier.

Rundio, A. (2016). *The nurse manager's guide to budgeting & finance* (2nd ed.). Indianapolis, IN: Sigma Theta Tau International.

Sorbello, B. (2008). Finance: It's not a dirty word. *American Nurse Today*, 3(8), 32–35.

Chapter 24

American Association of Colleges of Nursing (AACN). (2013). *Competencies and curricular expectations for clinical nurse leader education and practice.* Washington, DC: Author. Retrieved from http://www.aacn.nche.edu/cnl/CNL-Competencies-October-2013.pdf.

American Nurse Today. (2011). *Nursing peer review: Principles and practice.* Retrieved from https://americannursetoday.com/nursing-peer-review-principles-and-practice/.

Buckingham, M., & Goodall, A. (2015). Reinventing performance management. *Harvard Business Review, 93*, 40–50.

Budworth, M., Latham, G. P., & Manroop, L. (2015). Looking forward to performance improvement. *Human Resource Management, 54*, 45–54.

Coens, T., & Jenkins, M. (2000). *Abolishing performance appraisals.* San Francisco, CA: Berrett-Hoehler Publishers.

Decramer, A., Audenaert, M., Van Waeyenberg, T., Claeys, T., Laes, C., Vandevelde, S., et al. (2015). Does performance management affect nurses' well-being? *Evaluation and Program Planning, 49*, 98–105.

DeNisi, A. S., & Sonesh, S. (2011). The appraisal and management of performance at work. In S. Zedeck (Ed.), *APA handbook of industrial and organizational psychology* (Vol. 2., Chapter 9). Washington, DC: APA Press.

Heathfield, S. M. (2016). *Performance improvement plan: Contents and sample form.* Retrieved from https://www.thebalance.com/performance-improvement-plan-contents-and-sample-form-1918850.

Kluger, A. N., & DeNisi, D. (1996). The effects of feedback interventions on performance: A historical review, a meta-analysis, and a preliminary feedback intervention theory. *Psychological Bulletin, 119*, 254–284.

Performance. (n.d.). *Merriam-Webster* online. Retrieved from http://www.merriam-webster.com/dictionary/performance.

Performance appraisal. (2016). *BusinessDictionary.com.* Retrieved from http://www.businessdictionary.com/definition/performance-appraisal.html.

Scullen, S. E., Mount, M. K., & Goff, M. (2000). Understanding the latent structure of job performance ratings. *Journal of Applied Psychology, 85*, 965–970.

Smither, J. W., London, M., & Reilly, R. R. (2005). Does performance improve following multi-source feed- back? A theoretical model, meta-analysis, and review of empirical findings. *Personnel Psychology, 58*, 33–66.

Tziner, A. (1999). The relationship between distal and proximal factors and the use of political considerations in performance appraisal. *Journal of Business and Psychology, 14*, 217–231.

Chapter 25

Agency for Healthcare Research and Quality (AHRQ). (2012). *Allocation of scarce resources during mass casualty events.* Retrieved from http://www.effectivehealthcare.ahrq.gov/search-for-guides-reviews-and-reports/?pageaction=displayproducts&productID=1152.

American College of Emergency Physicians (ACEP). (2011). *Health care system surge capacity recognition, preparedness, and response.* Retrieved from https://www.acep.org/Clinical—Practice-Management/Health-Care-System-Surge-Capacity-Recognition,-Preparedness,-and-Response/.

American Nurses Association (ANA). (2008). *Adapting standards of care under extreme conditions: Guidance for professionals during disasters, pandemics, and other extreme emergencies.* Silver Spring, MD: Author. Retrieved from http://nursingworld.org/MainMenuCategories/WorkplaceSafety/Healthy-Work-Environment/DPR/TheLawEthicsofDisasterResponse/AdaptingStandardsofCare.pdf.

American Organization of Nurse Executives (AONE). (2016). *AONE guiding principles: Role of the nurse leader in crisis management.* Retrieved from http://www.aone.org/resources/role-of-the-nurse-leader-in-crisis-management.pdf.

Arnand, K. (2014). *Cyber attacks—Definition, types, prevention.* Retrieved from http://www.thewindowsclub.com/cyber-attacks-definition-types-prevention.

California Hospital Association. (2011). *Emergency preparedness: Hazards vulnerability analysis.* Retrieved from http://www.calhospitalprepare.org/hazard-vulnerability-analysis.

CBS News. (2016). *60 Minutes investigates medical gear sold during Ebola crisis.* Retrieved from http://www.cbsnews.com/news/60-minutes-investigates-medical-gear-sold-during-ebola-crisis/.

Centers for Disease Control and Prevention (CDC). (2007). *Ethical guidelines in pandemic influenza.* Retrieved from https://www.cdc.gov/od/science/integrity/phethics/panFlu_Ethic_Guidelines.pdf.

Centers for Disease Control and Prevention (CDC). (2001). *Biological and chemical terrorism: Strategic plan for preparedness and response.* Retrieved from https://www.cdc.gov/mmwr/preview/mmwrhtml/rr4904a1.htm.

Centers for Disease Control and Prevention (CDC). (2014). *Disaster epidemiology: Frequently asked questions (FAQs).* Retrieved from https://www.cdc.gov/nceh/hsb/disaster/faqs.htm.

Corporation for National & Community Service. (n.d.). *What is FEMA Corps?* Retrieved from https://www.nationalservice.gov/programs/americorps/americorps-programs/fema-corps/fema-corps-faqs#12439.

Coyle, G., Sapnas, K., & Ward-Presson, K. (2007). Dealing with disaster. *Nursing Management, 38*(7), 24–29. http://dx.doi:10.1097/01.NUMA.0000281132.18369.bd.

Drenkard, K., & Rigotti, G. (2002, updated 2016). *Inova Health System survey.* Falls Church, VA: Inova Health System.

Drenkard, K., Rigotti, G., Hanfling, D., Fahlgren, T., & LaFrancois, G. (2002). Healthcare system disaster preparedness, part 1: Readiness planning. *Journal of Nursing Administration, 32*(9), 461–469.

Federal Emergency Management Agency (FEMA). (2015a). *Emergency planning exercises.* Retrieved from https://www.fema.gov/emergency-planning-exercises.

Federal Emergency Management Agency (FEMA). (2015b). *Fact sheet: Incident management assistance teams.* Retrieved from http://www.fema.gov/media-library-data/1440617086827-f6489d2de59dddeba8bebc9b4d419009/IMAT_July_2015.pdf.

Federal Emergency Management Agency (FEMA). (2016). *National incident management system.* Retrieved from http://www.fema.gov/national-incident-management-system.

Federal Emergency Management Agency (FEMA). (2017). *Incident management assistance teams.* Retrieved from https://www.fema.gov/incident-management-assistance-teams.

FEMA Emergency Management Institute. (2014). *Academic emergency management and related courses (AEMRC) for the higher education program: Comparative emergency management book.* Retrieved from https://training.fema.gov/hiedu/aemrc/booksdownload/compemmgmtbookproject/.

Harvin, D., Caplan, N., & Kivlehan, S. M. (2014). *EMS response to pediatric disasters.* Retrieved from http://www.emsworld.com/article/11519841/pediatric-disaster-response.

Hick, J. L., & O'Laughlin, D. T. (2006). Concept of operations for triage of mechanical ventilation in an epidemic. *Academic Emergency Medicine, 13*(2), 223–229. http://dx.doi:10.1197/j.aem.2005.07.037.

Hodge, J. G., Jr., Hanfling, D., & Powell, T. (2013). Practical, ethical, and legal challenges underlying crisis standards of care. *Journal of Law, Medicine, and Ethics*, Volume 41, pp. 50–55, 2012. Public Health Law Conference: Practical Approaches to Critical Challenges, Spring 2013.

Institute of Medicine (IOM). (2012). *Crisis standards of care—A systems framework for catastrophic disaster response.* Washington, DC: National Academics Press. Retrieved from http://www.nationalacademies.org/hmd/Reports/2012/Crisis-Standards-of-Care-A-Systems-Framework-for-Catastrophic-Disaster-Response.aspx.

International Federation of Red Cross and Red Crescent Societies (IFRC). (2016). *Biological hazards: Epidemics.* Retrieved from http://www.ifrc.org/en/what-we-do/disaster-management/about-disasters/definition-of-hazard/biological-hazards-epidemics.

Joint Commission Resources. (2008). *Emergency management in health care: An all-hazards approach.* Oakbrook Terrace, IL: Author.

Joint Commission Resources. (2016). *Emergency management in health care: An all-hazards approach* (2nd ed.). Retrieved from http://www.jcrinc.com/emergency-management-in-health-care-an-all-hazards-approach-second-edition/.

Kraus, C. K., Levy, F., & Kelen, G. D. (2007). Lifeboat ethics: Considerations in the discharge of inpatients for the creation of hospital surge capacity. *Disaster Medicine and Public Health Preparedness, 1*(1), 51–56. http://dx.doi:10.1097/DMP.0b013e318065c4ca.

McLean, Margaret R. (2013). Allocating resources—A wicked problem. *Health Progress, 94*(6), 60–67.

New York State Department of Health Task Force on Life and the Law. (2007). *Allocation of ventilators in an influenza pandemic.* Albany, NY: Author. Retrieved from www.health.state.ny.us/diseases/communicable/influenza/pandemic/ventilators/.

Phillips, S. J., & Knebel, A. (Eds.). (2007). *Mass medical care with scarce resources: A community planning guide.* (Prepared by Health Systems Research, Inc., an Altarum company, under contract No. 290-04-0010. AHRQ Publication No. 07–0001). Rockville, MD: Agency for Healthcare Research and Quality. Retrieved from http://archive.ahrq.gov/research/mce/mceguide.pdf.

Powell, T., Christ, K. C., & Birkhead, G. S. (2008). Allocation of ventilators in a public health disaster. *Disaster Medicine and Public Health Preparedness, 2*(1), 20–26.

Ready.gov. (2016). *Chemical threats.* Retrieved from https://www.ready.gov/chemical-threats.

The Joint Commission (TJC). (2008). *Accreditation program: Hospital emergency management.* Oakbrook Terrace, IL: Author. http://www.calhospitalprepare.org/resources/JointCommissionAccProg-EmergencyManagement.

The Joint Commission (TJC). (2012). *Comprehensive accreditation manual for hospitals 2012: Emergency management accreditation standards.* Oakbrook Terrace, IL: Author.

Tillman, P. (2011). Disaster preparedness for nurses: A teaching guide. *The Journal of Continuing Education in Nursing, 42*(9), 404–408. http://dx.doi:10.3928/00220124-20110502-02.

US Department of Defense. (2015). *DOD dictionary of military terms.* Retrieved from http://www.dtic.mil/doctrine/dod_dictionary/.

US Department of Health & Human Services. (2012). *Emergency management and the incident command system.* Retrieved from https://www.phe.gov/preparedness/planning/mscc/handbook/chapter1/Pages/emergencymanagement.aspx.

US Department of Homeland Security. (2011). *NTAS public guide.* Retrieved from https://www.dhs.gov/xlibrary/assets/ntas/ntas-public-guide.pdf.

US Department of Homeland Security. (2016). *National incident management system (NIMS).* Retrieved from https://www.fema.gov/national-incident-management-system.

World Health Organization (WHO). (2013). *Emergency response framework.* Geneva, Switzerland: WHO. Retrieved from http://apps.who.int/iris/bitstream/10665/89529/1/9789241504973_eng.pdf.

Wright State University. (2016). *Emergency preparedness.* Retrieved from https://www.wright.edu/police/emergency-preparedness.

Chapter 26

Agency for Healthcare Research and Quality (AHRQ). (2016). *What is comparative effectiveness research.* Retrieved from http://effectivehealthcare.ahrq.gov/index.cfm/what-is-comparative-effectiveness-research1/.

American Nurses Association (ANA). (2012). *ANA recognized terminologies that support nursing practice.* Retrieved from http://www.nursingworld.org/MainMenuCategories/Tools/Recognized-Nursing-Practice-Terminologies.pdf.

American Nurses Association (ANA). (2015a). *Nursing informatics: Scope and standards of practice* (2nd ed.). Silver Spring, MD: Nursesbooks.org.

American Nurses Association. (2015b). *4 health care trends that will affect American nurses.* Retrieved from http://nursingworld.org/MainMenuCategories/Career-Center/Resources/4-Health-Care-Trends-That-Will-Affect-American-Nurses.html.

American Organization of Nurse Executives (AONE). (2015). *Nurse executive competencies.* Retrieved from http://www.aone.org/resources/nurse-executive-competencies.pdf.

Austin, C. (1979). *Information systems for hospital administration.* Ann Arbor, MI: Health Administration Press.

Bakken, S., Warren, J., Lundberg, C., Casey, A., Correia, C., Konicek, D., & Zingo, C. (2001). An evaluation of the utility of the CEN categorical structure for nursing diagnoses as a terminology model for integrating nursing

diagnosis concepts into SNOMED. *Studies in Health Technology and Informatics, 84*(Pt 1), 151–155.

Ball, M. J., Douglas, J. V., Walker, P. H., DuLong, D., Gugerty, B., Hannah, K. J., Kiel, J., Newbold, S. K., Sensmeier, J. E., Skiba, D. J., & Troseth, M. R. (Eds.). (2011). *Nursing Informatics: Where caring and technology meet* (4th ed.). London: Springer-Verlag.

Bartgis, J., & Bigfoot, D. (2010). *Evidence based practice and practice based evidence: What are they? How do we know if we have one?* Retrieved from http://www.ncuih.org/krc/D_bigfoot_EBP_PBE.

Bell, B., & Thornton, K. (2011). From promise to reality achieving the value of an EHR. *Healthcare Financial Management, 65*(2), 51–56.

Berner, E. S. (2009, June). *Clinical decision support systems: state of the art.* AHRQ Publication No. 09-0069EF. Rockville, MD: Agency for Healthcare Research and Quality.

Brokel, J. (2007). Creating sustainability of clinical information systems. *Journal of Nursing Administration, 37*(1), 10–13.

Brokel, J. M., Cole, M., & Upmeyer, L. (2011b). Longitudinal study of symptom control and quality of life indicators with patients receiving community-based case management services. *Applied Nursing Research, 25*(3), 138–145. doi:10.1016/j.apnr.2011.02.002.

Brokel, J. M., Schwichtenberg, T. J., Wakefield, D. S., Ward, M. M., Shaw, M. G., & Kramer, J. M. (2011a). Evaluating clinical decision support rules as an intervention in clinical workflows with technology. *Computers, Informatics, Nursing, 29*(1), 36–42.

Burnes-Bolton, L. (2009, April 6). *SSNI-505 - Innovation and trends in technology: Exploring the nursing workflow of the future.* Chicago, IL: Nursing Informatics Symposium.

Calhoun, C., Hall, L. K., & Kemper, D. (2016). Patient engagement: Engaging patients in the care process by leveraging meaningful use goals. In D. B. Nash, R. J. Fabius, A. Skoufalos, J. L. Clarke, & M. R. Horowitz (Eds.), *Population health: Creating a culture of wellness* (2nd ed., Chapter 7). Burlington, MA: Jones and Bartlett Learning.

Centers for Medicare & Medicaid Services (CMS). (2010). Medicare and Medicaid programs: Electronic health record incentive program. *Federal Register, 75*(144), 44314–44588.

Centers for Medicare & Medicaid Services (CMS). (2011). *Overview of accountable care organizations (ACOs).* Retrieved from https://www.cms.gov/ACO/.

Centers for Medicare & Medicaid Services (CMS). (2016a). *ICD-10-CM/PCS myths and facts.* https://www.cms.gov/medicare/coding/icd10/downloads/icd-10mythsandfacts.pdf.

Centers for Medicare & Medicaid Services (CMS). (2016b). *Hospital-acquired conditions.* Retrieved from https://www.cms.gov/medicare/medicare-fee-for-service-payment/hospitalacqcond/hospital-acquired_conditions.html.

Centers for Medicare & Medicaid Services (CMS). (2017). *Quality measures, reporting and performance standards.* Retrieved from https://www.cms.gov/medicare/medicare-fee-for-service-payment/sharedsavingsprogram/quality-measures-standards.html.

Clark, J. L., & Lang, N. (1992). Nursing's next advance: An internal classification for nursing practice. *International Nursing Review, 39*(4), 109–111.

Coenen, A., Marin, H., Park, H., & Bakken, S. (2001). Collaborative efforts for representing nursing concepts in computer-based systems: International perspectives. *Journal of the American Medical Informatics Association, 8*(3), 202–211.

Cummins, M. R. (2014). Nursing informatics and learning health system. *Computers, Informatics, Nursing, 32*(10), 471–474.

Das, M., & Eichner, J. (2010). *Challenges and barriers to clinical decision support (CDS) design and implementation experienced in the Agency for Healthcare Research and Quality CDS Demonstrations.* AHRQ Publication No. 10-0064-EF. Retrieved from https://healthit.ahrq.gov/sites/default/files/docs/page/CDS_challenges_and_barriers.pdf.

Donabedian, A. (1986). Criteria and standards for quality assessment and monitoring. *Quarterly Review Bulletin, 12*(3), 99–100.

Fisher, E. S., McClellan, M. B., & Safran, D. G. (2011). Building the path to accountable care. *New England Journal of Medicine, 365*(26), 2445–2447.

Fuller, R. L., McCullough, E. C., Bao, M. Z., & Averill, R. F. (2009). Estimating the costs of potentially preventable hospital acquired complications. *Health Care Financing Review*, *30*(4), 17–32.

Furukawa, M. F., Raghu, T. S., & Shao, B. B. (2011). Electronic medical records, nurse staffing, and nurse-sensitive patient outcomes: Evidence from the national database of nursing quality indicators. *Medical Care Research & Review*, *68*(3), 311–331.

Garcia, A., Caspers, B., Westra, B., Pruinelli, L., & Delaney, C. (2015). Sharable and comparable data for nursing management. *Nursing Administration Quarterly*, *39*(4), 297–303.

Gartner, Inc. (2016). *Data warehouses. IT glossary*. Retrieved from http://www.gartner.com/it-glossary/.

Gee, P. M., Greenwood, D. A., Kim, K. K., Perez, S. L., Staggers, N., & DeVon, H. A. (2012). Exploration of the e-patient phenomenon in nursing informatics. *Nursing Outlook*, *60*(4), E9–E16.

Hannah, K., Ball, M., & Edwards, M. (2006). *Introduction to nursing informatics*. New York, NY: Springer.

Harrington, L., Porch, L., Acosta, K., & Wilkens, K. (2011). Realizing electronic medical record benefits: An easy-to-do usability study. *Journal of Nursing Administration*, *41*(7/8), 331–335.

Häyrinen, K., Sarantoa, K., & Nykänen, P. (2008). Definition, structure, content, use and impacts of electronic health records: A review of the research literature. *International Journal of Medical Informatics*, *77*, 291–304.

HealthIT.gov. (2014a). *What is HIE?* Retrieved from https://www.healthit.gov/providers-professionals/health-information-exchange/what-hie.

HealthIT.gov. (2014b). *Data analytics update*. Retrieved from https://www.healthit.gov/facas/sites/faca/files/HITSC_Data_Analytics_Update_2015-04-22.pdf.

HealthIT.gov. (2015a). *Meaningful use definition & objectives*. Retrieved from https://www.healthit.gov/providers-professionals/meaningful-use-definition-objectives.

HealthIT.gov. (2015b). *Interoperability*. Retrieved from https://www.healthit.gov/policy-researchers-implementers/interoperability.

Horn, S. D., & Gassaway, J. (2010). Practice based evidence: Incorporating clinical heterogeneity and patient-reported outcomes for comparative effectiveness research. *Medical Care*, *48*(6 Suppl.), S17–S22.

Huber, D. G., Delaney, C., Crossley, J., Mehmert, M., & Ellerbe, S. (1992). A nursing management minimum data set: Significance and development. *Journal of Nursing Administration*, *22*(7–8), 35–40.

Huber, D., Schumacher, L., & Delaney, C. (1997). Nursing management minimum data set (NMMDS). *Journal of Nursing Administration*, *27*(4), 42–48.

Huston, C. (2013). The impact of emerging technology on nursing care: Warp speed ahead. *The Online Journal of Issues in Nursing*, *18*(2), Manuscript 1.

IMIA Special Interest Group on Nursing Informatics. (2016). *Nursing informatics*. Retrieved from https://www.amia.org/programs/working-groups/nursing-informatics.

Institute of Medicine (IOM). (2004). *Keeping patients safe: Transforming the work environment of nurses*. Washington, DC: National Academies Press.

Institute of Medicine (IOM) Committee on Crossing the Quality Chasm: Adaptation to Mental Health and Addictive Disorders. (2006). Increasing workforce capacity for quality improvement. In *Improving the quality of health care for mental and substance-use conditions: Quality Chasm Series*. Washington, DC: National Academies Press.

Institute of Medicine (IOM). (2011). *The future of nursing: Leading change, advancing health*. Washington, DC: National Academies Press.

Institute of Medicine (IOM). (2012). *Best care at lower cost: The path to continuously learning health care in America*. Washington, DC: National Academies Press.

International Organization for Standardization (ISO). (2002). *Health informatics: Integration of a reference terminology model for nursing* (Committee Document No. ISO/TC 215/N 142). Geneva, Switzerland: Author.

Kalisch, B. J., & Xie, B. (2014). Errors of omission: Missed nursing care. *Western Journal of Nursing Research*, *36*(7), 875–890.

Kennedy, R. (2003). The nursing shortage and the role of technology. *Nursing Outlook*, *51*, S33–S34.

Kopp, B., Erstad, B., Allen, M., Theodorou, A., & Priestley, G. (2006). Medication errors and adverse drug events in an intensive care unit: Direct observation approach for detection. *Critical Care Medicine*, *34*(2), 415–425.

Malloch, K. (2015). Measurement of nursing's complex health care work: Evolution of the science for determining the required staffing for safe and effective care. *Nursing Economic$*, *31*(1), 20–25.

Manyika, J., Chui, M., Brown, B., Bughin, J., Dobbs, R., Roxburgh, C., & Byers, A. H. (2011). *Big data: The next frontier for innovation, competition, and productivity. McKinsey Global Institute*. Retrieved from http://www.mckinsey.com/business-functions/business-technology/our-insights/big-data-the-next-frontier-for-innovation.

Minthorn, C., & Lunney, M. (2010). Participant action research with bedside nurses to identify NANDA-International, Nursing Interventions Classification, and Nursing Outcomes Classification categories for hospitalized persons with diabetes. *Applied Nursing Research*, *25*(2), 75–80. doi:10.1016/j.apnr.2010.08.001.

Moerbe, M., & Kelemen, A. (2014). Turning electronic health record data into meaningful information using SQL and nursing informatics. *Computers, Informatics, Nursing*, *32*(8), 366–377.

Moss, J., Andison, M., & Sobko, H. (2007). An analysis of narrative nursing documentation in an otherwise structured intensive care clinical information system. In *Proceedings of the American Medical Informatics Association Annual Symposium* (pp. 543–547). Chicago, IL: American Medical Informatics Association.

Muller-Staub, M. (2009). Study to the implementation of NANDA-1 nursing diagnosis, interventions and nursing sensitive patient outcomes. *Pflegewissenschaft*, *11*(12), 688–696.

National Institute of Standards and Testing (NIST). (2011). *Health IT at NIST*. Retrieved from http://www.nist.gov/healthcare/hit/upload/Health-IT-Fact-Sheet-09FEB11.pdf.

Ochylski, S., McDonald, T. F., Brokel, J., Zimmerman, D., Forzley, G., Banas, C., et al. (2012). Meaningful use: Changing physician documentation in the hospital setting. *Journal of Healthcare Information Management*, *26*(1), 58–63.

Office of the National Coordinator for Health Information Technology (ONC for Health IT). (n.d.). *Standards and interoperability framework*. Retrieved from https://www.healthit.gov/sites/default/files/pdf/fact-sheets/standards-and-interoperability-framework.pdf.

Osheroff, J. (Ed.). (2009). *Improving medication management, safety and other outcomes with CDS: A practical guide*. Chicago, IL: HIMSS.

Pathak, J., Wang, J., Kashyap, S., Basford, M., Li, R., Masys, D. R., & Chute, C. G. (2011). Mapping clinical phenotype data elements to standardized metadata repositories and controlled terminologies: The eMERGE Network experience. *Journal American Medical Informatics Association*, *18*, 376–386. doi:10.1136/amiajnl-2010-000061.

Petersen, L., Woodard, L., Urech, T., Daw, C., & Sookanan, S. (2006). Does pay-for-performance improve the quality of health care? *Annals of Internal Medicine*, *145*(4), 265–272.

Piscotty, R. J., & Kalisch, B. (2014). The relationship between electronic nursing care reminders and missed nursing care. *Computers, Informatics, Nursing*, *32*(10), 475–481.

Pruinelli, L., Delaney, C. W., Garcia, A., Caspers, B., & Westra, B. L. (2016). Nursing Management Minimum Data Set: Cost-effective tool to demonstrate the value of nurse staffing in the Big Data science era. *Nursing Economic$*, *34*(2), 66–71, 89.

Raghupathi, W., & Raghupathi, V. (2014). Big Data analytics in healthcare: Promise and potiential. *Health Information Science and Systems*, *2*(3). Retrieved from http://www.hissjournal.com/content/2/1/3.

Roth, C., Payne, P. R. O., Weier, R. C., Shoben, A. B., Fletcher, E. N., Lai, A. M., et al. (2016). The geographic distribution of cardiovascular health in stroke prevention in healthcare delivery environments (SPHERE) study. *Journal of Biomedical Informatics*, *60*(1), 95–103.

Salsberg, E. (2009). *State of the national physician workforce.* Paper presented at Annual Meeting of the Association of American Medical Colleges, Boston, MA.

Sampaio Santos, F. A., de Melo, R. P., & deOliveira Lopes, M. V. (2010). Characterization of health status with regard to tissue integrity and tissue perfusion in patients with venous ulcers according to the nursing outcomes classification. *Journal of Vascular Nursing,* 28(1), 14–20.

SAS Institute Inc. (n.d.). *Big Data: What it is and why it matters.* Retrieved from http://www.sas.com/en_us/insights/big-data/what-is-big-data.html.

Scherb, C. A., Head, B. J., Maas, M. L., Swanson, E. A., Moorhead, S., Reed, D., et al. (2011). Most frequent nursing diagnoses, nursing interventions, and nursing-sensitive patient outcomes of hospitalized older adults with heart failure, part 1. *International Journal of Nursing Terminologies & Classifications,* 22(1), 13–22.

Sensmeier, J. (2015). Big Data and the future of nursing knowledge. *Nursing Management,* 46(4), 22–27.

Sewell, J., & Thede, L. (2013). *Informatics and nursing. Opportunities and challenges* (4th ed.). Philadelphia, PA: Wolters Kluwer Lippincott Williams & Wilkins.

Shaljian, M., & Nielsen, M. (2013). *Managing populations, maximizing technology: Population health management in the medical neighborhood. Patient-Centered Primary Care Collaborative.* Washington, DC: Patient-Centered Primary Care Collaborative.

Sir, M. Y., Dundar, B., Barker Steege, L. M., & Pasupathy, K. S. (2015). Nurse-patient assignment models considering patient acuity metrics and nurses' perceived workload. *Journal of Biomedical Informatics,* 55, 237–248.

Sitterding, M. C., & Broome, M. (2015). *Information overload: Framework, tips and tools to manage in complex healthcare environments.* Silver Spring, MD: American Nurses Association.

Staggers, N., Bagley Thompson, C., & Snyder-Halpern, R. (2001). History and trends in clinical information systems in the United States. *Journal of Nursing Scholarship,* 33(1), 75–81.

Stetson, P., McKnight, K., Bakken, S., Curran, C., Kubose, T., & Cimino, J. (2001). *Development of an ontology to model medical errors, information needs, and the clinical communication space.* Paper presented at the AMIA Annual Symposium, Washington, DC.

Terry, K. (2015, April 29). Patient portals: Essential, but underused by physicians. *Medical Economics.* Retrieved from http://medicaleconomics.modernmedicine.com/medical-economics/news/patient-portals-essential-underused-physicians?page=full.

Topaz, M. (2013). The hitchhiker's guide to nursing informatics theory: Using the data-knowledge-information-wisdom framework to guide informatics research. *Online Journal of Nursing Informatics,* 17(3), 1–5.

US Department of Health and Human Services (HHS). (2011). *Partnerships for patients to improve care and lower costs for Americans.* Retrieved from https://www.cms.gov/Newsroom/MediaReleaseDatabase/Press-releases/2011-Press-releases-items/2011-04-12.html.

US Department of Health and Human Services (HHS). (2014). *HITECH and funding opportunities.* Retrieved from http://www.nihb.org/hitech/funding_opportunities.php.

Ward, M. M., Jaana, M., Bahensky, J. A, Vartak, S., & Wakefield, D. S. (2006). Clinical information system availability and use in urban and rural hospitals. *Journal of Medical Systems,* 30(6), 429–438.

Werley, H., & Lang, N. (Eds.). (1988). *Identification of the nursing minimum data set.* New York, NY: Springer.

Chapter 27

Aiken, L. H., Sloane, D. M., Bruyneel, L., Van den Heede, K., Griffiths, P., Busse, R., et al. (2014). Nurse staffing and education and hospital mortality in nine European countries: A retrospective observational study. *Lancet,* 383, 1824–1830.

American Nurses Credentialing Center. (2016). *Magnet Recognition Program®: Testimonials and case studies.* Retrieved from http://www.nursecredentialing.org/Magnet/ProgramOverview/WhyBecomeMagnet/MagnetTestimonials.

American Organization of Nurse Executives (AONE). (2015). *Nurse executive competencies.* Retrieved from http://www.aone.org/resources/nurse-executive-competencies.pdf.

Barro, J. (2015, December 11). Sorry, but your favorite company can't be your friend. *New York Times.* Retrieved from http://www.nytimes.com/2015/12/13/upshot/sorry-but-your-favorite-company-cant-be-your-friend.html?_r=0.

Berry, L. L., & Seltman, K. D. (2014). The enduring culture of Mayo Clinic. *Mayo Clinic Proceedings,* 89(2), 144–147.

Blegen, M. A., Goode, C. J., & Park, S. H. (2013). Baccalaureate education in nursing and patient outcomes. *Journal of Nursing Administration,* 43(2), 89–94.

Briginshaw, S. (2013, September 29). *Start with why—Simon Sinek TED talk—YouTube.* Retrieved from https://www.youtube.com/watch?v=sioZd3AxmnE.

Bureau of Labor Statistics. (2015). *Employment projections—2014-24* (BLS Publication No. USDL-15-2327). Retrieved from http://www.bls.gov/news.release/pdf/ecopro.pdf.

Byrnes, J. (2015). The value proposition in action. *Healthcare Financial Management,* 69(5), 106–107.

Chen, S.-Y., Wu, W.-C., Chang, C.-S., & Lin, C.-T. (2015). Job rotation and internal marketing for increased job satisfaction and organizational commitment in hospital nursing staff. *Journal of Nursing Management,* 23, 297–306.

Delina, G., & Raya, R. P. (2013). A study on work-life balance in working women. *International Journal of Commerce, Business and Management,* 2(5), 274–282.

Deloitte. *eVisits: The 21st century housecall.* (2014). Retrieved from https://www2.deloitte.com/content/dam/Deloitte/au/Documents/technology-media-telecommunications/deloitte-au-tmt-evisits-011014.pdf.

Depra, D. (2015, March 8). Having a goal in life may help extend lifespan. *Tech Times.* Retrieved from http://www.techtimes.com/articles/38096/20150308/having-a-goal-in-life-may-help-extend-lifespan.htm.

Ellison, A. (2015, April 8). 3 major challenges of healthcare price transparency. *Becker's Hospital CFO.* Retrieved from http://www.beckershospitalreview.com/finance/3-major-challenges-of-healthcare-price-transparency.html.

Evans, J. D. (2013). Factors influencing recruitment and retention of nurse educators reported by current nurse faculty. *Journal of Professional Nursing,* 29(1), 11–20.

Healthcare Financial Management Association. (2015). *Developing a blueprint for Accountable Care,* 69(11), 1–8.

Hotopf, M. (2013). How patients' review sites will change health care. *Journal of Health Services Research and Policy,* 18(4), 251–254.

Irish, K. (2014). Trends affecting the future of home healthcare. *Home Healthcare Nurse,* 32(9), 567–568.

Kavanagh, K. T., Cimiotti, J. P., Abusalem, S., & Coty, M. (2012). Moving healthcare quality forward with nursing-sensitive value-based purchasing. *Journal of Nursing Scholarship,* 44(4), 385–395.

Kemp, E., Jillapalli, R., & Becerra, E. (2014). Healthcare branding: Developing emotionally based consumer brand relationships. *Journal of Services Marketing,* 28(2), 126–137.

Kennedy, B., Craig, J. B., Wetsel, M., Reimels, E., & Wright, J. (2013). Three nursing interventions' impact on HCAHPS scores. *Journal of Nursing Care Quality,* 28(4), 327–334.

Kotler, P., & Keller, K. L. (2016). *Marketing management* (15th ed.). New York, NY: Pearson.

Kutney-Lee, A., Sloane, D. M., & Aiken, L. H. (2013). An increase in the number of nurses with baccalaureate degrees is linked to lower rates of postsurgery mortality. *Health Affairs,* 32(3), 579–586.

Landro, L. (2016, February 1). Hospitals find a way to say, 'I'm sorry'. *Wall Street Journal,* D1, D3.

Long, L. (2012). Impressing patients while improving HCAHPS. *Nursing Management,* 43(12), 32–37.

McCarthy, E. J. (1964). *Basic marketing: A managerial approach* (rev. ed.). New York, NY: McGraw-Hill.

McClelland, L. E., & Vogus, T. J. (2014). Compassion practices and HCAHPS: Does rewarding and supporting workplace compassion influence patient perception? *Health Services Research,* 49(5), 1670–1683.

Millenson, M. L., & Macri, J. (2012, March). Will the Affordable Care Act move patient-centeredness to center stage? Timely analysis of immediate health policy issues. *Urban Quick Strike Series*, 1–10. Retrieved from http://www.rwjf.org/en/library/research/2012/03/will-the-affordable-care-act-move-patient-centeredness-to-center.html?cid=XEM_A5765.

Moneke, N., & Umeh, O. J. (2013). Factors influencing critical care nurses' perception of their overall job satisfaction. *The Journal of Nursing Administration*, 43(4), 201–207.

Montoya, I. D., & Kimball, O. M. (2012). Nursing services: An imperative to health care marketing. *Journal of Nursing Education and Practice*, 2(4), 187–193.

Nelson, R., Joos, I., & Wolf, D. M. (2013). *Social media for nurses: Educating practitioners and patients in a networked world*. New York, NY: Springer Publishing Company.

Planetree. (2014). *Person-centered care designation*. Retrieved from http://planetree.org/designation-2/.

Radwin, L. E., Cabral, H. J., & Woodworth, T. S. (2013). Effects of race and language on patient-centered cancer nursing care and patient outcomes. *Journal of Health Care for the Poor and Underserved*, 24, 619–632.

Sanky, M., Berger, P. D., & Weinberg, B. D. (2012). A segmentation approach to patient health intervention. *Journal of Medical Marketing*, 12(4), 221–228.

Sheth, J. N., & Sisodia, R. (2012). *The 4 A's of marketing: Creating value for customer, company and society*. New York, NY: Routledge.

Sinek, S. (2009). *Start with why: How great leaders inspire everyone to take action*. New York, NY: Penguin Group.

Steege, L. M., & Pinekenstein, B. (2016). Addressing occupational fatigue in nurses. *Journal of Nursing Administration*, 46(4), 193–200.

Ten Hoeve, Y., Jansen, G., & Roodbol, P. (2014). The nursing profession: Public image, self-concept, and professional identify. *Journal of Advanced Nursing*, 70(2), 295–309.

Walker, L. (2014). Promoting nursing's professionalism. *Nursing New Zealand*, 20(3), 2.

INDEX

A

Ability, of follower, 12
Absenteeism, cost of, 161
Academic detailing
  definition of, 270
  for evidence-based practice, 272
Accents, in workplace diversity, 183
Acceptability, as marketing mix element, 452t, 453t
Accessibility
  lack of, in health record, 443
  as marketing mix element, 452t, 453t
Accommodating, problem-solving style, 170
Accountability
  definition of, 141
  delegator and delegatee, 143f
  imperative, patient engagement, 311–312
Accountable care organization (ACO), 62, 70
Accounting, creative, 77
Accuracy, rating, for performance appraisal, 404–405
Action
  enablement, 9
  plan, 217
Action items list, 417
Active listening, 39
Active shooter
  as example of collaboration by DHS, 337
  procedures, 337b
Activities, coordination of, 196
Activity-based costing (ABC), 396
Acuity, of patients, 396
Acute care hospitals, in economic external forces, 233
Acute care nursing CM models, 243
Ad hoc committee, 129
Ad hoc members, in emergency management committee, 412
Ad hoc team, 126
Adaptation, 121
Adapting, as leadership skill, 5
Adaptive capacity, 9
Administrative decisions, performance appraisal for, 401–402
Admission, discharges, and transfers (ADT), 371
Adopter frequency distribution, categories of, 42
Adult child, problem of, 94
Advanced practice nurses, project team leaders (partnering), 279
Advertising, nursing shortage, 358
Affidavit of merit, 90–91
Affordability, as marketing mix element, 452t, 453t
Affordable Care Act (ACA) of 2010, 44–45, 77, 179, 203, 236, 444
Agency for Healthcare Research and Quality (AHRQ)
  quality indicator, 318
  TeamSTEPPS, 313
  workforce characteristics review, 161
Aging patients, conditions/chronic diseases (increase), 323
All-hazards, definition of, 411

All-hazards disaster preparedness, 411
  action items list for, 417
  case study on, 424–425b
  command center and, development of, 419–421
  definition of, 410
All-hazards planning subgroup, creation of, 418–419
All-hazards preparedness
  issues and trends in, 422–426
  leadership and management implications, 421–422
  staff fear associated with, overcoming, 421
  transitioning theory for, 410–411
All-hazards preparedness plans
  external drills and, 420
  internal drills and, 420
  nomenclature, structure and role for writing, 417
  procedural annexes to, creation of, 417–418
  testing, 420
All-hazards preparedness task force, creation of, 411–412
Alternative dispute resolution (ADR), 167–169
Ambiguity, 183
American Academy of Nursing's Task Force on Nursing Practice in Hospitals, 52
American Association of Colleges of Nursing (AACN), *Salaries of Instructional and Administrative Nursing Faculty in Baccalaureate and Graduate Programs in Nursing*, 346
American Association of Critical-Care Nurses (AACN)
  Clinical Scene Investigator Academy, 80
  healthy work environments standards, 80, 80t
American Case Management Association (ACMA), Standards of Practice & Scope of Services for Health Care Delivery System Case Management and Transitions of Care (TOC) Professionals, 250
American Nurses Association (ANA)
  call to action, 354–355
  Guide to the Code of Ethics for Nurses with Interpretive Statements, 290
  nursing informatics in, 433
  Nursing's Agenda for the Future, 345, 354
  Nursing's Social Policy Statement: The Essence of the Profession, 85
  principles for nurse staffing, 373
  recognized terminologies, for nursing, 439–440
American Nurses Credentialing Center's Magnet Recognition Program, 217, 295
American Organization of Nurse Executives (AONE), 3, 216, 354, 373, 450
  all-hazards preparedness task force, 411–412
  Nurse Executive Competencies: Population Health, 257
  nursing informatics, 434
  Staffing Management and Methods, 373
American Osteopathic Association's Healthcare Facilities Accreditation Program (HFAP), 303
American Recovery and Reinvestment Act of 2009 (ARRA), 95, 281–282
Americans With Disabilities Act (ADA), 179–180
Annexes, procedural, creation of, 417–418
Annual workload, forecasted, 378

Page numbers followed by *b*, *t*, and *f* indicate boxes, tables, and figures, respectively

Appraisal, performance, 277, 401–409, 408–409b
    case study on, 409b
    employee development through, 405–407
    issues and trends in, 407–409
    issues in, 402–407
    leadership and management implications, 407
    measurements for, 402–404
        behaviors, 403
        competencies, 403
        results, 403–404
        traits, 402–403
    performance metrics for, 404
    purposes of, 401–402
    rating accuracy for, 404–405
Arbitration, 169
Assertiveness, influence tactics, 155
Assessing Progress on the Institute of Medicine Report: The Future of
    Nursing, 356, 356t
Assignment, 141
Association of American Colleges and Universities, 180
Association of periOperative Registered Nurses, 373–374
Attitude, inflexible, 183
Authentic leadership, 16
Authoritarian, as leadership style, 10
Authoritative decision making, 124, 124f
Authority, 155–156
    definition of, 141
    influence, contrast, 155t
Autonomy, 45, 87
    nursing shortage, 352
Average daily census (ADC), 371, 377, 392
Average length of stay (ALOS), 371
    calculated, 377
Awareness, as marketing mix element, 452t, 453t
Awareness-knowledge, creation of, 42

B
Baby boomers, 181–182
Baldrige National Quality Award (BNQA), performance
    standards, 295
Bargaining, 102
Behavioral norms, topics for, 127–128
Behaviors, in performance appraisal, 403
Benchmarking, definition of, 286
Beneficence, 87
Benefits, of workplace diversity, 180
Berwick, Donald M, 288–289
Best alternative to a negotiated agreement (BATNA), 169
Best practice, definition of, 269
Bias, in performance rating, 404
Big Data, 436
    outcomes and, 323–324, 324t
Biological disaster, 411
Biological terrorism, 418, 419
Biomedical ethics, 87
Biomedical technicians, 430–431
Biopsychosocial Individual and Systems Intervention Model,
    for case management, 246
Bioterrorism, preparedness for, 203
Blocking, influence tactics, 155
Bottoms-up approach, for evidence-based practice, 279–280
Boundaries, setting, in stress management, 79
Boundary spanning roles, 193
"Brain drain," 350

Brand, definition of, 448–449
Breach of contract, 88f
Brokerage model, for case management, 245, 248
Budget
    definition of, 389
    expenditures, evaluation of, 395, 398
    forms, completing, 390
    organizational, types of, 389
    preparation of, 389–390
    revenue, 393
    revision and resubmission, 390
    supply, 393
    tracking and monitoring of, 393–394
Budgeted salary expense flow sheet, 393t
Budgeting, 388–400, 399b, 400b
    background of, 388–389
    case study on, 400b
    definitions of, 389
    issues and trends in, 398–400
    leadership and management implications, 394–397
    process of, 389–393
Bullying, 166–167, 335
    workplace, 329
Bureau of Labor Statistics (BLS), in population and health
    trends, 256
Bureaucracy
    concept of, in historical context, 189
    modernist theories related to, 187–188
Bureaucratic theory, 189
Business
    plan, 217
    skills and principles of, 4
Business intelligence, 429
Butterfly effect, 26

C
Campaign for Nursing's Future, 351
Canadian Patient Safety Institute in Canada, safety innovations
    and, 204
Capital budget
    definition of, 389
    development of, 390–391
Care
    coordination of, for case management models, 243
    quality of, in workplace diversity, 178
Care coordinator, on population health management, 256
Care delivery, effective, 434
Care delivery model, 226
    culture and, 50
    types of, 230–234
Care management, leadership differentiated from, 2–3
Care of Mental, Physical and Substance Use Syndromes
    (COMPASS), 257
Carefronting, 167–168
CARF International, performance standards, 303
Carondelet St. Mary's model, 244
Case management (CM), 233–234, 242–254, 266b
    advocacy, 243
    assessment, 252
        questions, 253b
    case study on, 266b
    code of professional conduct, 251
    defined by the Case Management Society of America (CMSA), 375
    definition of, 240

Case management *(Continued)*
    financial gain, problems in, 254
    with human resources, 263
    individual suitability for, 263
    issues and trends in, 263–266
        branding and lack of universal definition, 263–264
        legislative and regulatory disruptors, 264
        non-clinical workers, influx of, 264
        outcomes, measuring and sharing, 264–265
        treatment adherence, 265
    key activities in, 243
    landmark legislation in, 242
    leadership and management implication of, 262–263
    models, 242–250
        competency-based models, 247–248
        gatekeeper model, 248–249
        government model, 250
        insurance models, 248
        interdisciplinary models, 245–247, 246b
        managed care models, 250
        practice models background, 242–243
        seminal nursing, 244
        social work models, 244–245
    outcomes, 253–254
    practice standards, 250
    process, 251, 252t
    program development, 251–253
Case Management Society of America (CMSA)
    case management defined by, 375
    case management process and, 251, 252t
    Standards of Practice for Case Management, 250, 251, 252
Case manager
    in population health management, 256
    role of, 242, 251–252
Case nursing, 231
Catastrophic illness or injury, case management in, 250
Cause-and-effect diagram, sample, 301f
Celebrations, evidence-based practice and, 278–279
Center for Quality Improvement and Safety in the United States,
        safety innovations and, 204
Centers for Disease Control and Prevention (CDC), in population
        and health trends, 256
Centers for Medicare & Medicaid Services (CMS), 444
    data submission programs, 305
    Hospital Value-Based Purchasing Program, 305–306
    provision 1533-F, 385
    QIOs, 305
    time and stress management, 76
Centrality, 161
    definition of, 159
Centralization, 194
    decision making, 206, 207f
    definition of, 206
    organizational philosophy, 207
Centralized staffing, 381
Champions, 274–275
Change, 32–48, 46–47b
    approaches or models of, 32–33
    background in, 33–34
    capacity to, 36
    case study on, 47–48b
    communication to facilitate, 113–114, 114b
    constancy, perception, 45–46
    cycles, types of, 37–38

Change *(Continued)*
    effectiveness of, 38
    emergence of, 36–37
    emotional responses to, 39
        strategies of, 39
    executives/administrators, impact in, 37
    human factor of, 38–39
    implementation of, 41
    implications of, 44–45
    interconnected transformations of, 45
    interpretations of, 37
    issues in, 45–46
    leadership
        relationship in, 40
        roles in, 40
    maintenance in, 39–40
    management, 37–38
        meaning of, 37
        small scale of, 37–38
    meaning of, 33
    moving, 35
    nurse experience, 39
    nursing process/problem solving, similarities of, 35t
    objectives, selection of, 36
    occurrence, 44–45
    perspective of, 35
    practices, development of, 36–37
    process (Lewin), 34–35
    recipients of, 37
    refreezing, 35
    resistance to, 38–39
    structural components of, 45
    successful, elements of, 35f
    theories/models of, 34–36
        process, comparisons of, 36t
    trends in, 45–46
    unfreezing, 35
    views, contrast of, 33t
Change agent, 33
    motivation/resources, assessment of, 36
    role, selection of, 36
Change fatigue, 74
Change process, 36–40
    flow of, 36
    management of, 37–38
    phases of, 36
Chaos theory, 26–28
Chaotic behavior, 26
Chemical disaster, 411
Chemical terrorism, 418, 419
Chief financial officer, in emergency management committee,
        413–414t
Chief information technology officer, in emergency management
        committee, 413–414t
Chief nursing officer (CNO), role of, 411–412, 413–414t, 416–417
Chief operating officer, in emergency management committee,
        413–414t
Chronic Care Model, for case management, 246
Chronic Care Professional (CCP) Certification, 257
Chronic health condition, in population health management (PHM),
        255–256
Cincinnati Children's Hospital Medical Center Interprofessional
        Practice Model, 211f
Civil Disobedience, 38–39

Civil law, 89–92
Civility, 340
Clarifier, 132
Classical management theory, 189–190
Classification systems, in data management, 440
Client, in nursing's data needs, 431
Client care activities, definition of, 141
Client population assessment, in case management program development, 252, 253b
Clinical data repository, 433
Clinical decision making, 61, 64–65
Clinical decision support systems (CDS), 429
Clinical documentation, electronic health record and, 437
Clinical ethics, 95–96
Clinical informatics, 428–446, 444–445b
    case study on, 445–446b
    issues and trends in, 443–446
    leadership and management implications, 442–443
    standardized clinical terminology in, 439–440
Clinical information systems (CIS), 429
Clinical judgment, 61
Clinical leadership, 16–17
Clinical practice
    fiscal responsibility for, 395
    guidelines, 229–230, 269
Clinical process management (CPM), 212
Clinical protocols, 229–230
Clinical reasoning, 61, 64
Clinical Scene Investigator Academy, 80
Clinical stress, 380
Coaching, 21
Coalitions, influence tactics, 155
Code of ethics, 96
Code of Ethics for Nurses with Interpretive Statements, 96
Code of professional conduct, in case management, 251
Coercive power, 156–157, 157b
Cognitive innovation-decision process, 41
Cohorts, generational group categorization, 181
COLLABORATE model, for case management, 248, 249t
Collaborating, problem-solving style, 170
Collaboration, 120
    in decision making, 69
    health care quality, nursing imperative, 290
    relationships, 290
    shared governance (impact), 212
Collaborative Care Model, for case management, 247
Collective bargaining agreements, 375–376
Collectivism, in workplace diversity, 183
Command center
    development of, 419–421
    processes in, development, 420
    room, setting up, 419–420
    testing, 420
Commission for Case Manager Certification (CCMC)
    case management process in, 251, 252t
    Code of Professional Conduct for Case Managers with Standards, Rules, Procedures, and Penalties, 251
Commitment, 12
Committee, 119, 128–129
    ad hoc, 129
    multidisciplinary, 129
    structures, 128
    types of, 128–129
Common data elements (CDEs), 318, 324

Communal relationships, 449
Communicating, as leadership skill, 5
Communication, 120
    background of, 102–103
    case study on, 117b
    definitions in, 102
    delegation and, 148
    as disease management program component, 260–261
    effective, tools for, 106–107
    electronic, social media and, 115–117
    in emergencies, 115
    to facilitate change, 113–114
    in group members, 121
    holistic and spiritual health care, 109–110
    ineffective, cures for, 105–106t, 105–107
    issues in, 114–117
    leadership, 7–8, 102–117, 116–117b
        implications, 110–113
    management
        approach in, 107
        implications, 110–113
    organizational culture and climate and, 108–109
    senior manager monitoring of, 37
    standardization of, 193
    teaching, 114–115
    team/group, 111–113
    theories and models in, 103–108, 104f
        evidence-based practice, 107–108
        intrapersonal and interpersonal communication, 104–107, 104f, 112f
        transformational leadership, 108
    trends in, 114
    workplace diversity, 181
    written, 115
Community, hospital's role in, establishing, 420–421
Community health, 255
Comparative effectiveness research (CER), 319, 430, 433
Compatibility, as planned change factor, 42
Competencies, 290b
    health profession competencies, 290
Competencies, in performance appraisal, 403
Competency-based models, 247–248
Competing, problem-solving style, 170
Competition
    definition of, 449–450
    in group process, 112
Competitive conflict, 162–163
Complete schedule, 379
Complexity, as planned change factor, 42
Complexity Compression, 76
Complexity leadership, 15
Complexity theory, 25–26, 190–191
Compliance, demonstration, 94
Comprehensive service center model, for case management, 245
Compromiser, 132
Compulsive talkers, 133
Conciliation, 169
Confidence, 12
Confidentiality, 87, 94
Conflict, 161–174, 173b
    accommodating, 167
    avoiding, 167
    bullying and, 166–167
    case study on, 173–174b

Conflict *(Continued)*
  cause of, 165–166
  collaborating, 167
  competing, 167
  competitive, 162–163
  compromising, 167
  conceptual framework of, 165f
  constructive effects of, 163, 163b
  core process of, 165–166
  definition of, 162
  destructive effects of, 163, 163b
  disruptive, 162–163
  disruptive behavior and, 166–167
  dysfunctional outcomes of, 166
  effects of, 163b, 165–166
  existence of, 166
  face negotiation therapy and, 169–170
  factors of, 162
  functional outcomes of, 166
  handling intentions, 168–169
  interactionist view of, 162
  intergroup, 164
  interpersonal, 164
  intragroup, 164
  Intragroup Conflict Scale, 167
  intrapersonal, 163–164
  job, 162
  leadership implications, 171–172
  models of, 164–166
  organizational, 162, 171–172
  Organizational Conflict Inventory-II, 171
  Perceived Conflict Scale, 167
  process, 164
  process models of, comparison of, 165t
  Rahim Organizational Conflict Inventory-I, design, 167
  relationship, 164
  resolution, 169–171
    alternative dispute, 167–169
    inventories, 171
    outcomes, 170, 170b
    strategies for, 171–172
  scales, 167
  task, 164
  traditionalist view of, 162
  trends, issues and, 172–174
  types of, 163–164
    illustration of, 164f
  unit performance and, 163f
  views of, 162–163
Conflict management, 167–169
  implications, 171–172
  styles, 167, 168t
  win-win resolution, 170
Connection power, 157–158
Conscious change leadership, 34
Constructive criticism, leadership strategy of, 35
Constructive group roles, 132–133
Consultation, in decision making, 69
Consultative decision making, 124, 124f
Contemporary approaches, in case management, 242
Context, in evidence-based practice, 276–279
Contingency theory, 24, 190
  technology as core concept in, 190
Continuous quality improvement (CQI), definition of, 286–287

Continuum of care, 255
Contracts, breach, 88f
Contrast, bias, 404
Control chart, 300f
Controlling, 22
  defined, 20
Conversations, crucial, performance appraisal and, 406–407
Cooperating, problem-solving style, 170
Coordinating, 21
Coordination
  of labor, 191–194
  mechanisms of, 194
  requirement of, 190
  types of, 193–194
Core coverage, 377–379
Core purpose
  definition of, 217
  usage, 218
Core values, 227–228
  definition of, 217
  expression for, 206
  usage, 218
Corporate strategy, 194
Cost, marketing and, 455
Cost containment, delegation and, 147–148
Cost management, 45
Costing out nursing services, 395–397
Council, 119–120
Creative accounting, 77
Criminal law, 92
Crisis standards of care, 411, 421
Critical Infrastructure Partnership Advisory Council (CIPAC), 336–337
Critical path, 229–230
Critical pathways, 229–230
Crosby, Philip B., 288, 290
Cross-examination, 86
Crossing the Quality Chasm: A New Health System for the 21st Century, 296
Crossing the Quality Chasm (IOM), 49, 234–235, 254, 345, 354
Crucial conversations
  performance appraisal and, 406–407
  as tool for effective communication, 107
Cultural and linguistic competency training, 179
Cultural diversity, definition of, 175
Cultural static, 176
Cultural tendencies, 175
Culture
  definition of, 175
  impact of, 176–178
  measurement of, 50
  representation, 50
Culture change, in long-term care, 56
Culture-climate link, 50–51
Curing Health Care: New Strategies for Quality Improvement, 288–289
CUS model, for effective communication, 107
Customer-oriented marketing mix, 453, 453t
Customer satisfactions, 235–236
Cyber disaster, 411

D
Damages, 86
Danger, fear of, 81–82

Data
   collecting and extracting, 433
   definition of, 433
   interoperability of, 443
Data analysis, 433
Data analysis systems, evolution and improvement, 306
Data analyst, 430–431
Data analytics
   in decision making, 68–69
   for nurse leaders, 444
Data collection sheet, sample, 300f
Data elements, in Nursing Minimum Data Set (NMDS),
   440–442
Data management, 428–446, 444–445b
   case study on, 445–446b
   classification systems in, 440
   effectiveness, 439
   issues and trends in, 443–446
   leadership and management implications, 442–443
Data normalization, 442
Data operations, 433
Data repository, 433
Data sources, 397–398
Data tables, 442
Data warehouse, 429–430, 433
Decentralization, 206–215, 213–214b
   case study on, 214b
   decision making, 207, 207f
   definition of, 206
   issues and trends in, 212–214
   leadership and management implications, 209–211,
      211f
   organizational philosophy, 207
DECIDE model, 62, 63t
Decision, powers, ranges of, 124f
Decision making
   case study on, 72b
   clinical, 61, 61f, 64–65
   data analytics in, 68–69
   decision support systems in, 68–69
   definitions of, 60–61
   environment, 60–61
   ethical, 66
   evidence-informed, 67
   group, 124–125, 124f
   group participation in, 130
   managerial, 60–73
   maze in, 64f
   meeting for, 130
   models of, 61–63, 63t
   organizational, 61, 61f, 65–66
   pilot projects in, 67–68
   policies, guide, 228
   process of, 64
   SBAR in, 68
   shared governance in, 67
   simulation in, 68
   strategies for, 69–70, 70f
   tools for, 67–69, 67t
Decision-making authority, 206
Decision process, power from, 159
Decision support systems, in decision making, 68–69
Deescalation, definition of, 332
De-implementation, definition of, 269

Delegated decision procedure, 124f, 125
Delegatee, 141
   accountability of, 143f
Delegation, in nursing, 140–152, 151b, 152t
   barriers to, 145–147, 146f
   case study on, 151–152b
   definition of, 141
   direct versus indirect, 148
   ethical and legal issues concerning, 147–149
   issues and trends in, 149–152
   leadership and management implications, 149
   prioritization in, 144–145
   process of, 142–144, 143f, 144f
Delegator
   accountability of, 143f
   definition of, 141
   types of, 146f
Demand management, 380–381
Deming, W. Edwards, 288, 290
Democratic, as leadership style, 10
Department chiefs, in emergency management committee,
   413–414t
Department of Homeland Security (DHS), 336–337
Departmentalization, of work, 193
Deposition, 86
DESC script, for effective communication, 107
Desired objectives analysis, 67t
Developed countries, health care systems in, 203
Development, performance appraisal for, 402
Diagnosing, as leadership skill, 5
Diagnosis-related group (DRG) reimbursements,
   395–396
Diagnosis-related groups (DRGs), 82
Differentiation, 189
   basis of, 451
   by function, 195
Diffusion of Innovations Model, 272
DIKW framework, 433
Direct-care costs, 395–396
Direct delegation, 148
Direct examination, 86
Direct intervention, 69
Directing, 21–22
   defined, 20
Disaster preparedness, 203
   all-hazards, 411
      action items list for, 417
      case study on, 424–425b
      command center and, development of, 419–421
      definition of, 410
Disasters
   biological, 411
   chemical, 411
   cyber, 411
   definition of, 411
   occurrence of, 410
   staff fear associated with, overcoming, 421
   types of, 411
Disease management (DM), 254–262
   background of, 254–256
   definition of, 240
   history of, 254–256
   implementation, 258
   Population Care Coordination Process in, 257–258

Disease management *(Continued)*
    process, 258
    program components, 258–262, 259f
        delivery, 260–261
        effectiveness evaluation, 261, 262t
        enrollment and engagement, 260
        identification, 258–260
        outcomes, 261
        population risk assessment, 258
        reporting, 261–262
        stratification, 260
    program development, 258
    transitions to population health management, 254–255
Disease-Specific Care (DSC) Certification, 257
Disruptive behavior, 166–167
    management of, 134
Disruptive conflicts, 124, 162–163
Disruptive innovation, 43
Distance practice, 92
Diversity, definition of, 175
Documentation, in clinical decision making, 64–65
Documents, legal, 93–95
Dominating, problem-solving style, 170
Duty to report, 98
Dyad team model, for case management, 245–246
Dynamic information exchange, 144, 144f

E
E4 framework, in case management, 248
Early adopters, adopter frequency distribution, 42
Early majority, adopter frequency distribution, 42
Ebola crisis, emergency preparedness and, 419
Economics, integration of, in clinical practice, 399–400
Education director, in emergency management committee, 413–414t
Educational capacity, productivity and, 398
Educational outreach, 270
    for evidence-based practice, 272
Effective change, 42
Effective groups, 120
Effective leadership, importance of, 2
Effectiveness
    communication for, 8
    of data management, 439
    implementation, 221
Effectiveness research, 430
Efficiency
    reliability and, balancing tensions between, 4
    scientific management and, 232
Electronic communication, social media and, 115–117
Electronic documentation systems, for evidence-based practice, 278
Electronic health records (EHRs), 436–438
    computerization with, 45
    implementation of, in evidence-based practice, 281–282
    purpose of, 437
Electronic medical records (EMRs), adoption of, 374
Emergence, 121
Emergencies, communication in, 115
Emergency department/medical director, in emergency management committee, 413–414t
Emergency management and preparedness, 410–427, 424b
Emergency management committee
    creation of, 412
    lead person in, 420
    membership responsibilities of, 413–414t

Emergency operations plan (EOP), 411–412
Emotional intelligence, leadership and, 5–6
Empathy, nonviolent communication, 111
Employee assistance programs (EAPs), 333–334
Employees
    empowerment and, 154
    performance appraisal and, 405–407
    selection of, 359–360
Employer, intense, in population health management, 265
Empowerment, 6, 45, 154–155
    employees and, 154
    nurse, 154
    physiological, 154
    for work-related stress, 80–81
Encouragement, leadership strategy of, 35
Encourager, 132
End-of-life care, 229–230
End-of-shift report, 130
Engagement
    as disease management program component, 260
    employees, shared governance (impact), 213–214
Engineering, in emergency management committee, 413–414t
Enrollment, as disease management program component, 260
Enterprise risk management (ERM), 312
    definition of, 287
    health care, 303–315
    process, 312
    program, 287, 312
Entry-level baccalaureate programs in nursing, enrollments in, 345
Environment, assessment of, 218–219
Environmental design, 335–336
Equal Employment Opportunity Commission (EEOC), 334–335
Equal opportunity employer, 358–359
Equilibrium, 35–36
Equity, WHO definition of, 177
Ethical components, 95–96
Ethical decisions, 98–99
    making, 66
Ethical dilemmas, 95
Ethical issues, 85–101, 100b
    case study on, 100–101b
    definitions, 87
    education and licensure, 87
    leadership and management implications, 96–99
Ethnocentrism, 183–184
Eustress, 74
Events, emergence of, 36–37
Evidence, 430
    hierarchy of, 270
Evidence-based care, 281
Evidence-based Magnet Recognition Program®, 357
Evidence-based management, implementation of, 4
Evidence-based practice (EBP), 283b, 433
    bottoms-up approach, use of, 279–280
    business case, articulation, 278
    case study, 283–284b
    communication and, 107–108
    context, 276–279
    definition of, 268–269, 286–287
    evaluation, 275–276
    exemplar, 274–276, 276f
    implementation, 271–272
        strategies, 274–275, 275f
    issues and trends, 280–282

Evidence-based practice *(Continued)*
  leadership and management implications, 280
  leadership roles, 279–280
  models, 270, 271t
  organizational infrastructure, 276–279
    building, strategies, 279
  performance expectations and appraisal, 277
  quality improvement and, 278
  reporting for, 278
  resources for, 278, 281
  rewards in, 278–279
  shared governance in, 277
  steps for performing, 270
  sustaining, 271–272
  value of, 277
Evidence-Based Practice Implementation Guide, 272, 273f
Evidence-informed decision making, 67
Evidenced-based algorithms, 229–230
Exchange, influence tactics, 155
Exchange relationships, 449
Executive administrator, in emergency management committee, 413–414t
Executive attorney, in emergency management committee, 413–414t
Executive leadership, responsibility of, 226–227
Executive summary, 221
Expenses, definition of, 389
Experience, of follower, 12
Expert power, 156–157, 157b
Expert testimony, 86
Expert witness, 86, 91
Explosives, 411
External drills, 420

F
Face negotiation therapy, 169–170
  revision, cross-cultural empirical tests, 170
Facework, 169
Facilitation, in decision making, 69
Facility design checklist, 336b
Fact witness, 86, 91
Fair and just culture
  concept of, 307
  definition of, 286–287
Family-centered care, 55, 234
Family dynamic, changing, legal issues and, 99
Fear
  of danger, 81–82
  staff, overcoming, 421
Federal Emergency Management Administration (FEMA) Corps, as community-based assistance program, 423
Feedback mechanisms, 193
Feedforward, 406
Feigenbaum, Armand V., 288
Feminist leadership perspective, 11
Fidelity, 87
Financial gain, problems in, case management, 254
Fiscal responsibility, for clinical practice, 395
Fiscal year, 391
Five Practices of Exemplary Leadership, 9
Five rights of delegation, 144
Fixed staffing, 378
Flat organizational structure, 198–199, 200f, 200t
Florence Nightingale International Foundation, 350

Flow stress, 380
Fluency, in workplace diversity, 183
Follower
  leadership and, 7
  types of, 17–18
Followership, 6, 7, 17–18
Formal policies, 228
Formal relationship, management determination, 187–188
Formalized questions, 359
Forming stage, in group development, 111–112
Fragmentation, offset of, 197
Full-time equivalents (FTEs), 378
  status, 357–358
Functional nursing, 232
Functions, isolation of, offset of, 197
Future loss, reduce or prevent, 312
Future of Nursing: Leading Change, Advancing Health, 1, 355–356, 434, 442
Future of Nursing, The (IOM), 41, 153, 281

G
Gap analysis
  performing, 412–416
  survey, hospital, 415–416b
Gatekeeper, 132
Gatekeeper model, 248–249
Geister, Janet, 231–232
General guardian, 93
Generation Why?, 182
Generation X, 182
  nurses, concerns, 56
Generation Y, 182
  nurses, 56
Generational diversity, 56, 181–182
Generational markers, 181
Geriatric workforce shortage, marketing and, 456
Global decision-making strategies, 69, 70f
Goals
  differences in, conflict factor, 162
  leadership process and, 8
Golden Circle, 458f
Good stress, 74
Governance, shared, 206–209, 213–214b
  case study on, 214b
  challenges, 208–209
  concept, 210
  in decision making, 67
  in evidence-based practice, 277
  history, 208
  implementation, 210
  implications, 211
  increase, 208
  issues and trends in, 212–214
    engagement, 213–214
    inter-professional education and collaboration, 212
    whole-system integration, 212–213
  leadership and management implications, 209–211, 211f
Government affairs director, in emergency management committee, 413–414t
Government model, 250
Graduates
  national baseline projections of, 343f
  retention, 361–364
    strategies, 362b

Group, 119
  adaptation in, 121
  advantages of, 122–123
  authoritative decision making in, 124
  background of, 120–121
  compulsive talkers in, 133
  consultative decision making in, 124
  decision making, 124–125, 124f
  definition of, 112
  delegated decision procedure in, 125
  disadvantages of, 123–124
  disruptive conflicts in, 124
  distracted or unreliable members in, 134
  emergence in, 121
  formation of, 121
  for greater knowledge and information, 122
  individual domination in, 123
  interactions, elements of, 120–121
  interrupters in, 133–134
  issues and trends in, 135–138
  joint decision making in, 124–125
  leadership and management implications, 134–135
  meetings, effectiveness of, 129–132
  members
    communication in, 121
    roles of, 121
  nontalkers in, 133
  orientation in, 121
  problem, approaches to, 122–123
  process, 120
  roles, constructive, 132–133
  solutions, acceptance of, 122
  squashers in, 134
  stages, 121
  working in, 121
Group decision-making power, 158
Group development, stages of, 111–112
Group nursing, 231–232
Guardian, 93
Guardian ad litem, 94
Guardianship, 93–94
Guide to the Code of Ethics for Nurses with Interpretive
  Statements, 290
Guidelines International Network, 281

H
Halo effect, 404
Handoff communication, 113
  implementation of, 307–308
Hardiness, impact of, 9
Harmonizer, 132
Hazard vulnerability analysis, 411
  performing, 412
Health care
  business of, 449
  change
    areas of, 44f
    reimbursement, impact, 45
  disruptive innovation, example of, 44b
  enterprise risk management, 303–315
  innovation in, 42–43
  performance, emerging models of, 293–296
  practice of, 449
  providers, responsibilities of, 380

Health care (Continued)
  quality management, emerging models of, 293–296
  safety, 303–315
    environment, nurse manager, 308
    program, components of, 306b
  trends in, 45
Health care management continuum, components of, 241, 241t
Health care organizations, liability of, 97–98
Health care professionals, in data management and clinical
  informatics, 443–444
Health care quality
  collaboration, nursing imperative, 290
  costs associated with poor, 296–297
  definition of, 287
  improvement, IOM aims, 289b
  indicators of, 287
  planning, 297–303
  structure, process, and outcomes, 291–292
  in twenty-first century, 288–290
Health care technology, nursing application and, 434–436
Health care workforce, communication and, 114
Health coach, on population health management, 256
Health disparities, 177–178
Health Enhancement Research Organization (HERO), 261–262
Health equity, 177–178
Health inequities, 177–178
Health information exchange (HIE), 430, 438–439
  networks, 443
Health information management (HIM), 430–431
Health Information Technology for Economic and Clinical Health
  (HITECH) Act, 95, 374
  enactment, 281–282
  funding, 438
Health information technology (HIT), 434–436
  tools, 435t
Health Insurance Portability and Accountability Act (HIPAA),
  37, 410
  provisions, 115
Health profession competencies, components, 290
Health Resources and Services Administration (HRSA), in
  population and health trends, 256
Health risk behaviors, in population, 265
Healthcare Effectiveness Data and Information Set (HEDIS),
  261, 304
Healthcare Facilities Accreditation Program (HFAP), performance
  standards, 303
Healthcare Failure Modes and Effects Analysis (HFMEA), 307,
  309–311
Healthy work environments, 53–54, 230, 230b
  standards, for work-related stress, 80, 80t
Heart, encouragement, 9
Heath Information Portability and Accountability Act (HIPAA), 94
  Privacy Rule, 95
Hierarchical centralization, 194
Hierarchy, 194–195
  formal structure of organization and, 198
  reporting structure and, 194–195
High-level decision making, participation in, 172
High-reliability organizations, 295, 307
High-risk predictions, 83
Historical projections, 393
Hold harmless agreement, 88f
Holistic health care, communication and, 109–110
Holistic orientation, 449

Home Health Quality Initiative (HHQI), 305
Homeostasis, stress and, 74
Horizontal violence, 329
Horn effect, 404
Hospital
    gap analysis survey, questions for, 415–416b
    measures, 305b
    nurse turnover, loss from, 364
Hospital-acquired conditions (HACs), 385
Hospital-based coaches, development of, 43
Hospital Compare website, hospital measures, 305b
Hospital Consumer Assessment of Healthcare Providers
        and Systems (HCAHPS), 216
Hospital-specific all-hazards gap analysis, creation of, 414–415
Hospital Value-Based Purchasing Program, 216
    CMS development, 305–306
Hospitalists, 292
Hostile work environment, 110
Hours per patient day (HPPD), 397
Human interaction issues, 103
Human relations school, 190
Human resources
    case management and, 263
    inputs from, emphasis on, 195–196
    management, policies, 333
    staffing strategy, 370
Hyperglycemia, stress-induced, 74

I

"I Pass the Baton," strategy for, effective communication, 107
Identification, participant, as disease management program
        component, 258–260
Implementation science, 269
Implementation strategies
    development of, 220
    for evidence-based practice, 274–275, 275f
Incident management assistance teams (IMATs), creation of, 423
Incident reports, 96, 312–313
Incivility, 340
Inclusive excellence, 179–180
Income, definition of, 389
Indemnity agreement, 88f
Indicators
    definition of, 318
    sets, development, 318
Indirect delegation, 148
Indirect intervention, 69
Individualism, 183
Infection prevention and control practitioner, in emergency
        management committee, 413–414t
Infectious disease medical director, in emergency management
        committee, 413–414t
Inflexible attitude, 183
Influence, 155–156
    assertiveness, 155
    authority, contrast, 155t
    blocking, 155
    coalitions, 155
    exchange, 155
    ingratiation, 155
    rationality, 155
    sanctions, 155
    tactics, 156t
    upward appeal, 155

Influence Behavior Questionnaire (IBQ), development of,
        156
Informal clinical leadership, 55
Informal leaders, 6
Informal nurse leaders, on work-related stress, 78
Informal policies, 228–229
Informal power, 201
Informal work group norms, influence of, 122
Informatics nursing specialists (INSs), 433
Information
    definition of, 433
    dissemination of, 130
    medical, access to, 94
    sharing of, 130
Information officer, in emergency management committee,
        413–414t
Information operations, 433
Information power, 158
Information systems, for evidence-based practice, 278
Information technology, productivity and, 398–399
Informed consent, 89
Ingratiation, influence tactics, 155
Initiator, 132
Innovation
    complexity and, 42
    decentralization, 207
    diffusion of, 42
    disruptive, 43
    existence/functions, knowledge of, 41
    group/social system adoption in, 42
    in health care, 42–43
    process of, 41
    required, amount of, 142
    review of, 43
    system-related views of, 43
    theory, 41–43
Innovation centers, 136
Innovation-decision
    process actions/behaviors/choices of, 41
    stages of, 41
Innovators, adopter frequency distribution, 42
Inpatient prospective payment system, 385
Institute for Healthcare Improvement, 281
Institute of Medicine (IOM), 153
    Crossing the Quality Chasm, 234–235, 254, 345
    Crossing the Quality Chasm: A New Health System for the
        21st Century, 296
    To Err Is Human: Building a Safer Health Care
        System, 296
    The Future of Nursing, 41, 153, 281
    The Future of Nursing: Leading Change, Advancing Health,
        1, 355–356, 434, 442
    health care quality, improvement aims, 289b
    Leadership by Example: Coordinating Government Roles in
        Improving Health Care Quality, 296–297
    six aims for improvement of, 1
Insurance models, 248
Integrating, problem-solving style, 170
Integration, by program, 195
Integrity, sense of, 9
Intelligence, emotional, leadership and, 5–6
Intensivists, 292
Intention, in work-related stress prevention, 77
Intentional torts, 88f, 89

Inter-professional education, shared governance (impact), 212
Inter-professional team, in case management, 247
Interaction and management, as disease management program component, 260–261
Interactive planning, as nursing leadership behavior, 20–21
Interdependence
 conflict factor, 162
 definition of, 154
Interdisciplinary Neighborhood Team project, team development and, 43
Interdisciplinary team model, for case management, 245
Interface terminologies, 440
Intergroup conflict, 164
Intergroup dissonance, in group process, 112
Internal drills, 420
Internal predisposing factors, in communication, 104f
Internal reporting, 313
International Council of Nurses (ICN)
 aging population, 345
 international recruitment, 350
International Health Terminology Standards Development Organisation (IHTSDO), 438
International Organization for Standardization (ISO), standardized clinical terminology, 440
International recruitment, 350, 350f
Internet Generation, 182
Internship programs, 360
Interoperability, of data, 443
Interoperable health information technology (HIT), 430
 aggregation and analysis of, 433
Interpersonal communication, 102, 104–107, 112f
Interpersonal conflict, 164
Interpersonal relationship skills
 importance of, 5
 as leadership skills, 103
Interpreters, workplace diversity, 185–186
Interprofessional care, prominence, 49
Interprofessional Education (IPE) and Core Competencies: A Literature Review, 247
Interprofessional shared governance, 210
Interrupters, 133–134
Interviewing, nursing shortage, 359
Intragroup conflict, 164
Intragroup Conflict Scale, 167
Intrapersonal communication, 104–107, 112f
Intrapersonal conflict, 163–164
"Invincible" nurse, 146, 146f
Ishikawa, Kaoru, 288

J
Joanna Briggs Institute, 281
Job conflict, 162
Job position, for committee structures, 129
Job satisfaction, communication and, 108–109
Job stress, 75. See also Work-related stress
Johnson & Johnson, Campaign for Nursing's Future, 351
Joint decision making, 124–125, 124f
Joint Statement on Delegation, 141
Journaling, for work-related stress, 79
Judicial risk, 89
Juran, Joseph M., 288, 290
Just culture, 54
Justice, 87

K
Keeping Patients Safe: Transforming the Work Environment of Nurses, 434
Knowledge
 definition of, 433
 of follower, 12
Knowledge operations, 433
Knowledge resources, 430
Knowledge translation, definition of, 269
Kotter's change process, 113–114, 114b
Kotter's model of change, 36

L
Labor, division and coordination of, 191–194
Laggards, adopter frequency distribution, 42
Laissez-faire leadership style, 10–11
Landmark legislation, in case management, 242
Language
 in communication, 105
 usage of, 36–37
Late majority, adopter frequency distribution, 42
Lateral violence, 329
Law, sources of, 87–92
Lay witness, 86
LEAD instruments, 18
Leaders, 280
 authentic, 16
 change agent and, 40
 change process, impact of, 39
 communication and, 102
 duties of, 131–132
 focus of, 34
 in leadership process, 7
 meeting checklist for, 131b
 nurse, best practice suggestions for, 46–48
 skill sets for, 5–6
 transactional, 13
 transformational, 13
Leadership, 1–31, 30b
 ability, 103
 adapting and, 5
 aspects of, 6–8
  communication, 7–8
  follower, 7
  goals, 8
  leader, 7
  situation, 7
 authentic, 16
 background related to, 6
 behavior in, study of, 190
 care management differentiated from, 2–3
 case study for, 30b
 change relationship in, 40
  role in, 40
 characteristics of, 8–9
 climate and culture and, 54–55
 clinical, 16–17
 communicating, 5
 communication, 102–117, 116–117b
 complexity, 15
 contemporary, 14–17
 continuum of, 10f
 critical thinking applied to, 8
 decision making and, 66, 69–70

Leadership *(Continued)*
  definitions in, 2
  diagnosing and, 5
  effective, 17
  evidence-based practice, 279–280
    management implications and, 280
  feminist perspective of, 11
  focus on, 6
  as function, 5
  implications of, 28
  importance of, 3
  issues and trends in, 28–30
  management implications and, 44–45
  management roles and, 18
  moment of, components of, 7f
  as multidimensional process, 8
  overview of, 3–6
  power and, 160–161, 160f
  quantum, 15
  relationship behavior and, 9
  role of, 5
  servant, 15–16
  skills for, 5–6
    emotional intelligence as, 5–6
    relationship management and relational coordination as, 6
  strategies, 35
  styles, 6
    authoritarian, 10
    defined, 9
    democratic, 10
    Laissez-Faire, 10–11
    theories for, 9–11
  task behavior and, 9
  teams, 126
  theories in, 8–14
    situational, 11–13
  trait theories on, 8–9
  transactional, 13–14, 13f
  transformational, 13–14, 13f
  trust and, 9
  vision and, 9
Leadership by Example: Coordinating Government Roles in Improving Health Care Quality, 296–297
Lean enterprise, 294–295
  definition of, 287
Learning
  environment for, creation of, 4
  organizations, 27
  practices for, 45
Legal compliance, 94
Legal issues, 85–101, 100b
  case study on, 100–101b
  and changing family dynamic, 99
  definitions, 86
  education and licensure, 87
  leadership and management implications, 96–99
Legal liability, 87, 88f
Legal system, 87–92
Legislative and regulatory disruptors, in case management, 264
Legitimate power, 156–157, 157b
Length of stay, 395–396
Leniency, bias, 404

Liability
  decreasing risk of, in workplace diversity, 180–181
  of health care organizations, 97–98
Liable, definition of, 86
Licensure portability, in case management, 264
Line position, 194–195
Linguistic competency training, 179
Listener, 132
Litigation, cost of, 161–162
Living wills, 93
Long-term care, culture change in, 56

M
Magnet-designated organizations, 52
Magnet designation, 295
  with work environments, 385
Magnet hospitals, 52
Magnet model, exemplary professional practice of, 227
Magnet Recognition Program, 1, 4, 52, 80, 208
  addresses organizational attributes, 227
  application for, 304
  evidence-based, 357
  health care organization, ANCC recognition, 295
  on performance appraisal, 408
  transformational leadership and, 14
Magnet research, 52
Magnetism
  concept of, 227
  forces of, 52
Malcolm Baldrige National Quality Award Program, 295
Malperformance, 229
Malpractice, 86, 88f, 90, 229
Managed care
  care coordination and, 233
  models, 250
  systems, in disease management, 254
Management, 1–31, 30b
  case study for, 30b
  of change process, 4
  contemporary theories for, 23–28
    chaos theory as, 26–28
    complexity theory as, 25–26
    contingency theory as, 24
    systems theory as, 24–25, 25t
  decision making and, 69–70
  definitions for, 18–19
  formal relationship determined by, 187–188
  implications, 28
    leadership, relationship, 44–45
  importance of, 3
  increase in layers of, 198–199
  issues and trends in, 28–30
  mind-sets in, 19
  in organizations, 22–28
  overview of, 18
  practice of, IOM focus on, 4
  process of, 19–22
    controlling, 22
    directing, 21–22
    organizing, 21
    planning, 20–21
  span of, 199–201
Management information systems (MIS), 430–431

Management time, cost of, 161
Managerial decision making, 60–73, 71b
  background of, 61–63
  case study on, 72b, 72f
  definitions of, 60–61
  issues and trends in, 70–72
  leadership and management implications, 69–70
  patient acuity and staffing in, 66
Managerial influence strategies, usage, 156t
Managerial leadership, 363
Managerial work, nature of, 22–23, 23f, 24f
Managers
  as coach, 406
  communication and, 102
  in data management and clinical informatics, 442
  decision-making data, outcomes research (usage), 321
  leadership and, 363
  relations with, 352
  roles of, 357–361
  span of control of, 198–199
Mandatory reporting, 98
Market
  definition of, 449
  research, 449
    approach, 450
Marketing, 447–459, 456–457b, 458f
  activities, 447–448
  background of, 450
  case study on, 457
  core concepts, 448–450, 448b
  definitions, 448–450
  issues and trends, 455–456
  leadership and management implications, 453–455, 454b
  lifestyle management, 456–457b
  mix elements, 451–453, 452t, 453t
  orientation, 449
  process, 451–453, 452t, 453t
  strategy, 450–451
    setting, 451
Marketing director, in emergency management committee, 413–414t
Marketplace, workplace diversity, competitive edge in, 180
Mass casualty incident, 411
Mass marketing, 450–451
Material fact, 86
Materials management director, in emergency management committee, 413–414t
Mature Generation, 181
Mayo Clinic value statements, 298t
Maze, decision-making, 64f
McKinsey Global Institute, Big Data in, 436
Meaningful use, 434
  three stages of, 434
Measurement, performance appraisal for, 402
Mediation, 169
Medical errors
  awareness and disclosure of, 204
  Institute of Medicine (IOM) and, 107
Medical home, patient-centered, 55–56
Medical information, access to, 94
Medical models, 243
Medical- social models, 243
Medicare Severity Diagnosis Related Groups (MS-DRGs), 374

Medication administration, in clinical decision making, 65
Medication nurse, 232
Medication reconciliation (improvement), multidisciplinary team-generated interventions (usage) to, 43
Meeting
  checklist for, 131b
  effectiveness of, 129–132
  leader duties during, 133–134
  preparation for, 130
  timed agenda in, 130
Memorandum of understanding (MOU), 422–423
Mental model, learning organization of, 45
Messages, reframing of, 39
Millennials, 56, 182
Minimum Data Set (MDS) program, 305
Missed care, 340
Mission
  development of, 277
  importance of, 206
  statements, 217–218, 227
    communication effectiveness, 297
Mistrust, in nonenrollment, 260
Modeling, in decision making, 69
Models of care delivery, 226
Modern perspective, 187–188
Moral distress, 76
Motivation, 12
  assessment, 36
  directing and, 21
  political, performance appraisal and, 405
Motivational interviewing (MI), 108
Moving, change stage as, 35
Multidisciplinary committee, 129
Multidisciplinary quality improvement teams, 136–138
Multidisciplinary team-generated interventions, impact, 43
Multifactor Leadership Questionnaire (MLQ), 18
Multigenerational workforce, retention factors related to, 363t
Mutual adjustment, coordination of work and, 193

N
National Association of Chronic Disease Directors, 258
National Association of Social Workers (NASW), for case management models, 244
National Center for Cultural Competence, 180–181
National Center for Patient Safety (NCPS), 307
National Citizens' Coalition for Nursing Home Reform (NCCNHR), 56
National Committee for Quality Assurance (NCQA)
  HEDIS outcomes, 304
  performance standards, 303
National Council Licensure Examination (NCLEX), 87
National Council of State Boards of Nursing (NCSBN), 85
  delegation and, tools for, 142
  Joint Statement on Delegation, 141
  Working With Others: A Position Paper, 142
National Database of Nursing Quality Indicators (NDNQI), 301–302
  development, 321–322
National Federation of Independent Business v. Sebelius case, 82
National Guideline Clearinghouse, 281
National Guidelines for Nursing Delegation, 142
National Health Expenditures (NHEs), 388
National Healthcare Quality and Disparities Report, 177

National Incident Management System (NIMS), creation of, 417
National Institute for Occupational Safety and Health (NIOSH)
    homicide report, 328–329
    recommendations from, 331
National Institute of Standards and Testing (NIST), 429
National Patient Safety Goals, 311
    TJC's Board of Commissioners approval, 311
National Quality Forum (NQF), 291–292
    health care quality and safety, 307–308
    nurse-sensitive performance measures, 301–302
    performance measurement evaluation criteria, 293b
National Sample Survey of Registered Nurses, 56
National Standards for Culturally and Linguistically Appropriate Services (CLAS), 178–180
National Terrorism Advisory System (NTAS), 422
Near miss, 312
Needs, definition of, 448
Negligence, 86, 88f, 89–90
Negotiations, 102, 169, 185
Network theory, 190–191
New England Medical Center (NEMC) model, 244
Nexters, 182
Niche marketing, 450–451
Nightingale, Florence, 140, 439
Non-clinical workers, in case management, 264
Non-verbal communication, 102
Nonabandonment, 96–97
Nonmaleficence, 87
"Nonproductive" time, 378
Nontalkers, 133
Nonviolent communication, 111, 111t
    in teaching communication, 114–115
Norming period, in group development, 111–112
Nuclear disaster, 411
Nurse Executive Competencies: Population Health, 257
Nurse leaders
    on outcomes, 320
    outcomes research and, 321
    participation in development of Big Data, 324
    responsibility of, 399
Nurse leadership
    differentiation of management from, 3
    interactive planning and, 20–21
Nurse Licensure Compact (NLC), 92
    in case management, 264
Nurse managers, 54
    in evidence-based practice, 279
    health care quality toolbox, 298–299, 299–300t
    responsibility of, 96–97
    standards, 304
    stress and, special considerations for, 81
Nurse manager's quality toolbox
    cause-and-effect diagram for, 301f
    control chart for, 300f
    data collection sheet for, 300f
    flowchart for, 301f
    Pareto chart for, 302f
    scatter diagram for, 302f
Nurse practice, environment, 51
Nurse practitioner (NP) time, cost of, 396
Nurse-sensitive performance measures, 301–302
Nurse-to-patient ratio, 76, 370
Nurse Work Index (NWI), 230

Nurses
    access to, 382
    barriers to gender diversity in, 351b
    burnout, provider-focused outcome, 320
    centrality, 161
    in data management and clinical informatics, 442–443
    delegators, types of, 146f
    empowerment, 154
    international recruitment of, 350
    as leaders, 4–5
    leadership positions, responsibility, 268, 276
    legal documents and, 93–95
    new, residency programs for, 78
    participation in development of Big Data, 324
    patient and, relationship of, 374
    performance measures, 301–302
    recruitment of, 357
    retention strategies for, 362b
    retirement, 398
    roles of, 4–5, 4f
    shortages of, 203
    spirituality in practice, 109–110
    staffing, 370
        American Nurses Association's principle, 373
        management plan, 370
    supplemental staffing resource guidelines of, 382
        operational metrics, 382
    vacancy, 352
    as witness, 91–92
    workforce participation, 398–399
    workplace
        diversity, 175
        violence, 328
Nursing
    case, 231
    change, areas in, 44f
    conflict management in, studies of, 168–169
    core mission of, 4
    data needs, 431–433
        domains, outcomes and variables in, 432t
    delegation in, 140–152, 151b, 152t
        barriers to, 145–147, 146f
        case study on, 151–152b
        ethical and legal issues concerning, 147–149
        issues and trends in, 149–152
        leadership and management implications, 149
        prioritization in, 144–145
        process of, 142–144, 143f, 144f
    direct-care hours, 370–371
    education, 346–347
    entry-level baccalaureate programs in, enrollments in, 345
    functional, 232
    group, 231–232
    innovativeness in, 47f
    knowledge-based work of, 398
    national policy initiatives, 385
    primary, 232–233
    private duty, 231–232
    process, 252t
        change/problem solving, similarities of, 35t
        components of, 217
    require policy formulation, 229
    staff adequacy, 379
    supply model, overview of, 343f

Nursing *(Continued)*
   surplus cycles and, 344f
   tasks, factors in, 142–143
   team, 232
   unit, 51
   work groups, 51
   workload, 370
     forecasted, 377–379
Nursing activities, definition of, 141
Nursing Alliance for Quality Care (NAQC), 314
Nursing assistant, cost of, 396
Nursing assistive personnel, 142
Nursing care
   costs of, 395–396
   organizational culture and, 51
Nursing care delivery models, 225–226, 374–375
   traditional, 231
Nursing documentation systems, 429
Nursing Home Quality Initiative (NHQI), 305
Nursing Home Reform Act legislation, 56
Nursing hours per patient day (NHPPD), 377
Nursing informatics, 431, 433–436
Nursing informatics specialists, 433–434, 439
Nursing intensity, 66
Nursing leader, role of, 54
Nursing licensure, delegation and, 148
Nursing management, definition of, 19
Nursing Management Minimum Data Set (NMMDS), 440–442
   elements, 440–442
   variables, 441f
Nursing Minimum Data Set (NMDS), 440–442
Nursing outcome databases, 439
Nursing outcomes research, 319
Nursing services
   costing out, 395–397
   delivery of, 3
Nursing shortage, 56, 340–368, 366–367b
   advertising in, 358
   background of, 341–344
   case study on, 367b
   compensation and, 353
   counseling and coaching in, 360
   cycles, 344f
     factors, 341
   definition of, 340
   demand and, 353–354
   demographic factors in, 347–351
   demographic nature, changing, 354
   events and predictions, time line of, 345–346b
   factors contributing to, 344–354
   graduates, national baseline projections of, 343f
   "graying" factor, 347
   health delivery system and, 354
   image of nursing, 351–352
   international recruitment and, 350
   interviewing in, 359
   issues and trends in, 365–367
   leadership and management implications, 364–367
   marketing and, 456
   nursing education and, 346–347
   orienting, 360
   performance evaluation in, 361
   position posting in, 357–358
   recruitment and, 356

Nursing shortage *(Continued)*
   retention and, 361–364
   screening and, 358–359
   selection, 359–360
   staff development in, 361
   staffing and, 353
   supply and, 346–353
   work environment factors in, 352–353
   workforce strategy map, 342f
   workload and, 353
Nursing-specific outcomes, metrics, 385
Nursing work redesign, 434
Nursing's Agenda for the Future, 345, 354
Nursing's Social Policy Statement: The Essence of the Profession, ANA, 85

O

Objective entity, organization approached as, 187–188
Objective perspective, 187–188
Objectives
   definition of, 217
   setting, 219–220
Objectivism, 187
   and subjectivism, polarization between, 188–189
Obliging, problem-solving style, 170
"Observability, " as planned change factor, 42
Occupational Safety and Health Administration
   general duty to protect workers under, 330–331
   violence prevention programs, 331
Occupational Safety and Health Review Commission (OSHRC)
   judge, 335
Offering, definition of, 448–449
Office of Infrastructure Protection (OIP), 336–337
Office of the National Coordinator for Health Information Technology, 438
Omnibus Budget Reconciliation Act of 1987 (OBRA), 229
Open system theory, 190
   contingency theory and, 190
Operating budget
   definition of, 389
   development of, 391–393
     projected volume of, 391–392, 392t
     salary calculation in, 393, 393t
     staffing calculation in, 392
     supply and revenue budgets in, 393
Opinion giver, 132
Opinion leaders, definition of, 270
Opinion seeking, meeting for, 130
Opportunity, structure of, 201
Order sets, 229–230
Organizational assessment, in case management program development, 252, 253b
Organizational budget, types of, 389
Organizational change, 34
   study of, 37
Organizational charts, 198, 206
Organizational climate, 49–59, 57b
   background of, 51
   case study on, 58b
   communication and, 108–109
   definition of, 49–50
   issues and trends in, 55–58
     culture change, 56
     generational diversity, 56

Organizational climate *(Continued)*
    nursing shortage, 56
    patient-centered care, 55–56
    patient-centered medical home, 55–56
    Quality and Safety Education for Nurses, 56–58
    leadership and management implications, 54–55
    research of, 51–54
        healthy work environments, 53–54
        just culture, 54
        Magnet Recognition Program®, 52
        professional practice environment, 52–53
        safety culture and climate, 53
Organizational configurations, continuum of, 195f
Organizational conflict, 162, 171–172
Organizational Conflict Inventory-II, 171
Organizational context, 269
Organizational culture, 49–59, 57b
    background of, 51
    case study on, 58b
    communication and, 108–109
    definition of, 49–50
    issues and trends in, 55–58
        culture change, 56
        generational diversity, 56
        nursing shortage, 56
        patient-centered care, 55–56
        patient-centered medical home, 55–56
        Quality and Safety Education for Nurses, 56–58
    leadership and management implications, 54–55
    research of, 51–54
        healthy work environments, 53–54
        just culture, 54
        Magnet Recognition Program®, 52
        professional practice environment, 52–53
        safety culture and climate, 53
Organizational decision making, 61, 65–66
Organizational design
    dimensions of, 192t
    division and coordination of labor in, 191–194
    key concepts of, 191–198
Organizational ethics, 95–96
Organizational forms, 195–198
    functional, 195–196, 196f
    matrix, 197–198
        simplified, 198f
    parallel, 197
    program, 196–197, 196f
        modified, 197
Organizational framework, 52
Organizational goals (achievement), power (usage), 158
Organizational governance, 182
Organizational infrastructure
    building, strategies, 279
    for evidence-based practice, 276–279
Organizational issues, delegation and, 147
Organizational mission, 217
Organizational performance, enhancement of, 189
Organizational position, 129
Organizational recommendations, for work-related stress, 79–81, 80b
Organizational shapes, 198–201
Organizational social structure, definition of, 187
Organizational structure, 187–205, 204b
    case study for, 205b
    definitions in, 187

Organizational structure *(Continued)*
    flat, 198–199, 200f, 200t
    issues and trends in, 203–205
    leadership and management implications, 201–203
    objective perspective and, 187–188
    postmodern perspective and, 188–189
    power of, 201
    subjective perspective and, 188
    tall, 198–199, 199f, 200t
Organizational subunit, shared consensus within, 159
Organizational transformation, transformational change (impact), 44
Organizational values, 55
Organizational vision, 217
Organization-directed prevention, of stress, 78
Organization-focused outcomes, 320
Organizations
    bureaucratic theory, 189
    classical management theory and, 189–190
    core purpose in, 218
    core values in, 218
    as entities, 187
    formal aspects of, subjective perspective focus on, 188
    formal structure of, hierarchy and, 198
    human relations school and, 190
    informal structure of, 198
    mission, 217, 297
    open system theory and, 190
    scientific management school and, 189
    social structure, formal aspects of, 190
    as social systems, key theories of, 189–191
    strategic plan
        implementation of, 222
        job responsibilities, relevance of, 158
    structure of, changes to, 202
    vision, 217, 297
    workforce of, social composition of, 201
Organization theory, 187–189
Organizing, 21
    defined, 20
Orientations, 121
    holistic, 449
    marketing, 449
    product, 449
    selling, 449
ORYX®, 304–305
Outcome and Assessment Information Set (OASIS), 305
Outcomes
    analyses of, 321
    Big Data and, 323–324, 324t
    case study, 326b
    definition of, 317
    influences on, 320
    issues and trends in, 322–326
    leadership and management implications, 321–322
    management of, 317–327, 326b
        definition of, 318
    measurement of, 317–327, 326b
    nurse leader role on, 320
    organization-focused, 320
    patient experiences and, 324–326, 325t
    patient-focused definition of, 317
    process and measures, 292

Outcomes *(Continued)*
  provider-focused, 320
  research, 319
    elements of, 320–321
    nursing, 319
  risk adjustment, 321
  standards and measures, 288, 292–293
  variable selection, 320–321
Outcomes-driven acuity system, 381
Outpatient Case Management for Adults With Medical Illness and Complex Care Needs, 264–265

P
"Pal, " leadership style, 146, 146f
Pandemics, preparedness for, 203
Pareto chart, example, 302f
Participative leadership, 208
Patient
  acuity, 66, 374
  assignments, 383
  diversity in, communication and, 114
  engagement, 287
    accountability imperative, 311–312
  interaction, level of, 143
Patient activation, definition of, 287
Patient care, synergy model for, 375
Patient care delivery models, 226
  current and evolving types of, 234
Patient-centered care (PCC), 55–56, 234, 234b
  growing demand for, 280
  marketing and, 455–456
Patient-centered medical home (PCMH), 55–56, 150, 235
Patient classification system (PCS), 396, 431
Patient experiences, outcomes and, 324–326, 325t
Patient Protection and Affordable Care Act (HR 3590), 150
Patient-reported experience measures (PREMs), 325
Patient-Reported Outcomes Measurement Information System (PROMIS), 324
Patient safety
  culture and climate, 53
  improvement, multidisciplinary team generated interventions (usage) and, 43
  practices, 287
Patient Safety Indicators (PSIs), 318
Patient-to-RN ratios, 357
Pay-for-performance, reimbursement systems, 323
Peer review, definition of, 401
Peer review organizations (PROs), 305
People
  level, 23
  time, blocking, 75b
Perceived Conflict Scale, 167
Perceptions, differences (conflict factor), 162
Performance
  definition of, 401
  evaluation, 361
  expectations, in evidence-based practice, 277
  gap assessment, 272
  pay-for, reimbursement systems, 323
Performance and quality improvement (PQI) tools, 298–299
Performance appraisal, 277, 401–409, 408–409b
  case study on, 409b
  employee development through, 405–407

Performance appraisal *(Continued)*
  issues and trends in, 407–409
  issues in, 402–407
  leadership and management implications, 407
  measurements for, 402–404
    behaviors as, 403
    competencies as, 403
    results as, 403–404
    traits as, 402–403
  performance metrics for, 404
  purposes of, 401–402
  rating accuracy for, 404–405
Performance improvement (PI)
  culture, organizational adoption, 297
  program, 287
    development, 293
  standards (TJC), 303–304
Performance improvement plan (PIP), 401, 406–407
Performance measure, definition of, 287
Performance measurement
  evaluation criteria, 293
  selection criteria, 293b
  system, 287
Performance Readiness® Level, 12
Performance review, employee development through, 405–407
Performance review system, elements of, 407
Performing period, in group development, 111–112
Person-as-customer, transformation, 45
Personal health, stress and, 74
Personal liability, 88f, 89
Personal management, journaling and, 79
Personal mastery, learning organization of, 45
Personal negligence, in clinical practice, 97
Personal power base, building, 172–173
Personnel budget, 389, 393t
Personnel services, 392
Persuasion, 102
Persuasive power, 158
Pew Health Professions Commission (PHPC), relationship-centered care, 290
Pharmacy director, in emergency management committee, 413–414t
Philosophy, 228
Physician leader, 274–275
Physician's Quality Reporting Initiative (PQRI), 305
Pilot projects, in decision making, 67–68
Pioneer Network, 56
Place, as marketing mix element, 452t
Plan, Do, Check, Act (PDCA), 291
Plan, Do, Study, Act (PDSA) cycle, 291f
  definition of, 287
Planetree, 455–456
Planned change, 33
  description of, 35
  determination of, 45
  term, creation, 37–38
Planning, 20–21
  defined, 20
  interactive, 20–21
  phases of, 20
  strategic, 20
  tactical, 20
Point-of-care nurses, 279–280

Policies, 228–229, 229b. *See also* Standard operating policies and procedures
formal, 228
informal, 228–229
procedures and, 228–229
Political action, 173–174
Political motivations, performance appraisal and, 405
Politics, power and, 40–41
Population
definition of, 255
demographic nature of, changing, 354
risk assessment, 258
Population-as-customer, transformation, 45
Population Care Coordination Process, 257–258
Population health, 255
Population Health Alliance Outcomes Guidelines,
Vol. 6, 257
Population Health Alliance (PHA), 261–262
Population health management (PHM)
chronic health condition in, 255–256
definition of, 240
disease management transitions to, 254–255
health information technology in, 434–435, 435t
practice approaches, 256–257
practice standards and guidelines, 257–258
shift to, 4–5
Position control, 379
Positioning
definition of, 449–450
product, 451
Positive communication outcomes, 102–103
Positive feedback, leadership strategy of, 35
Postmodern perspective, 188–189
Postmodernism, 187
Power, 153–161, 173b
from being irreplaceable, 159
case study on, 173–174b
centrality and, 161
coercive, 156–157, 157b
conceptualized as resource, 187–188
connection, 157–158
from decision process, 159
definition of, 153–155
from dependence, 159
dependency aspect of, 154
empowerment and, 154–155
expert, 156–157, 157b
French and Raven typology, problem with, 156
group decision-making, 158
individual sources of, 156–157
information, 158
leadership and, 160–161, 160f
implications, 160–161
legitimate, 156–157, 157b
management implications, 160–161
persuasive, 158
politics and, 40–41
from providing resource, 159
referent, 156–157, 157b
relational aspect of, 154
reward, 156–157, 157b
sanctioning aspect of, 154
from shared consensus, 159
sources (French and Raven), 157b

Power (Continued)
sources of, 156–158
other, 157–158
structural, 201
structural determinants of, 158–159
substitutability and, 161
of subunit, 158–159
theories, 159–160
with uncertainty, from coping, 159
Power distance, 183
Power of attorney, 93
Practice-based evidence (PBE), 433
Practice specialty, case management and, 242
Predictions, risk and, 82–84
Predictive modeling, 258
Present on admission (POA), 306, 385
Presenteeism, cost of, 161
Price, as marketing mix element, 452t
Primary key, 442
Primary nursing, 232–233
Primary therapist model, for case management, 245
Primary work teams, 126
Principled negotiation, 169
Prioritization, 65, 144–145
Privacy, 87
of patient, 115
Privacy Rule, HIPAA, 95
Private duty nursing, 231–232
advantages of, 231
Problem solving
change/nursing process, similarities of, 35t
purpose of, 130
required, amount of, 142
strategy, Six Sigma, 294t
styles of, 170
Procedural annexes, creation of, 417–418
Procedures, 229, 229b
policies and, 228–229
Process
conflict, 164
of group interactions, 120
improvement, 303–304
Product
differentiation, 451
as marketing mix element, 452t
orientation, 449
positioning, 451
Productivity, 388–398
background of, 388–389
case study about, 400b
issues and trends in, 398–400
leadership and management implications, 394–397
measures of, 397–398, 397t
Profession, 86
Professional judgment, 86
Professional liability, 90–91
Professional negligence, 86, 90
Professional practice environment, 52–53
Professional practice models (PPMs), 225–239, 237–238b, 237t
background of, 227
case study on, 238–239b
definition of, 226
evolving, 234
examples, 225

Professional practice models *(Continued)*
  framework, 225
  innovative and future, 234–236
  issues and trends in, 236–239
  leadership and management implications, 236
  mission statements and, 227
Professional safeguards, 90–91
Professionalism, 4
Proficiency, in communication, 103
Profitable, 450–451
Prognosis, 83
Program, design of, service delivery optimized by, 197
Program delivery, as disease management program component, 260–261
Program Measurement & Evaluation Guide: Core Metrics for Employee Health Management, 261–262
Programming devices, development of, 202
Project director, in evidence-based practice, 280
Project facilitator, role of, 412
Project team, 129
  leaders, advanced practice nurses, 279
Projected volume, of operating budget development, 391–392, 392t
Promotion, communication and, 452t
Proportion, structure of, 201
Protocols, 229–230
Provider
  continuity of, 45
  in nursing's data needs, 431
Provider-focused outcomes, 320
Psychological empowerment, 154
Pure matrix form, 197–198
Pure nursing models, 230–231

Q
Quality, 286–316, 314b
  accreditation, influences on, 303–304
  case study, 315b
  definition of, 287
  Deming's 14 points for, 292b
  educating nurses, 313–314
  fitness for use, definition, 291
  indicator (AHRQ development), 318
  indicators, development (ANA), 321–322
  industrial models of, 290–291
  issues and trends, 303–315
  leadership and management implications, 297–303
  outcomes, data collection and public reporting, 304–306
  outcome standards and measures, 288, 292–293
  policy and advancement, 314–315
  process standards and measures, 288, 292
  regulatory, influences on, 303–304
  on staffing evidence, 383–384
  standards of, 291–293
  structure standards and measures, 288, 292
Quality and Safety Education for Nurses (QSEN), 56–58, 313–314
Quality care, in disease management, 254
Quality improvement, 306–308
  culture, organizational adoption, 297
  in evidence-based practice, 278
  program, 287
    development, 293
Quality improvement organizations (QIOs), 305
Quality indicators, definition of, 287
Quality Initiative program, 305

Quality management, performance, emerging models of, 293–296
Quality of life, leaders and, 2
Quantum leadership, 15

R
Racial disparities, principles for eliminating, 177
Radiological/nuclear disaster, 411
Rahim Organizational Conflict Inventory-I, design, 167
Rapid cycle change, methodology of, 38
Rating accuracy, for performance appraisal, 404–405
Rationality, influence tactics, 155
"Rationalizer" leadership style, 146, 146f
Readiness, ability/willingness, 160
Recency, bias, 404
Recruitment, 356, 340
  advertising in, 358
  counseling and coaching in, 360
  human resources in, 357–361
  international, 350, 350f
  interviewing in, 359
  managerial roles in, 357–361
  orienting in, 360
  performance evaluation in, 361
  position posting in, 357–358
  screening in, 358–359
  selecting in, 359–360
  staff development in, 361
  staff roles in, 357–361
  strategies, 358b
  student-related and faculty-related strategies for, 355t
Referent power, 156–157, 157b
Refreezing, change stage as, 35
Regional Hospital Command Center (RHCC), establishment of, 422–423
Registered nurse
  distribution of
    by race/ethnicity, 349f
    by sex and age, 348f
  hiring cost of, 364f
  retention, 361–364
    strategies, 362b
  workforce, 341–344
    aging of, 347–348
    composition of, changing, 348–351
Registered Nurses' Association of Ontario, 281
Regulatory compliance, 94–95
Reiki, spiritual health care and, 109
Reimbursement, impact of, 45
Reinfusion, definition of, 269
Relational coordination, leadership and, 6
Relationship-based care (RBC), 375
Relationship building, performance appraisal for, 402
Relationship-centered care (PHPC), 290
Relationship conflict, 164
Relationship management
  centrality of, emphasis on, 6
  in leader skill set, 6
  leadership and, 6
Relationship-oriented leader, impact of, 11–12
Relationships, 8
Relative advantage, as planned change factor, 42
Relaxation, for work-related stress, 79
Reliability, efficiency and, balancing tensions between, 4

Reporting
   as disease management program component, 261–262
   for evidence-based practice, 278
Research, in nursing's data needs, 432
Research utilization, 268
Residency programs, 360
Resignation/voluntary turnover, 341
Resilience, 77
Resistance, 33, 38–39
   concept, understanding of, 38
   human factor of, 38–39
   perspective of, 38
   reframed, 38–39
Resource pool, 381–382
Resources
   distributed, 55
   for evidence-based practice, 278, 281
Responsibility, assignment of, 195
Restructuring, 202
Results, in performance appraisal, 403–404
Retention, 340, 361–364
   factors, 363t
   managerial leadership and, 363
   strategies, 362b
   student-related and faculty-related strategies for, 355t
Revenue
   definition of, 389
   management of, 45
Revenue budget, 393
Review system, performance, elements of, 407
Reward power, 157b
   usage, 156–157
Rewards, in evidence-based practice, 278–279
Risk, predictions and, 82–84
Risk adjustment, 321
   definition of, 287
Risk management, 312
   effort, integration of, 332
Risk manager, 312
Robert Wood Johnson Foundation, 153
   nurse-sensitive performance measures, 301–302
Rogers' innovation theory, 41–42
Role of the Nurse Leader in Crisis Management, AONE, 411–412
"Room and board" hospital charges, 385
Root Cause Analysis (RCA), 308
   formal RCA, submission of, 313
   purpose of, 309
Root Cause Analysis and Action, 310f

S

Safety, 286–316, 314b
   case study, 315b
   educating nurses, 313–314
   health care safety and health care enterprise risk management, 303–315
   issues and trends in, 303–315
   leadership and management implications, 297–303
   National Patient Safety Goals, 311
      TJC's Board of Commissioners approval, 311
   personnel management, 307
   policy, advancement, 314–315
Safety and security director, in emergency management committee, 413–414t

Safety climate, 53
Safety culture, 53
Salaries of Instructional and Administrative Nursing Faculty in Baccalaureate and Graduate Programs in Nursing, 346
Salary calculation, in operating budget development, 393, 393t
Salary expense flow sheet, budgeted, 393t
Sanctions, influence tactics, 155
Satisfaction, definition of, 448–449
SBAR (Situation, Background, Assessment, and Recommendation), in communication, 113, 113f
Scalar principle, 198–199
Scaling up, definition of, 269
Scatter diagram, example, 302f
Scheduling, 369–380, 386b
   case study, 386–387b
   issues and trends, 384–387
   leadership and management implications, 376–377
   procedures, assessment of, 379
Scientific management, concept of, 232
Scientific management school, 189
Scope of practice, 147
   definition of, 141–142
Screening, nursing shortage, 358–359
Second change, 35
Security measures checklist, 336b
Segmentation, 451
   definition of, 449–450
Selection, 340
Self-awareness
   authentic leadership and, 16
   followership and, 18
   in leader skill set, 5
Self-care, for work-related stress, 79
Self-construal (self-image), discussion of, 170
Self-direction, 45
Self-evaluation, definition of, 401
Self-management, in leader skill set, 6
Self-report rating, performance appraisal and, 405
Selling orientation, 449
Semantic interoperability, 429
Seminal nursing case management models, 244
Sentinel event, 308–311
   definition of, 287–288
   TJC definition, 308
Sentinel Event Database, TJC, 334
Servant leadership, 15–16
Service components, for case management models, 243
Service delivery, optimized by program designs, 197
Service Employees International Union (SEIU), 375
Service line, 193
Services, quality of, in workplace diversity, 178
Setting boundaries, for work-related stress, 79
Shared decision making, 45
Shared governance, 45, 206–209, 213–214b
   case study on, 214b
   challenges, 208–209
   concept, 210
   in decision making, 67
   in evidence-based practice, 277
   history, 208
   implementation, 210
   implications, 211
   increase, 208

Shared governance *(Continued)*
  issues and trends in, 212–214
    engagement, 213–214
    inter-professional education and collaboration, 212
    whole-system integration, 212–213
  leadership and management implications, 209–211, 211f
Shared meaning, engagement in, 9
Shared vision
  inspiration of, 9
  learning organization of, 45
Sharing, 130
Shewhart, Walter, 290
"Shining example" nurse, 146–147, 146f
Sigma Theta Tau International (STTI), 354
Silence Kills, 107
Silent Generation, 181
Similar-to-me effect, 404
Simulation, in decision making, 68
Situation, Background, Assessment, Recommendation (SBAR), in decision making, 68
Situation, in leadership process, 7
Situational Leadership® Model, 12–13
Situational leadership theories, 11–13
Six Sigma, 68–69, 136–137, 294, 294t
  problem-solving strategy, comparison, 294t
Skill
  domains of, 4
  of follower, 12
  level, 370
  mix, 370
Smoothing, problem-solving style, 170
Social awareness, in leader skill set, 6
Social capital, 191
Social casework, 244
Social determinants, of health, 246
Social media, electronic communication and, 115–117
Social Security Act (1935), in case management, 242
Social structure, postmodernists challenging assumption of, 189
Social systems, organizations as, key theories of, 189–191
Social work models, 244–245
Span of control, 198–199
Speaking up, tools for, 106–107
Specialists, 292
Specialization, 191–193
  advantages of, 193
Specification Manual for National Hospital Inpatient Quality Measures, 305
Spillover, 74
Spiritual health care
  communication and, 109–110
  requirements in, 109
Spirituality
  defined as, 109
  in practice, 109–110
Squashers, 134
Staff. *See also* Nursing
  authority, 197
  development, 361
    Magnet studies, 361
  empowerment, 208
  fear, overcoming, 421
  roles, 357–361
  turnover, 364
  vacancy, 340

Staff-leadership partnership, 208
Staff management
  collective bargaining agreements and, 375–376
  demand management in, 380–381
  framework for, 371, 372f
  legislative impact on, 376–377
  patient acuity and, 374
  plan, 377–383
  position control in, 379
  scheduling in, 379–380
  strategies for, 371–376
Staffing, 66, 369–387
  allocation, 381–382, 383b
  case study, 386–387b
  centralized, 381
  complexity compression and, 76
  computerized, 382
  definitions in, 370–371
  demand management in, 380–381
  effectiveness of, 370, 383
  evidence on quality, 383–384
  fixed, 378
  issues and trends, 384–387
  leadership and management implications for, 376–377
  legal and ethical aspects, 99–101
  lower, 321
  methods, 378
  nurse manager role, 81
  organizational outcomes of, 383–384
  patient assignment in, 383
  position control, 379
  recommendations by professional organizations, 373–374
  resource pool, 381–382
  scheduling and, 379–380
  variable, 378, 378b
Staffing calculation, in operating budget development, 392
Staffing/labor budget, 392
Staffing Management and Methods, 373
Staffing pattern, 370, 377–379
  sample, 378t
  staff calculation in, 378b
Standard operating policies and procedures, 228
Standardized clinical terminology, 439–440
Standards
  of care, 229–230
  definition of, 288
  of group's behavior, 120
  nurse managers, knowledge, 304
  of quality, 291–293
Standing committee, 128–129
State law, and nursing, 87
Status-based communications, 112
Statute of limitations, 90
Storming, in group development, 111–112
Strategic Contingency Theory, 159
Strategic management, 216–224, 223–224b
  case study on, 224b
  definitions of, 217
  external components of, 219
  issues and trends of, 222–223
  leadership and management implications, 222
  strategic planning process in, 217–221
Strategic objectives, 219

Strategic plan
    action plan, impact in, 222
    appendix materials of, 221
    definition of, 217
    development of, 277
    documents in, 221
    elements of, 221
    implementation of, 222
Strategic planning, 20, 450–451
    for evaluation, 221
    implementation of, 220–221
    process, 217–221, 217f
        questions in, 218
Strategies
    for decision making, 69–70
    definition of, 217
    implementation, 220
    organizational infrastructure, building of, 279
Strategy meeting, 130
Stratification, as disease management program component, 260
Strengths, weaknesses, opportunities, and threats (SWOT)
    analysis template, 219t
    methods of, 219
Strengths model, for case management, 245
Stress, 74–84, 83b
    case study on, 83–84b
    decrease
        institutional strategies for, 80b
        personal strategies for, 78b
        strategies for, 77–79, 78b
    definitions in, 75
    emotional support, strategies of, 39
    good, 74
    issues and trends in, 81–84
    leadership and management implications, 77–81
    management, 77–78
    moral distress and, 76
    nurse managers and, special considerations for, 81
    personal health and, 74
    predictions and risk in, 82–84
    resilience and, 77
    scarcity of evidence on, 81
    time and, 75–76
    uncertain situations and, 82
    work-related. See Work-related stress
Stress-induced hyperglycemia, 74
Strict liability torts, 88f
Structural power, 201
Structural team building, 127
Structure, definition of, 187
Structured care methodologies (SCMs), 229–230
Structured interview process, 359
Student clinical assistant (SCA) programs, 356–357
Stumbling on Happiness, 82
Subjective perspective, 188
Subjectivism, 187
    and objectivism, polarization between, 188–189
Substitutability, 161
    definition of, 159
Subunit power, 158–159
Suitability, individual, for case management, 263
Summarizer, 132
Supervision, 142
    direct, coordination of work and, 193

Supplemental staffing resources, 382
Supply budget, 393
Supressing, problem-solving style, 170
Surge capacity, 417–418
Sustainability
    definition of, 269
    for evidence-based practice, 272
System of Profound Knowledge, 25
System stress, 380
Systematic review, 269
Systematized Nomenclature of Medicine Clinical Terms
        (SNOMED CT), 438
Systems, modernist theories related to, 187–188
Systems theory, 24–25, 25t
Systems thinking, 20–21
    learning organization of, 45

T
Tactical planning, 20
Tactics, definition of, 217
Tall organizational structure, 198–199, 199f, 200t
Tangible resources, control over, 158
Targeted interview method, 359
Targeted selection process, 359
Targeting, 451
    definition of, 449–450
Task conflict, 164
Task forces, 119–120, 197
Task-oriented leader, impact of, 11–12
Tasks, 8
Taylor, Frederick W., 189
Team-based outcome measures and coaching, 127
Team building, 118–139, 137–138b
    background of, 120–121
    case study, 138b
    issues and trends in, 135–138
    leadership and management implications, 134–135
Team/group communication, 111–113
Team leader, 232
Team learning, learning organization of, 45
Team nursing, 232
Teams, 120
    ad hoc, 126
    articulated expectations of, 128
    case study on, 138b
    code of conduct of, 128
    committees, 128–129
    dynamics, 126–128
    issues and trends in, 135–138
    leadership, 126
    leadership and management implications, 134–135
    meetings, effective, 129–132
    norms, established, 127–128
    operating agreement, 128
    primary, 126
    project, 129
    types of, 126
    working with, 125–128
TeamSTEPPS (Team Strategies and Tools to Enhance Performance
        and Patient Safety), 112, 136, 313
TeamSTEPPS 2.0, 149
Team Strategies and Tools to Enhance Performance and Patient
        Safety (TeamSTEPPS), 112, 136, 313
Technological innovations, in informatics, 435

Technology, use of, 398–399
Temperature nurse, 232
10-Step Process for Quality Assurance, 303
Tension reliever, 132
Termination, 341
Terrorism, in workplace violence, 336
The 21st Century Black Death, 74
The Atlantic, 74
The Joint Commission (TJC), 331
    10-Step Process for Quality Assurance, 303
    on emergency preparedness, 410
    evolution, 303
    ORYX®, 304–305
    performance improvement standards, 303–304
    performance standards, 303
    Sentinel Event Database, 334
    spiritual care, requirements in, 109
    staffing effectiveness requirements, 383
    staffing regulation, 375
The Path to Continuously Learning Health Care in America, 442–443
The Persistence of Memory, 77
The Principles of Scientific Management, 189
"The Quandary of Job Stress Compensation," 74–75
The Silent Treatment, 107
Theory of Group Power, 159–160
Thomas-Kilmann Conflict Mode Instrument (TKI), 171
    norms, 168–169
Threat assessment teams, 333
Threat management, 333
360-degree feedback review, 405
Time, 74–84, 83b
    case study on, 83–84b
    definitions in, 75
    issues and trends in, 81–84
    leadership and management implications, 77–81
    management
        deliberative process in, 75
        journaling and, 79
        strategies for, 75b
    moral distress and, 76
    resilience and, 77
    stress and, 75–76
    uncertain situations and, 82
To Err Is Human: Building a Safer Health Care System, 296
Tools, in decision making, 67–69
Top-down change, promotion, 33–34
Tort, 88f, 89–90
Total operating expenses, 389
Total operating revenues, 389
Total patient care, 231, 232
Total quality management (TQM)
    definition of, 288
    initiatives, 136
Traditional nursing care delivery models, 231
Trait theories, on leadership, 8–9
Traits, in performance appraisal, 402–403
Transactional leadership, 13–14, 13f
Transactional managerial leadership, 363
Transfer, 341
Transformational change, impact, 44
Transformational leadership, 13–14, 13f, 108
    idea, introduction, 40
    style, 363
Transforming Care at the Bedside (TCAB), 37–38

"Transition shock," 78
Transitional care model (TCM), 235
Translational research, 269
Transparency, marketing and, 455
Transtheoretical Stages of Change Model (TTM), 39–40
Treatment adherence, in population health management, 265
Triage decisions, 65
"Trialability, " as planned change factor, 42
True team, 120
Trust
    for effective work teams, 127
    leadership and, 9
    sustaining and creating, 4
Turnover, 340–341
    cost of, 161
        strategies, 364
    formula, 365f
    management strategies, 364
    rates, 352
    voluntary, 341
"2030 problem," 28–29

U
Uncertainty
    coping, 159
    definition of, 159
Unfreezing, change stage as, 35
Uniform Licensure Requirements (ULRs), 92
Unit-based nurse managers, 54
Unit practice councils (UPCs), 208
United States Registered Nurse Workforce Report Card and Shortage Forecast, 341
Unlicensed Assistive Personnel (UAP), definition of, 142
Unreliable members, 134
Upward appeal, influence tactics, 155
US Census Bureau, in population and health trends, 256
US Department of Health and Human Services (HHS), 95

V
Value-based purchasing (VBP), 385
Values, 298
    core, 227–228
    definition of, 448–449
    Mayo Clinic statements, 298t
    organizational, 55
    proposition, 455
    statements, 227–228
Variable selection, 320–321
Variable staff calculation, 378b
Variable staffing, 378
Variance
    analysis of, 318–319
    definition of, 389
Variety, as Big Data characteristics, 324t
Velocity, as Big Data characteristics, 324t
VERA framework, in teaching communication, 115
Veracity, 87
    as Big Data characteristics, 324t
Verbal communication, 102
Veterans Affairs (VA), National Center for Patient Safety, 307, 309b
Vicarious liability, 88f, 89
Violence. *See also* Workplace violence
    definition of, 328–329
    horizontal, 329

Violence *(Continued)*
  lateral, 329
  parameters of, 330
  prevalence of, 329
  prevention of workplace, 328–339
  regulatory background of, 330–334
  risk factors for, 330
  sources, variation, 330
  workplace violence, definition, 328–329
Vision
  development of, 277
  importance of, 206
  leadership and, 9
  statements, 217–218, 227
    communication effectiveness, 297
  strategies, 355
Volume, as Big Data characteristics, 324t
Volume budget flow sheet, 392t

W
Wants
  definition of, 448
  satisfying, 448–449
"Watchdog" nurse, 146–147, 146f
Watchful waiting, in decision making, 69
Weber, Max, 189
Wellness programs, for work-related stress, 78–79
Whole-system integration, shared governance (impact), 212–213
Willingness, 12
Wisdom, definition of, 433
Withdrawing, problem-solving style, 170
Words, in communication, 105
Work
  allocation, 374
  coordination of, with direct supervision, 193
  departmentalization of, 193
  environment factors, 352–353
  excessive fragmentation of, 189
  managerial, nature of, 22–23, 23f, 24f
  outputs from, standardization of, 193
  processes of, standardization of, 193
Work-arounds, 53–54
Work environments
  establishment/sustaining (AACN standards), 80t
  healthy, 53–54, 230, 230b
  Magnet designation, associated with, 385
Worker skills, standardization of, 193
Work flow, 292
Workforce characteristics, systematic review (AHRQ) of, 161
Work groups, 120
  disrupted, 122
  true team and, 120
Working, 121
Working With Others: A Position Paper, 142
Work-life balance, marketing and, 456, 456b
Workload
  adjustment, 377
  forecasted, 377–379
  nursing shortage, 353

Workplace
  bullying, definition of, 329
  safety/health guidelines (OSHA), 330–331
Workplace diversity, 175–186, 185–186b
  background, 176
  business benefits of, 180
  case study, 186b
  communication, 181
  competitive edge in marketplace, 180
  culture, impact of, 176–178
  generational diversity, 181–182
  health benefits of, 180
  high context and low contexts, 184
  issues and trends in, 184–186
  leadership and management implications, 182–184
  liability, decreasing risk of, 180–181
  multicultural teams, 176–177
  social benefits of, 180
Workplace violence
  background of, 329–330
  case study on, 338–339b
  checklist of, 332b
  collaboration in, 336–337
  definition of, 328–329
  environmental design of, 335–336
  issues and trends in, 335–337
  leadership and management implications, 334–335
  legal implications of, 334–335
  management of, 331–332
    policy recommendations, 330–331
  NIOSH, recommendations from, 331
  Occupational Safety and Health Administration for, 330–331
  parameters of violence in, 330
  prevention of, 328–339, 338b
  regulatory background of, 330–334
Workplaces, healthy, 135–136
Work-related stress, 74
  getting started with, 77
  organizational recommendations for, 79–81, 80b
    empowerment in, 80–81
    healthy work environments standards as, 80, 80t
  prevention and addressing, 77–81
  special considerations for nurse managers in, 81
  strategies for, 77–79
    institutional, 80b
    journaling for, 79
    personal, 78b
    relaxation for, 79
    self-care for, 79
    setting boundaries for, 79
    stress management for, 77–79
    wellness programs in large context in, 78–79
Worksite analysis, 331
World Health Organization, social determinants of health defined by, 246
Written communication, 115